Care of the acutely ill adult – an essential guide for nurses

Edited by

Fiona Creed

Senior Lecturer,
School of Nursing and Midwifery,
University of Brighton, UK

and

Christine Spiers

Principal Lecturer,
School of Nursing and Midwifery,
University of Brighton, UK

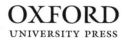

OXFORD
UNIVERSITY PRESS

OXFORD

UNIVERSITY PRESS

Great Clarendon Street, Oxford OX2 6DP

Oxford University Press is a department of the University of Oxford.
It furthers the University's objective of excellence in research, scholarship,
and education by publishing worldwide in

Oxford New York

Auckland Cape Town Dar es Salaam Hong Kong Karachi
Kuala Lumpur Madrid Melbourne Mexico City Nairobi
New Delhi Shanghai Taipei Toronto

With offices in

Argentina Austria Brazil Chile Czech Republic France Greece
Guatemala Hungary Italy Japan Poland Portugal Singapore
South Korea Switzerland Thailand Turkey Ukraine Vietnam

Oxford is a registered trade mark of Oxford University Press
in the UK and in certain other countries

Published in the United States
by Oxford University Press Inc., New York

© Oxford University Press 2010

The moral rights of the author have been asserted
Database right Oxford University Press (maker)

First published 2010

British Library Cataloguing in Publication Data
Data available

Library of Congress Cataloging in Publication Data
Care of the acutely ill adult : an essential guide for nurses / edited by Fiona Creed and Christine Spiers.
     p. ; cm.
  Includes bibliographical references and index.
  ISBN 978-0-19-956438-5
1. Intensive care nursing. I. Creed, Fiona. II. Spiers, Christine.
  [DNLM: 1. Acute Disease—nursing. 2. Adult. 3. Critical Illness. 4. Nursing Assessment—methods. WY 154
C2708 2010]
  RT120.I5C366 2010
  610.73'6—dc22   2009053050

Typeset in Minion by Glyph International, Bangalore, India
Printed in Great Britain on acid-free paper by Ashford Colour Press, Gosport, Hampshire

ISBN 978–0–19–956438–5

10 9 8 7 6 5 4 3 2 1

Care of the acutely ill adult – an essential guide for nurses

WITHDRAWN

Foreword

The recognition of deterioration in the acutely ill patient and timely referral for treatment has been, and remains, a 'hot topic' for acute care services and the educators of the nurses who work there. Recent advances aim to prevent rather than manage deterioration to forestall the escalation of patients' conditions into critical status. The purpose of recent guidance (see Chapter 1) is to enable the recognition and referral sooner for effective and timely care. This text serves to empower nurses, through the acquisition of core knowledge and competencies, to make a significant contribution to these outcomes.

Since the work of McQuillan *et al.* (1998), who contributed the term 'suboptimal care' to the lexicon of healthcare workers, a series of interventions have been put in place to improve the recognition of deterioration in the acutely ill patient. Interventions include the introduction of emergency care teams and critical care outreach services (see Chapter 12), who respond to calls from acute care nurses for assistance, and the introduction of early warning scores (see Chapter 11) to enable ward teams to identify signs of deterioration sooner and make referrals to these teams. Despite these initiatives, further work remains to be done to support acute care staff in the recognition of clinical signs of cascade sooner and make appropriate and timely referrals to specialist teams to instigate advanced treatment. This text serves to provide detailed information on how to assess various body systems, recognize the significance of those assessment findings, and plan to implement thoughtful, timely, and compassionate care (Chapters 2–10).

The term 'failure-to-rescue' is an indicator to measure or track error at an individual or organizational level (Talsma *et al.* 2008). Critical incident analyses examine documentation alongside an audit of the clinical events that lead to the outcome, normally sadly related to a patient's unexpected death. The importance of accurate documentation and how this might be improved is emphasized (see Chapter 16). Although such approaches seek to learn from mistakes and redress omissions in the organization or delivery of care, one fact remains: the capacity to recognize and respond to acute deterioration, formulate salient decisions and take appropriate action resides in the knowledge and clinical wisdom of the practitioner. We may create systems to facilitate better communication between clinical teams, tools to prompt a reaction, or data to inform the effectiveness of emergency care pathways, but without the relevant 'know how' exercised by the carer at the patient's bedside the problem will remain.

This book is an invaluable text to enable nurses to aquire knowledge and assessment skills but it can also serve as an invaluable reference book to those who wish to refresh their thinking about what to look for, and how to respond, to the early signs of physiological change. However, there can be no substitute for the rehearsal of those skills to ensure theory can be applied to practice. The learning outcomes and clear identification of competences gives the reader the material to take with them into supervised practise or, better still, a simulation environment where they can truly test out their applied knowledge without risk to the patient. Furthermore, the structure of the chapters will be invaluable to those who support or supervise clinicians to think about what to consider when assessing competencies in their colleagues.

I am particularly proud that the authors of this text are educators and clinicians, all in the front line of delivering services and training to those who work in the acute care setting, yet linked to the University of Brighton. I have had the privilege of working with the authors as a fellow clinician, teacher and researcher. Beyond the personal, this book is evidence of strong collegiate relationships and partnerships working between the clinical environment and the higher education sector. This group of authors come together as a 'community of practice' dedicated to addressing 'failure to rescue'. This demonstrates the importance of working together to achieve the same outcome: creating a safer environment for our patients. The book celebrates the expertise of both the academic and the clinician in achieving the same goal. All the authors are aware of the issues and complexities of recognizing deterioration and have disassembled the vast array of theory into easily accessible yet challenging learning chapters that can then be applied to practice and close the theory–practice gap. Thus, as the authors have worked together to inform the generation of the book, invaluable learning has taken place for all those who have been involved and myths have been dispelled about the relative value of knowledge from the 'ivory tower' of academia or clinical know how. In this book we see fusion, and this can only serve to inform the application of knowledge and improve the care we provide to all our patients in acute care services.

In summary, I believe this is an outstanding book that will be a constant source of reference for educators and clinicians. I am honoured to have been asked to review this manuscript and write this foreword. I commend it to you.

Professor Julie Scholes
Centre for Nursing and Midwifery Research University of Brighton
Co-editor: *Nursing in Critical Car.*

References

Talsma, A., Bahl, V., and Campbell, D.A. (2008) Exploratory analyses of the 'failure to rescue' measure: evaluation through medical record review. *J. Nurs. Care Qual.* **23**(3), 202–10.

Acknowledgement

'This book is dedicated to our ever-patient families and the immense support they offered us throughout the preparation of this book. We are also indebted to all our contributors who gave their time and expertise so willingly'.

The editors wish to thank Clare Gochmanski for taking the photographs included in Chapter 13.

Fiona Creed and Christine Spiers

Permissions

Critical Care Outreach Team: Eastbourne District Hospital for allowing us to use their track-and-trigger scoring chart.

Keith Young, Department of Health for permission to quote the new competence framework (2009) *Competencies for recognising and responding to acutely ill adults in hospital*. Department of Health, HMSO, London.

Iain Moir at NICE for permission to quote from the NICE (2007) Guidelines *Acutely ill patients in hospital: recognition of and response to acute illness of adults in hospital*. HMSO, London.

Resuscitation Council for permission to use

Resuscitation Council (UK) (2006) *Immediate Life Support*, 2nd edn. Resuscitation Council (UK), London.

Resuscitation Council (UK) (2006) *Advanced Life Support*, 5th edn. Resuscitation Council (UK), London.

Resuscitation Council (UK) (2008) Anaphylaxis Algorithm.

Contents

Glossary of terms and abbreviations

AAGBI	Association of Anaesthetists of Great Britain and Ireland
ABC	(mental health) Affective, behaviour, cognition
ABCDE	Airway, Breathing, Circulation, Disability, Exposure
ACE	Angiotensin-converting enzyme
ACS	Acute coronary syndromes
ADH	Antidiuretic hormone
ADP	Adenosine diphosphate
A&E	Accident and Emergency
AED	Automated external defibrillator
AHP	Allied health professionals
AIM	Acute illness management
AKI	Acute kidney injury
AKIN	Acute kidney injury network
ALERT	Acute Life-threatening Events Recognition and Treatment
ALP	Alkaline phosphatase
ALS	Advanced life support
ALSG	Advanced life support group
ALT	Alanine aminotransferase
ANS	Autonomic nervous system
ANTT	Aseptic non-touch technique
A/P	Anterior:posterior (position)
APEL	Accreditation of Prior Experiential Learning
APL	Accreditation of Prior Learning
APTT	Activated partial thromboplastin time
ARF	Acute renal failure
AST	Aspartate aminotransferase
ATN	Acute tubular necrosis
ATLS	Advanced trauma and life support
ATP	Adenosine triphosphate
AV	Atrioventricular (node)
AVPU	Method of quickly assessing consciousness (A= awake, V= awake to speech (verbal commands), P = awake to painful stimuli, U = unconscious)
BAPEN	British Association of Parenteral and Enteral Nutrition
BE	Base excess
BEE	Basal energy expenditure
BIPAP	Biphasic positive airway pressure
BMI	Body mass index
BNF	British National Formulary
BP	Blood pressure
BTS	British Thoracic Society
BVM	Bag valve mask
Ca	Calcium
CAM	Confusion assessment method
CCFNI	Critical care family needs inventory
CCP	Critical Care Paramedic
CO$_2$	Carbon dioxide
COPD	Chronic obstructive pulmonary disease
CPE	Continuing professional education
CPAP	Continuous positive airway pressure
CPP	Cerebral perfusion pressure
CPR	Cardiopulmonary resuscitation
CRP	C-reactive protein
CSF	Cerebral spinal fluid
CT	Computerised tomography
CURB	Confusion, urea elevation, respiratory rate, blood pressure
CVP	Central venous pressure
CVS	Cardiovascular system
Cx	Circumflex
CXR	Chest X ray
CTZ	Chemoreceptor trigger zone
C3, C4	Cervical vertebrae
DIC	Disseminated intravascular coagulopathy
DKA	Diabetic ketoacidosis
DLB	Dementia with Lewy bodies
DNAR	Do not attempt resuscitation
DTs	Delirium tremens
DVT	Deep vein thrombosis
ECF	Extracellular fluid
ECG	Electrocardiogram
e-GFR	Estimated glomerular filtration rate
EME	Electronic medical engineer

EPAP	Expiratory positive airway pressure	ICD	Internal cardiac defibrillator
EPUAP	European Pressure Ulcer Advisory Panel Classification System	ICF	Intracellular fluid
		IMCA	Independent mental capacity advocate
ERC	European Resuscitation Council	ICS	Intensive Care Society
ET	Endotracheal	IDDM	Insulin-dependent diabetes mellitus
ESR	Erythrocyte sedimentation rate	ILCOR	International Liaison Committee on Resuscitation
ESRF	End stage renal failure		
ENT	Ear nose and throat	IMPACT	Ill Medical Patients Acute Care and Treatment
EWS	Early warning scores		
FBC	Full blood count	IPAP	Inspiratory positive airway pressure
FDP	Fibrin degradation products	ICNARC	Intensive Care National Audit Research Committee
FEV_1	Forced expiratory volume in 1 second		
FiO_2	Fractional inspired oxygen	ICU	Intensive Care Unit
FTD	Fronto temporal dementia	INR	International normalised ratio
FVC	Forced vital capacity	IO	Intraosseous
GCS	Glasgow coma scale	ITU	Intensive therapy unit
G force	Gravitational force	IV	Intravenous
GFR	Glomerular filtration rate	JVP	Jugular venous pressure
GGT	Gamma glutamyl transferase	K^+	Potassium
g/L	Grams per litre	kPa	Kilopascals
g/dL	Grams per decilitre	LAD	Left anterior descending (coronary artery)
GI	Gastrointestinal system	LBBB	Left bundle branch block
GIP	Glucose-dependent insulinotrophic peptide	LMA	Laryngeal mask airway
		LMWH	Low molecular weight heparin
GP	General practitioner	LPA	Lasting Power of Attorney
GP11b/111a	Glycoprotein11b/111a receptor	LVF	Left ventricular failure
Hb	Haemoglobin	MALT	Mucosa-associated lymphoid tissue
$HbCO_2$	Carbaminohaemoglobin	MAP	Mean arterial pressure
H_2O	Water	MAU	Medical assessment unit
HbA1c	Glycated haemoglobin A1	MC&S	Microbiological culture and sensitivity
HCAI	Health care associated (or acquired) infection	MCV	Mean cell volume
		MDRT	Modified diet renal disease
HCl	Hydrochloric acid	MDT	Multi-disciplinary team
HCO_3	Bicarbonate	MET	Medical emergency team
H_2CO_3	Carbonic acid	MEWS	Modified early warning system
HCSS	Health care support staff	MI	Myocardial infarction
HCT	Haematocrit	Mg^{2+}	Magnesium
HDL	High-density lipoproteins	MONA	Morphine oxygen nitrates aspirin
HDU	High dependency unit	MODS	Multi-organ dysfunction syndrome
HEI	Higher education institution	MRI	Magnetic resonance imaging
HHS	Hyperglycaemic Hyperosmolar syndrome	MRSA	Methicillin-resistant *Staphylococcus aureus*
HIT	Heparin-induced thrombocytopaenia	MMC	Migratory motility complex
HR	Heart rate	mmol/L	Millimols per litre
HRT	Hormone replacement therapy	MUST	Malnutrition universal screening tools
IABP	Intra-aortic balloon pump	Na^+	Sodium

NaCl	Sodium chloride		RBBB	Right bundle branch block
NCEPOD	National Confidential Enquiry into Patient Outcome and Death		RCUK	Resuscitation Council (UK)
NHS	National Health Service		RCA	Right coronary artery
NHSLA	National Health Service Litigation Authority		RCN	Royal College of Nursing
			RBC	Red blood cell
NH_2	the amino group on an amino acid		RIFLE	Risk Injury Failure Loss End stage renal failure
NH_3	Ammonia		ROSC	Return of spontaneous circulation
NIDDM	Non-insulin dependent diabetes mellitus		RRT	Renal replacement therapy
NICE	National Institute for Health and Clinical Excellence		RRVVII	Reperfusion rhythm vital signs volume inotropes intra-aortic balloon pump
NIV	Non-invasive ventilation		r-PA	Recombitant plasminogen activator
NKHS	Non-ketotic hyperosmolar states		RVMI	Right ventricular myocardial infarction
NMC	Nursing and Midwifery Council		SA	Sino-atrial (node)
NPSA	National Patient Safety Agency		SALT	Speech and language therapy
NSF	National Service Framework		SaO_2	Saturation of oxygen
NSTEMI	non-ST segment elevation myocardial infarction		SARS	Severe acute respiratory syndrome
Nu DESC	Nursing delirium scale		SBAR	Situation background assessment recommendation tool
O_2	Oxygen		SI	Small intestine
ODP	Operating department practitioner		SIGN	Scottish Intercollegiate Guidelines Network
$PaCO_2$	Partial pressure of carbon dioxide		SIRS	Systemic inflammatory response syndrome
PaO_2	Partial pressure of oxygen		SNA	Sympathetic nervous system
PARS	Patient at risk scores		SOPRA	System of patient-related activity
PART	Patient at risk teams		STEMI	ST-segment elevation myocardial infarction
PCV	Packed cell volume			
PE	Pulmonary embolus		SV	Stroke volume
PEA	Pulseless electrical activity		SVR	Systemic vascular resistance
PEEP	Positive end expiratory pressure		SVT	Supraventricular tachycardia
PEFR	Peak expiratory flow rate		S_1	Sound 1 (heart sound 1)
PCI	Percutaneous coronary intervention		S_2	Sound 2 (heart sound 2)
Ph	Power of hydrogen		S2, S3, S4	Sacral vertebrae
PICC	Peripherally inserted central catheter		TB	Tuberculosis
PID	Pelvic inflammatory disease		t-PA	Tissue plasminogen activator
PID	Prolapsed inter vertebral disc		TnC	Troponin C
P-PCI	Primary-percutaneous coronary intervention		TnI	Troponin I
PO_4	Phosphate		TnT	Troponin T
PPE	Personal protective equipment		TNK	Tenecteplase
PT	Prothrombin time		T5, T6	Thoracic vertebrae
PTH	Parathyroid hormone		U&E	Urea and electrolytes
PTSD	Post-traumatic stress disorder		UK	United Kingdom
Q	Perfusion		UTI	Urinary tract infection
RAS	Reticular activating system		V	Ventilation
RAWL	Recognition and accreditation of work-related learning		VF	Ventricular fibrillation
			VT	Ventricular tachycardia

VIP	Visual intravenous phlebitis	WPW	Wolff-Parkinson-White (syndrome)
VLDL	Very low density lipoproteins	2 3 BPG	2 3 Biphosphoglycerate
VTE	Venous thromboembolism	2 3 DPG	2 3 Diphosphoglycerate
WBC	White blood cell	5HT	5-Hydroxytryptamine
WCC	White cell count	$5HT_3$	5-Hydroxytryptamine receptor
WHO	World Health Organisation		

Contributors

Heather Baid
Senior Lecturer,
School of Nursing and Midwifery,
University of Brighton,
Brighton, UK

Kevin Barrett
Senior Lecturer,
School of Nursing and Midwifery,
University of Brighton,
Brighton, UK

Annie Chellel
Principal Lecturer,
School of Nursing and Midwifery,
University of Brighton,
Brighton, UK

Ruth Creasy
Critical Care Outreach Team,
Eastbourne District General Hospital
NHS Trust,
Eastbourne,
East Sussex, UK

Fiona Creed
Senior Lecturer,
School of Nursing and Midwifery,
University of Brighton,
Brighton, UK

Gary Creed
Laboratory Operations Manager/
Chief Critical Care Physiologist,
Department of Intensive Care and
Critical Care Medicine,
Guy's & St Thomas Foundation NHS Trust,
London, UK

Jackie Dawson
Lead Nurse,
Sussex Critical Care Network,
Lewes,
East Sussex, UK

Lorna East
Cardiology Audit Co-ordinator,
Western Sussex University Hospital
NHS Trust,
Worthing, West Sussex, UK

Corinne Elliott
Critical Care Outreach Team,
Eastbourne District General Hospital
NHS Trust,
Eastbourne,
East Sussex, UK

Sylvia Hedges
Critical Care Outreach Team,
Eastbourne District General Hospital
NHS Trust,
Eastbourne East Sussex, UK

Denise Hinge
Nurse Consultant Critical Care,
Brighton and Sussex University Hospitals
NHS Trust,
Chair Sussex Critical Care Outreach Forum,
Brighton, UK

Kaye Looker
Sister Critical Care Outreach team,
Eastbourne District General Hospital
NHS Trust,
Eastbourne,
East Sussex, UK

Kathy Martyn
Principal Lecturer,
School of Nursing and Midwifery,
University of Brighton,
Brighton, UK

Cristina Osorio
Matron for Renal Services,
Sussex Kidney Unit,
Brighton and Sussex University Hospital
NHS Trust,
Brighton, UK

Christine Spiers
Principal Lecturer,
School of Nursing and Midwifery,
University of Brighton,
Brighton, UK

Helen Stanley
Principal Lecturer,
School of Nursing and Midwifery,
University of Brighton,
Brighton, UK

Joanna Thorpe
Critical Care Outreach Team,
Eastbourne District General Hospital NHS
Trust,
Eastbourne,
East Sussex, UK

Chapter 1

Introduction to acute care

Fiona Creed

Chapter contents

The delivery of acute care has changed considerably over the last decade, leading to an increased acuity of patients nursed in the ward environment. At the same time a number of reports have focused on problems with care delivery for these acutely ill patients (Robson 2002). The publication of the National Institute for Health and Clinical Excellence (NICE) guidelines (2007) and the publication of competencies for recognizing and responding to acutely ill patients in hospital (Department of Health 2009) will impact on services provided for acutely ill patients. In order to understand why these recommendations have been made by the Department of Health, it is important to understand the background to these changes, why they have been recommended, and ultimately how these changes affect nurses working in acute care areas. This chapter will examine:

- the introduction to acute care
- the background to these changes
- policy drivers for acute care
- classifications of acute care
- the effects on care/suboptimal ward care
- contemporary guidance on delivery of acute care
- the drive for assessment of competence in acute care delivery
- how this book may help the acute care nurse.

Learning outcomes

This chapter will enable you to:

- understand the effects of reorganization on acute care delivery
- examine national developments in acute care delivery
- discuss how changes have impacted on care delivery in acute wards
- understand how acutely ill patients are classified
- analyse the concept of suboptimal care
- explore commonly ignored warning signs of deterioration
- examine current recommendations surrounding acute care delivery
- analyse the need to develop competent practitioners
- understand the Department of Health's framework for competence (2009).

Introduction to acute care

Nursing the acutely ill patient in the hospital environment has changed considerably over the past decade and this is reflected in the types of patients seen in acute hospital wards and the need for the development of acute nursing knowledge and skills. This change of focus of care has been driven by a number of factors and it is essential that the nurse is able to understand the context of these changes, drivers for these changes, and how this will ultimately affect care. This chapter will focus on the background and need for changes in acute care, highlighting the significance of the NICE guidelines (2007) and the Department of Health competencies (2009). It will emphasize the need for a timely and appropriate recognition of acute illness and identify how the practising nurse can use this book to enable the development of knowledge and skills that will enhance the delivery of care to the acutely ill patient.

In discussing these issues an overview of the findings of several reports will be highlighted. It should be remembered that the causes of these problems are multifactorial in nature and there is no intent in this chapter to criticize care, merely to highlight the problems that have been found.

Background to changes in acute care delivery

A number of factors have been influential in changing how and where acute care is delivered in hospital. Over the last two decades it has become increasing clear that changes in technology and treatment, and an aging population have increased the numbers of acute patients in wards (Coad & Haines 1999; NICE 2007). At the same time, changes to discharge patterns have meant earlier planned discharge, further increasing the acuity of patients in wards. The more recent changes to community care delivery have yet to impact on care but it is likely that these will further increase the acuity levels of patients, as those patients who are relatively well will be nursed at home under the context of care in a 'virtual hospital'.

As the level of acuity increased, it became apparent that the wards did not seem to be able to cope with the increased demands on their services. In the mid- to late-1990s there was a growing body of concern that patients' deterioration prior to admission to the intensive therapy unit (ITU) may not have been identified sufficiently quickly enough (Robson 2002). The need for timely recognition of deterioration and appropriate delivery of acute care has become a recurring message of research papers and government policy (Jevon 2007).

Government documentation

One of the most significant documents in relation to acute care was *Comprehensive Critical Care: A Review of Adult Critical Care Services* (Department of Health 2000). This document marked the end of traditional boundaries associated with acute care. It highlighted the need for a hospital-wide approach to the delivery of acute care, emphasizing the need for care to be based on need rather than geographical location. The vision was that hospitals should aim to meet the needs of all patients who are critically ill, rather than just those who are in beds designated as ITU/high dependency unit (HDU), introducing the concept of 'critical care without walls'. It highlighted the need for NHS trusts to rationalize the resources required to care for acutely ill patients in accordance with the workload generated by the patients' care needs (Sheppard & Wright 2005). Comprehensive critical care highlighted the characteristics of a modern critical care service, including:

+ integration of services throughout the hospital beyond the physical boundaries of ITU/HDU beds to allow optimum use of the resources available
+ the development of critical care networks, linking trusts in similar geographical locations to ensure common standards and protocols were developed

♦ workforce development, to ensure that all staff caring for acutely ill patients are educated and skilled to provide timely and appropriate care.

It also stressed the need to move away from systems that classified patients according to their geographical location, e.g. ITU/HDU patient, and to focus more on the level of treatment required (see Table 1.1).

The report also recognized the need to move away from rigid staffing ratio systems to a system based on the needs assessment of the nursing workload. It suggested implementation of a system of patient-related activity (SOPRA) that would enable calculation of nurse:patient ratios dependent on patient workload rather than other factors.

One of the most influential factors from the comprehensive critical care report (Department of Health 2000) was the recommendation of teams to support acutely ill patients in the ward. The report recommended the development of outreach teams to enable the concept of 'critical care without walls'. The main remits of outreach were:

♦ to avert admissions into higher levels of care (ITU/HDU) by detection of early signs of deterioration

♦ to enable discharge from ITU by providing support to ensure continued recovery of patients discharged to the ward

♦ to share critical care skills through training programmes.

The report also recommended the development of early-warning scoring systems based on physiological changes that would allow the nurse to quickly identify the patient who is deteriorating. The aim of these 'track-and-trigger' scoring systems was to capture deterioration or potential critical changes, to prevent further deterioration, and to enable the patient to be moved to a higher level of care if appropriate.

The implementation of this report was reviewed in the document *Beyond Comprehensive Critical Care* (Department of Health, 2005). This review highlighted some of the successes of comprehensive critical care, including:

♦ the successful implementation of outreach

♦ the development of more level 3 beds throughout the UK

♦ the implementation of track and trigger scores.

It recognized, however, the need to continue to develop:

♦ outreach to provide 24-h cover, 7 days a week

♦ effective track-and-trigger scoring systems

Table 1.1 Level of care definition

Level	Descriptor of level
Level 0	Patients whose needs can be met through normal ward care in an acute hospital
Level 1	Patients at risk of their condition deteriorating or those recently relocated from higher levels of care whose needs can be met on an acute ward with advice and support
Level 2	Patients requiring more detailed observation or intervention, including support for single organ failure, post-operative care, and those stepping down from higher levels of care
Level 3	Patients requiring advanced respiratory support or basic respiratory support and support of at least two organs, including all complex patients requiring support for multi-organ failure

Department of Health (2000)

- knowledge and skills in ward nurses
- education programmes
- services for those patients discharged from higher levels of care
- roles to support and optimize patient care.

More worryingly, however, it identified a number of problems that were not new and had not improved, despite the widespread acceptance of comprehensive critical care. The review highlighted that sometimes patient observations were not recorded and this led to acutely ill patients not always being assessed appropriately. It identified that even where observations were recorded there was sometimes an inadequate understanding of critical illness and its presentation that may have prevented the instigation of timely interventions. It again acknowledged the concept of suboptimal care in some ward patients.

The concept of suboptimal care

The concept of suboptimal care is not new and over the last decade a number of studies have examined whether ward patients, whose conditions deteriorated, received suboptimal care prior to cardiac arrest/ITU admission (McArthur Rousse 2001).

The term suboptimal care is used to relate to the multifactorial issues regarding the significance of clinical changes in patients causing potential misdiagnosis, inappropriate management, or lack of timely and appropriate care delivery. Studies suggest that suboptimal care commonly relates to airway/breathing/circulatory problems that are sometimes ignored, misdiagnosed, or inappropriately managed on ward areas (McArthur Rousse 2001).

One of the most frequently cited studies is McQuillain *et al.* (1998). This study identified that approximately 54% of patients had received 'suboptimal' care prior to admission to ITU that had a substantial impact on patient mortality and morbity. It highlighted that a large proportion of ITU admissions may have been avoidable if the patients' deterioration in condition had been diagnosed/treated earlier. The study identified several potential problems, including:

- lack of knowledge/experience of staff
- failure to appreciate the urgency of the patient's changing condition
- failure to seek advice about the patient's condition
- lack of medical staff/supervision of medical staff
- organizational failings that prevented appropriate assessment and treatment of the patient who was deteriorating.

Worryingly, the study highlighted a fundamental problem related to inadequate assessment of their breathing and circulation, which could quickly lead to patient death if not treated appropriately. Approximately 50% of the patients had received suboptimal assessment of their airway, and inadequate assessment of their respiration and circulatory systems. Additionally, several had not received sufficient monitoring or appropriate oxygen therapy.

A similar study (McGloin *et al.* 1999) also acknowledged that patients had shown clinical signs of deterioration that had not been recognized and had received inappropriate treatment. They concluded that patients with obvious clinical indicators of acute deterioration were sometimes overlooked and may have received inappropriate treatment. A number of changes were suggested to overcome these problems, including:

- changes in the structure of the organization to recognize the need for training and support when caring for acutely ill patients
- changes to the supervision of junior staff

- improved recognition of serious illness symptoms, especially those related to changes in airway, breathing, and circulation
- the need for the development of medical emergency teams.

It was anticipated that adoption of these and other recommendations would decrease suboptimal care on acute wards.

However, the publication of the National Confidential Inquiry into Patient Outcome and Death (2005) highlighted that detection and management of the acutely ill patient remained problematic despite measures to improve care. It highlighted a continuing problem with the delivery of acute care, indicating continuing problems with the assessment and management of acute illness.

Patient assessment

The National Confidential Enquiry into Patient Outcome and Death (2005) report importantly acknowledged that there were positive improvements in patient assessment. It identified that nursing staff did record observations and the frequency of these appeared to increase as the patient's condition worsened.

However, it recognized a number of critical areas, including prolonged periods of physiological instability prior to ITU admission. The report identified that 66% of patients had exhibited physiological instability for more than 12 h. Assessment therefore remained an issue, especially omission of part/parts of the assessment.

The most frequently omitted assessment was respiratory rate assessment, and oxygen saturation appeared to be recorded in preference to respiratory rate. Although pulse oximetry monitoring was increasing, staff were sometimes unfamiliar with the use, limitations, and interpretation of results, leading to potentially serious errors in interpretation. The report additionally highlighted problems with the qualifications of those recording observations, identifying that observations were frequently recorded by healthcare assistants who may not fully understand the implications of changes in physiological measurements.

Although there appeared to be an increase in the amount and frequency of observations, there were still limitations related to plans for observation and acting on these observations. Patients' notes seldom contained detail related to the type and frequency of observations. In addition, instructions giving parameters that should trigger patient review were rarely documented. These issues often led to problems with patient assessment and delay in appropriate management.

Patient management

The National Confidential Enquiry into Patient Outcome and Death report acknowledged that 90% of patients' notes documented adequate history and examination. However, the remaining 10% of the patients had incomplete history and physical examination, and no clear treatment plan. In addition, appropriate treatment was often delayed and up to 42% of the patients had received either inappropriate or delayed treatment. Common problems were lack of appropriate oxygen therapy and delayed fluid resuscitation. Medical referral and assessment remained problematic and 50% of patients were reviewed by very junior medical staff; only 39% of the patients had been reviewed by a consultant within 24 h of admission. The report also highlighted delays in the medical decision to admit a patient to ITU and admission to ITU. Lack of staff/beds was the cause in 36% of delayed admissions. Patients were often not referred to ITU in a timely manner and in 22% of cases the referral was deemed too late.

The report highlighted that on some occasions more timely and appropriate care may have prevented admission to ITU. It also highlighted admissions where ITU care was inappropriate and palliative care may have been a more appropriate option. It emphasized the need for appropriate treatment, Do not attempt resuscitation (DNAR) orders, and ceilings for treatment in patients who were unlikely to respond to intensive care. Worryingly, the study still noted some problems with the appreciation of urgency, ability to seek advice from senior doctors, and lack of supervision of junior staff.

Among the recommendations from the National Confidential Enquiry into Patient Outcome and Death report, a number have been made in relation to assessment and management following this audit (see Table 1.2).

Following publication of this report, the National Patient Safety Agency (2007a) published statistics of failures in care relating to patient safety issues in acute care. The aim of these is to highlight areas where acute care is failing and provide solutions to recurrent problems. The last National Patient Safety Agency report (2007a) highlighted specific management issues that had resulted in the death of patients. Sixty-four deaths in 2005 were found to be related to 'patient deterioration not recognized and not acted upon'.

In 14 reports it was found that there was a failure to measure basic observations:

> 'Outreach nurse attended cardiac arrest. . . . On review of MEWS chart, no observations performed for 2 days and therefore no early warning scores available'
>
> National Patient Safety Agency (2007a)

In 30 reports the importance of clinical deterioration had not been recognized and no action taken:

> 'Patient transferred, handover given. Routine observations showed low oxygen saturations 80%—no oxygen prescribed . . . no information given at handover re oxygen'
>
> National Patient Safety Agency (2007a)

Table 1.2 NCEPOD recommendations

Assessment recommendations	Management recommendations
Clear physiological monitoring plan for every patient	Consultants should review all patients within 24 h of hospital admission
Documented explicit parameters that should prompt medical review	Consultants should be involved in the decision to admit the patient to ITU
Importance of respiratory recording should be highlighted	Training should be provided to junior doctors in the recognition and management of fluid and oxygen therapy
Education regarding use and limitation of pulse oximetry	Junior doctors should seek senior advice more readily
It should be emphasized that oxygen saturation recording should not replace respiratory rate monitoring	Junior doctors should be closely supervised
More attention paid to those patients exhibiting physiological abnormalities	Resuscitation status should be clearly documented in patients who are at risk of clinical deterioration
Development of robust track-and-trigger systems	Delays in ITU admission should be recorded as a clinical incident and referred to clinical governance
Implementation of formal outreach teams	

ITU, intensive therapy unit.

In 17 reports it was noted that although deterioration had been identified, there was a delay in medical treatment. These reports highlighted that although nurses had noted deterioration they could not get medical help quickly enough:

'The doctor was very indecisive and the patient's condition was deteriorating, staff member suggested the doctor speak to the ITU outreach team . . . the patient's condition was still deteriorating and crashed'

National Patient Safety Agency (2007a)

Examination of these recurrent problems suggests there is a still a problem with suboptimal care and, whilst clearly a lot of progress has been made, there is a need to provide greater guidance, develop more services, and improve education for all staff caring for acutely ill patients.

The National Patient Safety Agency report again acknowledged the need for changes in the delivery of acute care. Its key recommendations in relation to recognition and timely treatment were:

♦ better recognition of patients at risk of deterioration or who have deteriorated

♦ appropriate monitoring of vital signs

♦ accurate interpretation of clinical findings

♦ calling for help early and ensuring it arrives

♦ training for junior doctors to enable them to recognize and respond to acutely ill patients quickly

♦ junior doctors to seek support from senior staff more readily

♦ training and skills development

♦ ensuring appropriate drugs and equipment are available.

It also emphasized the need for national guidelines relating to the management of acute care.

A subsequent study by the National Patient Safety Agency (2007b) highlighted practitioners' perceptions of contributory factors that affect the management of the patient whose condition is deteriorating. Overwhelmingly this study highlighted communication problems as the biggest problem area within incidents. It identified:

♦ poor communication between ward and medical staff

♦ lack of clarity/detail when communicating concerns about patients

♦ lack of detail regarding the patient, a factor that was particularly problematic when medical staff were covering areas out of hours

♦ poor written communication.

The study identified the need to use effective communication tools (see Chapter 12).

Contemporary guidance on delivery of acute care

The NICE guidelines *Acutely Ill Patients in Hospital: Recognition of and Response to Acute Illness in Adults in Hospital* (2007) have arisen because of the problems associated with acute care and the continuing recurrence of suboptimal care.

The aim of the guidelines is to make evidence-based recommendations on the recognition and management of acute illness in acute hospitals. The philosophy behind the guidelines is to ensure a timely and rapid response to the acutely ill hospital patient. The NICE guidelines set out key priorities relating to acute care delivery focusing on:

♦ monitoring the acutely ill patient

♦ use of track-and-trigger systems

+ graded responses to the patient who is deteriorating
+ accepting a patient back from level 3/ITU care
+ development of acute care competencies.

To avoid confusion all recommendations made by NICE are quoted verbatim.

Monitoring the acutely ill patient

NICE acknowledged that physiological abnormalities are a marker for clinical deterioration and that the number of physiological abnormalities impacts greatly on mortality (21.3% risk of death if there are three changes in physiological parameters Goldhill & McNarry 2004). They recommend the following:

+ Physiological observations should be recorded on admission or initial patient assessment.
+ There should be a clear monitoring plan that specifies which physiological signs should be recorded and how often. This plan should take account of the patient's diagnosis, presence of comorbities, and agreed treatment plan.
+ Physiological observations should be recorded and acted on by staff who have been trained in the procedure and understand the clinical relevance of the recording.
+ As a bare minimum the following should be recorded:

  • heart rate
  • respiratory rate
  • systolic blood pressure
  • level of consciousness
  • oxygen saturation
  • temperature.

Use of track-and-trigger systems

NICE identified a number of problems surrounding the evidence base relating to track-and-trigger systems. They suggested that there were inherent flaws with the design of the systems, and that as yet there was not one system robust enough to detect changes in all patient groups. However NICE recommended that:

+ physiological track-and-trigger systems should be used for all adult patients in acute hospital settings
+ track-and-trigger systems should use multi-parameter or aggregate weighting scoring systems
+ physiological observations should be recorded at least every 12 h unless a decision has been made at senior level to increase or decrease the frequency for an individual patient
+ the frequency of monitoring should increase if any abnormal physiological response is detected (further detail is included in Chapter 11).

Graded response to the patient who is deteriorating

NICE stressed the need for two levels of response to the deteriorating ward patient. Firstly, at ward level the response may be increased in terms of frequency of observations or a call to the medical team responsible for the patient care. The second level response is at hospital level, and involves the use of a dedicated hospital team who are skilled at managing the acutely ill patient. They recommended a graded response strategy for patients identified as being at risk of deterioration. It should be agreed locally but would consist of three levels:

♦ low score group

♦ medium score group

♦ high score group.

More detail about graded response is included in Chapter 11.

Transfer of patients from critical care areas

NICE highlighted the evidence against unplanned discharge from ITU, identifying that transfer of patients from ITU at night is associated with an increased mortality rate and a higher ITU re-admission rate. They recommended that:

♦ the patient should be transferred out of ITU (once the decision to discharge is made) as early in the day as possible

♦ transfer out of ITU between 22:00 and 07:00 should be avoided where possible, and documented as an adverse incident if it occurs.

Alongside this, NICE also stressed the need to support the ward staff when discharging a patient from ITU. Evidence suggests that care of patients post ITU discharge is complex, but four areas are important:

♦ continuity of care between ward and ITU staff

♦ help with managing physical and emotional experiences

♦ help with managing transition from one-to-one care to lower staffing levels on a ward

♦ information on condition and the recovery process.

More detail about caring for a patient post ITU can be found in Chapter 15.

Development of acute care competencies

In the original documentation, NICE do not provide an evidence base for the development of competence. However they recommend that:

♦ staff caring for patients in acute hospital settings have competencies in monitoring, measurement, interpretation, and prompt response to acutely ill patients appropriate to the level of care they are providing

♦ education and training should be provided to ensure staff have these competencies, and they should be assessed to ensure they can demonstrate them.

Since the publication of the NICE guidelines the Department of Health (2009) have now released competencies for recognizing and responding to acutely ill patients in hospital. The development of these competencies is timely, recognizing the increased acuity of patients nursed in ward areas and the need to ensure that staff are able to recognize deterioration and manage patients who are at risk of deterioration competently and efficiently (Department of Health 2008).

A chain of response approach

The key principle behind the development of competence is to ensure that all staff that care for the acutely ill patient are competent to respond within their own sphere of competence, and to ensure rapidly escalating levels of intervention if a patient's condition deteriorates.

The competencies stress the need for a team approach to the patient who is deteriorating. Team members need to be competent in (Department of Health 2009):

- recording and documentation of vital signs
- recognition of abnormal values and the ability to interpret these in the context of the individual patient
- provision of clinical intervention in a timely manner that reflects the risk of further patient deterioration
- recognition when a higher level of assistance is required
- effective communication to ensure patient receives optimum care.

The competencies identify and define the knowledge, skills, and attitudes required for safe and effective care. They acknowledge that acute care is a team responsibility and identify differing team roles using a 'chain of response'. Each member of the chain has identified roles and limitations; it is acknowledged that there may be some crossover in roles for some team members.

The roles are organized on a continuum:

Non-clinical staff	Recorder	Recognizer	Primary responder	Secondary responder	Tertiary responder (critical care)

The guidelines only really identify that members of the team who are tertiary responders will be staff with expert critical care experience. They have, however, provided role descriptors for each of the levels of staff. It is likely that there will be some individual interpretation of these roles by local NHS trusts.

- *Non-clinical staff*: may be 'the alerter'. This could include the patient or a relative/visitor.
- *The recorder*: undertakes designated measurements, records observations and information.
- *The recognizer*: monitors patient's condition, interprets measurements, observations and information. Adjusts frequency of observations and level of monitoring.
- *The primary responder*: goes beyond recording and interprets measurements and implements a clinical plan, e.g. commencement of oxygen, insertion of airway, selection of intravenous fluid and administration of fluid bolus.
- *The secondary responder*: is likely to be called to attend when a patient fails to respond to primary intervention to formulate a diagnosis, refine the management plan, initiate a secondary response, and have the skills/knowledge to recognize when referral to critical care is indicated.
- *Tertiary responder*: this role will be undertaken by staff who have advanced critical care skills, e.g. advanced airway management, resuscitation, clinical examination, and interpretation of critically ill patients.

Alongside these roles the Department of Health (2009) recognizes the need for complementary generic competencies, including:

- effective record keeping
- interpersonal skills
- the ability to work as a team member
- clinical decision making.

The need for effective and timely communication in the recognition and management of the acutely ill patient is stressed in the conceptualization of the chain of response.

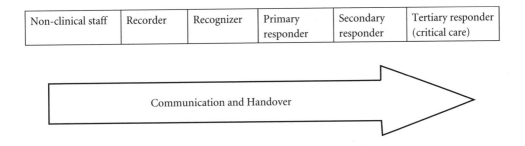

| Non-clinical staff | Recorder | Recognizer | Primary responder | Secondary responder | Tertiary responder (critical care) |

Communication and Handover

The competencies have been designed to provide consistent standards for hospital and ward staff involved in the care and management of acutely ill patients. They have been designed so that each member of 'the chain of response' has clearly articulated roles and competence.

The competencies identified as essential are organized into groups using subheadings for the groups of competencies identified. These include:

♦ airway, breathing, ventilation, and oxygenation

♦ circulation

♦ transport and mobility

♦ acute neurological care

♦ patient-centred care, team working, and communication.

Each of these subheadings has a number of skills identified and competence is described in relation to the 'chain of response'. One example, for a ward nurse assessing respiration, is provided below (Table 1.3). The ward nurse, depending on local protocol/experience and level of assessed competence, will act as a recorder, a recognizer, or a primary responder.

Roles and competence levels are also identified for secondary/tertiary responses. These are likely to be roles carried out by outreach nurses/senior medical staff. The tertiary response must be adopted by staff with critical care expertise (see Table 1.4).

The full guidelines and list of competencies can be found on the Department of Health website (http://www.dh.gov.uk) and covers a wide range of skills and associated knowledge required to effectively manage the acutely ill patient.

Table 1.3 Clinical example demonstrating the chain of response

Competency group	Recorder sphere of competence	Recognizer sphere of competence	Primary responder sphere of competence
Respiratory rate	Measures respiratory rate, records result, and assigns trigger score Has knowledge of what constitutes an abnormal value	Interprets trigger in context of patient and responds in accordance with escalation protocols Adjusts frequency of observations in keeping with trigger	Identifies inadequate respiratory effort and institutes clinical management therapies

Department of Health (2008 draft guidelines)

Table 1.4 Role descriptors/chain of response

Secondary responder	Tertiary (ITU) response
Evaluates effectiveness of treatment, refines treatment plan if necessary, formulates a diagnosis, and recognizes when referral to critical care is indicated	Refer to critical care core competencies, but main aim is to provide an 'expert' critical care response and appropriate intervention

ITU, intensive therapy unit.

Alongside publication of this chain of response, the Department of Health has also stressed the need for a number of other changes to facilitate the development of competence, including:

♦ workforce planning and design

♦ role design

♦ role appraisal

♦ education, training, and development.

♦ education commissioning, planning, and provision.

♦ design of professional and vocational qualifications

♦ clinical supervision

♦ professional revalidation/registration.

The document emphasizes the need for the development of competence and, for the first time, makes explicit the need for hospitals to take ownership and responsibility in ensuring all staff are competent in early recognition and treatment of acutely ill patients. As this process is still in its developmental stages it is difficult to comment on implementation of the competency framework. It is clear, however, that additional education will be an important tool in developing these competencies.

How can this book contribute to the development of competence?

The authors of this book acknowledge the need for safe and competent care when nursing acutely ill patients. They support the view that assessment of competence is integral if safe and effective care is to be delivered. They suggest that the publication of the NICE guidelines and the competence framework is an important first step but more input is needed. Recommendations, although highlighting the drive for improvement of acute care delivery, will do little to support the development of competence in acute care without other interventions. There is a need to provide practising nurses with the knowledge and evidence base to care for acutely ill patients as well as providing guidelines for care and frameworks for assessment.

It is clear from examination of the literature that several 1-day or short courses are available relating to acute care (e.g. basic life support, acute life-threatening events recognition and treatment (ALERT™) course, advanced life-support, and ill medical patients acute care and treatment (IMPACT)). These are useful in providing short courses on recognizing and treating acutely ill patients.

Most higher education institutions have developed acute care modules/pathways to support the drive for acute care education. This is an important development and should be viewed as the 'gold standard' for nursing acutely ill patients. However, these courses have limited numbers and may not be immediately accessible to all nurses.

Several short books have been recently published offering 'quick guides' to the rapid assessment and treatment of acutely ill patients. Again this is an important step, as often these books allow rapid diagnosis and treatment for the patient who is deteriorating. However, many of these books do not offer sufficient depth to allow nurses to explore and develop understanding of the knowledge and skills required to enable them to effectively care for this very complex group of patients.

The authors of this book fundamentally believe knowledge and practice skills need to be developed so that competence can be achieved in practice. They acknowledge the complexities associated with caring for this growing group of patients, where performing skills alone is insufficient. It is fundamentally important for nurses to understand why (knowledge) and how (evidence-based skills) these patients should be cared for. Effective acute care cannot be provided unless staff have the:

♦ associated knowledge

♦ psychomotor skill/evidence based practice

♦ need for continuous development of competence/lifelong learning.

This view is supported by educationalists. As early as the 1950s Bloom (1956) identified a number of components to effective learning, stressing the need for education to cover all components of learning. He identified three components or domains, including:

1 cognitive domain (knowledge)

2 psychomotor domain (practical skills)

3 affective domain (attitude/professional approach).

Because all of these domains are of significance in caring for the acutely ill patient, each chapter of this book will cover each of these domains to ensure an in-depth approach to the complex subject of acute care. The necessity to test all of these domains when assessing competence is recognized. Each chapter will conclude with a competence-based assessment that focuses on testing appropriate knowledge, skills, and attitudes when delivering care to acutely ill patients. Each competence assessment includes elements of the Department of Health (2009) competence framework. Completion of all of the assessments will ensure that most elements of the 2009 competence framework are assessed.

Using this book in clinical practice

The knowledge and practice discussed in each chapter will ensure that this book is an extremely useful resource for nurses working in the ward area or in high-dependency units.

It is aimed at nurses who will be identified at trust level as recognizers and primary responders. It may also be useful for lower levels, e.g. recorders. and for higher levels, e.g. secondary responders, as a teaching resource.

Initial chapters in the book will focus on body systems and each chapter will include the following:

♦ In-depth knowledge of the physiology and pathophysiology to enable the ward nurse to understand the complexities of caring for the acutely ill patient. Knowledge of physiology/pathophysiology will allow nurses to understand why the patient has become unwell and how the patient may present. It will also allow exploration of how treatments may be effective/how treatments relate to physiology/pathophysiology.

♦ Discussion of assessment of each body system. Particular attention will be paid to patient assessment, as this is a fundamental tool in caring for patients with acute illness. Signs and symptoms of patient deterioration and the nurse's role in identifying these will be stressed.

♦ Explanation of the recommended management of patients who are acutely ill, providing the rationale for management/treatment options. The treatment options are evidence-based general guidelines and staff should be aware that local protocols may be used instead.

Treatment and management will focus on generic issues for each system and also include management of common conditions.

♦ Application of theory to practice through the use of acute-care scenarios.

♦ Allow the student to 'test' their own competence at the end of a chapter, using a competence-based testing tool that examines theory, knowledge, and skills related to a specific aspect of acute care. It is recognized that other assessment tools may be used in clinical areas that are trust-specific.

Later chapters will relate to particular management issues of acute illness and will explore current issues relevant to acute care, including:

♦ the role of outreach

♦ patient assessment tools/track-and-trigger systems

♦ care of the patient post ITU

♦ peri-arrest/cardiac arrest management

♦ the need for continuing education.

References

Bloom, B. (1956) *The Taxonomy of Educational Objectives: the Classification of Educational Goals, Handbook 1.* McKay, New York.

Coad, S. and Haines, C. (1999) Supporting staff caring for critically ill patients in acute care. *Nurs. Crit. Care.* **4,** 245–8.

Department of Health (2000) *Comprehensive Critical Care, a Review of Adult Critical Care Services.* HMSO, London.

Department of Health (2005) *Beyond Comprehensive Critical Care.* HMSO, London.

Department of Health Foreword, Beasley, C. (2008) In: *Competencies for Recognising and Responding to Acutely Ill Adults in Hospital.* Draft guidelines for consultation. HMSO, London.

Department of Health (2009) *Competencies for Recognising and Responding to Acutely Ill Adults in Hospital.* Draft guidelines for consultation. HMSO, London.

Goldhill, D. and McNarry, A. (2004) Physiological abnormalities in early warning scores are related to mortality in adult patients. *J. Roy. Coll. Anaesthetists.* **92,** 882–4.

Jevon, P. Foreword, Endacott, R. (2007) In: *Treating the Critically Ill Patient.* Blackwell, Oxford.

McArthur Rousse, F. (2001) Critical care outreach services and early warning scores: a review of the literature. *J. Adv. Nurs.* **36,** 396–704.

McGloin, H., Adam, S., and Singer, M. (1999) Unexpected deaths and referrals to ITU of patients on wards. Are some cases potentially avoidable?. *J. Roy. Coll. Physicians Lond.* **33,** 255–9.

McQuillain, P., Pilkington, S., Allan, A.*et al.* (1998) Confidential inquiry into quality of care before admission to ITU. *BMJ.* **316,** 1853–8.

National Confidential Enquiry into Patient Outcome and Death (2005) *An acute problem? A Report of National Confidential Enquiry into Patient Outcome and Death.* National Confidential Enquiry into Patient Outcome and Death, London.

National Patient Safety Agency (2007a) *Safer Care for the Acutely Ill Patient: Learning from Serious Incidents.* National Patient Safety Agency, London.

National Patient Safety Agency (2007b) *Recognising and Responding Appropriately to Early Signs of Deterioration in Hospitalized Patients.* National Patient Safety Agency, London.

NICE (2007) *Acutely Ill Patients in Hospital: Recognition of and Response to Acute Illness of Adults in Hospital.* HMSO, London.

Robson, W. (2002) An evaluation of the evidence base related to critical care outreach teams—2 years on from comprehensive critical care. *Intensive Crit. Care Nurs.* **18,** 211–8.

Sheppard, M. and Wright, M. (2005) *Principles and Practice of High Dependency Nursing.* Elsevier, Edinburgh.

Chapter 2

Respiratory assessment and care

Annie Chellel

Chapter contents

The purpose of this chapter is to increase your confidence in recognizing, assessing, and managing patients with respiratory impairment. It will enable you to develop the knowledge, skill, and understanding to fulfil your nursing role, which is threefold: firstly it is to ensure patient safety by assessing patients using your knowledge and understanding of the respiratory system, secondly it is to co-ordinate and support the medical management, and thirdly it is to reassure and comfort the patient, who will inevitably be distressed and frightened. The chapter will examine:

- the anatomy and physiology of respiration
- ventilation perfusion ratios: type I and type II respiratory failure
- lung dynamics
- the transport of gases
- the principles of arterial blood gas analysis
- the prevalence and cost of respiratory disease
- the causes of breathlessness
- assessing respiratory function
- three common respiratory pathophysiologies
- oxygen therapy
- drug therapy
- the principles of non-invasive ventilation
- management of patients with chest drains
- nursing the patient with acute respiratory impairment.

Learning outcomes

This chapter will enable you to:

- recognize and interpret the signs and symptoms of respiratory impairment
- carry out a nursing assessment of respiratory function
- identify the most likely cause of respiratory impairment
- interpret the clinical significance of arterial blood gas analysis
- differentiate between the modes of action of bronchodilators
- manage the care of the patient undergoing non-invasive ventilation

- manage the safe delivery of oxygen therapy
- manage the care of patients with a chest drain.

Anatomy and physiology of respiration

The purpose of breathing is to move oxygen from the air into the lungs (external respiration), where it can enter the blood for transport to the tissues. The tissues need oxygen from the blood (internal respiration) for cell metabolism and the production of energy. The anatomy of the respiratory system consists of upper airways from the nose, mouth, and oropharynx to the larynx, leading to the lower airways, i.e. trachea, bronchi, bronchioles, and alveoli. The lungs are contained in the thoracic cavity and protected by the spine, manubrium, and sternum, and the springy 'cage' of the 12 pairs of ribs and their costal cartilages (see Figure 2.1). Note that, anteriorally, the apices of the lungs extend above the clavicle and the bases are curved around the hemispherical dome of the diaphragm. Their position relative to the ribs varies with inspiration and expiration (see Figure 2.2). The trachea, bronchi, and bronchioles are for the conduction of air to the alveoli, and the air in them, which is not involved in gaseous exchange, is known as the anatomical dead space. The diameters of the trachea and bronchi are maintained by cartilaginous rings and the trachea, bronchi, and bronchioles are lined with a ciliated epithelium coated with mucus. The synchronous wafting movement of the cilia results in an upward movement of the mucus and is known as the mucociliary escalator. This removes small inhaled particles from the lungs (see Figure 2.3).

Ventilation

Ventilation means getting oxygen from the air into the lungs by inspiration and getting the waste carbon dioxide out of the body by expiration. It is essentially a mechanical process, governed by the laws of physics. The lungs are divided into lobes, with three on the right but only two on the left because of the space taken up by the heart (see Figure 2.4). They are contained in the thorax by the pleura. The parietal pleura adhere to the ribs and intercostal muscles, while the visceral

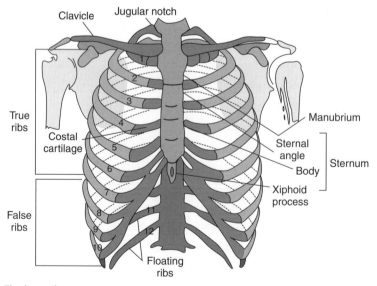

Figure 2.1 The bony thorax.

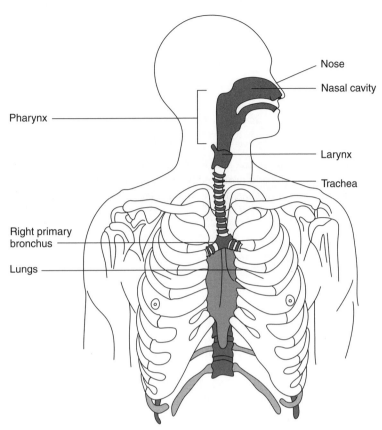

Figure 2.2 The anatomy of the respiratory system.

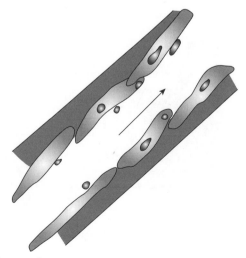

Figure 2.3 The mucociliary escalator.

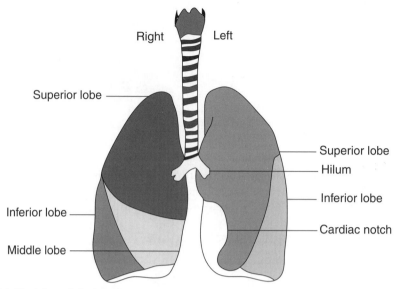

Figure 2.4 The lobes of the lungs.

pleura adhere to the lungs. This ensures that on inspiration, as the ribs are actively moved upwards and outwards by the intercostal muscles and the diaphragm moves downwards, the lungs are 'stretched' as the thoracic cavity enlarges (see Figure 2.5). This results in a lowering of intrathoracic pressure and the inhalation of air. Expiration is normally passive, as the intercostal muscles are relaxed, the diaphragm rises, the ribs move back downwards and inwards, reducing the size of the thoracic cavity, enabling elastic recoil of the lungs so that air is exhaled. Inspiration is active and unlike the heart, the muscles of respiration have no intrinsic activity.

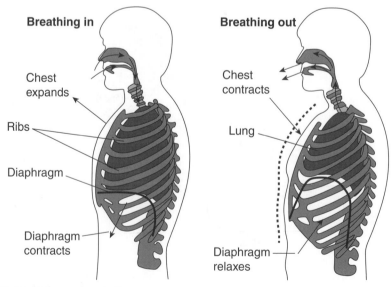

Figure 2.5 Inspiration and expiration.

Inspiration and expiration are governed by laws of physics that state that gases move from areas of higher pressure to areas of lower pressure to create equilibrium. It is the changes in pressure that bring about the changes in lung volume between inspiration and expiration. If atmospheric and intrathoracic pressures were to remain the same there would be no movement of air and therefore the work of breathing lies in moving the ribs and diaphragm to increase thoracic capacity, reduce intrathoracic pressure, and draw air into the lungs.

External respiration (gaseous exchange in the lungs)

External respiration refers to the gaseous exchange that takes place in the alveoli of the lungs across the thin alveolar capillary membrane (see Figure 2.6). There are approximately 300 million alveoli available for gaseous exchange. There are two types of cell within the alveoli. Type I cells line the alveoli and have few organelles while there is a much smaller number of type II cells, which are rounded, have large nuclei, and produce and store surfactant. Gaseous exchange in the alveoli is governed by Dalton's law, which relates to the partial pressure of gases. Diffusion takes place because of the concentration gradient between alveolar and capillary partial pressures of oxygen and carbon dioxide. Venous blood has a higher carbon dioxide and a lower oxygen content than alveolar air, resulting in diffusion to create an equilibrium. Oxygen moves into the blood and carbon dioxide moves into the alveoli. Carbon dioxide is able to diffuse more readily than oxygen as it is a more soluble gas (Henry's law).

Internal respiration (gaseous exchange in the tissues)

The cells need oxygen to drive metabolism. This is the intracellular process, which takes place in the mitochondria of the cell nucleus. Glucose and oxygen are used in Kreb's citric acid cycle to produce energy in the form of energy-rich phosphate bonds by converting adenosine diphosphate (ADP) to adenosine triphosphate (ATP), see Figure 2.7.

The waste products of cell metabolism are water and carbon dioxide. This means that, at the tissues, where oxygen is consumed by the requirements of cell metabolism and carbon dioxide is produced, the situation is reversed. Carbon dioxide moves into the capillaries and oxygen moves into the cells (see Figure 2.8). This exchange of gases in the tissues is referred to as internal respiration.

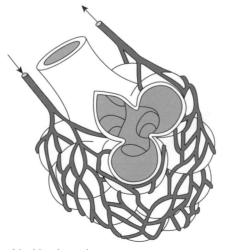

Figure 2.6 An alveolus and its blood supply.

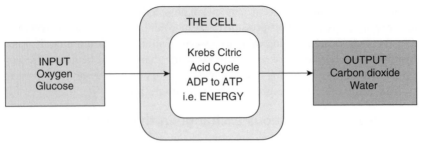

Figure 2.7 Cell metabolism.

The control of breathing

Clinical presentation is the basis for diagnosing respiratory failure, which is confirmed by arterial blood gas analysis. However, the most significant clinical indicator is breathlessness. No matter what the cause may be, respiratory failure can be defined as a fall in the level of oxygen in the blood, giving rise to the clinical presentation of breathlessness. This can be explained by the physiological control of respiration, which is mediated by the central nervous system in a very complex interaction of neural, chemical, and muscular stimuli, which is still not entirely understood. Breathing is largely voluntary, with no intrinsic driving system like the heart, and it is therefore dependent on an external neural drive from specialized collections of neurons in the central nervous system. These are the respiratory control centres in the brain, which are located in both the medulla and the pons. In the medulla, the dorsal respiratory group controls inspiration and the ventral respiratory group controls expiration. Normally, expiration is passive through recoil of the respiratory muscles, but becomes active on exertion or respiratory distress.

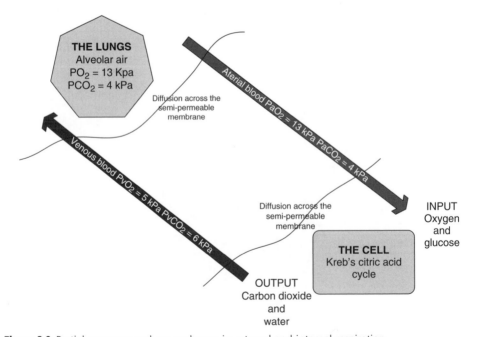

Figure 2.8 Partial pressures and gas exchange in external and internal respiration.

In the pons, the apneustic centre and the pneumotaxic centre control the depth and rhythm of breathing. Together these centres co-ordinate the muscles of respiration to bring about changes in the rate, depth, and rhythm of breathing in response to stimuli from three main influences:

♦ mechanical receptors

♦ the cerebral cortex

♦ central and peripheral chemoreceptors.

Mechanical receptors include irritant receptors in the upper airways, juxtacapillary or j receptors in the alveoli, which respond to increased interstitial volume, and bronchial and pulmonary stretch receptors. These mechanisms ensure that the lungs are, to some extent, protected from barotrauma and overinflation. Pyrexia can also stimulate the respiratory centres while pain can cause inhibition via the mechanical receptors (West 2005).

The *cerebral cortex* can act on the respiratory centres, which is why heightened emotion such as fear can affect respiratory rate and depth.

Chemoreceptors lie centrally on the ventral surface of the medulla, and peripherally in the aortic arch and in the carotid bodies at the bifurcation of the common carotid arteries (West 2005). They lie within the central and peripheral nervous system (Davies & Moores 2003). They are sensitive to changes in the pH, carbon dioxide, and oxygen levels in the blood, and to cerebrospinal fluid. When the level of carbon dioxide in the blood rises (causing a fall in pH) and/or the oxygen content of the blood falls, the chemoreceptors stimulate the respiratory centres, which in turn stimulate the muscles of respiration, causing an increase in the rate and depth of breathing, giving rise to the sensation of breathlessness. This is shown diagrammatically in Figure 2.9.

Ventilation perfusion ratios: type I and type II respiratory failure

The two core components of respiratory function are ventilation and perfusion:

♦ ventilation (V)—getting the air into the alveoli for gaseous exchange to take place

♦ perfusion (Q)—getting blood to the alveoli for the diffusion of oxygen into the blood.

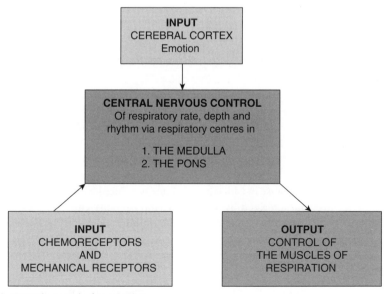

Figure 2.9 Central control of respiration.

The ratio of ventilation to perfusion is important and describes the relationship between the volume of air in the lungs and the volume of blood available in the lungs for gaseous exchange. The output of the right ventricle goes to the lungs, providing pulmonary perfusion at about 5 L/min. Alveolar ventilation is about 4 L/min, giving a V/Q ratio of 0.8:

$$\frac{\text{alveolar ventilation (V)} = 4\ \text{litres per minute}}{\text{pulmonary perfusion (Q)} = 5\ \text{litres per minute}}, \ \text{V:Q ratio} = 0.8$$

This ratio varies a little throughout the lungs because of the effects of gravity, with greater perfusion at the bases and greater ventilation at the apices. Changes in the V/Q ratio give rise to an increased physiological shunt or venous admixture, in which deoxygenated blood enters the arterial circulation and lowers the overall oxygen concentration of the blood. This might be because ventilation is reduced, giving a low ratio, or because perfusion is reduced, giving a high ratio, as illustrated in the following examples:

- If ventilation were reduced to 2 L but perfusion remained at 5 L the V/Q ratio would be low at 0.4. A clinical example of a low V/Q ratio is atelectasis
- If ventilation remained at 5 L but perfusion were reduced to 3 L, the V/Q ratio would be high at 1.7. A clinical example of a high V/Q ratio is pulmonary embolism.

In either case the effect would be to lower the oxygen content in the blood and this is called *type I respiratory failure*. It is characterized by a normal pH and arterial carbon dioxide ($PaCO_2$), but a low arterial oxygen (PaO_2) of less than 8 kPa. This is because the hypoxaemia triggers the chemoreceptors, resulting in an increased respiratory rate that increases the expired CO_2. This compensation cannot be maintained indefinitely and, left untreated, will lead to alveolar hypoventilation as the patient tires, the arterial carbon dioxide rises, and the pH consequently falls (see section on the principles of arterial blood gas analysis). This is called *type II respiratory failure* and it is characterized by both hypoxaemia and hypercapnia (raised arterial CO_2) and a fall in pH (respiratory acidosis).

The other significant component of respiratory function is lung dynamics, which are concerned with the flow of air into the lungs and the resistance to it created by the airways.

Lung dynamics

Compliance

Compliance refers to the distensibility of an elastic structure (such as the lung) and is defined as the change in volume of that structure produced by a change in pressure across the structure: in other words, stretchiness or elasticity of the lung tissue is essential in allowing the chest to expand and draw in air. It is important to understand that the lungs will not increase in size if the pressure within and around them is increased equally at the same time. It is the difference between the pressure within the lungs and the outside air that causes air to be drawn in, but it is the stretchiness of the lungs that allows the chest to expand and alter the pressure. It therefore follows that abnormally stiff, non-compliant lungs cause a restriction of lung expansion, giving rise to ventilatory deficit.

Restrictive lung diseases are those in which lung volume is reduced without reduction of flow in the airways. They are characterized by a reduced vital capacity caused by diseases of the lung parenchyma such as fibrosis, neuromuscular conditions, and mechanical or pathological disruption of pleura.

Resistance

Airway resistance is the opposition to flow caused by the forces of friction. It is a function of the ratio of inspiratory pressure to the rate of air flow. While a single small airway provides more resistance than a single large airway, resistance to air flow depends on the number of parallel pathways present. For this reason, the large and particularly the medium-sized airways actually provide greater resistance to flow than the more numerous small airways.

Obstructive lung diseases are those in which there is increased resistance caused by an obstruction to inspired airflow, leading to a reduction in exhaled volume, air trapping, and a consequent retention of CO_2.

Surface tension

This is a tendency for the molecules on the surface of a liquid to pull together. This is why, when water lies on a surface, it forms rounded droplets, and why bubbles tend to be spherical. The higher the surface tension the lower the compliance.

Surfactant

A surfactant is a mixture of phospholipids that is produced by type II alveolar cells and reduces the surface tension within the alveoli. This increases alveolar stability by inhibiting alveolar collapse as they shrink.

Alterations in lung dynamics affect respiratory function by bringing about changes in lung volumes.

Lung volumes

Measures of lung volume using spirometry are used clinically to assess respiratory function. Some are measured and some are calculated in order to assess some of the changes that take place in the common respiratory pathologies, although for most clinical purposes in acute care, the vital capacity (i.e. the maximum volume that can be inhaled and exhaled) and the tidal volume (i.e. the volume breathed in and out in one normal breath) are the most useful. The forced expiratory volume 1 (FEV1), i.e. the forced expiratory volume in 1 second, should be about 80% of the forced vital capacity (FVC), and the ratio of the FEV1 to the vital capacity is used as an indicator of severity in obstructive lung disease. The ratio normally declines with age and so actual and predicted measures are used in assessment by spirometry.

The transport of gases

The effective transport of gases from the lungs to the tissue and from the tissue to the lungs is essential and dependent on a number of factors involved in the carriage of gases and maintenance of adequate cardiac output. The majority of oxygen (98.5%) is transported on the haemoglobin (Hb) molecule, while a small amount is dissolved in plasma (approximately 1.5%). A number of factors affect the uptake of oxygen at lung level and the release of oxygen at tissue level.

The main factor that affects oxygen carriage at the lungs is the concentration of oxygen at alveoli level. If the concentration is high, more oxygen will be available for diffusion. If the concentration is low, blood oxygen levels will be reduced. At the lungs oxygen binds to the haemoglobin molecule to facilitate its delivery to the tissue. Each haemoglobin molecule has the capacity to carry four molecules of oxygen, so if four molecules of oxygen are attached to a haemoglobin molecule it is fully saturated. Once the haemoglobin molecule is fully saturated, increased levels of inspired oxygen will not improve oxygen carriage.

At tissue level, oxygen will dissociate from the haemoglobin molecule and enter into the cells because of the decreased intracellular oxygen concentration. A number of factors, usually present when the cell is very active, will facilitate this release. These factors include the presence of hydrogen ions and an increase in cellular temperature. These factors facilitate the release of oxygen

.rom the haemoglobin molecule and ensure that cells that are actively metabolizing receive an increased supply of oxygen.

The carriage of carbon dioxide from the tissue is more complex. When it binds with cellular water, carbon dioxide forms carbonic acid. This has the potential to increase the acidity within the blood and may be detrimental to cellular function. It is essential carbon dioxide is 'buffered' to prevent dramatic changes in blood pH. Carbon dioxide is carried in three ways:

1 a small amount of carbon dioxide is dissolved in plasma (7%)

2 23% combines with globin portion, forming carbaminohaemoglobin ($HbCO_2$)

3 70% is transported in plasma as bicarbonate ions.

At the lungs the complex chemical reactions reverse and CO_2 diffuses into the alveoli to be excreted.

The principles of arterial blood gas analysis

Arterial blood gas measurement

Arterial blood is required to assess with greater accuracy than the pulse oximeter the levels of oxygen and carbon dioxide in the blood. The sample analysis also provides important data concerning the patient's blood pH and other parameters for the estimation of acid–base balance.

The sample is normally taken from the radial artery unless the patient is very poorly peripherally perfused, in which case one of the femoral arteries may be used. Arterial sampling is painful and analgesia should normally be used (British Thoracic Society 2008a). A 'pulsator' syringe should be used, which means that the arterial pressure will fill the syringe without the need to withdraw the piston manually. The syringe should also be pre-heparinized to prevent the blood sample from clotting. Following removal of the needle, firm pressure should be applied for at least 5 min to prevent bleeding and bruising. Air should be removed from the sample and the needle replaced with a cap for safe transport. The sample should be taken immediately to the analyser and it is important to note the patient's name, date of birth, and hospital number as well as the level of inspired oxygen at the time of sampling. It is commonly believed that inspired oxygen should be removed prior to taking arterial blood, but this is unnecessary so long as the inspired oxygen level is recorded with the results, and indeed in the acutely sick patient it may be dangerous to do otherwise.

What is the pH?

The pH is a scale that measures the relative acidity or alkalinity of a substance, ranging from 0 (most acidic) to 14 (most alkaline). It is a measurement of hydrogen ion concentration and the higher the hydrogen ion concentration, the lower the pH. It is calculated as a negative logarithm, which simply means that a change of 1 on the pH scale represents a tenfold change in hydrogen ion concentration. A normal blood pH is 7.35–7.45; the life-supporting range allows very little deviation from the normal and is believed to be between 6.8 and 7.8. The pH matters because a change in pH will alter the structure and function of protein. At more extreme hydrogen ion concentrations a protein's structure may be completely disrupted and the protein is said to be 'denatured'. Enzymes are proteins and the body's cell chemistry depends on enzymes as biological catalysts. Enzymes cannot function physiologically outside this narrow pH range.

Acids, bases, and buffers

An acid is a substance that has the ability to donate a hydrogen ion. A base is a substance that has the ability to accept a hydrogen ion and remove it (the buffer) from the circulation. In health the amount of acid and base is carefully regulated. However, in illness the acid–base regulation may become disturbed. It may be useful to think of the buffer as being like a sponge. When hydrogen ions are in excess, the sponge 'mops up' the extra ions. Conversely, when in short supply, the sponge can be squeezed out to release more hydrogen ions. Any excess of acids or bases in the blood may be prevented from altering the blood pH by using buffers to correct the acid–base balance. Buffers allow the harmful effects of acids/bases on the pH to be reduced but they are unable to remove the substances from the blood and are only a temporary measure. The principal buffers are:

◆ plasma proteins, e.g. haemoglobin

◆ bicarbonate buffer system

◆ phosphate buffer system.

Buffers also enable the hydrogen that builds up from cell metabolism to be transported safely to the organs of excretion for permanent removal and so to maintain the pH within normal limits. The reaction in the following equation takes place in the tissues, moving from left to right, because of the build up of carbon dioxide from cell metabolism. The hydrogen is buffered by haemoglobin for safe transport to the organs of excretion, i.e. the kidneys and the lungs. At the lungs the haemoglobin gives up the hydrogen as it takes on oxygen and in the presence of more hydrogen, the carbon dioxide is excreted into the alveoli:

$$CO_2 + H_2O \rightarrow H_2CO_3 + HCO_3^- + H^+$$
$$\text{carbon dioxide} + \text{water} \rightarrow \text{carbonic acid} + \text{bicarbonate} + \text{hydrogen}$$

The end products of cellular metabolism are water and carbon dioxide. When these combine in the plasma they form carbonic acid. This needs to be buffered to prevent the blood becoming acidic. One hydrogen ion is buffered by the haemoglobin molecule, leaving bicarbonate circulating in the blood and allowing safe transport to the organs of excretion. A similar process occurs in the kidneys, where hydrogen is excreted by the proximal and distal convoluted tubules using phosphate as a buffer.

Acid–base disturbances

The classification of acid–base disturbances is dependent on the cause of the disorder and its net effect on the acid–base balance. They may be respiratory or metabolic in nature, and in some incidences of very acute illness they may have both metabolic and respiratory causes. The patient will present with either an acidosis or an alkalosis.

Respiratory acidosis

Respiratory acidosis occurs when there is an accumulation of carbon dioxide in the blood. Carbon dioxide is not acidic in nature until it combines with the water in the plasma to form carbonic acid. Respiratory acidosis commonly occurs as a result of decreased alveolar ventilation and prevention of carbon dioxide removal by the lungs. It may be caused by a number of respiratory disturbances, such as atelectasis, lung infection, neuro muscular dysfunction, chronic obstructive pulmonary disease (COPD), or respiratory failure (see section on respiratory pathophysiologies). It may also be seen post-operatively in patients whose breathing is shallow due to drugs, pain, or anaesthetic. The accumulation of carbon dioxide creates an overall increase in the hydrogen ion concentration in the blood, causing acidity and a fall in the pH. Respiratory acidosis is characterized by high carbon dioxide concentration and a low pH—less than 7.35.

Respiratory alkalosis

Respiratory alkalosis occurs when the lungs remove too much carbon dioxide. The rate and depth of respiration has a direct influence on the excretion of carbon dioxide from the blood. If the respiratory rate or depth of respiration is increased, excessive amounts of carbon dioxide will be removed. A reduction in carbon dioxide causes the overall acid nature of the blood to become alkaline. Respiratory alkalosis is commonly seen in states that may cause the patient to hyperventilate. One of the most common causes is anxiety and this is often seen in patients who are extremely frightened. Other causes are excessive pain that triggers hyperventilation, high temperature that increases the metabolic demand for oxygen, alkalosis, and iron-deficiency anaemia. This increases the respiratory rate and this may in turn cause excessive amounts of carbon dioxide to be removed and result in an alkalosis. Iatrogenic respiratory alkalosis may be caused by excessive mechanical ventilation. Respiratory alkalosis is characterized by a pH of less than 7.45 and a low carbon dioxide concentration.

The parameters on arterial blood gas analysis which indicate respiratory disorders are the oxygen and the carbon dioxide levels.

Metabolic acidosis

Metabolic acidosis occurs if there is an excessive build up of metabolic-acid-based waste products in the blood or failure of the kidney to regulate substances that buffer acids in the blood. Excessive metabolic acid is always indicative of disease processes. Typical acids that may be accumulated are lactic acid (lactate) and ketones. Lactate is produced as an end product of anaerobic metabolism. This is usually caused by poor perfusion to cells. It occurs in most shock states, where lack of blood flow means that demand for oxygen exceeds supply. If cellular metabolism occurs without oxygen then lactate is produced.

Ketones are produced as an end product of fat metabolism in place of glucose and whilst this may occur in moderate amounts in severe dieting, excessive ketones are usually linked to poorly controlled diabetes mellitus. In this condition, lack of insulin prevents metabolism of glucose by the cells and fat is broken down to provide energy.

Patients with renal failure may be unable to produce sufficient amounts of bicarbonate and be unable to excrete hydrogen ions in urine. Both of these factors will cause an increase in hydrogen ion concentration and cause the blood to become acidic. Metabolic acidosis is characterized by a pH less than 7.35 and a low bicarbonate level.

Metabolic alkalosis

This is not seen often in clinical practice. It occurs either if there is an excessive loss of hydrogen ions from the body or if there are excessive amounts of base substances. There are only a very small number of reasons for metabolic alkalosis and each should be quickly excluded. The loss of acid can be caused by excessive vomiting, nasogastric aspiration, or the excessive use of diuretics. Excess base can be caused by the ingestion of large amounts of antacids or by the infusion of sodium bicarbonate. Metabolic alkalosis is characterized by a pH greater than 7.45 and a high bicarbonate.

The parameters on arterial blood gas analysis which indicate metabolic disorder are the base excess and the standard bicarbonate.

Compensation

When an acid–base disturbance exists, the body will attempt to correct the disturbance and maintain homeostasis. This is referred to as 'compensation' and may be respiratory or metabolic in origin.

Respiratory compensation

Respiratory compensation can happen very quickly and the body is therefore able to compensate for metabolic acidosis very quickly. The lungs remove carbon dioxide from the blood in order to lower the overall concentration of acids. The lungs are unable to excrete the offending acids (ketones and lactate) as these are non-volatile and require excretion via the kidneys. However, carbon dioxide is a volatile acid (it is able to move from a fluid to a gaseous state) and therefore removal via the lungs is possible. The lungs are unable to compensate for an acid–base disturbance if the origin is respiratory in nature.

Metabolic compensation

Normally the kidneys excrete hydrogen ions to maintain homeostasis but renal compensation to correct acidosis is much slower than respiratory compensation and works by:

♦ facilitating the removal of hydrogen ions via the kidneys

♦ increasing the production of bicarbonate ions to raise plasma bicarbonate levels

♦ facilitating the removal of bases secreted in the urine.

The renal compensation mechanism takes a considerable time to be effective and the pH may take days to return to normal.

To recap, the body will try to compensate for an acid–base disturbance by trying to create the opposite disorder. For example, if a metabolic acidosis is present the body will attempt to create a respiratory alkalosis to return the pH to normal. If a respiratory acidosis is present the body will try to create a metabolic alkalosis. Compensation will only ever return the pH to its normal or near-normal value; over-correction will never occur.

Assessing a patient's arterial blood gas

The use of arterial blood gases to inform clinical decision-making on wards has become increasingly frequent, necessitating the ward nurse having a basic understanding of acid–base-balance physiology and the basic skills of blood gas interpretation in the context of the patient.

It must be stressed that arterial blood gases must always be considered in the context of the individual patient and their presenting symptoms. It is not useful to interpret in isolation, as factors that may explain the changes in arterial blood gases must be considered. It is useful to use a systematic tool to assess blood gases to ensure each element of the gas is given consideration.

When measuring blood gases you will receive the following information:

pH	a measure of hydrogen ion concentration
PaO_2	partial pressure of oxygen dissolved in the plasma
$PaCO_2$	partial pressure of carbon dioxide dissolved in plasma
HCO_3	amount of bicarbonate in plasma
SBC	standardized bicarbonate (a derived value)
BE	the base excess, preceded by a + (indicating alkalosis) or a – (indicating acidosis)
SaO_2	the amount of oxygen bound to the haemoglobin molecule.
	Normal values for these measures are:
pH	7.35–7.45
PaO_2	11.5–13 kPa (kilopascals)
$PaCO_2$	4.5–6 kPa

HCO_3 22–26 mmol/L

BE   −2 to +2

SaO_2 >95%

Systematic tools

Many tools are available to assist interpretation of blood gases. Most use a stepwise process. Variations occur in which variable is examined first. A useful tool by Simpson (2004) includes six important steps:

1 Assess oxygenation.

2 Determine status of pH.

3 Assess the respiratory component ($PaCO_2$).

4 Assess metabolic component (HCO_3).

5 Assess for mixed problems.

6 Assess for compensation.

Step 1: Assess oxygenation The PaO_2 and SaO_2 should be examined for signs of hypoxia. It is essential that these values are also considered in the light of the inspired oxygen concentration. If the oxygen levels are low, more oxygen may be required. High oxygen levels usually necessitate a reduction in oxygen administration as it is preferable to keep inspired oxygen concentrations as low as possible to minimize the adverse consequences of oxygen administration.

Step 2: Assess pH The pH should be checked to see if it is in the normal range or whether there is an acidosis (< than 7.35) or an alkalosis (>7.45). A normal pH may also indicate problems that have been corrected by compensation, so it is essential to examine the rest of the arterial blood gas result as either the HCO_3 or the $PaCO_2$ will be deranged if compensation has occurred.

Step 3: Assess the respiratory component The $PaCO_2$ should be checked to see if it is high, low, or within normal range. A high $PaCO_2$ indicates a respiratory problem and is usually accompanied by an acidic pH unless renal compensation has occurred. A low $PaCO_2$ indicates either a respiratory alkalosis (high pH) or partial or full compensation for a metabolic acidosis (low or normal pH).

Step 4: Assess the metabolic component The bicarbonate level should be assessed to see if it is high, low, or normal. If a metabolic acidosis is present the bicarbonate level will be low. If a metabolic alkalosis is present the bicarbonate will be high. The bicarbonate may also be high if there is compensation for a respiratory problem; in this instance the high bicarbonate will be accompanied by a high $PaCO_2$ level.

Step 5: Assess for mixed problems Extremely ill patients may present with a mixed acidotic profile. For example, a patient with severe sepsis who is tiring may present with a low bicarbonate level because of the sepsis (metabolic acidosis) and a high $PaCO_2$ because they are becoming increasing tired (respiratory acidosis). These patients require urgent medical intervention.

Step 6: Assess for compensation
A patient's blood results may be:

♦ uncompensated

♦ partially compensated

♦ fully compensated.

An uncompensated result will present with an abnormal pH and an abnormal parameter indicating the cause/causes of the problem, for example a low pH (acidosis) accompanied by high $PaCO_2$.

A partially compensated result will present with an abnormal pH, an abnormal parameter indicating the cause of the problem, and a change in the other parameter in an attempt to compensate for the abnormal result. For example, a patient with a partially compensated respiratory acidosis will present with a low pH, a high $PaCO_2$ and increasing bicarbonate in an attempt to compensate for the respiratory acidosis. In partial compensation results there is insufficient compensation to return the pH to a normal value.

A fully compensated result will present with a normal pH but other two parameters will be deranged in opposite directions. For example, a patient with a fully compensated metabolic acidosis will present with a normal pH but a low bicarbonate level and a lower than normal $PaCO_2$. Other clinical data will be required to determine which parameter is compensating for a deranged value.

Practice and experience alongside an expert practitioner is always useful when developing blood gas interpretation skills and further reading to support interpretation this increasingly common blood test is recommended. Some clinical examples are included in Clinical links 2.1a–c. The answers to these scenarios are given in the appendix.

Clinical link 2.1a (see Appendix for answers)

Patient A is a 56-year-old lady admitted to your ward postoperatively. She has been given some intravenous morphine and she is quite sleepy. Analyse the blood gas results and discuss further management.

◆ pH: 7.30
◆ PaO_2: 10 kPa
◆ $PaCO_2$: 6.5 kPa
◆ HCO_3: 24
◆ BE: –3
◆ SaO_2: 94%

Clinical link 2.1b (see Appendix for answers)

Patient B is a 34-year-old diabetic patient who is admitted to the medical assessment unit with a diabetic keto acidosis. He is breathing very quickly and deeply and is quite sleepy. Analyse his blood gas results and discuss further management:

◆ pH: 7.31
◆ PaO_2: 9 kPa
◆ $PaCO_2$: 3.3 kPa
◆ HCO_3: 20
◆ BE: –4
◆ SaO_2: 94%

Clinical link 2.1c (see Appendix for answers)

Patient C is a 65-year-old admitted to a medical ward with an acute exacerbation of COPD. She is complaining of severe breathlessness and is expectorating green sputum. Analyse her blood gas result and discuss further management:

- pH: 7.32
- PaO_2: 8 kPa
- $PaCO_2$: 8.5 kPa
- HCO_3: 31
- BE: –4
- SaO_2: 88%

The prevalence and cost of respiratory disease

The British Thoracic Society, in their publication *The Burden of Lung Disease* (2006), have provided some interesting figures on the morbidity, mortality, and costs of respiratory disease which need to be considered by practitioners. Here are few key points to consider from the summary (British Thoracic Society 2006).

Mortality

- More people die from respiratory disease (117,456 deaths in 2004) than from ischaemic heart disease (106,081).
- Respiratory disease now kills one in five people.
- Lung cancer kills more women than breast cancer.
- 27,478 people died as a result of COPD in 2004.
- The number of deaths from occupational lung disease rose by 15% between 1998 and 2004.
- Social inequality causes a higher proportion of deaths from respiratory disease than any other disease area—44% of all deaths from respiratory disease are associated with social class inequalities compared with 28% of deaths from ischaemic heart disease.
- The standardized mortality ratio for respiratory diseases shows a threefold difference across all social classes.

Morbidity

- The most commonly reported long-term illnesses in children and babies are conditions of the respiratory system.
- Lung cancer is the second most common cancer in both men and women.
- Survival rates for lung cancer are very low—the 5-year survival rate is 6.3% for men and 7.5% for women.
- In 2004, nearly 1 in 5 males and 1 in 4 females consulted their family doctor for a respiratory complaint.
- In 2003/2003 nearly 25 million certified sickness absence days related to respiratory disease (not including days lost from self-certified illness).

◆ Respiratory disease is the second most common illness responsible for emergency admission to hospital.

◆ Cases of COPD take up more than one million (1,099,440) hospital bed days a year in England.

◆ More than 62 million prescriptions were used in the prevention and treatment of respiratory disease in 2004.

Cost

◆ Respiratory disease cost the UK £6.6 billion in 2004: £3.0 billion in NHS care costs, £1.9 billion in mortality costs, and £1.7 billion in morbidity costs.

◆ The prevalence of respiratory disease means that many patients in acute care will present with a respiratory pathophysiology as a primary reason for seeking health care or as a co-morbid or complicating condition.

The causes of breathlessness

In order to understand and prioritize the management of respiratory impairment, it is essential to understand the cause. There are many reasons for breathlessness and these determine its clinical management: clearly the priorities in the treatment of asthma are quite different from those in treatment of respiratory failure, which is secondary to heart failure or infection. To get back to basics we need to remember that the reason we breathe is to get oxygen from the air into the blood so that it can be transported to the cells. Mapping out the process requirements for getting oxygen from the air to the cells enables us to visualize the principal causes of respiratory impairment and breathlessness (see Figure 2.10). Each essential component of the air-to-cell journey for oxygen must be in place and operational in order for normal respiratory function to occur. Problems in any area will trigger the feedback and control mechanisms, resulting in impaired respiratory function and breathlessness.

It is not possible to list all the possible causes of breathlessness, but the cause may lie in impaired ventilation or altered internal or external respiration secondary to a variety of primary conditions as outlined briefly below.

The brain and spinal cord

Anything which raises the intracranial pressure (haemorrhage, cerebral oedema, tumour, trauma, abscess, encephalitis, or meningitis) will act directly on the respiratory centres and may cause changes in the rate pattern and depth of respiration.

The airways and lungs

Mechanical obstruction of airflow may be caused by foreign bodies, tumour, inflammation, anaphylaxis, heat or chemical injury, trauma, or disease. Obstructive lung disease is characterized by increased resistance to the inspiratory flow caused by diffuse narrowing of the airways. This results in a reduction in peak expiratory flow rate and FEV1. Consequently the FEV1:vital capacity ratio is also reduced (see section on lung volumes). The mechanism is occlusive, with reduction of the lumen through chronic inflammation as in chronic bronchitis, accompanied by thickening of the wall by oedema or hypertrophy. Further reduction of the lumen of the airways can be caused by excessive secretions or muscle spasm, resulting in the characteristic wheeze of asthma and COPD.

1. BRAIN AND SPINAL CORD
Raised intracranial pressure
Tumour
Infection
Drugs
Trauma

2. AIRWAYS AND LUNGS
Laryngospasm
Bronchospasm
　　Asthma, COPD, Anaphylaxis
Oedema
　　Infection
　　Chemical or heat burn
Mechanical obstruction
　　Sputum
　　Tumour
　　Trauma
　　Pneumothorax
　　Restrictive lung disease

3. MUSCLES OF RESPIRATION
Neuro muscular disorders (eg Multiple Sclerosis, Motor
Neurone Disease, Myasthenia Gravis, Guillain Barré)
Spinal injury
Inhibition by pain
Splinting of the diaphragm (eg pregnancy or acites)

4. SEMI PERMEABLE ALVEOLAR CAPILLARY MEMBRANE

| Emphysema | Atelectasis | Pulmonary oedema | Consolidation | Fibrosis | Sputum |

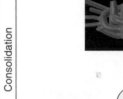

THE CELL
Anerobic
metabolism
Glucose lack

5. BLOOD AND HAEMOGLOBIN
Anaemia
Hypovolaemia

6. HEART AND PULMONARY PERFUSION
Left ventricular failure
Mitral valve disease
Septal defects
Congestive heart failure
Pulmonary hypertension
Pulmonary Embolism
Cor pulmonale

7. METABOLIC ACIDOSIS
Renal failure
Diabetic Keto Acidosis
Tissue hypoxia / ischaemia
Sepsis

VENTILATION = V
(Air to alveoli for gas exchange)

PULMONARY PERFUSION = Q
(Blood to lungs for gas exchange)

Figure 2.10 Diagram summarizing the causes of breathlessness.

The muscles of respiration

There are many muscles involved in respiration, most notably the diaphragm and the internal and external intercostal muscles. Any neuromuscular condition such as motor neurone disease, muscular dystrophies, multiple sclerosis, or Guillain–Barré syndrome will impair inspiration. Splinting of the diaphragm by tumour, pregnancy, or ascites will also impair inspiration, as will pain from surgery or thoracic pain from fractured ribs. Reduced muscle function will result in restrictive lung disease with impaired lung expansion, alveolar hypoventilation, reduced air entry, and reduced vital capacity and residual volume. This will cause a type II respiratory failure with hypoxia and hypercapnoea.

The semi-permeable alveolar capillary membrane

Intrinsic lung diseases of the alveoli that damage the alveolar capillary membrane will also cause restrictive lung disease by inhibiting diffusion and gaseous exchange. This will result in type II respiratory failure. The interstitial lung diseases affect the alveoli and parenchyma and are characterized by inflammation (alveolitis) and fibrosis. These restrictive lung diseases are caused by the inhalation of fibrogenic or carcinogenic dusts, e.g. asbestos, drugs such as amiodarone, sarcoidosis, and connective tissue diseases, such as systemic lupus erythematosis or scleroderma. Cryptogenic fibrosing alveolitis is fibrosis without a recognizable cause. The inflammation and fibrosis is progressive, leading to reduced compliance and restricted capacity. Gaseous exchange is impaired, resulting in a progressive hypoxia, initially on exertion or sleep, and then to hyper-capnoea and peripheral oedema.

Other conditions of the alveolar capillary membrane which reduce gaseous exchange are those in which there is an increased capillary permeability, resulting in diffuse pulmonary oedema such as anaphylaxis, adult respiratory distress syndrome, or initiation of the systemic inflammatory response syndrome as in sepsis.

Pulmonary perfusion

Any condition which alters pulmonary perfusion will impair gaseous exchange and lead to a ventilation perfusion mismatch, for example interrupted blood flow by pulmonary embolism and hypovolaemia. Pulmonary hypertension, however, will lead to pulmonary oedema as the mechanism for impairment of gaseous exchange.

Heart failure

Left-sided heart failure through mitral valve disease or left ventricular hypertrophy will result in pulmonary oedema. Increasing breathlessness is often a sign of deteriorating heart failure and may precede other signs and symptoms.

Blood disorders

Any blood disorder that results in a reduction in haemoglobin, such as leukaemia or anaemia, will lead to a reduction in the oxygen content of the blood.

Disorders of acid–base balance

Metabolic acidosis caused by ischaemia (producing a lactic acidosis as a waste product from anaerobic metabolism, or ketones as a waste product from non-glucolytic pathways) will result in a compensatory increase in respiratory rate. The lungs are the 'rapid response' to changes in pH (see section on the principles of arterial blood gas analysis).

Assessing respiratory function

The assessment of respiratory function is neither difficult nor complex, requiring intelligent observation and common sense rather than complex investigation and equipment. The sequence of taking a history, inspection, palpation, percussion, and auscultation is normally followed, but percussion and auscultation will not be included in this chapter for two reasons. Firstly, because the acquisition of these practical skills cannot be achieved by reading alone but requires a great deal of practice, and, secondly, because acute respiratory failure can be assessed and diagnosed using good nursing skills and common sense without the use of a stethoscope. If you feel that in your nursing practice you need to acquire the skills of chest auscultation and percussion, it is recommended that you undertake a physical assessment module and develop the skills in practice under the supervision of a suitably qualified mentor.

Patient consent should be obtained before beginning an examination of respiratory function and the patient's privacy, dignity, and comfort ensured throughout. Normal infection control measures should be taken and the patient positioned comfortably to allow maximum visibility of the head and thorax. Enquiry about pain should be made before commencing and appropriate control measures taken to ensure that the patient is able to cooperate if possible. In acute care, the severity of the patient's condition may influence assessment, which may have to be rapid if medical review is the clinical priority.

History

The foundation of any assessment is the history and in respiratory assessment this is especially so because of the wide range of possible causes. A subjective history includes the patient's account and understanding of their problem, and you should remember that the experience of breathlessness is subjective and highly variable. However, in the acutely ill patient suffering from dyspnoea it may not be appropriate or possible to obtain this data. The medical notes or nursing documentation can provide the necessary information about the patient's history, including the presenting problem or reason for admission. Verbal information can also be obtained from nursing and medical colleagues or family members if necessary. The absence of this information should in no way delay your assessment. The more immediate concern is the patient's current respiratory function and severity of illness. The respiratory presentation may range from slight breathlessness to acute cyanosis, tachypnoea, and a peri-arrest situation. Do not be misled by the patient who appears only slightly breathless as they may actually be acutely ill, exhibiting the early signs of sepsis, and require admission to intensive care (see Chapter 8 on sepsis and the Chapter 11 on track-and-trigger systems).

The history in acute care should include the reason for admission or the chief complaint, length of admission, history or precursors to the current respiratory presentation, and other relevant medical or surgical history. Smoking history is clearly significant and its impact may be calculated as pack years, i.e. the number of cigarettes smoked per day, multiplied by the number of years smoked, divided by 20. Thus, if the patient has smoked 10 per day for 10 years the number of pack years is 5. Employment history may also be significant, indicating risk of occupational respiratory disease (Douglas *et al.* 2005). This is related to the inhalation of toxic chemicals or particles, which can cause fibrosis or are carcinogenic. Miners, bakers, carpenters, builders, and those who have worked in the printing or dyeing industries are susceptible to chronic respiratory disease and this information would usually be available in the medical notes.

If the patient is able to give a full history you should enquire about coughing, to include its nature (dry or productive) and any precipitating or relieving factors. If the patient does produce sputum the frequency, amount, and nature should be sought. Sputum can be described as:

◆ frothy

◆ watery

◆ viscous (thick and tenacious).

The colour may be:

◆ pink throughout with blood

◆ red, in haemoptysis, with fresh blood

◆ rusty (flecks) in old blood

◆ clear

◆ creamy or yellow

◆ green, when infected.

In pulmonary oedema, sputum may be watery, pink, and frothy, while in infection it may be viscous and green.

Exercise tolerance should be included in the history, along with any other lifestyle inhibitions caused by respiratory impairment. The impact of chronic respiratory disease can be devastating, leaving patients housebound, socially isolated, dependent on others, and depressed.

Wheezing requires investigation of the precipitating and relieving factors, frequency and severity, and any medication taken for prevention or alleviation. Other significant details include anorexia and weight loss, which may indicate malignancy or chronic infection and sleep disturbance. Night sweats may indicate chronic infection such as tuberculosis, and snoring with daytime somnolence may suggest obstructive sleep apnoea. (Boon *et al.* 2006) Prolonged hoarseness may be indicative of malignancy causing damage to the laryngeal nerve (Bickley & Szilagyi 2007).

Inspection of the respiratory rate and breathlessness

Observation is the most useful tool in assessing respiratory function, but the breathless patient is also anxious and requires a gentle, calm, and reassuring manner. Breathlessness is extremely frightening and distressing for both the patient and their relatives, but the patient's perception of breathlessness is subjective and variable according to their normal level of respiratory function. Patients with chronic respiratory disease who may seem acutely breathless and cyanosed will often describe themselves as having a good day or feeling much better than they were. In this situation it is always a good idea to ask the patient if they feel more or less breathless than usual to provide you with a starting point for your assessment. The Medical Research Council (2009) dyspnoea scale for grading the degree of a patient's breathlessness can be a useful tool, but in acute situations this may be of limited value (see Table 2.1).

The respiratory rate is the simplest and possibly the most neglected of vital signs (Chellel *et al.* 2002). It has been known for some time that tachypnoea is one of the most significant predictive indicators of both in-hospital cardiorespiratory arrest and admission to intensive care (Stenhouse *et al.* 2000). It is now an important component of both the multiple parameter and aggregate-weighted-scoring track-and-trigger systems used by critical care outreach teams and recommended in NICE guidelines for *Acutely Ill Patients in Hospital* (2007) (see Chapter 11). It is the respiratory rate that indicates the work of breathing and severity of illness. A severely breathless patient is acutely ill and requires urgent medical review. The respiratory rate should be counted for one full minute and the pattern and depth of respiration observed. Any irregular or

Table 2.1 Medical Research Council dyspnoea scale (2009)

Grade	Degree of breathlessness related to activities
1	Not troubled by breathlessness except on strenuous exercise
2	Short of breath when hurrying or walking up a slight hill
3	Walks slower than contemporaries on the level because of breathlessness or has to stop for breath when walking at own pace
4	Stops for breath after about 100 m or after a few minutes on the level
5	Too breathless to leave the house or breathless when dressing or undressing

asymmetrical pattern of respiration should be noted. However, there are some distinctive patterns of respiration:

- Cheyne–Stokes respiration consists of waxing and waning ventilation, sometimes with periods of apnoea, which occur in cycles.
- Kussmaul's breathing is deep sighing respiration caused by diabetic keto acidosis.
- Hyperventilation may be caused by anxiety. It is an abnormally increased pulmonary ventilation, being both deep and rapid. This condition results in a reduction of carbon dioxide tension and, if persistent, can lead to the development of a respiratory alkalosis and carpopedal spasm.
- Biot's breathing, or ataxic breathing, is irregular in timing and depth, and may be indicative of meningitis or medullary lesions.
- Paradoxical respiratory movement occurs when the abdominal wall is sucked in during inspiration (it is usually pushed out), giving a see-saw appearance to the chest and abdomen. It is due to inhibition of the diaphragm.
- Sleep apnoea is a condition affecting the obese and patients with fleshy faces and short necks. The airways collapse when the patient falls asleep, resulting in a period of apnoea followed by a sudden and noisy intake of air that wakes the patient, although not fully. The patient may suffer extreme drowsiness during the day as sleep apnoea can wake the patient hundreds of times in the night, resulting in sleep deprivation.
- Paradoxical movement of the ribs may occur in chest injury, with multiple rib fractures resulting in a free-floating or flail segment that is sucked inwards on inspiration, while the rest of the thorax moves upwards and outwards.

The ability to speak is a significant indicator of the degree of breathlessness. Normally, speech and breathing can be managed easily and simultaneously. However, as breathlessness increases, speech comes in staccato bursts with breaks for the patient to take a number of deep breaths. *In extremis*, the patient may be unable to speak at all and this indicates a severe and dangerous level of breathlessness.

Inspection of the head, thorax, and hands

Inspection of the patient's head, neck, and thorax is necessary to identify any physical abnormalities that might impair ventilation or lung expansion. Deformity of the mouth, jaws, airways or neck should be noted. Scars may signal previous surgery of relevance and bruising of the thorax may suggest fractured ribs or pain inhibition of respiratory function. Other observations of the thorax might include curvature of the spine or kyphosis, which may occur naturally with aging but which can be excessive (see Figure 2.11).

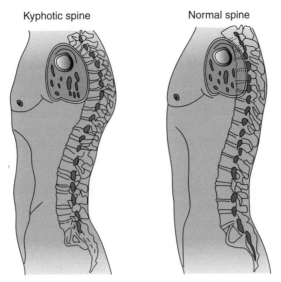

Figure 2.11 Kyphosis.

Scoliosis is an S-shaped deviation of the spine (see Figure 2.12), which can best be observed by looking horizontally along the patient's back as they lean forward at the waist, although in acutely sick patients this may not be possible. Either separately or in combination, as kyphoscoliosis, spinal deformity can inhibit respiration, restricts lung capacity and make X-ray examination difficult to interpret.

Other abnormalities of the thorax include the increased anterior–posterior diameter, giving rise to the barrel chest of COPD. This is caused by the chronic increase in residual volume, which gradually alters the shape of the thorax, making it appear square rather than rectangular with

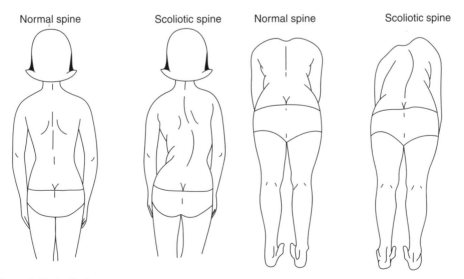

Figure 2.12 Scoliosis.

horizontal ribs on X-ray. The lungs are also over-inflated because the patient has to make an increased inspiratory effort against the resistance of airway obstruction and because, on passive expiration, not all the air is exhaled.

Inspection and observation should also encompass an assessment of the patient's colour. Central cyanosis indicates a high level of reduced (deoxygenated) haemoglobin. However, peripheral cyanosis may indicate poor peripheral perfusion rather than hypoxia. Central cyanosis, in the oral mucosa, lips, or tongue, is a more reliable indicator of hypoxia and it denotes an advanced stage of respiratory impairment and suggests desaturation to below 85%. In black or dark-skinned patients, cyanosis may not appear in the skin and the oral mucosa should be examined (Esmond 2001). In severe anaemia cyanosis may be absent because of the lack of haemoglobin in the presence of acute hypoxia (Davies & Moores 2003).

The use of the accessory muscles of ventilation is another obvious sign of respiratory distress. When the patient experiences hypoxia the work of breathing is increased and, in an effort to increase pulmonary ventilation, additional muscles are brought into use. The accessory muscles are those controlled by the eleventh cranial nerve and the spinal accessory nerves, which are the trapezius, sternocleidomastoid, and scalenes. Increased effort of the intercostal and abdominal muscles may also be observed and there may be nostril flaring (Bickley & Szilagyi 2007).

Inspection of the hands should also be included in the assessment of respiratory impairment. As already stated, peripheral cyanosis should be noted but interpreted with caution in the case of poor peripheral perfusion. The nails should be examined for finger clubbing. This is a flattening of the angle at the nail bed between the finger and the nail. The nails become curved and the ends of the fingers enlarged, giving the characteristic sign. A simple check is to ask the patient to hold the nails of the middle finger against each other up in front of you: in unaffected patients you should be able to see a diamond shape gap between them. In finger clubbing this gap disappears and the nails will bend away from each other (see Figure 2.13). This is a sign of chronic hypoxia from respiratory or heart disease but it may also be present in liver or gastrointestinal pathologies.

The presence of koilonychia or spoon-shaped nails, i.e. concave rather than convex, can indicate iron deficiency anaemia (Kumar & Clark 2005), which may be significant in the breathless patient. While observing the hands and feet for peripheral cyanosis, the presence of oedema may indicate a cardiac origin for breathlessness (see Chapter 3 on cardiovascular care).

Palpation of the thorax and respiratory excursion

The bony structures of the thorax should be gently palpated, noting the location of any tenderness. Fractured ribs may be detected. The spine, clavicles, scapulae, sternum, and ribs should be palpated for signs of bony injury and the location of any pain identified. The supra, infraclavicular, and axillary lymph nodes should be palpated. Lymph nodes become palpable and feel like tiny

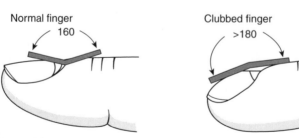

Figure 2.13 Finger clubbing.

nodules under the skin in the presence of infection and malignancy. Any lumps or surgical emphysema should be noted.

Chest expansion can be assessed by spreading the hands over the ribs on either side of the chest, with the thumbs along the costal margin. Ask the patient to take a deep breath and, on inspiration, the thumbs should separate and chest expansion be detected under the hands (Douglas *et al.* 2005). This indicates that the patient is able to ventilate the lungs. In patients with splinting of the diaphragm, neuromuscular disorders, or restrictive lung disease there may be little or no chest movement. Shallow, rapid breathing can also indicate fatigue, the transition from type I to type II respiratory failure, and a rise in arterial carbon dioxide signalling deterioration in the patient's condition. Finally, the index and middle fingers should be placed gently either side of the trachea just above the suprasternal notch to palpate for centrality of the trachea. Tracheal deviation may indicate a mediastinal mass, pleural effusion, or pneumothorax. The trachea deviates toward the affected side in a collapsed lung and away from the affected side in pneumothorax and large pleural effusion (Bickley & Szilagyi 2008).

The breathless patient will also be tachycardic and hypertensive as a result of the sympathetic stress response mediated by adrenaline acting on the β_1-receptors in the heart.

Pulse oximetry

Pulse oximetry is a simple non-invasive method of monitoring the percentage of haemoglobin (Hb) that is saturated with oxygen (see section on the transport of gases). It is known as 'the fifth vital sign' (British Thoracic Society 2008a) and should be checked in all acutely ill patients. The findings should be recorded on the patient's chart along with the level of inspired oxygen. The pulse oximeter consists of a probe attached to the patient's finger or ear lobe, which is linked to a computerized unit. The unit displays the percentage of haemoglobin saturated with oxygen together with an audible signal for each pulse beat, a calculated heart rate, and, in some models, a graphical display of the blood flow past the probe. In the form of a graph it is called the plethysmograph.

The pulse oximeter works by emitting a source of light from the probe at two wavelengths. The light is partly absorbed by haemoglobin, by amounts which differ depending on whether it is saturated or desaturated with oxygen. By calculating the absorption at the two wavelengths the processor can calculate the proportion of haemoglobin that is oxygenated. The computer within the oximeter is capable of distinguishing pulsatile flow from other more static signals (such as tissue or venous signals) to display only the arterial flow. The oximeter is dependent on a pulsatile flow and produces a graph of the quality of flow. It is important to remember that when flow is sluggish, as in hypovolaemia or vasoconstriction, the pulse oximeter may give low readings that do not reflect poor saturation but poor peripheral perfusion. The simple way to distinguish between true desaturation and poor perfusion is to take an apical heart rate for 1 min. If the apical rate corresponds with the heart rate reading on the pulse oximeter, it may be considered accurate, but a significantly lower reading suggests poor peripheral perfusion. In the following situations the pulse oximeter readings may not be accurate:

♦ A reduction in peripheral pulsatile blood flow produced by peripheral vasoconstriction (hypovolaemia, severe hypotension, cold, cardiac failure, some cardiac arrhythmias) or peripheral vascular disease. These result in an inadequate signal for analysis.

♦ Venous congestion, particularly when caused by tricuspid regurgitation, may produce venous pulsations, which may produce low readings with ear probes. Venous congestion of the limb may affect readings.

♦ Bright sunlight or overhead lights in theatre may cause the oximeter to be inaccurate.

♦ The signal may be interrupted by surgical diathermy.

♦ Shivering may cause difficulties in picking up an adequate signal.

♦ Pulse oximetry cannot distinguish between different forms of haemoglobin. Carboxyhaemo-globin (haemoglobin combined with carbon monoxide, which may be seen in smokers) results in overestimation of the saturation. Methaemoglobin (a form of haemoglobin that is unable to carry oxygen and results from toxicity or injury) results in underestimation of the saturation.

♦ Nail varnish and false nails may cause falsely low readings.

As a tool for assessing respiratory function, pulse oximetry offers a rough estimate of the effectiveness of breathing as part of an interrelated triad:

1 respiratory rate: the work of breathing

2 saturation: the effectiveness of breathing

3 inspired oxygen: the support for breathing.

These three components must be considered together in order to evaluate the severity of the patient's respiratory impairment. Clearly the patient who is desaturated to 85% on air, with a respiratory rate of 30, is less at risk that a patient who is desaturated to 85% on 60% oxygen with a respiratory rate of 40.

In clinical practice the patient's history and presentation in terms of the triad above are all that is required to assess respiratory function. It should be remembered, however, that the respiratory rate is also a key 'red flag' indicator of advanced critical illness from other causes (see Chapter 11 on track-and-trigger systems).

↓ News 2 → by Royal college of physicians

Peak expiratory flow rate

Peak expiratory flow rate (PEFR) is the maximum flow rate achieved in rapid forced expiration following maximum inspiration measured. It depends on patient effort and technique but is widely used in acute care as a measure of the effectiveness of inhaled bronchodilators by pre and post testing. The PEFR varies with gender and age and it is generally the trend that is significant. The best of three readings is normally recorded and patients who use PEFRs to monitor their asthma will know what their normal range should be. In patients who are so severely breathless that they are unable to achieve a measurable PEFR, urgent medical review should be sought.

Three common respiratory pathophysiologies

Asthma revision

Asthma is characterized by increased responsiveness of the airways to a variety of stimuli and chronic airway inflammation, leading to a variable narrowing of the airways and the symptoms of wheeze, cough, and chest tightness (West 2003; Boon *et al.* 2006). The aetiology is complex and research continues to develop knowledge in this area. There is evidence of environmental and genetic factors and early onset asthma is largely atopic. Early exposure to childhood infections and animals appears to offer some protection, leading to the 'hygiene hypothesis', which suggests that the increasing prevalence of asthma is a result of a cleaner housing environment than in the past. Mature onset asthma may be triggered by pollution, exercise, viral infections, or some drugs, such as aspirin and β-blockers. Hyper-responsiveness and airway inflammation are the dominant features and these are initiated by the release of mediators such as leukotrienes, histamine, cytokines, prostaglandin, and platelet-activating factor. Eosinophils, mast cells, neutrophils, and macrophages have all been implicated in the complex pathology of asthma. Bronchoconstriction is reversible, although remodelling of the airways occurs with hypertrophy of smooth muscle and mucous glands, resulting in abnormally thick mucus and fixed narrowing (see Figure 2.14).

Presentation may vary, but wheezing, cough, tightness of the chest, and breathlessness are the main features. Patients may be asymptomatic between attacks because the airway obstruction is reversible. The British Thoracic Society have developed the stepwise approach, in which treatment is stepped up with increasing disease severity, in order to guide optimal and evidence-based treatment (British Thoracic Society 2008b). Denial is common in patients who do not wish asthma to affect their lives; this can lead to a failure to monitor their own PEFR and poor compliance with treatment plans, resulting in a failure to manage the disease effectively. The British Thoracic Society (2008b) include the management of acute asthma in their guidelines and state clearly the seriousness of this condition, with emphasis on the significance of psychosocial factors:

> 'Health care professionals must be aware that patients with severe asthma and one or more adverse psychosocial factors are at risk of death.'

Assessment is based on the clinical presentation, PEFR, saturations, and arterial blood gas analysis. β_2-agonist bronchodilators remain the first-line treatment. According to Kumar and Clark (2005), patients with acute severe asthma (previously named status asthmaticus):

- are unable to speak in complete sentences
- are tachypnoeic at 25 or more breaths per minute
- are tachycardic with a pulse of 110 or more
- have a PEFR that is less than 50% of predicted or best.

The British Thoracic Society guidelines for the management of acute asthma recommendations include:

- Give high-flow oxygen to all patients with acute severe asthma.

Use high-dose inhaled β_2-agonists as first-line agents in acute asthma and administer as early as possible. Reserve intravenous β_2-agonists for those patients in whom inhaled therapy cannot be used reliably.

- β_2-agonist bronchodilators should be driven by oxygen.
- In severe asthma (PEF less than 50% of normal, best, or predicted) and asthma that is poorly responsive to an initial bolus dose of β_2-agonist, consider continuous nebulization.
- Give steroids in adequate doses in all cases of acute asthma.

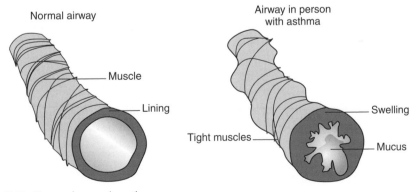

Figure 2.14 Airway changes in asthma.

Clinical link 2.2 (see Appendix for answers)

Patient 1 is a 45-year-old female admitted from the accident and emergency (A&E) department into the medical assessment unit. She is very breathless and her speech is coming in short bursts. She wants you to phone her husband at work because she is very anxious about not being able to pick up the children from school. She came to hospital following an asthma attack while doing some cleaning at home. Nebulized β_2-agonist was given in A&E with nebulized ipatropium.

She is distressed and frightened and peripherally cyanosed. There is an audible respiratory wheeze and she is using the accessory muscles of respiration. She is on oxygen at 35% via a yellow Venturi mask at 8 L/min. She is unable to give a history but her medical notes state that she is a known asthmatic with an allergy to dust and house mites. She is prescribed alternating salbutomol and ipatroprium via nebulizers, which are in progress but she keeps removing the mask and asking you to get her the phone. There is no evidence of thoracic abnormality or finger clubbing, and her vital signs are as follows:

- respiratory rate: 36
- temperature: 37.0°C
- peripheral pulse: 110
- blood pressure: 145/90
- SpO_2: 85%

Her chest X-ray is clear and her arterial blood gas analysis taken in A&E 1 h ago shows:

- pH: 7.35
- PaO_2: 9.8 kPa
- $PaCO_2$: 3.5 kPa
- SBC: 26 mmol/L
- BE: +2 mmol/L

Consider the following questions:

- What type of respiratory failure does this patient have and what is the most likely cause?
- What are your main priorities and why?
- What clinical actions should you take and why?

- Add nebulized ipratropium bromide (0.5 mg, 4–6 hourly) to β_2-agonist treatment for patients with acute, severe, or life-threatening asthma or those with a poor initial response to β_2-agonist therapy.

- Intravenous magnesium therapy may also be prescribed if the patient fails to respond to normal therapy or is having a life-threatening exacerbation of their asthma.

In patients with a deteriorating PEFR, failure to respond to therapy, exhaustion, and hypoventilation, worsening hypoxia or hypercapnoea, increasing acidosis, drowsiness, confusion, or coma should be referred to intensive care (British Thoracic Society 2008b).

Chronic obstructive pulmonary disease revision

Chronic obstructive pulmonary disease is a generic term describing the effects of two main conditions with which it is associated: emphysema and chronic bronchitis. It means that the patient is suffering from chronic and poorly reversible airway obstruction (Selby 2002). Patients experience increasing breathlessness, poor exercise tolerance, chronic cough with sputum production, over-inflated lungs, and impaired gas exchange (West 2003). Pursed lip breathing may be present in which the patient closes the lips on expiration to increase the pressure in the airways and by splinting prevent their collapse. The principal cause of COPD is smoking, which accounts for 95% of cases in the UK (Boon *et al.* 2006) and it causes the death of 30,000 people per year in the UK. Chronic obstructive pulmonary disease is a slowly progressive disease, characterized by airway obstruction and increasing breathlessness, initially on exertion and then at rest. Acute intermittent exacerbations that may be infective occur. Structural changes arising from emphysema result in reduced compliance and collapse of the small airways on expiration, which causes air trapping and hyperinflation. The PEFR, FEV1, and FEV1:VC ratio are reduced (Bourke 2007).

The FEV1 as a percentage of the predicted value is used to classify the severity of the disease as mild, moderate, or severe (see Table 2.2).

In chronic bronchitis there is an increased number of goblet cells in the larger airways, resulting in increased sputum production and a productive cough for most days over 3 months in more than two successive years. There is also a loss of elastic tissue in the smaller airways, with diffuse airway narrowing and fibrosis. In emphysema there is destruction of the alveolar wall and dilation of the airspaces in the lungs, with loss of alveolar capillary surface area. Elastic recoil is reduced and the airways are more prone to collapse and increase the work of inspiration. Emphysema may also be associated with an inherited deficiency of α_1-antitrypsin. The traditional classification of COPD patients as 'blue bloaters' or 'pink puffers' is unreliable. 'Blue bloaters' refers to patients with chronic bronchitis who are chronically hypoxic, resulting in increased haemoglobin and who are therefore cyanosed, but who have a poor respiratory drive with oedema due to cor pulmonale. 'Pink puffers' is the description of patients with emphysema who maintain a good respiratory drive and are very breathless but are not cyanosed until the late stages of the disease (Bourke 2007). Recent improvements in understanding and investigation of COPD indicate that most patients experience elements of both conditions, making these rather crude distinctions obsolete.

Persistently high carbon dioxide levels lead to a reduced responsiveness and hypoxia becomes the dominant respiratory drive so that the administration of oxygen can worsen respiratory failure and increase the level of carbon dioxide (Kumar & Clark 2005). NICE Guidelines (2004) state that airflow obstruction is defined as:

♦ FEV1 < 80% predicted

♦ FEV1/FVC < 0.7

The key aspects of management are:

♦ diagnosis

♦ smoking cessation

♦ effective inhaler therapy, using long-acting bronchodilators and steroids (see section on inhaler therapy)

Table 2.2 Classification of chronic obstructive pulmonary disease

Chronic obstructive pulmonary disease category	FEV1 (percentge of predicted value)
Mild	60–80
Moderate	40–59
Severe	Below 40

FEV1, forced expiratory volume 1.

- pulmonary rehabilitation for all who need it
- use of non-invasive ventilation (see section on the principles of non-invasive ventilation)
- management of exacerbations to minimize impact
- multidisciplinary working.

Differentiation between asthma and COPD is not always clear and some of the guidelines are shown in Table 2.3.

Patients are increasingly encouraged to manage their own COPD and, in primary care, case management by community matrons aims to support patients at home to avoid repeated admissions (Department of Health 2005).

In hospital management of acute exacerbations, the following investigations are required:

- chest X-ray and electrocardiogram (ECG)
- arterial blood gas analysis
- full blood count urea and electrolytes
- theophylline level if appropriate
- sputum culture and sensitivity.

Treatment is with oxygen so as to maintain saturations at 88–94% (see section on oxygen therapy), bronchodilators, oral antibiotics as indicated, and oral steroids (30 mg prednisolone daily for 7–14 days). Mucolytic therapy should be considered and in patients with oedema and/or a raised jugular venous distention or other signs of heart failure, cor pulmonale should also be considered and diuretics used as indicated. The guidelines recognize the possibility of depression and anxiety for patients with COPD, which should be treated. Restricted activity, social isolation, and the fear of dying with each exacerbation and admission to acute care are aspects of this disease that require sensitive and compassionate nursing care. Multidisciplinary care, including physiotherapists, dietitians, and primary care practitioners, is essential and discharge planning should include consideration of patient education and the involvement of the primary care team for future management of acute exacerbations (NICE 2004).

Pneumonia revision

Pneumonia is an acute lower respiratory tract infective illness causing parenchymal lung inflammation and alveolar filling with exudate (West 2003). Risk factors include age, chronic disease of heart, lungs or kidneys, immunological supression, aspiration, and environmental factors such as recent travel, exposure to birds, and farm animals. It is estimated that 1 in 1000 of the UK population are admitted to hospital with pneumonia each year and mortality is in the region of 10%

Table 2.3 NICE summary of differentiating features between chronic obstructive pulmonary disease and asthma

Feature	Chronic obstructive pulmonary disease	Asthma
Smoker or ex-smoker	Nearly all patients	Possibly
Symptoms began under 35 years of age	Rare	Common
Chronic and productive cough	Common	Not common
Patient is breathless	Progressive	Variable
Night waking/wheeze	Not common	Common
Day-to-day variability	Not common	Common

Clinical link 2.3 (see Appendix for answers)

Patient 2 is a 74-year-old male, admitted to a medical ward from A&E yesterday. He is very thin, with a marked barrel chest. He uses oxygen at home and since his wife died 6 months ago he has needed help with shopping and housework from his daughter, who lives nearby. He has had three admissions in the last year for acute exacerbation of his COPD. He is peripherally and centrally cyanosed and his fingers are clubbed. His speech is wheezy and staccato, and he is breathing through his mouth, which is dry. His tongue is coated. He looks ill and tired and, although he is not using the accessory muscles, he is clearly having to make an effort to breathe. He is sitting slumped in the bed and he says he is fed up and can't be bothered with anything. His fluid chart indicates a poor oral intake and low urine output for that 6 hours. He has been catheterized and the urine in the bag appears dark in colour. His vital signs are:

- respiratory rate: 28
- temperature: 37.8°C
- peripheral pulse: 110
- blood pressure: 180/95
- SpO_2: 85%

He is on oxygen at 2 L via nasal specs and is producing viscous green sputum. His chest X-ray shows consolidation of the left base and his arterial blood gas analysis shows:

- pH: 7.2
- PaO_2: 8.7 kPa
- $PaCO_2$: 6.3 kPa
- HCO_3: 32 mmol/L
- BE: +7 mmol/L

Consider the following questions:

- What type of respiratory failure does this patient have and what is the cause?
- What are your main priorities and why? What clinical actions should you take and why?

(Bourke 2007). Clinically significant factors are the age of the patient, their previous health, the causative organism, and the severity. Pneumonia presents with breathlessness, cough, pleuritic chest pain, and pyrexia. Fever may be severe with rigors, anorexia, and vomiting may also be present (Boon *et al.* 2006). Cyanosis may occur, chest expansion may be reduced on the affected side, and chest X-ray usually shows signs of consolidation (Esmond 2003). The severity of illness and prognostic indicators are indicated by the CURB score (Boon *et al.* 2006), which allocates 1 point for each of the following features: *BTS*

- confusion
- urea elevation
- respiratory rate >30
- blood pressure <90 systolic.

Investigation is by chest X-ray, sputum culture to identify the causative organism, blood cultures, full blood picture, urea, and electrolytes. Arterial blood gas analysis will show a type I respiratory failure with hypoxia, which may be severe. If the patient's condition worsens and they

Clinical link 2.4 (see Appendix for answers)

Patient 3 is a 45-year-old male on a surgical ward following resection of large bowel and formation of a temporary colostomy for perforated diverticular disease. He looks pale and is listless and complaining of feeling 'really rotten'. He is speaking with difficulty because of his respiratory rate but there is no central or peripheral cyanosis and no use of accessory muscles. He is pain free and there is no thoracic abnormality or finger clubbing. His vital signs are:

- respiratory rate: 40
- temperature: 39.5°C
- peripheral pulse: 120
- blood pressure: 100/70
- SpO_2: 88%

He is without oxygen and his chest X-ray is clear and he is not producing any sputum. His skin feels warm and dry and arterial blood gas analysis shows:

- pH: 7.2
- PaO_2: 10.8 kPa
- $PaCO_2$: 3.2 kPa
- HCO_3: 15 mmol/L
- BE: −8 mmol/L
- lactate: 8

Consider the following questions:

- What type of respiratory failure does this patient have and what is the most likely cause?
- What are your main priorities and why?
- What clinical actions should you take and why?

begin to tire, they may also show type 2 respiratory failure with hypoxia and hypercapnia. Treatment is with oxygen, analgesia, and antibiotics (Bourke 2007), in accordance with local policy, until the culture and sensitivity findings identify the causative organism. Hospital-acquired or nosocomial pneumonia are caused by different organisms. Gram-negative bacteria are more prevalent in hospital infections, while in the community, droplet infection in winter-time of previously well patients is most commonly caused by streptococcus pneumonia, mycoplasma, legionella and chlamydia. Hospital-acquired pneumonia includes that caused by aspiration as well as by opportunistic pathogens, including escherichia, pseudomonas, klebsiella and multi-drug resistant *Staphylococcus aureus* (Boon *et al.* 2006). In severe cases it may be complicated by empyema or lung abcesses (Kumar & Clarke 2005).

General nursing treatment for the breathless patient

Positioning the patient

Appropriate positioning of the breathless patient is a fundamental yet often overlooked aspect of care. The patient should be sitting and well supported by pillows (British Thoracic Society 2008a). An upright position is not appropriate for patients who are critically ill or hypotensive. However, ventilation is facilitated by a more upright position and good support with plenty of pillows.

Tilting the foot of the bed upwards can prevent the patient slipping down the bed and time taken to make the patient comfortable is well invested in order to assist their breathing. Use of profiling beds is beneficial when nursing the breathless patient.

The need to reposition the patient should also be considered. Field (2005) highlights the benefits of repositioning for enhancing oxygenation by altering the ventilation/perfusion ratio and also enabling the mobilisation of secretions. It is vital, however, that the patient's response to position change is assessed, as it may adversely affect oxygenation. If this is the case the patient should be returned to their previous position.

Oxygen therapy

Oxygen therapy is an important adjunct in the treatment of type I and type II respiratory failure, but it is of little use in the patient whose breathlessness is not caused by hypoxia. It is delivered at low flow rates (<6 L/min) via simple face masks or nasal cannulae, or high flow rates via Venturi systems or a reservoir mask at 10–15 L/min. Nurses should ensure that pulse oximetry is used to monitor patients receiving oxygen therapy. The flow rate of oxygen, the delivery system/inspired oxygen percentage and saturations should be recorded on the patient's observation chart. It is the responsibility of the nurse to ensure that the prescribed oxygen is delivered to the patient and if the target saturations are not achieved, that the medical team are informed.

The British Thoracic Society Guidelines (2008a) state that oxygen should be prescribed to achieve a target saturation of 94–98% in the acutely ill patient and 88–92% in patients with COPD or a risk of hypercapnoea. The target saturation should be stated on the prescription, which should be signed on each drug round. While breathlessness can be caused by hypoxia, not all breathless patients are hypoxic and oxygen is not always needed. Pulse oximetry should be used to monitor oxygen administration and both should be recorded. Humidification is not required for low-flow or short-term oxygen administration (<24 h), but may be useful in loosening viscous sputum. Oxygen can induce hypercapnoea and should be used cautiously in patients with COPD. In summary:

- Initial oxygen therapy is via nasal cannulae at 2–6 L/min or a simple face mask at 5–10 L/min.
- If there is no risk of hypercapnoea, 10–15 L/min via a reservoir mask should be used if saturation is less than 85%.
- The recommended target saturation is 94–98%.
- If the target range cannot be achieved with nasal cannulae or simple face mask, change to a reservoir mask and ensure medical review.
- In patients with COPD who are at risk of hypercapnoea, target saturation should be 88–92% until arterial blood gas analysis is available and a Venturi mask at 4 L/min should be used.
- Patients over 50 years old, whose diagnosis is unknown but with a history of smoking or chronic breathlessness, should be treated as COPD patients and a risk of hypercapnoea assumed.

When using a simple face mask with flow rates below 5 L/min there is a risk of rebreathing carbon dioxide and the flow rate should be 5–10 L/min. While nebulizers for patients with asthma should be driven by high-flow oxygen, nebulizers for patients with COPD should be driven by air, not oxygen, although supplementary oxygen via nasal cannulae at 2–4 L/min may be needed to prevent desaturation below 88%. Nurses should be vigilant to ensure that the oxygen does not become disconnected or the tubing occluded. High-flow oxygen for more than 24 h requires humidification but this should be nebulized as 'bubble bottles' are ineffective (British Thoracic Society 2008a).

Physiotherapy

Breathless patients will require specialist assessment and intervention by the physiotherapist. The physiotherapist has an important role to play in management of the breathless patient. Physiotherapy treatment will include interventions that will aim to enhance ventilation and perfusion. Full discussion of physiotherapy intervention is beyond the scope of this book but treatment may include:

- effective positioning
- deep breathing and coughing exercises
- postural drainage
- chest percussion
- suctioning if appropriate.

Drug therapy

Inhaled bronchodilator medication for obstructive lung disease is the main treatment. Bronchodilators are often used in conjunction with steroids (systemic or inhaled) and antibiotics. Administration directly to the lungs allows lower dosage and minimizes unwanted systemic effects (Kumar & Clarke 2005). There are four different modes of action, which are outlined below.

Selective β$_2$-adrenergic agonists

Selective β$_2$-adrenergic agonists are the most widely used bronchodilators. A typical example is salbutamol. They are sympathomimetic in action (i.e. they act like adrenaline, stimulating the sympathetic nervous system) and cause relaxation of the smooth muscle in the airways, providing symptomatic relief. They are delivered by handheld metered-dose inhalers, spacer devices, or, in hospital, by nebulization. They may be short or long acting and the long-acting drugs are used in primary care in the maintenance of symptom control. Metered-dose inhalers only deliver 15% of the content and most of the dose is deposited in the mouth and oropharynx and swallowed (Kumar & Clarke 2008). Technique is important and very young and elderly patients may need a spacer device, which requires less co ordination. Nebulizers use high pressure gas (air or oxygen) to convert liquid into a fine spray, which is inhaled. Because the particles are so small they are able to reach the bronchioles. They have effect within 15 min and the duration of action is 4–6 h. In asthmatic patients, oxygen is used to drive nebulizers, but in patients with COPD who retain carbon dioxide, air is used.

Antimuscarinic bronchodilators

Antimuscarinic bronchodilators such as ipratropium act on the neuromuscular junction. They work by inhibiting the acetylcholine-mediated transmission of the nervous impulse across the neuromuscular junction. By blocking the muscarinic receptors of the autonomic nervous system in the respiratory tract, smooth muscle in the airways is relaxed, relieving bronchoconstriction.

Leukotriene receptor antagonists

Cysteinyl leukotrienes are one of the chemical mediators of the allergic response. They are released from mast cells and basophils. They stimulate smooth muscle and cause bronchoconstriction. Drugs such as montelukast block this action, causing bronchodilation (Rang *et al.* 2003).

Theophylline

Theophylline inhibits the enzyme phosphodiesterase in the smooth muscle wall of the airways, resulting in relaxation and the relief of bronchospasm. It also has an anti-inflammatory effect similar to corticosteroids. It is given by slow intravenous infusion as aminophylline and requires close monitoring of plasma levels because the therapeutic range is small and the toxic dose is close to the therapeutic dose.

Non-invasive ventilation (NIV)

When patients are experiencing type I or type II respiratory impairment, non-invasive ventilation (NIV) is now commonly used to provide support. It is important to understand that there are only two ways to increase the PaO_2 in patients with type I respiratory impairment:

1 increase the inspired oxygen

2 increase the expiratory positive airway pressure (EPAP) with continuous positive airways pressure (CPAP) in spontaneously ventilated patients or positive end expiratory pressure (PEEP) in ventilated patients.

Equally, there are only two ways to decrease the $PaCO_2$ in patients with type II respiratory impairment:

1 increase the tidal volume so that more carbon dioxide is exhaled

2 increase the rate in patients who are ventilated, but this is obviously not an option in spontaneously ventilating patients in whom a rapid respiratory rate is already initiated as a normal physiological response.

Non-invasive ventilation works by using a fan to create a rapid flow of air, which generates high pressure. This requires a tightly fitting mask that is held in place with head straps. The tubing is wide bore but has a smooth lining so that the flow and pressure are not impeded. Oxygen may be added to the circuit to increase the fractional inspired oxygen (FiO_2) and it is a bit like breathing with your head out of the window of a car travelling at 70 mph, i.e. minimal respiratory effort is boosted to give higher tidal volumes. If tidal volume is increased, the effort of breathing is reduced and more CO_2 is expired, reducing the $PaCO_2$. Alveolar collapse is prevented by the end expiratory pressure and collapsed alveoli are recruited, leading to an increase in alveolar ventilation and gaseous exchange. The increase in pressure can be also be used as a treatment for pulmonary oedema. NIV can be carried out on the ward without admission to the high-dependency unit and the hazards of intubation and ventilation are avoided.

The inspiratory pressure is set on the machine in order to increase the tidal volume and this is called inspiratory positive airway pressure (IPAP). The increased inspiratory pressure will increase the tidal volume according to the airway resistance. The end expiratory pressure can also be held above zero to create a positive EPAP, which will increase oxygenation. If both are used it is called bilevel positive airway pressure or BiPAP, and this is frequently required because patients often present with type II respiratory impairment with a low pH, high $PaCO_2$, and low PaO_2 (see Figure 2.15).

Although each machine varies, they are sensitive to slight changes in flow and pressure, which means that a very slight inspiratory effort by the patient is used to trigger the machine. The flow is increased to produce a breath at the preset inspiratory pressure. The machine can usually be set to deliver the preset pressure very rapidly or in a slower, gentler rise. In patients with high airway resistance such as asthma or COPD the rapid pressure rise may be less effective than a slower rise because the resistance will mean that the preset pressure is achieved too quickly to increase the tidal volume. In pressure-cycled machines, the tidal volume will vary according to the airway resistance. In volume-cycled machines, the pressure will vary according to the airway resistance.

It is the responsibility of nurses who care for patients using NIV to ensure that they are familiar with the machines and adhere to local guidelines. The decision to use NIV is usually made by the medical specialist registrar following chest X-ray and arterial blood gas analysis to assess respiratory function and exclude pneumothorax, which is a contraindication. The British Thoracic

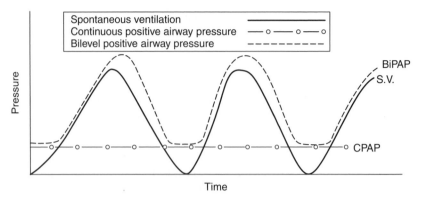

Figure 2.15 Differences between CPAP and normal ventilation.

Society (2008b) have updated their 2002 guidelines for the use of NIV in COPD. These are based on best practice as indicated by their analysis of the research evidence. They are the gold standard that will inform trust protocols and advise that full medical therapy should be initiated, i.e. oxygen (to maintain saturations at 88–92%), antibiotics, and inhaled bronchodilators and steroids as indicated before initiating NIV.

Inclusion criteria

The effective use of NIV will be determined by a number of factors, including:

- primary diagnosis of COPD exacerbation (known diagnosis or history and examination consistent with diagnosis)
- able to protect airway
- conscious and cooperative
- potential for recovery to quality of life acceptable to the patient
- patient's wishes considered.

It is important that the medical team responsible for the patient make a decision about the ceiling treatment. In other words, a clear treatment plan should be communicated in the notes, identifying what should happen if the patient's condition continues to deteriorate. If admission to intensive care is indicated, anaesthetic review will be necessary because they are responsible for the admission and discharge of intensive care patients and will co-ordinate the transfer of patients.

NIV may be used in heart failure or pneumonia in patients with COPD if intubation and ventilation are not deemed appropriate. In the unconscious patient, NIV should be considered if endo-tracheal intubation is deemed inappropriate or NIV is to be provided in a critical care setting. There is evidence to support the use of NIV in patients who are comatose, secondary to COPD-induced hypercapnoea (British Thoracic Society 2008b).

Contraindications to NIV include (British Thoracic Society 2008b):

- life-threatening hypoxaemia
- co-morbidity
- confusion/agitation/severe cognitive impairment
- facial burns/trauma/recent surgery on face or upper airway
- vomiting

- fixed upper airway obstruction
- undrained pneumothorax
- upper gastrointestinal surgery
- inability to protect the airway
- copious respiratory secretions
- haemodynamic instability (except in intensive care)
- patient moribund
- bowel obstruction.

The guidelines recommend (British Thoracic Society 2008b):

- a full-face mask should be used for the first 24 h, followed by switching to a nasal mask if preferred by the patient
- an initial inspiratory positive airway pressure (IPAP) of 10 cm H_2O and expiratory positive airway pressure (EPAP) of 4–5 cm H_2O should be used
- IPAP should be increased by 2–5 cm increments at a rate of approximately 5 cm H_2O every 10 min, with a usual pressure target of 20 cm H_2O or until a therapeutic response is achieved or patient tolerability has been reached
- oxygen, when required, should be entrained into the circuit and the flow adjusted to achieve the target saturation, usually 88–92%
- bronchodilators, although preferably administered off NIV, should as necessary be entrained between the expiration port and face mask
- if a nasogastric tube is in place, a fine-bore tube is preferred to minimize mask leakage.

Nursing considerations

NIV is uncomfortable and unpleasant because of the tight fitting mask and the constant high flow of gases. Poor fitting masks can result in leaks that cause rapid drying of the eyes and the machine will alarm frequently as it fails to reach the preset pressure. For the breathless and frightened patient, anything on the face can feel more restrictive than supportive of their breathing and it may require a great deal of nursing time, reassurance, and patience to initiate NIV. Low initiation pressures, short trials of the mask without the airflow from the machine, and feeling the flow of gas against the skin of the arm can help the patient to prepare for a brief initial trial. It is extremely important that the patient retains control and can ask for the mask to removed, until they become accustomed to it. Patient compliance can be low and indeed many refuse it. NIV cannot, of course, be used without the patient's full cooperation and consent. NIV is frequently nurse-managed and regular monitoring of its effectiveness is required. Ideally a cardiac monitor with facility for respiratory rate and pulse oximetry recording should be used but the following nursing considerations should also be addressed:

- Monitoring and recording vital signs, including pulse oximetry, is essential for the first 12 h (British Thoracic Society 2008b); after this, monitor in accordance with local guidelines or as indicated by the patient's condition.
- NIV should be discontinued if patient's condition or saturations deteriorate.
- Oral intake is restricted and therefore hydration and nutritional needs must be met.
- The advantages are lost very rapidly as soon as the mask is removed, therefore until the patient can tolerate periods off NIV, intravenous fluids may be needed.

- Correct and timely administration of concomitant drug therapy is equally important.
- Nurses must be trained in the use of the machine.
- Nurses must know how to fit the mask.
- Leaks result in a loss of pressure and volume, and consequently of therapeutic effect.
- Nurses must keep the medical team informed of progress and ensure that arterial blood gas analysis is carried out in accordance with local guidelines to monitor the effectiveness of NIV.
- Nurses should ensure that they receive appropriate education and training to maintain their knowledge and skills in the use of NIV.
- Local protocols for the clinical management of NIV should be followed to ensure patient safety and optimal care.
- Above all, nurses should support and encourage the patient to relieve their anxiety and in doing so, promote patient cooperation and the consequent effectiveness of NIV.

Management of patients with chest drains

Chest drains are tubes inserted into the pleural space to drain air, blood, or pus (empyema) and facilitate re-expansion of the lung. The end of the drain is placed below the surface of water in a bottle to create an underwater seal and so ensure that there is a one-way flow of air or fluid out, while preventing air from flowing back into the pleural space (see Figure 2.16). The end of the drain should be immersed by no more than 3 cm to minimize resistance to drainage (Sullivan 2008). A one-way flutter valve may also be used. Chest drain insertion uses a large trochar and is a painful procedure requiring premedication and local anaesthetic (Laws *et al.* 2003). The indications for chest drain insertion are (Laws *et al.* 2003):

- pneumothorax
- malignant pleural effusion
- empyema
- traumatic haemo pneumothorax
- post-operatively following thoracotomy.

The drain may be positioned apically to drain air or basally to drain fluid. A wide or small bore drain may be used. Small bore drains are more comfortable but a wide bore may be required to

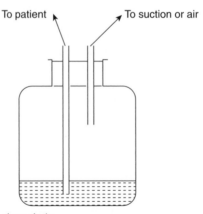

Figure 2.16 Underwater seal chest drain.

drain acute haemothorax and monitor blood loss. The drain is secured by two sutures, one to close the incision and one to secure the drain. Purse string sutures should not be used (Laws *et al.* 2003). A chest X-ray is performed after insertion to confirm an appropriate position and the drain. The drain should not be 'milked' or clamped during general care. However, chest drains may be clamped when the bottle is being changed, when two clamps should be used, one above and one below the junction between the drain in the patient and the tubing leading to the bottle (Sullivan 2008). Bubbling in the bottle will occur while air is draining from a pneumothorax in the pleural space and the drain will stay in place until the bubbling has ceased. It is very important that the bottle should remain below the level of the patient's chest and remain upright at all times to prevent backflow into the pleural space or breaking the seal. Either would cause collapse of the lung and rapid desaturation. The water in the tubing should swing with respiration and bubbling and drainage should be recorded. Low-pressure suction may be used at 10–20 cm H_2O and this requires a special low suction unit; normal wall suction cannot be used. Complications include:

- infection
- surgical emphysema at the insertion site
- damage to internal structures
- accidental breaking of the underwater seal by knocking the bottle over.

Removal requires two nurses, one to remove the retaining suture and the drain during expiration, and one to tie the closure suture as the drain is removed to prevent air entering the pleural cavity. Analgaesia is required because the drain is uncomfortable and the dressing must be changed using an aseptic technique. Clamps should be available at all times in case of accidental detachment from the bottle. Patients should be managed in specialist wards where nursing staff have appropriate training (Laws *et al.* 2003).

Nursing considerations

Infection control issues

- Aseptic technique when changing the dressing.
- Aseptic technique when changing the bottle.

Safety issues

- Ensure that the drain does not get knocked over.
- Ensure that the drain is always below the chest.
- Ensure that the drain does not become disconnected from the bottle.
- Ensure that clamps are available at all times.

Ensure that analgesia is prescribed and administered as required.

Nursing the patient with acute respiratory impairment

There is nothing more frightening than not being able to breathe and no matter what the cause, these patients are acutely sick. Fear of dying is in the mind of every patient who is experiencing difficulty with breathing and they need to feel safe and supported by considerate and caring nursing. They need to be reassured by a calm and sympathetic manner in an environment where the 'confidence creators' identified by Moore (Department of Health CNO Directorate 2008) are present:

- a calm, clean, safe environment
- a positive, friendly culture

Clinical link 2.5 (see Appendix for answers)

Patient 4 is a 30-year-old male admitted to the medical assessment unit by his family doctor following sudden onset of right-sided chest pain and breathlessness. He has previously been fit and well, with no history of chest infection or other respiratory problems. He is tall and thin, and very anxious. Saturations on arrival were 85% but have improved to 92% on high-flow oxygen 40% via a red Venturi mask at 12 L/min.

He is breathless with halting speech but is not using the accessory muscles of ventilation and there is evidence of peripheral cyanosis. He is awaiting a portable chest X-ray but A&E are busy and there has been a delay. His vital signs are:

- respiratory rate: 32
- temperature: 36.5°C
- peripheral pulse: 95
- blood pressure: 120/70
- SpO_2: 92%

Arterial blood gas analysis shows:

- pH: 7.35
- PaO_2: 9.8 kPa
- $PaCO_2$: 3.5 kPa
- SBC: 25 mmol/L
- BE: +1 mmol/L

Consider the following questions:

- What type of respiratory failure does this patient have and what is the most likely cause?
- What are your main priorities and why?
- What clinical actions should you take and why?

- good team working and good relationships
- well-managed care and efficient delivery
- personalized care for and about every patient.

Compassion is recognized as a key feature of high-quality nursing care and is one of the nursing metrics (quality indicators) identified by Griffiths (2008). Its importance is confirmed in the Dazi Report as an important value for NHS staff (Department of Health 2008 P70).

> We find the time to listen and talk when it is needed, make an effort to understand, and get on and do the small things that mean so much—not because we are asked to but because we care.

Respiratory distress is inevitably accompanied by anxiety, and nurses should be calm and reassure the patient that they are being closely observed. The patient should not be unobserved or left alone behind curtains and frequent monitoring demands a nursing presence. Respiratory impairment indicates critical illness and the next of kin should be informed of the seriousness of the patient's condition. Relatives at the bedside while the patient is acutely ill may be comforting, especially on a busy ward where nursing contact may be limited to the time taken to observe and record vital signs. The level of breathlessness may inhibit speech and it is important to be patient and allow time for the patient to express their needs. A family member can assist in this by sitting quietly with the patient if appropriate and offering comfort. This is not always possible in acute care and not all relatives can remain calm but it is important to keep relatives informed if the patient's condition is deteriorating or if admission to critical care becomes likely. Comfort for the respiratory patient also includes positioning (see earlier section).

Tachypnoea, pyrexia, and mouth breathing will increase the risk of dehydration and careful monitoring of fluid balance is essential. Oral hygiene is important and patients may need frequent help with mouth care when weak, ill, and dehydrated. The production of sputum should also be managed with care and attention. Pots and tissues should be at hand and the containers changed frequently. Infection control considerations in accordance with local policy should be observed assiduously for the protection of both staff and other patients.

In severely ill patients, timely administration of prescribed medication, secure oxygen delivery and frequent monitoring of vital signs and pulse oximetry are the responsibility of nursing staff. Patients with respiratory impairment need intelligent and thoughtful nursing, underpinned by knowledge, understanding, and skills. A combination of the art and science of nursing is essential to achieve the quality of nursing care which patients, relatives, and medical staff have a right to expect.

End of chapter test

It is important that you understand both the theory related to respiratory care and the practice of specific respiratory skills to safely care for patients with respiratory problems. To test your knowledge and apply this knowledge to clinical practice you should undertake the following assessment with an appropriately trained member of staff in clinical practice. If you are unable to answer any question it may be helpful to revisit the section in this chapter.

Knowledge assessment

Work with your mentor/supervisor in practice and ask them to test your knowledge in relation to the following areas. Incorrect answers/lack of knowledge will require further reading of this chapter.

- Discuss normal physiology and critically examine altered physiology in relation to patient's clinical condition.
- Analyse groups of patients at risk of respiratory deterioration and discuss why patients with chronic conditions are especially vulnerable.
- Critically evaluate need for respiratory assessment and discuss methods of respiratory assessment.
- Critically discuss causes and treatments of breathlessness in the acutely ill patient.
- Discuss indications for oxygen.
- Critically evaluate the effectiveness of differing oxygen delivery systems.
- Critically evaluate the need for oxygen supplementation and examine factors that may affect this.
- Analyse the differing types of humidification systems.
- Critically examine the value of oxygen saturation monitoring and highlight the limitation of saturation recording.
- Analyse the role of the physiotherapist in the management of respiratory impairment.

- Discuss different methods of spirometry and when these should be used.
- Discuss pharmacological actions of bronchodilators.
- Critically evaluate the role of arterial blood gas measurement in patient assessment.
- Interpret arterial blood gas data and debate appropriate management.
- Distinguish between type I and type II respiratory failure.
- Discuss indications/contraindications for CPAP and BiPAP.
- Discuss advantages and disadvantages of NIV.
- Critically evaluate situations in which advanced respiratory support is not appropriate.

Skills assessment

Work with your mentor/supervisor in practice and ask them to assess your ability to care for patients with respiratory impairment using the following criteria where appropriate. Note that you may not be able to demonstrate all these skills. Ask your mentor/supervisor to give you feedback on areas where you did well and areas that may require improving.

- Utilizes ALERT framework (see Chapter 11) to make initial assessment of airway patency, taking emergency action and summoning help if required.
- Monitors respiratory rate and utilizes the appropriate track-and-trigger system to facilitate reporting of concerns.
- Observes for abnormal patterns of respiration.
- Increases rate of respiratory monitoring as per trigger score.
- Observes for signs of respiratory distress and reports appropriately.
- Auscultates chest if appropriately trained and reports changes.
- Recognizes factors that may impede ventilation and reports/takes appropriate action.
- Ensures patient positioned appropriately.
- Monitors oxygen saturation, explaining potential limitations.
- Identifies any potential causes of hypoxia and takes appropriate action.
- Utilizes spirometry as required to enhance assessment.
- Administers oxygen as prescribed, selecting appropriate delivery system and concentration.
- Selects appropriate humidification.
- Administers medication, e.g. nebulizers, as prescribed and monitors this.
- Refers to physiotherapist as appropriate.
- Recognizes the need for arterial blood sampling and demonstrates ability to interpret blood gas result accurately.
- Evaluates patient's response to changes made and communicates concerns to medics/outreach team.
- Assists with implementation of NIV where local policy allows.
- Monitors effectiveness of NIV (if used).
- Documents changes and hands over plan of care appropriately.

References

Bickley, L. and Szilagyi, P. (2008) *Bate's Guide to Physical Examination and History Taking*, 10th edn. Lippincott Williams and Wilkins, Philadelphia.

Boon, N., Colledge, N., Walker, B., and Hunter, J. (2006) *Davidson's Principles and Practice of Medicine*, 20th edn. Churchill Livingstone Elsevier, London.

Bourke, S. (2007) *Lecture Notes on Respiratory Medicine*, 7th edn. Blackwell, Oxford.

British Thoracic Society (2006) *The Burden of Lung Disease*, 2nd edn. British Thoracic Society, London.

British Thoracic Society (2008a) *Guideline for Emergency Oxygen Use in Adult Patients*. British Thoracic Society, London.

British Thoracic Society (2008b) *British Guidelines on the Management of Asthma: Quick Reference Guide*. British Thoracic Society, London.

Chellel, A., Fender, V., Fraser, J., and Higgs, D. (2002) Nursing observation on ward patients at risk of critical illness. *Nurs. Times.* **98**, 36–39.

Davies, A. and Moores, C. (2002) *The Respiratory System*. Churchill Livingstone, London.

Department of Health (2005) *Supporting people with long-term conditions.* Department of Health, London.

Department of Health CNO Directorate (2008) *Confidence in Caring.* Department of Health, London.

Douglas, G., Nichol,F., and Robertson,C. (2005) *Macleod's Clinical Examination* 11th edn. Churchill Livingstone Elsevier, London.

Esmond G., ed. (2003) *Respiratory Nursing*. Bailliere Tindall, London.

Field, D. (2005) In: Sheppard, M., Wright, M. (eds), *Principles and Practice of High Dependency Nursing*. Bailliere Tindall, Edinburgh.

Griffiths, P., Jones, S., Maben, J., and Murrells, T. (2008) *State of the art metrics for nursing: a rapid appraisal.* National Nursing Research Unit King's College, London.

Kumar, P. and Clark, M. (2005) *Clinical Medicine* 6th edn. Elsevier Saunders, London.

Laws, D., Neville, E., and Duffy, J. (2003) British Thoracic Society Guidelines for the Insertion of a Chest Drain. *Thorax.* **58** (suppl I), ii53–59.

Medical Research Council (2009) Dyspnoea scale. Available at: http://www.nice.org.uk/usingguidance/commissioningguides/pulmonaryrehabilitationserviceforpatientswithcopd/mrc_dyspnoea_scale.jsp accessed 21/10/09 (accessed 15/03/09).

NICE (2004) *Chronic Obstructive Pulmonary Disease: Management of COPD in Adults in Primary and Secondary Care Quick Reference Guide.* National Institute for Health and Clinical Excellence, London.

NICE (2007) Acutely ill patients in hospital: recognition of and response to acute illness of adults in hospital. HMSO, London.

Selby, C. (2002) *Respiratory Medicine: An Illustrated Colour Text*. Churchill Livingstone, Edinburgh.

Stenhouse, C., Coates, S., Tivey, M., Allsop, P., and Parker, J. (2000) Prospective evaluation of modified early warning scores to aid earlier detection of patients at risk of developing critical illness on a general surgical ward. *Br. J. Anaesth.* **84**, 659–92.

Simpson, H. (2004) Interpretation of arterial blood gases: a clinical guide for nurses. *Br. J. Nurs.* **13**, 522–528.

Sullivan, B. (2008) Nursing management of patients with a chest drain *Br. J. Nurs.* **17**, 388–393.

Rang, H.P., Dale, M.M., Ritter, J.M., and Moore, P.K. (2003) *Pharmocology*. Elsevier, London.

West, J. (2003) *Pulmonary Pathophysiology: The Essentials.* 6th edn. Lippincott Williams and Wilkins, Philadelphia.

West, J. (2005) *Respiratory Physiology: The Essentials.* 7th edn. Lippincott Wiliams and Wilkins, Philadelphia.

Bibliography

Bourke, S. (2003) *Respiratory Medicine*, 6th edn. Blackwell, Oxford.

British Thoracic Society (2008c) *Non*-invasive *ventilation in chronic obstructive pulmonary disease: management of acute type 2 respiratory failure*, British Thoracic Society, London.

Department of Health (2007) Supporting People with Long Term Conditions. Department of Health, London.

Goldhill, D. and McNarry, A. (2004) Physiological abnormalities in early warning scores are related to mortality in adult inpatients. *Br. J. Anaesth.* **92**, 882–4.

McQuillain, P., Pilkington, S., Allan, A., *et al.* (1998) Confidential inquiry into quality of care before admission to ITU. *BMJ.* **316**: 1853–8.

Tortora, G. and Derrickson, B.H. (2008) Principles of anatomy and physiology: maintenance and continuity of the human body volume 2. 12th edn. Wiley, New Jersey.

Ward, J. (2006) *The Respiratory System at a Glance*, 2nd edn. Blackwell, Oxford.

Chapter 3

Cardiovascular assessment and care

Christine Spiers

Chapter contents

Cardiovascular disease remains the main cause of death in the UK. An understanding of cardiovascular anatomy and physiology is essential in understanding how to assess and manage patients with potential cardiovascular problems and complications. This chapter will examine:

♦ the normal anatomy of the heart and vascular system

♦ physiological mechanisms which control the cardiovascular function

♦ cardiovascular assessment

♦ cardiovascular monitoring

♦ cardiovascular management of the patient with:

  • chest pain

  • acute coronary syndromes

  • heart failure

  • cardiogenic shock

♦ overview of different types of shock.

Learning outcomes

This chapter will enable you to:

♦ review the normal structure and function of the cardiovascular system

♦ develop an understanding of the physiological mechanisms which control cardiovascular function

♦ consider the assessment, diagnosis and management of the patient with cardiovascular disorders

♦ identify the critically ill cardiac patient and know when to refer to senior/medical staff

♦ understand the impact of cardiovascular problems on the patient and carers

♦ use a skills assessment tool to assess your clinical practice.

Introduction

The cardiovascular system is a sophisticated transport system that serves to distribute essential substances to the cells of the body and to remove unwanted by-products of metabolism for elimination from the body. The cardiovascular system that completes this function is made up of a pump (the heart), a collection of distribution and collecting tubes (the arteries and veins), and

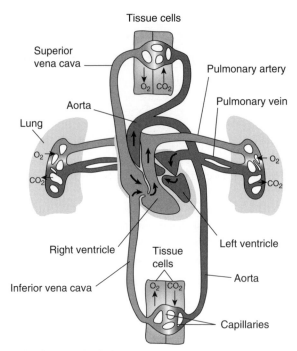

Figure 3.1 Systemic and pulmonic circulations.

a series of extensive thin-walled vessels that permit interchange between the vascular system and the tissues of the body (the capillaries).

The closed transport circuit that achieves this action comprises a vascular system and two pumps in series. The heart itself is described as a double-sided muscle pump, comprising a low- and a high-pressure system. The low-pressure output from the right ventricle sends blood into the pulmonary vasculature, where gaseous exchange between the blood and the alveoli in the lungs occurs. Oxygenated blood returns to the left side of the heart via the pulmonary veins. The relatively high pressure generated by the left ventricle propels blood into the systemic circulation and a series of arterial vessels distributes the blood to the tissues of the body. Exchange of nutrients and metabolic by-products takes place at the capillary level and de-oxygenated blood then drains back into small venules and veins and eventually back into the major veins (superior and inferior vena cava), which drain into the right atrium of the heart (Figure 3.1).

To fully understand the care and management of patients with cardiovascular problems, knowledge of the anatomy and blood flow through the heart is essential.

The anatomy of the heart

The adult heart is cone-shaped and lies between the lungs in a space called the mediastinum. It is approximately the size of a person's fist, weighing between 220 and 350 g. The top of the heart is referred to as the base and the pointed lower section the apex. Anatomically the base lies beneath the sternum, with two-thirds of the heart located to the left of the sternum. The base of the heart is aligned with the second intercostal space and the apex can be located in the fifth intercostal space in the mid-clavicular line. This can be palpated in a healthy adult and is known as the 'apex beat'. The location of the apex beat is an important clinical assessment and if the apex beat is displaced leftwards this can be an indication of cardiac enlargement.

Functionally the heart comprises a right heart and a left heart separated by a septum. Vessels bring blood into the upper two chambers, the atria, and leave the heart via outflow tracts from the lower ventricular chambers. The two sets of valves (atrioventricular and semilunar) ensure directional flow of blood through the heart.

Deoxygenated blood returns to the right side of the heart via the large capacitant veins, the superior and inferior vena cava. This is often referred to as the venous return. Blood flows passively through the tricuspid valve into the right ventricle. The right ventricle pumps the blood into the pulmonary artery via the pulmonary valve. The pulmonary artery takes the blood to the lungs, where gaseous exchange takes place. The oxygenated blood then returns to the left atrium via the four pulmonary veins (two from each lung). The blood flows through the mitral valve into the left ventricle where it is then ejected from the heart via the aortic valve into the aorta and the systemic circulation (Figure 3.1).

The heart is protected by the pericardium, which is a tough sac surrounding the heart with attachments to adjacent structures. There are two layers of pericardial tissues (parietal and visceral) and a narrow space between the two layers is filled with pericardial fluid. The pericardium allows the heart to contract smoothly within the thorax.

The myocardium comprises cardiac muscle, which can be classified into two types. The majority of cardiac cells are myocytes, which are striated involuntary muscle cells that have the capacity to contract due to specialized contractile proteins. The other cells are electrical cells or automatic cells, which form the specialized conduction system discussed later in this chapter.

Cardiac muscle cells contain cross-striated myofibrils, which have contractile properties and extensive numbers of mitochondria for the production of the energy source adenosine triphosphate (ATP); the contractile units are known as sarcomeres.

The endocardium is the smooth lining of the chambers of the heart and is continuous with the lining of the blood vessels (tunica intima). It consists of a lining of endothelial cells and allows the smooth passage of blood flow through the heart. The heart valves are created from folds of endocardium thickened by fibrous tissue. There are four heart valves: the tricuspid and pulmonary valves on the right side and the mitral and aortic valves on the left side. The two atrioventricular valves separate the atria from the ventricles (tricuspid and mitral valves) and the two semilunar valves are situated at the exit point of both ventricles (aortic and pulmonary valves). The atrioventricular valves have chordae tendineae, which are strong cord-like structures attached to papillary muscles within the ventricular chambers. The chordae tendineae prevent inversion and incompetence of the valves during ventricular systole.

At the junction of the upper third of the heart, a deep oblique atrioventricular groove runs around the heart. This atrioventricular groove separates the atria from the ventricles. Two other grooves run anteriorly and posteriorly towards the apex of the heart: the anterior and posterior interventricular grooves. These grooves mark the position of the interventricular septum, which separates the right and left ventricles and the grooves also form a route for the coronary artery circulation.

Physiological mechanisms of the cardiovascular function

The coronary circulation

The heart receives its blood supply from the coronary arteries, which arise from the sinuses of Valsalva, just above the semilunar cusps of the aortic valve. The right coronary artery arises from the anterior cusp and the left coronary artery from the left posterior sinus (see Figure 3.2).

The left coronary artery comprises the left main stem which rapidly divides into two components: the left anterior descending coronary (LAD) artery and the left circumflex (Cx). The LAD

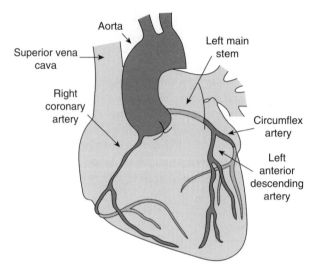

Figure 3.2 Coronary artery circulation.

coronary artery runs down the interventricular groove towards the apex of the heart and provides septal and diagonal branches. The diagonal branches of the LAD supply the anterior, apical, and lateral walls of the left ventricle. The septal branches supply the interventricular septum and the right bundle branch and part of the left bundle branch. The Cx runs down the posterior atrioventricular groove to supply the posterolateral aspect of the left ventricle (LV). The right coronary artery (RCA) runs down the anterior atrioventricular groove, supplying the right side of the heart, the inferior and posterior surface of the heart, the sino-atrial node, and the atrioventricular node.

Most of the venous drainage of the heart is via the cardiac veins. The great, middle, and small cardiac veins drain blood into the coronary sinus, which is situated on the posterior wall of the left ventricle. The coronary sinus drains into the right atrium. Venous blood from the anterior cardiac veins drains directly into the right atrium and the remaining blood drains directly from the Thebesian veins into the cardiac chambers.

As the coronary arteries lie on the epicardial (outside) surface of the heart, the epicardium receives more blood than the endocardium, which is more vulnerable during periods of reduced blood flow.

The heart is therefore a double-sided pump, which maintains a constant circulation of blood to the body. At rest, the heart pumps at approximately 70 beats per minute and maintains a cardiac output of 5 L/min. The cycle of blood flow through the heart is referred to as the cardiac cycle.

The conduction system

An understanding of the conduction system and the association with the electrocardiogram (ECG) is essential for any practitioner working with acutely ill patients. Most acute units have facilities to monitor the patient's cardiac rate and rhythm, and increasingly sophisticated technology makes the continuous recording of 12-lead ECGs a possibility.

The cardiac conduction system consists of specialized electrical or 'automatic' cells, which contain specific properties that allow the generation, propagation, and conduction of electrical impulses from the atria and into the ventricles in order to produce myocardial contraction (Figure 3.3).

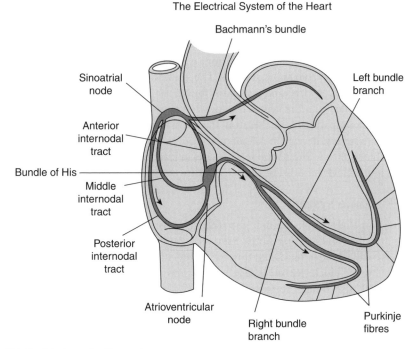

Figure 3.3 Electrical conduction system.

The cardiac conduction system comprises:

- the sino-atrial (SA) or sinus node
- the atrioventricular (AV) node or junction
- the bundle of His
- the right bundle branch
- the left bundle branches (anterior and posterior fascicles)
- the Purkinje fibres.

The sino-atrial node

The sino-atrial node, sometimes referred to as the cardiac pacemaker, is located on the posterior wall at the junction of the right atrium with the superior vena cava. It is crest-shaped and approximately 25 mm long and 3 mm wide. It is heavily innervated with autonomic nerve fibres and the predominant influence on the SA node is the parasympathetic branches of the right vagus nerve.

The SA node has the property of *intrinsic automaticity*, which means that the SA node spontaneously depolarizes at a rate determined by the autonomic nervous system in order to cause atrial contraction. The co-ordination and transmission of right and left atrial activity is by specialized conducting pathways, the most well defined of these being Bachmann's bundle, which links the right and left atria. The blood supply to the SA node is from the nodal artery, which arises from the right coronary artery in 60% of adults and the left coronary artery in the remaining 40%.

The atrioventricular node

In health, the atrioventricular (AV) node is the only electrical connection between the atria and the ventricles. The annulus fibrosus (atrioventricular fibrous ring) creates an electrical insulator between the atria and the ventricles. The AV node is situated at the junction between the interatrial septum and the tricuspid valve annulus. The AV node creates a delay in transmission of electrical stimuli to the ventricles and this allows for atrial systole to occur, which allows the atrial contents to be expelled into the ventricles prior to ventricular systole. The AV node is richly innervated by parasympathetic branches from the left vagus nerve and it receives its blood supply from the AV nodal artery, derived in 90% of cases from the RCA and in 10% of cases from the Cx. Reduction in blood flow to the AV node, as occurs in inferior wall infarction (RCA infarction), often results in AV block (or heart block).

The His-Purkinje system

The transmission of electrical stimuli to the ventricular tissue is via the bundle of His, right and left bundle branches, and Purkinje fibres. Failure of conduction through the bundle branches is referred to as bundle branch block and this may affect either the right or the left bundle branch. Right bundle branch block (RBBB) is relatively common and may occur in a structurally normal heart as well as secondary to pathological processes. Left bundle branch block (LBBB) is never normal and is generally the result of severe cardiac disease such as myocardial infarction, hypertensive heart disease, or cardiomyopathy (Goldberger 2006).

Autonomic nervous system

Whilst the heart has the intrinsic nervous system described above, the conduction system itself is regulated by the autonomic nervous system. Control of the autonomic nerves is via the cardiac centre in the medulla oblongata in the brain stem. The sympathetic nerve supply to the heart is to the sino-atrial node, atrio-ventricular node, His-Purkinje system, and the atrial and ventricular myocardium. The parasympathetic nerves to the heart (the vagus nerve) supply mainly the sino-atrial and atrio-ventricular nodes and, to a much lesser extent, the atrial and ventricular myocardium. Sympathetic nerve activity is mediated via adrenaline (epinephrine) and nor-adrenaline (nor-epinephrine) and the β-receptors. Increased sympathetic activity increases heart rate and stroke volume. Stroke volume is defined as the amount of blood ejected from the ventricle per beat. Increased parasympathetic stimulation mediated via acetylcholine decreases heart rate and probably myocardial contractility.

Cardiac cycle

The cardiac cycle can be defined in terms of the mechanical events which occur from the beginning of one heart beat to the beginning of the next. This cycle is characterized by a series of pressure changes, which results in blood flowing from areas of high pressure to areas of low pressure. The cyclical contraction (systole) and relaxation of the heart (diastole) of the cardiac cycle is divided into four phases.

Ventricular filling

During mid to late diastole the pressures in the heart are low and blood returns passively to the atria and into the ventricles via the open atrioventricular valves; this is known as *passive ventricular filling* and 70–80% of ventricular filling occurs at this stage. The semi-lunar valves are closed at this stage due to the pressure in the pulmonary artery and aorta being higher than the pressure in the respective ventricles. Towards the end of diastole, *active ventricular filling* occurs as a result of atrial contraction initiated by stimulation from the sino-atrial node (P wave on the ECG). Atrial contraction (systole) forces the remaining 20–30% of blood into the ventricles.

Ventricular contraction

Atrial relaxation now occurs and the ventricles are depolarized (QRS complex on the ECG), resulting in ventricular contraction. As the ventricles start to contract, the pressure within the ventricles starts to rise, causing the atrioventricular valves to close. At this stage the volume of blood in the ventricles is constant, all four heart valves are closed, and the ventricles contract causing the pressure within the ventricular chambers to rise; this is known as *isovolumetric contraction*.

Ventricular ejection

As the pressure in the ventricles continues to rise, the pressure in the ventricles exceeds the pressure in the major arteries and the semilunar valves are forced open; this is the *ventricular ejection phase*. During the ejection phase blood is ejected into the pulmonary artery and aorta.

Isovolumetric relaxation

Repolarization of the ventricles occurs resulting in relaxation (diastole) of the ventricles (T wave on the ECG). The pressure falls in the ventricles allowing the aortic and pulmonary valves to close again. Once again, the ventricles are closed chambers; all four valves are closed. During this time the atria are filling with blood (passive venous return) and once the pressure within the atria is higher than the pressure in the ventricles, the AV valves open and blood flows into the ventricles again (*ventricular filling phase*). The pressure changes in the ventricles, and corresponding ECG waveforms and heart sounds are indicated in Figure 3.4.

Heart sounds

The normal heart sounds (lub-dup) arise from the closure of the heart valves during the cardiac cycle. The first heart sound (S_1) is principally the sound of the simultaneous closure of the mitral and tricuspid valves at the onset of ventricular systole (lub). The sound is loudest at the apex or may also be heard at the lower left sternal border. The second heart sound (S_2) is due to closure of the aortic and pulmonary valves at the end of ventricular systole and it forms the 'dup' component of lub-dup. It is heard at the upper left sternal border and both sounds are best heard with the diaphragm of the stethoscope. Familiarizing yourself with normal heart sounds is a useful skill, as once you are used to recognizing normal heart sounds you are more likely to be able to

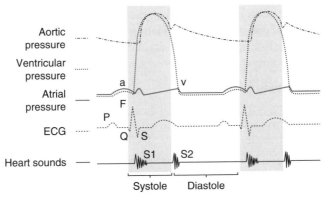

Figure 3.4 Cardiac cycle, including ECG waveforms and heart sounds.

identify added sounds and murmurs. Added sounds and murmurs are usually due to turbulent blood flow through the heart, across the valves or the great vessels. There are many causes of murmurs that are beyond the scope of this chapter.

Cardiac output

Cardiac output is defined as the total volume of blood ejected by the heart into the systemic circulation in L/min. This is normally calculated as:

$$\text{cardiac output (CO)} = \text{heart rate (HR)} \times \text{stroke volume (SV)}$$

The stroke volume is the amount of blood ejected from the ventricles per beat. In the resting adult, the cardiac output is approximately 5 L/min. The average heart rate (70 beats per minute) multiplied by an average stroke volume (70 mL of blood) is equal to 4.9 L/min. Cardiac output can vary between at rest values of 4.5 L/min and 25 L/min during vigorous exercise. Increases in heart rate or stroke volume or both can increase the cardiac output, whereas profound bradycardia or reduced stroke volume can decrease the cardiac output.

Cardiac output is therefore dependent on the relationship between the stroke volume and the heart rate.

Heart rate

In normal circumstances the heart rate is regulated by the activity of the sino-atrial node and its innervation from the autonomic nervous system (ANS) described above. Impulses from the sympathetic branches of the ANS have a *positive chronotropic* effect, which increases the heart rate; a similar chronotropic effect is produced by drugs such as β-adrenergic stimulants, such as salbutamol, and caffeine or nicotine.

The parasympathetic innervation to the SA node is via the vagus nerve and this acts as a 'brake' on the heart rate, causing it to slow. *Negatively chronotropic* effects may be caused by increased vagal stimulation as seen in extreme intense visceral pain or stimulation of baroreceptors in the carotid sinus or aortic arch. Negatively chronotropic drugs include β-blockers and digoxin.

Stroke volume

Three significant factors affect stroke volume and thus cardiac output; 'preload', 'myocardial contractility' and 'afterload'.

Preload

Preload can be defined as the tension exerted on the cardiac muscle at the end of diastole. The principle determinant of preload is the venous return and this is often referred to as 'ventricular filling'. The heart is able to adapt to varying loads of inflowing blood and it is partly this capacity which alters the cardiac output.

Myocardial contractility

Contractility is a property of myocardial fibres and essential for the effective pumping action of the heart; the strength of myocardial contraction is influenced by a number of factors. Sympathetic nervous stimulation, adrenaline (epinephrine) and nor-adrenaline (nor-epinephrine) and cardiac stimulants (such as caffeine) may increase the speed and strength of myocardial contraction. This is referred to as a *positive inotropic effect* and can be augmented by positive inotropic drugs such as dobutamine and digoxin. *Negative inotropic* effects (reduced contraction) may be induced by myocardial hypoxia or ischaemia or negatively inotropic drugs such as β-blockers.

Within physiological limits, cardiac muscle may be stretched to achieve increases in stroke volume and this is known as the Frank–Starling mechanism. Starling's law of the heart states that the myocardial fibres respond with a more forceful contraction when they are stretched. An example of this is to consider how an elastic band can be stretched to increase the elastic recoil when the elastic band is released. If an elastic band is continually overstretched, it will eventually lose its recoil and elasticity. Pathological processes such as cardiomyopathy and uncontrolled hypertension over a period of time may result in overstretching of the myofibrils and a subsequent reduction in cardiac stretch and hence reduced stroke volume. Reduction in the effectiveness of the contraction results in heart failure.

Afterload

Afterload is the force opposing the ejection of blood from the ventricles, and is a function of the resistance offered by peripheral (systemic) blood vessels and the size of the left ventricle. Pathologic conditions which increase afterload are either those which increase peripheral resistance (systemic or pulmonary hypertension) or conditions which obstruct outflow from the ventricles (aortic stenosis, pulmonary stenosis, or coarctation of the aorta).

Blood pressure

Blood pressure is defined as the force or the pressure the blood exerts upon the vessel walls and it is a function of cardiac output and systemic vascular resistance, hence the equation below is sometimes used:

$$\text{blood pressure (BP)} = \text{cardiac output} \times \text{systemic vascular resistance}$$

Clinically, however, the blood pressure is essentially the arterial pressure in the systemic circulation and the systolic pressure occurs as a result of systole and the diastolic pressure results from diastole in the cardiac cycle. The *pulse pressure* is the difference between systolic and diastolic blood pressure and the *mean arterial pressure* is the pressure in the large arteries averaged over time (Berne & Levy 2001). The mean blood pressure depends on the mean blood volume in the system and on the compliance of the arterial vessels. Mean arterial pressure is an important value, and whilst not directly measured in acute care settings it is a value given on the automated blood pressure machines in practice. It is widely accepted that a mean arterial pressure of 60 mmHg is needed to sustain perfusion pressure to vital organs.

Blood pressure is maintained by a number of factors, including:

♦ cardiac output

♦ blood volume

♦ elasticity and tone of the blood vessels.

Cardiac output

As described above, cardiac output is the amount of blood ejected from the heart measured in litres per minute. In the resting adult heart, the cardiac output is equal to the product of the heart rate and the stroke volume. In healthy individuals, this is equivalent to 4.5–5.5 L/min at rest, and up to a maximum of over 20 L/min during exercise.

Blood volume

Blood pressure is also affected by the volume of blood in the circulation and this is dependent on fluid and electrolyte balances and their controls (see Chapter 7).

Elasticity and tone of blood vessels

The arteries distribute blood to the cells and tissues of the body. Arteries are elastic vessels that help to maintain the forward (driving) pressure in the circulation. They also offer a variable resistance to blood flow. Arteries branch in a similar way to trees and become smaller arteries and eventually arterioles. Small arteries and arterioles have a greater proportion of elastic tissue within their walls and this enables them to alter their internal diameter. *Vasoconstriction* reduces the internal diameter of the vessel and *vasodilation* increases the vessel diameter. Normally the vessels are in a state of partial constriction and are said to have *tone*. Vasoactive substances such as neurotransmitters, hormones, and local factors can alter the arterial tone and these are listed in Table 3.1.

Arterial pressure needs to be maintained at a regular level; insufficient blood pressure can reduce the blood flow to the brain and heart and may result in loss of consciousness. Conversely, consistently raised blood pressure can cause irrevocable damage to internal organs and tissues.

Blood pressure is monitored and regulated by:

* neural mechanisms (baroreceptors, reflexes, and control centre)
* hormonal factors
* renal controls.

Neural mechanisms

Pressure sensors (baroreceptors) situated in the aortic arch and carotid sinus monitor changes to blood pressure and send afferent impulses to the cardiovascular centre in the brain stem. Baroreceptors are excited by stretch; impulses are transmitted from the receptors along the sensory nerve fibres to the spinal cord.

Reflexes

A fall in blood pressure is sensed by the baroreceptors; this stimulus acts reflexly via the control centres in the brain stem to increase cardiac output and arterial resistance to blood flow.

Table 3.1 Vasoactive substances in the control of blood pressure

Vasoactive substance	Vasoconstriction	Vasodilation
Neurotransmitters		
noradrenaline	Yes (α-receptors)	
acetylcholine		Yes
adrenaline	Yes (α-receptors)	Yes (β-receptors)
Hormones		
angiotensin	Yes	
serotonin	Yes	
bradykinin		Yes
Local metabolites		
carbon dioxide		Yes
hypoxia		Yes

This is mediated via the sympathetic nervous system. Adrenaline released by the adrenal gland acts via the α-receptor sites in the blood vessel walls to cause vasoconstriction. In addition, adrenaline mediates an increase in heart rate via the sino-atrial node and an increase in cardiac contractility by direct effect on the myocardium. The subsequent increase in heart rate and contractility contributes to an increase in cardiac output.

Hormonal factors

A number of hormones released by endocrine glands are vasoactive. The release of catecholamines (adrenaline and noradrenaline) from the adrenal medulla influences blood pressure by effects on the heart rate, cardiac output, and integrity of blood vessels. Other hormones such as bradykinin act as local regulators of blood flow in the circulation. Hormones which influence renal function and blood volume such as renin, angiotensin, aldosterone, and anti-diuretic hormone also affect blood pressure (see Chapter 5 for an extensive overview).

Local metabolites

Many local metabolites, such as carbon dioxide, hydrogen ions and low levels of oxygen, may act as vasodilators. The vasodilation activity of the metabolites counteracts the vasoconstriction effects of the sympathetic nervous system. This therefore allows local blood flow to active tissue to be maintained, despite increased activity by the sympathetic nervous system.

Renal controls

Extensive discussion is outwith the scope of this chapter, but the predominant effect of renal control of blood pressure is to maintain blood volume through direct or indirect release of the above hormones. Diuretics reduce excessive fluid retention by the kidney and are used to lower blood pressure, whilst the effect of angiotensin converting enzyme (ACE) inhibitors such as ramipril are well known for their effect on the renin-angiotensin-aldosterone mechanism and their effect in treating long-standing hypertension (Opie & Gersch 2004).

Pathophysiology of atherosclerosis

A common pathological process affecting the cardiovascular system is atherosclerosis, which is a chronic progressive disorder affecting the intimal layer of artery walls. It evolves from the complex interaction of the blood elements, vessel wall changes and alterations in blood flow. It is characterized by the proliferation of smooth muscle cells and the accumulation of elevated white lesions known as plaques. The plaques consist of a soft lipid-rich core and a hard fibrous cap and the term 'atherosclerosis' derives from the Greek 'athere', meaning 'gruel' or 'porridge', pertaining to the lipid rich core, and also the Greek 'skleros' meaning 'hard' referring to the hard fibrous cap which encases the lipid-rich core.

Atherosclerosis may cause coronary heart disease (angina, acute coronary syndrome, or myocardial infarction), cerebrovascular disease (transient ischaemic attack or stroke) or peripheral vascular disease (limb claudication or acute limb ischaemia). For a discussion of cerebrovascular disease see Chapter 4.

The extent of arterial plaques appears to increase with advancing age and with the number of risk factors. It is, however, a misnomer that atherosclerosis is entirely age-related, as a number of studies have demonstrated that atherosclerotic plaques occur at a very early age in those with cardiovascular risk factors. The role and importance of risk factors for coronary heart disease has been well demonstrated in epidemiological and interventional trials and many key factors have emerged. Non-modifiable risk factors include age, gender, particular ethnic groups, and family history. The authors of the Interheart Study (Yusuf *et al.* 2004) identify nine modifiable risk factors that contribute to the risk of heart disease:

- smoking
- hypertension
- lipid levels
- diabetes mellitus
- lack of exercise
- lack of dietary fruit and vegetables
- abdominal obesity
- psychological factors
- alcohol intake.

These risk factors are synergistic and thus the possession of a number of risk factors significantly increases the risk of developing atherosclerotic disease. Other factors have also emerged that are referred to as protective factors and appear to confer some degree of risk protection for individuals. These include:

- physical activity (20 min, two to three times per week)
- alcohol (moderate intake of 1–2 units daily)
- diet rich in antioxidants (particularly onions and garlic) and the inclusion of five fruit and/or vegetable portions daily
- diet rich in omega-3 rich fish oils (two to three portions of oily fish weekly)
- vitamin C and vitamin E rich foods.

The reader is referred to the British Heart Foundation for useful health promotional literature.

Finally there is emerging evidence that atherosclerosis is not a degenerative disease, but an active inflammatory process triggered by an infective process. Various theories have emerged to link *Chlamydia pneumoniae* (a common respiratory pathogen) to atherogenesis. Antibiotic trials are ongoing to assess the role of anti-chlamydial agents as a preventive treatment (Katz & Purcell 2006).

There is incontrovertible evidence that the five conventional cardiac risk factors of smoking, hypertension, diabetes, lack of physical exercise, and abnormal lipids account for the majority of the risk of an initial heart attack. Public health promotion campaigns including health professionals and governmental measures utilize a two-pronged approach to coronary heart disease prevention. The 'high-risk' (risk factor management) strategy includes the identification and aggressive treatment of those at 'high risk' of heart disease, such as patients with hyperlipidaemia or diabetes. The 'population' approach is aimed at healthy messages (lifestyle modification), media campaigns, and fiscal strategies directed at the population as a whole. The two approaches are utilized in combination to produce an effective risk reduction strategy and the reader is referred to the National Service Framework for Coronary Heart Disease (Department of Health 2000) for further information.

Nursing management of cardiovascular disorders

Nursing management of patients with cardiac problems has some common features. Specific management of different disorders will be detailed under specific subheadings. Cardiovascular disease may present acutely or chronically. However, in many situations the presentation is acute and requires urgent, prompt assessment and management by the nursing staff. The phrase 'time is myocardium' was introduced during the 1980s to reflect the importance of urgent intervention—the phrase is still relevant today. Care should be aimed at:

♦ accurate and timely cardiovascular assessment

♦ relief of immediate life-threatening and distressing symptoms (this will prevent further deterioration and is of course essential for ensuring patient comfort)

♦ timely nursing/medical intervention.

Cardiovascular assessment

Cardiovascular disease may manifest in a variety of ways, dependent on whether there is mechanical dysfunction, coronary artery insufficiency, or cardiac arrhythmias. Nevertheless the cardiac history is the most important part of the investigative process and requires skilful elucidation. It is often stated that 90% of the diagnosis is elicited from good history-taking. The aim of history-taking is to enable the patient to give a clear description of the presenting symptoms, to uncover any precipitating or relieving factors and to identify any pattern to symptom episodes. Past medical history, medication and risk factor identification, social factors, and occupational status may support the process. The most common cardiovascular symptoms include:

♦ breathlessness

♦ palpitations

♦ dizziness and syncope

♦ claudication

♦ fatigue

♦ chest pain.

Breathlessness

Breathlessness is nearly always caused by cardiac or respiratory illness (see Chapter 2). In cardiac disease, breathlessness is principally caused by reduced cardiac output, cardiac arrhythmias, or pulmonary oedema (Newby & Grubb 2005).

Breathlessness may be a chronic symptom (as in biventricular heart failure), may occur with an acute exacerbation of a chronic problem (ventricular tachyarrhythmia in cardiomyopathy), or may present as the principal symptom in an acute illness (acute pulmonary oedema secondary to myocardial infarction). Whatever the cause, the patient will be extremely anxious and distressed and will require urgent intervention. Some patients may only experience breathlessness when lying down (*orthopnoea*) or may be woken during the night with sudden episodes of breathlessness relieved by sitting upright (*paroxysmal nocturnal dyspnoea*). The symptoms of orthopnoea and paroxysmal nocturnal dyspnoea are often an indication of heart failure.

Palpitations

Palpitations are a common, but distressing, symptom. Palpitations can be defined as an abnormally perceived heartbeat. The term 'palpitation' may be erroneously used by patients to describe a number of symptoms such as an irregularity, a forceful heartbeat, or even chest pain or breathlessness. It is thus crucial to find out exactly what a patient means and accurate history-taking may elicit a missed beat, heart racing, or even an abnormally slow heart rate (Wolff & Cowan 2009). The patient may be able to tap out the rhythm of the palpitations with their hand.

An irregular heart beat may be caused by atrial or ventricular extrasystoles and periods of palpitations may be commonly experienced during periods of stress or anxiety. Extrasystoles or 'extra beats' may be triggered by caffeine, alcohol, or even chocolate. Atrial fibrillation, which is less benign, commonly presents with irregular and chaotic bouts of tachycardia and may be associated with episodes of breathlessness and syncope. Occasionally atrial fibrillation may be triggered by alcohol or be present in a normally healthy person (lone atrial fibrillation), although it is generally caused by cardiac disease (NICE 2006).

Occasionally, a pounding or forceful heart beat at a moderate rate (90–120/min) may reflect normal cardiac function in the presence of exercise, stress, anxiety, or a hyperdynamic state such as pregnancy or hyperthyroidism.

Dizziness or syncope

Dizziness and syncope are common symptoms and may have cardiac or neurological causes. Neurological causes include epilepsy, cerebrovascular ischaemia, and neoplasms (see Chapter 4).

Potential cardiac causes of syncope include cardiac arrhythmias (bradycardia and tachycardia), left ventricular outflow obstruction (aortic stenosis or hypertrophic cardiomyopathy), and postural hypotension (associated with autonomic dysfunction or induced by cardiac drugs such as vasodilators and diuretics). Cardiac syncope requires further investigation, which may include 12-lead ECG, ambulatory ECG and event recording, ambulatory blood pressure, echocardiography, tilt testing, and electrophysiological studies.

Claudication

Claudication, or ischaemic pain affecting the calf and other leg muscles, is described as peripheral vascular disease and is generally due to widespread atherosclerosis. Pain occurs on exercise and is relieved by rest. The best medical therapy for peripheral vascular disease includes risk factor management (as described above), in particular smoking cessation, management of lipid disorders, and the institution of antiplatelet therapy. Regular exercise may relieve the symptoms of claudication due to the development of collateral circulation.

Fatigue

Fatigue and lethargy are the most widespread symptom experienced by patients with chronic heart failure. It can be a debilitating symptom, which severely affects the patient's quality of life (Nicholson 2007). Reduced cardiac output causes low blood pressure. In order to maintain perfusion to vital organs, blood is diverted away from skeletal muscles and this contributes to fatigue and lethargy. The fatigue may be further exacerbated by skeletal muscle atrophy due to immobility. Anaemia is another common cause of fatigue, particularly in patients with chronic heart failure, and anaemia may also trigger anginal type chest pains. Fatigue may also lead to depression, especially in patients where the chronic condition reduces their daily activities.

Chest pain

Chest pain is one of the most common reasons for a consultation at the general practitioner and in addition it is a leading cause of emergency hospital admission. It is one of the most frightening symptoms experienced by patients, many of whom will know that it may herald an acute cardiac event such as a 'heart attack' or 'cardiac arrest'. Use of a mnemonic such as the PQRST (Albarran 2002) may serve to provide a useful framework for history taking:

P – **p**recipitating factors

Q – **q**uality

R – **region** and radiation

S – associated **symptoms**

T – **t**iming of symptoms and **t**reatments to relieve symptoms.

There are many causes of chest pain, some of which are life-threatening and many others which are less serious. The causes of chest pain from non-cardiac causes are considered in Table 3.2.

The causes of chest pain are therefore many and varied and the underlying problem may be life-threatening or trivial. A strategy of caution is, however, always adopted in assessing and managing chest pain in order to rule out life-threatening causes and to investigate possible cardiac causes.

Cardiac causes of chest pain include:

- acute coronary syndromes (angina, non-ST-segment elevation myocardial infarction and ST-segment myocardial infarction)

- myocarditis, pericarditis, and endocarditis

Table 3.2 Differentiation of chest pain from non cardiac causes

Cause of chest pain	Nature of pain	Other symptoms
Pulmonary		
Pneumonia Chest infection Pleurisy Pneumothorax Pleural effusion	Sharp, stabbing	Cough Wheeze Breathlessness Sputum production Haemoptysis Circulatory collapse
Musculoskeletal		
Blunt injury acquired from: contact sport, road traffic accident, physical assault	Sharp, diffuse or stabbing	Pain is often positional and exacerbated by deep breathing, turning or arm movement
Inflammatory, or autoimmune conditions; costochondritis, ankylosing spondylitis	Widespread and diffuse	Pain is associated with localized tenderness and/ or swelling
Acute oesophago-gastric disorders		
Oesophageal rupture (Boerhaave's syndrome)	Severe, burning	Excruciating retrosternal pain radiating to the back, chest or abdomen Associated symptoms include breathlessness, hypotension, poor peripheral perfusion and peripheral cyanosis
Gastro-oesophageal reflux	Upper or lower retrosternal, burning	Pain may be related to dietary intake, intermittent dysphagia or pain on bending forwards
Chest pain due to pulmonary embolism	Substernal, may be pleuritic in nature	Pain is not the major presenting feature; sudden onset of breathlessness is common Massive PE presents clinically with shock, hypotension, gallop rhythm (tachycardia with an added S3) and raised JVP.

JVP, jugular venous pressure.

Table 3.3 Differentiation of cardiac chest pain from non-cardiac chest pain

Features of chest pain	Cardiac chest pain	Non-cardiac chest pain
Characteristics	Heavy Dull Gripping Pushing Gripping Constricting	Dull Sharp Shooting Burning
Location	Central chest Retrosternal Back	Right chest
Radiation	Arms (particularly left arm, ulnar aspect) Neck and throat Upper epigastrium Lower jaw Back	Nil significant radiation
Precipitating factors	Exercise Stress and anxiety Cold weather	Movement Tender to palpation

Based on data from Newby & Grubb (2005).

- ♦ acute aortic dissection
- ♦ syndrome X (microvascular coronary artery disease)
- ♦ aortic stenosis
- ♦ cardiac arrhythmias
- ♦ takotsubo cardiomyopathy ('broken heart' syndrome) (Kelly 2007)
- ♦ hypertrophic obstructive cardiomyopathy.

Once again, the importance of the history is highlighted; patients should be encouraged to give the history of their symptom in their own words. Cardiac chest pain may be distinguished from non-cardiac chest pain by assessing the character, location, radiation, and precipitating factors (see Table 3.3). The management of chest pain will be explored later in this chapter.

Cardiovascular tools

Of the assessment tools available to the nurse, the most important is monitoring of the vital signs, oxygen saturations, peripheral perfusion, cardiac rate, and rhythm. These will be discussed in detail as it is a fundamental part of cardiac care.

Early identification of problems will lead to timely treatment that may reduce the impact of cardiac damage. It is essential that all staff should understand how to perform cardiac assessment correctly so that early changes can be identified and treated promptly.

Vital signs

Heart rate

Heart rate may be estimated by measuring and recording radial, carotid, femoral, or apical pulses. When the heart rate is irregular, the rate should be counted for 1 min and preferably identified by listening to the apex beat (fifth intercostal space, midclavicular line). An irregular pulse may be due to atrial or ventricular ectopics or atrial fibrillation and can be further assessed by counting the heart rate and the radial pulse concomitantly.

Blood pressure

Blood pressure is the force exerted by the volume of blood on the arterial walls and is a function of cardiac output and systemic vascular resistance. It is a dynamic and constantly changing pressure and varies by up to 30 mmHg throughout the day. It can be influenced by a variety of factors: blood volume, time of the day, anxiety, pain, and various drugs. It is important to note that anxiety alone may raise the blood pressure by 30 mmHg and this should be taken into account when patients are very frightened or anxious.

Measurement of blood pressure using a sphygmomanometer involves the occlusion of an artery using a cuff and either detection of Korotkoff sounds (auscultatory method) or monitoring by using oscillometry. The most common method employed in acute areas is the oscillometric method (Dynamap), which measures blood pressure by sensing arterial pulsations or oscillations (Clinton 2003). The sphygmomanometer, stethoscope, and cuff method detects turbulent blood flow within the artery, which is heard as Korotkoff sounds (named after the Russian army surgeon who first identified them in 1905).

The cuff should be located at heart level and a variety of cuff sizes should be available to accommodate variations in patient size. Incorrect cuff sizes can give false readings, as can incorrect location of the cuff site. Automated recordings should be instituted in patients who need regular observation or continuous tracking, although practitioners should note that automatic cuff inflations can be painful and disturbing to patients. Automated blood pressure can be set to trigger an alarm when the systolic blood pressure falls—various early-warning systems utilize different ranges, although a systolic blood pressure of <100 mmHg should alert the acute care practitioner to early intervention. Many cardiac patients do, however, have relatively low blood pressure, partly due to their reduced cardiac output and also related to commonly used cardiac drugs such as β-blockers and angiotension-converting enzyme inhibitors (ACE), which lower the blood pressure.

Respiratory rate

Variations in respiratory rate are the single most important physiological indicator in identifying the critically ill patient. Changes in respiratory rate, whilst not always an indicator of acute cardiac deterioration, may nonetheless indicate acute hypoxia secondary to acute onset pulmonary oedema, reduced myocardial perfusion, and reduced cardiac output. Monitoring and tracking the respiratory rate is thus just as vital in assessing cardiac patients as it is in respiratory patients (see Chapter 2). A respiratory rate of >15 should trigger further investigations from the nurse.

Oxygen saturation

Oxygen saturation indicates how much arterial oxygen is combined with haemoglobin and is expressed as a percentage. For a detailed description of the benefits and usage of oxygen saturation in acute care settings see Chapter 2. It is important to remember that pulse oximeter readings alone are of limited value and thus should be used in conjunction with other physiological assessments. Oxygen saturation levels may be low in pulmonary oedema, heart failure, myocardial infarction, and cardiogenic shock.

Peripheral perfusion

Peripheral fingers and toes should be examined for evidence of pallor and cyanosis. It is good practice to remove any nail varnish in order to establish nail bed colour and perfusion. The capillary refill is measured by placing the patient's hand at heart level and compressing the nail bed of a finger for 5 s. Pressure is released and the time to regain normal colour is measured. The normal capillary refill time should be 2 s although 2–3 s is considered normal in the elderly (Epstein *et al.* 2003).

Cardiac monitoring

Most acute-care settings have facilities for single-lead, triple-lead, and occasionally continuous 12-lead recordings of the heart rate and rhythm. The electrocardiogram (ECG) is a graphic representation of the electrical events generated by the cardiac conduction system described earlier in this chapter.

Monitoring electrodes placed on the body's surface can detect these electrical events and transmit, via monitoring leads, to an oscilloscope, where the events are amplified and displayed as a series of waveforms.

The basic ECG waveforms are labelled PQRST (and U) and reflect the electrical events which should trigger mechanical contraction within the heart (see Figure 3.5).

Additionally the PR interval, QT interval, and ST segment provide further information about the heart. The correlation of the ECG waveforms, intervals, and segments to the electrical and mechanical events is identified in Table 3.4.

ECG paper

ECG paper is marked out as graph paper in squares and the paper speed is usually 25 mm/s. Each small square on the horizontal axis is equivalent to 1 mm representing 0.04 s or 40 ms. One large square (marked with a darker line on the ECG paper) is 5 mm, representing 0.20 s or 200 ms. The vertical axis represents amplitude or voltage, thus 1 small square is 1 mm, equivalent to 0.1 mV. One large square (marked with a darker line on the paper) is 0.5 mV and 2 large squares represent 1.0 mV. Using standard ECG paper allows standardization and measurement of ECG waveforms and enables the accurate measurement of heart rate, regularity, and amplitude. Normal ranges of durations (in milliseconds) and amplitudes (in volts) of waveforms is given in Table 3.5. When there is no electrical activity present the ECG will show a flat (isoelectric) line. It is normal, for example, to see an isoelectric line between the P wave and the QRS (PR segment), between the S wave and the T wave (ST segment) and the T wave and the P wave (TP segment).

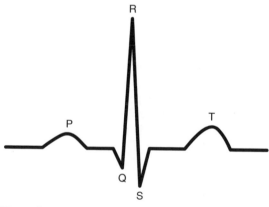

Figure 3.5 Normal ECG waveforms.

Table 3.4 ECG waveforms

Waveform	Electrical event	Mechanical event
P wave	Sino-atrial node	Atrial depolarization
P-R interval (measured from the beginning of the P wave to the beginning of the QRS complex)	Atrio-ventricular node	Ventricular filling following atrial systole
QRS complex	His-Purkinje activation	Ventricular depolarization
ST segment	Recovery	Ventricular repolarization Coronary perfusion
T wave	Recovery	Ventricular repolarization
QT interval (measured from the beginning of the Q wave to the end of the T wave)	His-Purkinje activation and recovery	Ventricular ejection

Recording the ECG—acquiring a good trace

Application of the ECG electrodes varies with different practice areas, although generally three electrodes are placed on the patient's trunk (two below the clavicles and one in the left chest area) and attached via leads to the monitor. Acquiring a good quality trace is imperative for effective rhythm identification, and attention should be paid to ensuring good skin/electrode contact to prevent artefact. It is also important to avoid placing too much emphasis on the technology—the old adage 'look at the patient, not at the monitor' is very true as patients (and their relatives/carers) will often focus on the trace on the monitor and may feel very anxious when the inevitable variations in rate and baseline occur during patient movement and breathing.

Sinus rhythm

Normal cardiac rhythm is identified when P waves, PR interval, QRS complexes, and T waves are present in a regular rhythm at a rate between 60 and 100/min (see Figure 3.6). Variations in cardiac rate and rhythm occur in normal health and rate changes in particular are precipitated in response to exercise, emotion, temperature, and exposure to stimulants such as caffeine and nicotine. Cardiac rhythm variations can occur in association with the respiratory pattern (sinus arrhythmia), although this is generally only seen in the very young and the elderly. In addition the heart rhythm may be either regular or irregular in both benign and malignant cardiac arrhythmias.

Table 3.5 Normal waveforms—duration and amplitude

Waveform/interval	Duration	Amplitude
P wave	80–120 ms	0.1–0.25 mV
PR interval	120–200 ms	N/A
QRS complex	60–100/120 ms	0.8–2.5 mV
ST interval	Varies with heart rate	N/A
T wave	Varies with heart rate	0.5 mV
QT interval	300–430 ms (variable with heart rate)	N/A

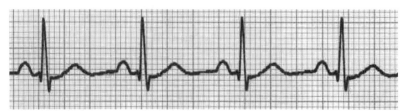

Figure 3.6 Sinus rhythm.

Rhythm interpretation

A simple approach to rhythm interpretation should be employed for all patients monitored on an acute ward. Rate, rhythm, P-QRS ratio, P-R interval, QRS complex, ST segment, and T waves all require evaluation.

♦ Rate: Bradycardia (less than 50 to 60 per minute), normal (50 or 60–100 per minute), tachycardia (more than 100 per minute). Rate may be measured by counting the number of small squares between two R waves and dividing the number into 1500 (the R-R interval method).

♦ Rhythm: Is it regular or irregular? Sinus rhythm may not be completely regular (heart rate may vary with inspiration as in sinus arrhythmia for example). On the other hand, various arrhythmias may be regular, for example ventricular tachycardia, atrial flutter, and supraventricular tachycardia (SVT) are usually regular. Atrial fibrillation usually produces an irregular rhythm.

♦ P-QRS ratio: There should always be a one-to-one relationship—one P wave to each QRS complex. Arrhythmias which produce more P waves to QRS complexes include heart block. Arrhythmias which have missing P waves to QRS complexes include atrial fibrillation, atrial flutter, junctional rhythm, and ventricular tachycardia (Khan 2004).

♦ P-R interval: A short P-R interval may be an indication of ventricular pre-excitation, such as Wolff-Parkinson-White (WPW) syndrome. A lengthened or variable P-R interval may be caused by AV node ischaemia (post acute myocardial infarction), drug-induced (β-blockers or digoxin), or age-related.

♦ QRS complex: The shape and duration of the QRS complex should be evaluated by closer inspection of the 12-lead ECG. However, a widened or bizarre-shaped QRS complex may indicate ventricular hypertrophy or bundle branch block (Goldberger 2006). A widened QRS complex in the absence of P waves with a fast rate may indicate ventricular tachycardia.

♦ ST segment: The ST segment should be flat on the isoelectric line; any deviation above or below the isoelectric line of more than 1 mm is strongly indicative of myocardial infarction or ischaemia respectively (Owens *et al.* 2006). A wandering baseline (induced by patient movement or breathing) may also cause apparent ST segment deviation.

♦ T waves: This is the most unstable aspect of the cardiac rhythm complex and abnormality in either the ST segment or the T waves usually indicates coronary artery ischaemia. The 'rule of thumb' for ECG interpretation is that it is normal for the T wave to follow the same polarity as the QRS complex. Hence if the QRS complex is positive (above the isoelectric line) then the T wave should also be positive. Conversely, when the QRS complex is negative (as is commonly seen in lead aVR) then it is normal for the T wave to be inverted. A negative T wave in the presence of a positive QRS complex may be indicative of myocardial ischaemia and requires further investigation. A hyperacute (tall) T wave may be indicative of early myocardial infarction or hyperkalaemia (potassium level greater than 5.5 mmol/L) (Goldberger 2006).

Table 3.6 Origin and classification of arrhythmias

Site of origin	Arrhythmia	QRS complex
Atrial (supraventricular)	Sinus arrhythmia Sinus bradycardia Sinus tachycardia Sinus arrest Atrial ectopics Atrial fibrillation Atrial flutter	Narrow
Junctional (AV nodal)	Junctional ectopics Junctional tachycardia Supraventricular tachycardia Atrioventricular re-entry tachycardia (WPW syndrome) AV blocks (heart blocks)	Variable
Ventricular	Ventricular ectopics Ventricular tachycardia Torsades des pointes Ventricular fibrillation	Wide

Many acutely ill patients will require cardiac monitoring and the purpose is to identify any abnormalities known as cardiac arrhythmias (in some textbooks referred to as dysrhythmias). Continuous ECG monitoring allows early identification of arrhythmias and should prompt immediate intervention. It is, however, important to analyse the arrhythmia in the context of the patient's overall clinical situation. For example a stressed, frightened patient may present with sinus tachycardia and similarly a patient who is prescribed β-blockers is likely to have a bradycardia; in the context of their clinical situation, the arrhythmia is not significant.

Arrhythmias are often classified according to the site of origin (Table 3.6). In general atrial arrhythmias produce narrow QRS complexes, as the ventricles are depolarized normally via the AV node and bundle of His. Ventricular arrhythmias produce broad, bizarre QRS complexes because the ventricles are activated via an abnormal pathway. Junctional arrhythmias may manifest as narrow or broad morphology.

Cardiac arrhythmias may cause unpleasant symptoms for patients such as palpitations, chest pains, syncope, or breathlessness. Many malignant arrhythmias may cause circulatory collapse, although occasionally patients may be asymptomatic in the presence of a serious arrhythmia. It is essential that an acute care nurse is able to recognize common cardiac arrhythmias, understand when to refer to senior/medical staff and be able to anticipate and understand appropriate treatment. A description of all cardiac arrhythmias is outside the range of this chapter, although the common arrhythmias will be presented. The reader is referred to a suitable textbook on cardiac arrhythmias.

Sinus arrhythmia

Sinus arrhythmia is a common (and normal) phenomenon in the very young and the elderly. It is characterized as an irregular sinus rhythm where the rate varies in relation to inspiration and expiration. Heart rate slows on inspiration and speeds up during expiration. The R-R interval will vary in relation to the respiratory rate. It is a normal arrhythmia and requires no intervention.

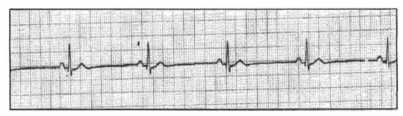

Figure 3.7 Sinus bradycardia.

On the monitor, sinus arrhythmia looks like an irregular sinus rhythm that appears to speed up and slow down during the cardiac cycle.

Sinus bradycardia

This is sinus rhythm with a rate less than 50 to 60 min. The characteristic P wave, PR interval, QRS complexes, ST segment, and T waves are present but the R-R interval is lengthened (Figure 3.7). In many patients they will be asymptomatic, although development of sudden bradycardia may result in circulatory collapse.

Causes Sinus bradycardia is a normal physiological phenomenon in athletes and is usually evident during sleep in healthy individuals. It is, however, pathologically associated with inferior myocardial infarction, hypothyroidism, raised intracranial pressure, hypothermia, and obstructive jaundice. It is induced by a number of commonly used drugs, including β-blockers, calcium channel blockers and digoxin. It may also be precipitated by iatrogenic procedures which cause vagal stimulation such as suctioning, instrumentation of the gastrointestinal tract, including suppository and enema insertion, and many gynaecological procedures. It may also be induced by deep pain and painful procedures such as femoral arterial sheath removal.

Treatment Treatment is rarely needed unless the patient is compromised by a low blood pressure. The underlying cause should be treated if possible and in cases of circulatory collapse Atropine may be administered intravenously.

Sinus tachycardia

The P wave, PR interval, QRS complexes, ST segment and T waves are normal but occur at a rate faster than 100 per minute (Figure 3.8). Thus the R-R interval is reduced and the diastolic filling time of the heart (including the coronary arteries) is reduced.

Causes Sinus tachycardia is a normal response to adrenergic stimuli, hence it is a physiological response to exercise and emotional stress. It is pathological in fever, hyperthyroidism, cardiac disease, respiratory disease, hypovolaemia, and all shock and low cardiac output states. It is also induced by a number of stimulants, including alcohol, nicotine, caffeine, amphetamines, and cocaine, and may also result from prescribed drugs such as salbutamol and aminophylline.

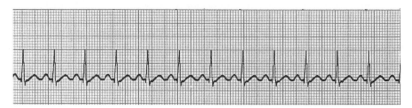

Figure 3.8 Sinus tachycardia.

Treatment This is aimed at finding the cause and managing it. Hence a hypovolaemic patient may require volume replacement. Cardiac patients are particularly susceptible to sinus tachycardia as coronary artery filling time is reduced and sinus tachycardia may induce chest pain. Occasionally sinus tachycardia requires treatment to slow the rate and drugs such as β-blockers (atenolol) or digoxin are useful.

Extrasystoles

Extrasystoles ('ectopic beats') may arise from ectopic foci in the atria, junctional region, or ventricles. A premature stimulus arises early and stimulates the surrounding tissue, resulting in abnormal conduction to the rest of the heart. The resulting waveform occurs early and is followed by a 'compensatory pause'. Atrial ectopics have an abnormal P wave, but a normal QRS, junctional ectopics have no P wave, but a normal QRS and ventricular extrasystoles may either have an absent P wave or an abnormally placed one with wide, bizarre QRS complexes and T waves facing in the opposite direction to the main QRS complex (Woodrow 2004).

Causes Atrial, junctional, and ventricular ectopic beats occur in normal hearts and may be precipitated by adrenergic stimuli such as exercise and stress (Figure 3.9). They may also be induced by stimulants such as caffeine, alcohol, cocaine, and β-adrenergic drugs. In cardiac disease they may result from myocardial ischaemia and hypoxaemia and, if frequent, may require treatment. Hypokalaemia is a common precipitant and maintaining the blood potassium above 4.0 mmol/L will often prevent ectopic formation.

Treatment Atrial and junctional arrhythmias are nearly always benign and require no intervention. Ventricular extrasystoles may be more malignant and are often associated with cardiac disease. If the ectopics are frequent or occur every other beat then intervention may be needed. Ventricular bigeminy is defined as a ventricular extrasystole occurring every other sinus beat and is occasionally the result of digoxin toxicity. Frequent ectopics may result from hypokalaemia (potassium less than 3.5 mmol/L), which is easily treated. There is little evidence that anti-arrhythmic therapy is useful and indeed Class 1 anti-arrhythmic drugs such as flecainide may increase the mortality of patients with ventricular ectopics following myocardial infarction (Opie & Gersch 2004; Julian *et al.* 2005).

Supraventricular tachycardia

Strictly speaking the term 'supraventricular tachycardia' (SVT) refers to all tachycardias that originate above the level of the AV junction. In practice, however, atrial fibrillation and atrial flutter are excluded from this description.

SVT presents as a rapid, regular rhythm, with a rate between 140 and 250 beats per minute (Figure 3.10). P waves are generally absent, the QRS is narrow and the T wave may be inverted or normal. It is often paroxysmal in its presentation and the patient will generally be aware of the

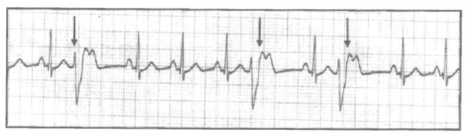

Figure 3.9 Ventricular ectopics (extrasystoles).

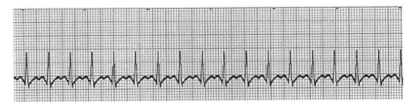

Figure 3.10 Supraventricular tachycardia.

rapid heart beat, complaining of palpitations, breathlessness and dizziness. SVT may reduce the cardiac output and the patient may be pale, clammy and hypotensive. SVT will often start suddenly and terminate equally abruptly.

Causes SVT may occur in normal, healthy individuals and may be precipitated by alcohol, stimulants, and hormonal disturbances. SVT may also occur in serious cardiac disease, in particular in relation to WPW syndrome, when the arrhythmia is known as atrioventricular re-entry tachycardia and requires specialist treatment (for further information see Goldberger (2006).

Treatment Termination of the arrhythmia may be achieved in a number of ways, but all require medical support. In a normal, healthy person the use of carotid sinus massage or the Valsalva manoeuvre may reverse the arrhythmia. Alternatively adenosine given as a fast intravenous bolus is also very effective. Occasionally, more persistent SVT requires an amiodarone infusion or electrical cardioversion. Clinically you should be aware that adenosine can cause nasty symptoms for patients, including severe chest pain, flushing, and anxiety; patients should be warned prior to its administration.

Atrial fibrillation

Atrial fibrillation is the most commonly encountered arrhythmia in acute care (Banner 2008). In an acute setting, where the onset is sudden, it is generally a fast arrhythmia with a variable rate from 90 to 160 beats per minute (Figure 3.11). It is characterized by erratic, chaotic re-entry circuits within the atria. This causes the atria to beat in an irregular and uncoordinated manner, resulting in ineffective atrial contraction and the fast transmission of impulses through the AV node to the ventricles. Reduced atrial contraction (atrial 'kick') reduces preload to the ventricles and subsequently reduces cardiac output by up to 25%. The resulting effect on the patient is to cause palpitations, breathlessness and potentially circulatory collapse, especially if the onset is sudden. In patients with pre-existing coronary artery disease, chest pain may develop and in patients with poor ventricular function, it may precipitate acute left ventricular failure. Patients will be distressed and frightened by this arrhythmia especially as they will be aware of the fast irregular heartbeat. If the arrhythmia persists there is the potential for thrombus formation due to atrial stasis and this puts the patient at risk of thromboembolic events such as embolic stroke or pulmonary embolism.

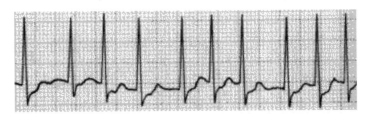

Figure 3.11 Atrial fibrillation.

Causes Atrial fibrillation may be described as paroxysmal (intermittent and self-terminating usually lasting less than 48 h), persistent (termination only achieved by electrical or pharmacological cardioversion), or permanent (unresponsive to the above therapies).

In most patients, atrial fibrillation is an indication of underlying heart disease (e.g. cardiomyopathy, ischaemic, valvular, or hypertensive heart disease), although it is also the result of advancing age. However, paroxysmal atrial fibrillation may occur in structurally normal hearts and this entity is termed 'lone atrial fibrillation'. Adrenergic atrial fibrillation may be precipitated by alcohol, stress, and exercise, and is most common in those over 50 years old without structural heart disease (Fuster *et al.* 2006).

Treatment The management of atrial fibrillation is complex and dependent on the cause, nature, and duration of the arrhythmia. Sudden onset atrial fibrillation requires urgent referral to the medical team. Numerous guidelines have been produced in recent years to assist clinicians, including the Department of Health (2005), NICE (2006) and Fuster *et al.* (2006) (Table 3.7). The urgency of treatment depends on the patient's symptoms and any underlying pre-existing heart disease that may exacerbate the physiological response. The aims of treatment include management of the patient's symptoms, ventricular rate control, restoration of sinus rhythm, and prevention of thromboembolic events.

Atrioventricular (heart) block

In atrioventricular (AV) block there is a delay or absence of conduction between the atria and the ventricles. AV block is divided into first, second, and third degree block. The main significance of first and second degree AV block lies in the potential for the patient to develop complete AV block or asystole (Julian *et al.* 2005).

Table 3.7 Treatment of atrial fibrillation

Aims of treatment	Treatment strategy
Management of patient's symptoms	Reassure patient and accompanying family to minimize distress Institute 15-min monitoring of heart rate, rhythm, blood pressure, respiratory rate, oxygen saturation If breathless sit upright and administer prescribed oxygen If hypotensive, semi-prone position to maintain blood pressure and conscious level
Ventricular rate control	This is used prior to cardioversion whilst awaiting anticoagulation therapy to achieve therapeutic levels Drugs used include β-blockers (atenolol), calcium channel blockers (diltiazem), cardiac glycosides (digoxin)
Restoration of sinus rhythm	Restoration of sinus rhythm may be achieved by electrical or pharmacological cardioversion Electrical cardioversion under short-term general anaesthetic is used if the arrhythmia is less than 48 h in duration. 200 J monophasic or 120 J biphasic waveforms delivered via the chest wall Antiarrhythmic therapy is used following the procedure to maintain sinus rhythm Pharmacological cardioversion is also used in the first 48 h; various antiarrythmic agents may be administered intravenously. including amiodarone, flecainide and sotalol
Prevention of thromboembolic events	The risk of thromboembolism increases after the arrhythmia has been present for 48 h Transoesophageal echocardiogram can be used to identify intracardiac thrombus in patients at risk Intravenous heparin is used acutely followed by adjustable dose anticoagulation

Based on data from Fuster *et al.* (2006) and NICE (2006).

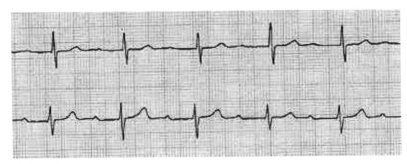

Figure 3.12 First degree AV block.

In *first degree AV block* all sinus impulses reach the ventricles, but there is a delay at the AV node resulting in a prolonged P-R interval, which will measure more than 0.2 s or 200 ms. The QRS duration and shape is normal.

First degree AV block is a normal variant in the elderly and also occurs in athletes (Figure 3.12). It may also be induced by drugs that slow conduction through the AV node such as β-blockers and digoxin. It requires no treatment unless it occurs in association with acute myocardial infarction, when it may be a precursor to second and third degree AV block. In this case, careful monitoring should be instituted.

Second degree AV block occurs when some impulses reach the ventricles and others do not. There are two types of second degree block: Mobitz type 1 (Wenckebach) and Mobitz type 2.

Wenckebach block (Mobitz type 1) is usually relatively benign and rarely progresses to third degree block (Figure 3.13). It is characterized by progressive prolongation of the P-R interval followed by a failure of conduction to the ventricles (resulting in a 'dropped beat'). The whole process is then repeated and generally follows a pattern (i.e. fourth or fifth beat dropped). The P-R interval becomes progressively lengthened, whilst the QRS complex remains normal. Treatment is not normally required, although careful monitoring should be maintained to ensure that the block does not progress further.

Mobitz type 2 block is more likely to progress to third degree heart block. There is a varying ratio of conduction to the ventricles (i.e. two P waves to one QRS, three P waves to one QRS, etc.). The P-R interval remains constant and the QRS is normal (Figure 3.14). Mobitz type 2 block indicates disease in the conduction system and is often associated with inferior myocardial infarction. If the block is 2:1 then the patient's rate may be very slow and their blood pressure significantly compromised. Temporary transvenous pacing may be needed.

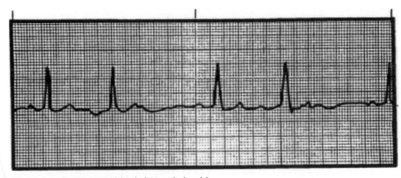

.13 Mobitz Type 1 AV block (Wenckebach).

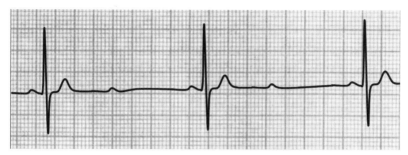

Figure 3.14 Mobitz Type 2 AV block.

Third degree (complete) AV block occurs suddenly following acute myocardial infarction, an episode of myocarditis or cardiac surgery, or alternatively may present in a chronic form in elderly patients when the underlying pathology is progressive fibrosis of the conduction system. There is complete failure of conduction from the atria to the ventricles at the AV node. An escape pacemaker generates a ventricular rhythm and the QRS is generally wide and bizarre and at a rate between 20 and 50, dependent on where the escape pacemaker originates from (AV junction, His-Purkinje system) (see Figure 3.15).

Treatment depends on the patient's haemodynamic compromise. In acute anterior myocardial infarction the presence of third degree AV block indicates extensive infarction and urgent temporary pacing is required. Temporary pacing may be instituted either externally (transthoracic) or via the transvenous route.

Ventricular tachycardia

All ventricular arrhythmias are serious and potentially life-threatening and require urgent intervention. Further guidance on the management of patients with ventricular arrhythmias is given by the ACC/AHA/ESC guidelines (ACC/AHA/ESC 2006). Ventricular tachycardia generally occurs in patients with serious underlying heart disease. An ectopic focus in the ventricles stimulates a fast and regular rhythm that overrides the normal conduction system and results in a fast regular rate. There are no discernible P waves; the QRS complexes are wide and bizarre, the rate is between 120 and 250 beats per minute.

Causes This commonly arises following myocardial infarction but may also result from digoxin toxicity.

Treatment Treatment should be initiated urgently as the arrhythmia will result in severe haemodynamic compromise. Medical emergency teams should be alerted and emergency equipment made available at the bedside. Ventricular tachycardia is a cardiac arrest rhythm and should be treated according to current resuscitation protocols (see Chapter 13). Emergency treatment may include electrical cardioversion or anti-tachycardia therapy such as amiodarone infusion. Underlying hypokalaemia, ischaemia, or acidosis should also be treated.

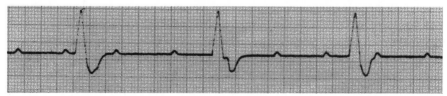

Figure 3.15 Third degree AV block.

Ventricular fibrillation

This is a cardiac arrest scenario and should be treated according to current resuscitation protocols (Chapter 13). It is easily identifiable on the monitor as rapid, chaotic irregular waveforms with no discernible P waves or QRS complexes. There are no effective cardiac contractions and consequently no cardiac output; the patient will require immediate cardiopulmonary resusitation (CPR).

Causes Ventricular fibrillation occurs following myocardial infarction, hypoxia, metabolic disturbances, drug overdose, electrocution, and drowning.

Treatment Immediate defibrillation is the only treatment and should be administered as early as possible in the cardiac arrest scenario (see Chapter 13).

Asystole

Sometimes referred to as ventricular standstill; this is another cardiac arrest scenario. There is effectively no electrical activity evident on the monitor and a 'flat line' will be evident. This may also occur when electrodes are detached from leads and thus is worth checking before calling arrest teams. The patient will collapse suddenly and have no cardiac or respiratory activity. Immediate CPR should be commenced and emergency equipment organized at the bedside.

Causes Causes are the same as for ventricular fibrillation, although the prognosis is much worse and patients rarely survive an asystolic arrest.

Treatment Treatment is as per current resuscitation protocols (see Chapter 13).

Pulseless electrical activity

Pulseless electrical activity (PEA) was previously defined as 'electromechanical dissociation'. It occurs when there is electrical activity that does not result in mechanical contraction of the heart. P waves, QRS complexes and T waves are evident on the monitor, although the rhythm will look slightly abnormal and may be slow. There will be no discernible pulses and the patient will be collapsed. It should be treated as a cardiac arrest scenario and early CPR should be initiated (see Chapter 13).

Causes Causes are classified under the easy to remember '4Hs and 4Ts' identified by the UK Resuscitation Council guidelines (2005):

- hypoxia
- hypovolaemia
- hyper/hypokalaemia (and other metabolic disorders)
- hypothermia
- tension pneumothorax
- tamponade
- toxic/therapeutic disturbances
- thromboembolism.

Treatment Treatment is directed at finding the cause, although PEA is difficult to manage and rarely successfully treated.

The clinical consequences of cardiac arrhythmias

Most cardiac arrhythmias are easily recognizable if a systematic approach is undertaken. The clinical consequences of cardiac arrhythmias are variable but are generally more pronounced in

Clinical link 3.1 (see Appendix for answers)

Mrs Jones, a 65-year-old lady, was admitted to the medical admissions unit for investigation of palpitations and breathlessness. In A&E her admission 12-lead ECG was 'unremarkable'. She is complaining of palpitations and says she feels dizzy. Her monitor shows the following:

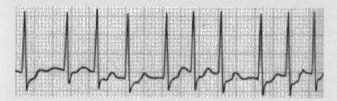

Examine the arrhythmia identified above and consider:

♦ systematic analysis of the arrhythmia, including diagnosis

♦ nursing actions for the next 10 min

♦ possible medical intervention.

patients with pre-existing heart disease. The majority of cardiac arrhythmias will affect cardiac output and subsequently will affect the patient's haemodynamic state. Tachycardias are particularly serious as they lead to a reduction in ventricular filling time, with a concomitant drop in cardiac output. Tachycardias also reduce diastolic coronary artery filling time and lead to reduced myocardial perfusion. Cardiac arrhythmias thus cause many deleterious symptoms for patients, including chest pain, breathlessness, palpitations and syncope.

Common cardiovascular problems

There are many potential causes of chest pain from benign problems such as indigestion or musculoskeletal pain to serious causes such as pneumothorax and oesophageal rupture. The many causes of chest pain were discussed earlier in this chapter but highlight the difficulty of diagnosis when a patient's presentation can be so different. A key priority for patients with chest pain is to rule in or rule out acute coronary syndrome (ACS) in order to prioritize timely care. ACS is an umbrella term first introduced in 2000 to encompass a range of ischaemic heart disease presentations (Fox 2004)

Acute coronary syndromes

ACS describes a spectrum of cardiac conditions ranging from ST-segment elevation myocardial infarction (STEMI) and non-ST-segment elevation myocardial infarction (n-STEMI) to unstable angina. These definitions replace previously used terminology: full thickness or Q wave MI, partial thickness or non-Q wave MI and unstable angina (Fox 2004).

Coronary heart disease (CHD) remains the single most common cause of death in the UK with 1 in 5 men and 1 in 6 women dying from the disease. CHD causes around 110,000 deaths in the UK each year (British Heart Foundation 2007). This chapter will focus upon the assessment and management of STEMI in the first 12 h, other acute coronary syndromes will also be briefly discussed.

A third of patients with STEMI die within the first 24 h of symptom onset and the highest mortality is seen in patients who have sustained an anterior wall myocardial infarction or left bundle branch block (Antman et al. 2004).

Table 3.8 Pathological process in different acute coronary syndromes

Type of acute coronary syndrome	Pathological processes	Myocardial damage/cardiac marker raised
Unstable angina	Occlusion of coronary artery with platelet rich thrombus	Nil necrosisTroponin T/I nil
N-STEMI	Occlusion of coronary artery with platelet-rich thrombus and vasoconstriction	Necrosis to subendocardial layer of myocardium/partial thickness. Positive troponin T/I levels.
STEMI	Occlusion of coronary artery with fibrin-rich thrombus and vasconstriction	Necrosis to epicardial to subendocardial layer of myocardium.Positive troponin T/I levels.

The consequences of ACS are not benign either; death rates are high in the 6 months following diagnosis. The GRACE registry (Global Registry of Acute Coronary Events 2008) identifies the following mortality statistics for acute coronary events:

♦ 12% of patients with STEMI will die within the first 6 months

♦ 13% of patients with n-STEMI die in the first 6 months

♦ 8% of patients with unstable angina die in the first 6 months.

It is therefore evident that prompt response and early diagnosis forms the cornerstone of the management of patients with suspected ACS. The sudden onset of chest pain is a critical situation and requires time-dependent interventions and the need for emergency medical specialist care from the outset.

Pathophysiology

ACS is the clinical manifestation of rupture or erosion of the atheromatous plaque (described earlier in this chapter), followed by coronary artery occlusion with intraluminal thrombus and/or distal embolization. The severity of the presentation is determined by the volume of the myocardium affected and the subsequent myocardial necrosis (Fox 2004). Whilst the underlying cause of ACS is similar (coronary arterial disease) the occlusive nature of the thrombus and the damage to the myocardium varies with the three types of ACS (Fox 2004) (see Table 3.8).

Acute ST-segment elevation myocardial infarction

Clinical presentation

STEMI may present with the following clinical features:

♦ chest pain—retrosternal, radiation to left (or less commonly right) arm, jaw, throat, back

♦ anxiety—some patients have a sense of 'impending doom'

♦ increased parasympathetic (vagal) activation – nausea/vomiting

♦ increased sympathetic activation—sweating, pallor, tachycardia and slightly raised blood pressure.

It is important to note that not all patients will present with the above symptoms; indeed fewer than 50% of patients may present with classic features of myocardial infarction and it is wise to be cautious with patients who fall into the following groups:

erly patients

betic patients

nale patients.

Patients in the above groups may have less or no pain (particularly diabetic patients), less autonomic disturbance, and less or more nausea or vomiting. Pain may vary in individuals who present at a younger age, and breathlessness may be the primary symptom rather than chest pain (Pope *et al.* 2000). There are significant gender differences; women tend to present with more subtle and less specific symptoms than men (Albarran 2007).

High-risk patients may present with tachyarrhythmias, hypotension, or breathlessness, and these symptoms indicate a larger area of myocardial necrosis, which may form a penumbra for serious ventricular arrhythmias or acute left ventricular failure.

All patients with suspected ACS should be managed as an emergency and early medical intervention is required. Most hospitals should have fast-tracking procedures to ensure timely intervention within an acute care or critical care environment.

Clinical diagnosis

The diagnosis of STEMI is made on the basis of a combination of:

♦ clinical presentation and patient history

♦ 12-lead ECG

♦ cardiac markers.

The gold standard for diagnosis of STEMI in the acute situation is the 12-lead ECG.

12-lead ECG The diagnosis of STEMI is indicated by the following criteria (Thygesen *et al.* 2007):

♦ ST-segment elevation >1 mm in two or more adjacent limb leads or V4–V6

♦ ST-segment elevation >2 mm in leads V2 and V3 (men) or

♦ ST-segment elevation >1.5 mm in leads V2 and V3 (women)

♦ new or presumed new left bundle branch block (LBBB).

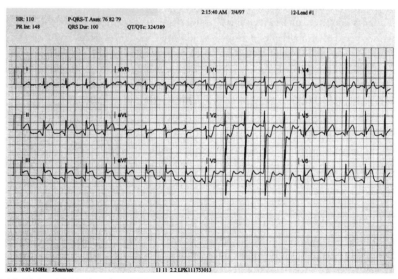

Figure 3.16 12-lead ECG showing STEMI.

An example of an ST segment elevation myocardial infarction (STEMI) is shown in Figure 3.16. Note the ST segment elevation in leads II, III, aVF (inferior wall) and the reciprocal ST segment depression in leads aVL, V1-V3.

Cardiac markers (biochemistry) The damaged myocardium will release enzymes or proteins into the bloodstream that can be measured within minutes/hours of presentation with chest pain. The two commonly used markers of cardiac injury are troponin T or I, a cardiac-specific protein found on the contractile mechanism of the cardiac myocyte, and CK-MB, a myocardial specific enzyme. Both are released into the blood within 4 h of cardiac damage and reach their optimum level within 12 h. Thus, although these markers are diagnostic of the cardiac event, their use in the acute setting is limited to confirming the diagnosis 12–24 h after the patient presented to an acute care facility (Collinson 2006).

Management

The main aims of treatment for the patient with a suspected STEMI are to:

♦ relieve pain

♦ relieve anxiety

♦ restore patency in the infarct-related artery.

A consensus document from the Resuscitation Council in 2000 suggested the use of *MONA* (*m*orphine, *o*xygen, *n*itrates and *a*spirin) as an aide-memoir for the acute management of suspected myocardial infarction. Pain relief is at the centre of this emergency management, and patients may require more than one analgesic agent in order to achieve pain relief.

Pain relief Early relief of pain is absolutely essential and many patients will find the pain both severe and frightening. The severity of the pain may result in a sympathetic response, which may further exacerbate the ischaemia and the potential for cardiac arrhythmias. Early intervention is therefore essential and morphine or diamorphine should be administered intravenously with an anti-emetic. Intravenous nitrates and oxygen may also improve perfusion to the myocardium. Supplemental oxygen is generally given even if the oxygen saturation levels are normal. Opiates should be used with care with patients with chronic obstructive pulmonary disease as respiratory depression may occur.

Nitrates have an established role in the management of persistent chest pain after STEMI and their advantage is that they can be given quickly and easily via the sublingual or intravenous route. Nitrates reduce preload and after-load as well as dilating coronary arteries and thus their effect is to reduce the myocardial oxygen demand and enhance myocardial perfusion. Care should be taken with intravenous administration as they do reduce systemic blood pressure and should be carefully titrated against the patient's blood pressure.

Unless contraindicated by hypotension or bradycardia, intravenous β-blockers are also given in the early phase of treatment. β-blockers reduce myocardial oxygen demand, relieve pain, and may prevent myocardial rupture.

Heart rate and blood pressure should be monitored regularly and continuous cardiac monitoring instituted. Many acute care areas have facilities for monitoring the 12-lead ECG continuously or for continuous vector-derived ST-segment monitoring (Greenfield 2008). Alternatively, monitoring from a single lead is perfectly acceptable and generally lead 11 is the chosen ECG lead for this purpose.

Anxiety management Anxiety is often linked to the pain and to the patient's perception of the severity of the situation. Some patients do describe a sense of 'impending doom' and require constant reassurance from the healthcare professionals. The morphine or diamorphine will not only relieve the pain, but also relieve the anxiety stimulated by catecholamine release.

Constant reassurance and explanation for patients is essential and skilled nurses with enhanced communication skills are the cornerstones of good nursing care.

Most patients who have sustained a STEMI should be managed in a designated coronary care unit where staff have advanced skills of communication and highly honed technological skills to monitor the patient safely.

Restore patency in the occluded artery The underlying pathophysiology in a STEMI is the occlusion of a major coronary artery with a fibrin-rich thrombus. This intracoronary thrombus may lead to a large area of infarction and potential necrosis, and this mandates early and rapid coronary artery reperfusion.

The fundamental treatment approach for STEMI therefore is to restore the blood flow to the occluded artery. All patients who are suspected of having sustained an acute coronary event should be given low dose aspirin as soon as possible. An acute coronary event is associated with enhanced platelet activity and increased production of thromboxane A2, a powerful vasoconstrictor. Aspirin is a powerful platelet antagonist (thromboxane A2 inhibitor) and also prevents platelet aggregation in the acute phase. Aspirin has a proven role in the early intervention strategy in all acute coronary events and should be given to all patients unless contraindicated (Anti-platelet Trialists' Collaboration 1994).

Two approaches to coronary artery reperfusion are currently adopted in the UK: thrombolysis and primary percutaneous coronary intervention (P-PCI). Both are recommended by the European Society of Cardiology (Van de Werf *et al.* 2003) and the American College of Cardiology/ American Heart Association (Antman *et al.* 2004).

Thrombolysis

The work which underpins the use of thrombolytic therapy for acute STEMI encompasses more than three decades of research, although the introduction of the National Service Framework for Coronary Heart Disease was a catalyst for the provision of evidence-base care (Castle 2006). Meta-analyses of the thrombolysis trials performed in the 1990s indicate that thrombolysis decreases overall mortality by 18–25% (Fibrinolytic Therapy Trialists Group 1994). The benefits are even more striking when the drugs are administered early and Boersma *et al.* (1996) described this as the 'golden hour' and demonstrated a 48% reduction in mortality in patients who were treated within an hour of symptom onset. This underpins the current NSF target for thrombolytic agents to be administered within 20 min of diagnosis in the hospital—the so called 'door-to-needle time' (Department of Health 2000). The mantra 'time is myocardium' is frequently quoted. The benefits of thrombolytic therapy decrease over time and it is not recommended beyond 12 h of symptom onset.

Whilst P-PCI is the gold standard for the management of an acute STEMI, the current management approach in the UK continues to include the use of intravenous thrombolysis. Thrombolytic agents (also known as fibrinolytic agents) catalyse the conversion of plasminogen to plasmin, thus lysing the fibrin thrombus. There are three types of thrombolytic agents available in the UK:

- streptokinase—first generation
- tissue plasminogen activator (t-PA) (alteplase)—second generation
- tenecteplase (TNK) and reteplase (r-PA)—third generation.

The second and third generation drugs are more fibrin-specific and more expensive. Streptokinase does have an increased risk of bleeding complications but remains the first-line treatment for a patient who has sustained a first acute STEMI (NICE 2002). Streptokinase does

Box 3.1 Contraindications to thrombolysis

Contraindications to thrombolysis are:

♦ previous cerebral haemorrhage

♦ surgery within the last 4–6 weeks

♦ recent trauma

♦ prolonged resuscitation

♦ recent gastrointestinal bleed

♦ neoplasm, particularly intracranial neoplasm

♦ major arterial puncture or biopsy within the last 2–4 weeks (this includes dental extraction)

♦ aortic dissection or aortic aneurysm

♦ pregnancy

♦ systemic hypertension SBP >180 mmHg DBP >110 mmHg.

also have the potential to evoke an antigen-antibody reaction in susceptible patients and its use is becoming superseded by the newer synthetic agents of TNK and r-PA. There are a number of absolute and relative contraindications to thrombolysis and you should consult your local trust protocol as these do vary (Box 3.1).

Nursing management of a patient receiving thrombolysis

Streptokinase is administered by a continuous intravenous infusion, whereas reteplase and tenecteplase are given by intravenous bolus injections. Nursing care is directed to maintaining the patient's safety throughout administration of the drug and to careful monitoring for potential complications associated with the therapy. These complications include:

♦ bleeding complications

♦ reperfusion arrhythmias

♦ anaphylactic reaction (streptokinase only).

Evaluating the efficacy of thrombolysis

It is essential that the efficacy of the treatment is assessed to ensure that coronary artery perfusion has been achieved. Various criteria are used to assess the efficacy of thrombolysis, including resolution of chest pain, evidence of reperfusion arrhythmias, and ECG criteria However the ECG criteria are the most robust and a 12-lead ECG should be performed to ensure that the ST-segment elevation is returning to the baseline. Individual NHS trusts will have guidelines of how much ST-segment elevation resolution is required; most require at least 50% resolution of ST-segment 90 min after treatment (Spiers 2003). There is evidence that when thrombolysis is not successful at 90 min, rescue PCI is beneficial (Silber *et al.* 2005).

Primary percutaneous coronary intervention

The alternative treatment for acute STEMI is primary percutaneous coronary intervention (P-PCI), and the evidence suggests that this treatment strategy is more effective than thrombolysis (Keeley *et al.* 2003). Percutaneous coronary intervention is a technique used to reopen a narrowed coronary artery to restore blood flow to the heart muscle. When the procedure is used for first-line treatment for patients suffering from STEMI it is referred to as primary PCI (P-PCI). P-PCI is also time-dependent and the target 'door-to-balloon time' is 60 min, although it is suggested that a P-PCI needs to be performed within 120–150 min of the patient's symptom onset (Department of Health 2008). The procedure involves the insertion of a balloon tipped catheter into the occluded coronary artery and the deployment of a stent to maintain the integrity of the coronary artery.

The National Infarct Angioplasty Project (Department of Health 2008) is investigating the feasibility of introducing P-PCI across the country. Whilst P-PCI is clinically the better treatment, issues other than clinical outcomes can affect the feasibility of this project, including:

- availability of cardiac catheterization facilities
- availability of a skilled team of nurses, radiographers, cardiac technicians, 24 h per day, 7 days per week
- evidence that cardiologists are skilled in interventional therapies
- availability of on-site (or nearby) cardiac surgical centre in case emergency cardiac surgery is required.

P-PCI is particularly useful for patients in whom severe heart failure, haemodynamic instability, or continuing ischaemic pain is evident (Antman *et al.* 2004).

Other acute coronary syndromes

Non-ST elevation ACS and unstable angina

Patients with non-ST elevation ACS may present in a similar way to patients with STEMI, with similar history and clinical presentation. The chest pain may be severe and the autonomic response similar to that seen in patients with STEMI. The biochemical analysis (troponin T/I) test may reveal only a minimal rise in n-STEMI and a normal recording in unstable angina.

The ECG changes reveal a number of subtle changes (Owens *et al.* 2006), which are far less easy to identify than the 'barn door' ST-segment changes seen in STEMI. Possible ECG changes seen in non-STEMI include:

- horizontal ST segment depression
- ST-segment deviation of less than 0.5 mm
- T wave inversion
- a normal ECG
- biphasic T waves in the anterior leads, V1-V3, indicating a critical proximal lesion in the left anterior descending coronary artery (Conover 2007).

Current guidelines recommend that n-STEMI patients are treated with the following groups of drugs:

- antiplatelet therapy
- antithrombin therapy
- nitrates
- β-blockers.

Intracoronary thrombus consists of fibrin and platelets and inhibition and dissolution forms the mainstay of this treatment approach.

Anti-platelet therapy

Aspirin, clopidogrel, and glycoprotein IIb/IIIa (GP IIb/IIIa) receptor blockers (tirofiban and abciximab) all affect platelet reactivity and aggregation. Patients who are allergic or who may suffer

Clinical link 3.2 (see Appendix for answers)

A 55-year-old patient has been admitted to hospital with chest pain and breathlessness. He presented to A&E with a 3-h history of chest pain, increasing in severity and described as 'heavy and numbing'. In A&E, 12-lead ECG was inconclusive and a peripheral line was inserted. Blood tests were taken and he is transferred to the medical assessment unit for further investigations and review.

Your initial assessment reveals a blood pressure of 90/50 mmHg, heart rate 120 beats/min irregular, respirations 22 breaths/min, temperature 36.8°C and O_2 saturations 95%. He is awake and orientated to person, time and place but he is still complaining of a dull ache in his chest and left arm, and he appears visibly scared and anxious.

His hands and feet are cool and pale and his capillary refill is 3 s. Results from investigations undertaken in A&E reveal blood results as follows:

glucose: 8 mmol/L

Na^+: 135 mmol/L

K^+: 3.2 mmol/L

♦ What would your priorities be for this patient? Justify your actions.

♦ What interventions from the doctors would you anticipate?

♦ What type of assessment and monitoring will you continually undertake?

♦ What are the potential differential diagnoses for this presentation? Give rationales for your answers.

---

aspirin-induced bronchospasm may be prescribed clopidogrel. Currently GPIIb/IIIa receptor blockers are reserved for high-risk patients undergoing early coronary angiography and intervention.

Antithrombin therapy

In addition to the activation of platelets there will also be production of thrombin from the unstable atherosclerotic plaque. Both intravenous unfractionated heparin and subcutaneous low molecular weight heparin (LMWH) are given for their anti-thrombin effects in combination with aspirin to further reduce the patient's risk. In high-risk patients anti-thrombin therapy should be continued until angiography can be undertaken (Van de Werf *et al.* 2002).

The addition of nitrates and β-blockers for patients considered to be high risk is also recommended.

Complications of acute coronary syndrome

Acute coronary syndromes are not benign and the potential for short-term complications is high, especially in patients in whom the area of myocardial ischaemia or infarction is extensive. High-risk patients include those where the ischaemia or infarction affects the anterior left ventricle or who develop LBBB. Cardiogenic shock or acute left or right ventricular failure may develop and require urgent assessment and management.

Heart failure

Heart failure can be defined as the inability of the heart to maintain sufficient output to meet the metabolic demands of the peripheral tissues. It is not a disease, but a clinical syndrome that includes a classic constellation of problems for the patient: breathlessness, tachycardia, hypotension, anxiety, and fatigue. The heart may fail in a number of ways: on the left side (left ventricular failure), on the right side (cor pulmonale or right heart failure), or both (biventricular failure). It may also fail acutely or chronically (Nicholson 2007). This chapter will initially focus on the presentation and management of acute left ventricular failure, which is a common acute emergency that occurs as a consequence of acute STEMI or other causes.

Left heart failure

Pathophysiology of left heart failure Acute left heart failure occurs as a response to factors that increase the workload of the heart or result in damage to myocardial tissue, reducing its ability to maintain stroke volume. Increased workload for the heart may be characterized as increases in volume load (preload) or pressure load (afterload).

Disorders that impose a greater volume load (preload) on the left heart include hyperdynamic states such as anaemia, hyperthyroidism, and aortic regurgitation. Increases in pressure load (afterload) are due to conditions that increase systemic vascular resistance to the heart, such as hypertension, which increases the resistance in the systemic arterioles, or aortic stenosis, which obstructs outflow from the left ventricle.

Acute left ventricular failure may also result from a tachycardia or a bradycardia, but it is, however, primarily caused by extensive damage to the left ventricular wall following acute myocardial infarction. This results in a number of compensatory measures designed to maintain cardiac output but which eventually embarrass the circulation.

Compensatory measures The body exhibits the following compensatory measures:

- The heart strives to maintain cardiac output and the heart rate increases.
- The heart dilates in response to the pressure and volume load. This increases the degree of myocardial fibre stretch to maintain stroke volume (Starling's law). However, following a myocardial infarction this expansion of the heart is known as *remodelling* and may result in ventricular hypertrophy, aneurysm, and tachycardia.
- Activation of the sympathetic nervous system increases the heart rate and contractility, but also increases systemic vascular resistance. Whilst this might appear to be helpful in maintaining blood pressure, the resistance to left ventricular output exacerbates the failing left ventricle and obstructs left ventricular emptying. Obstruction to left ventricular outflow results in back-flow to the lungs, causing pulmonary oedema and congestion.

Thus a vicious spiral of events results in the symptoms observed in the patient and constitutes a clinical emergency. Transudation of fluid into the pulmonary alveoli causes oedema of the pulmonary membranes and airway narrowing. This reduction in lung compliance makes breathing difficult and reduces gaseous exchange in the alveoli. This leads to breathlessness, arterial hyoxaemia, increased mucus production, and cough.

Clinical presentation Clinically the patient presents with the following signs and symptoms:

- acute breathlessness
- extreme anxiety
- tachycardia
- hypotension
- cough, wheeze
- pink, frothy sputum (pulmonary oedema).

The priorities of management include reassuring the patient, reducing volume and pressure overload, and enhancing fluid excretion.

Nursing measures to manage left heart failure The patient should be sat upright and given high concentration oxygen. Sitting the patient upright reduces venous return to the heart, thus reducing the formation of pulmonary oedema. High flow oxygen is important as it will improve arterial oxygen tension and reduce myocardial oxygen debt, thus improving myocardial function.

Diamorphine or morphine should be administered intravenously with an anti-emetic such as metoclopramide. *Opiates* have a number of useful effects in patients with acute heart failure. Diamorphine is an excellent anxiolytic and this helps to reduce the incipient tachycardia, which, if untreated, will exacerbate the myocardial ischaemia. It is also a powerful venous dilator and thus helps to reduce preload and thus workload for the heart. Morphine also dilates pulmonary vasculature and this helps to reduce pulmonary oedema formation (Opie & Gersch 2004). Intravenous metoclopramide prevents vomiting due to opiate usage.

A loop *diuretic* should be administered intravenously; typically 40 mg IV furosemide is given. This is a powerful diuretic and venodilator and will help the failing heart by reducing circulating blood volume and reducing preload. It will have an immediate effect on the patient's breathlessness by reducing pulmonary pressures (Julian *et al.* 2007). It is also a powerful diuretic and will cause water and sodium excretion reducing fluid retention.

Sublingual or intravenous *nitrates* have a dual effect in reducing preload (venous dilation) and afterload (arterial dilation), and should be administered if the patient's blood pressure can tolerate it. Careful titration to blood pressure should be maintained for continuous infusion.

Continuous positive airway pressure (CPAP) has been demonstrated as an invaluable treatment in the hypoxaemia associated with acute heart failure. CPAP is a mode of respiratory support that provides positive airway pressure during inspiration and expiration via a continuous flow of oxygen using a circuit. CPAP has beneficial effects on both the respiratory and cardiac function of a patient with heart failure. During continuous positive airway pressure, the pressure splints open the alveoli, preventing the small airways from collapsing under the high pressure of pulmonary vascular congestion. It also prevents further fluid from moving into the alveoli, improving hypoxaemia. Lastly, the increased intrathoracic positive pressure improves cardiac output by reducing left ventricular afterload (Nehyba 2007). CPAP offers a method of non-invasively supporting a patient's respiratory and cardiac function but is most commonly used in level 2 and level 3 care. See Chapter 2 for a discussion of the benefits and limitations of non-invasive ventilation techniques, including CPAP.

Patients with acute LVF may find it difficult to tolerate CPAP due to their extreme anxiety, copious pulmonary secretions, and dyspnoea. Patients need extensive reassurance and support particularly at the outset of the treatment and nurses should remain with the patient, particularly at the outset of the treatment. CPAP may be delivered via face mask, nasal mask, or helmet. Each method has its advantages but many patients find CPAP difficult to tolerate, as it limits their ability to speak, eat or drink and some patients find the face mask particularly claustrophobic. CPAP should be used with caution in patients who are hypotensive or who have cardiac arrhythmias. A patient who is to receive CPAP may benefit from transfer to the coronary care or high-dependency unit (Nehyba 2006).

Right heart failure

Pathophysiology of right heart failure Acute right heart failure is often related to a precipitating event, the most common reason being acute infarction of the right ventricle. Right ventricular myocardial infarction (RVMI) is a significant clinical entity. Its incidence is not common but early recognition is vital as there are a well-defined set of priorities for its management (Haji & Movahed 2000). The basic function of the right ventricle is to receive blood from the venous circulation and to pump it into the pulmonary circulation, where gaseous exchange occurs and onwards transmission to the left ventricle can be achieved. RVMI is most likely to occur in the presence of an inferior or posterior wall infarction; studies suggest that RVMI accompanies inferior wall myocardial infarction in approximately 25% of cases (Moye *et al.* 2005).

When RVMI occurs, the right ventricle becomes stiff and non-compliant. The right ventricle is unable to fill effectively and this results in decreased right-ventricular stroke volume. This reduces left-ventricular preload with diminished left-ventricular filling and reduced left-ventricular stroke volume. The net effect is to reduce cardiac output (Spiers 2006).

Compensatory measures The heart compensates by increasing its rate in order to maintain cardiac output. The tachycardia reduces diastolic (and thus coronary artery) filling time, making the reduced cardiac output worse and any pre-existing ischaemia critical. Right ventricular dilatation occurs and, as cardiac output decreases further, arterial vasoconstriction occurs and systemic vascular resistance increases; this further reduces left-ventricular output (Spiers 2006).

Clinical presentation This complex pathophysiology accounts for a classic triad of clinical signs: hypotension, elevated jugular venous pressure (JVP), and clear lung fields.

Clinically the patient will present with:

♦ tachycardia—this may be very rapid and weak

♦ hypotension—due to poor left ventricular output

♦ cool, clammy peripheries—due to reduced left-ventricular output and arterial vasoconstriction

♦ breathlessness and cyanosis—due to poor pulmonary perfusion

♦ fatigue due to poor left ventricular filling and reduced cardiac output and lactic acidosis

♦ elevated jugular venous pressure (JVP)—due to raised right ventricular pressure and backwards flow

♦ clear lung fields—initially there will be no pulmonary oedema.

Thus the patient with acute right heart failure will present with a picture of shock in the presence of acute inferior wall infarction. The typical absence of pulmonary oedema in the presence of breathlessness and a raised JVP should alert the practitioner to the possibility of acute right heart failure. The importance of early diagnosis is important as the haemodynamic consequences can be extreme for the patient and the management of RVMI is markedly different to an infarction and heart failure affecting primarily the left ventricle (Spiers 2006).

Electrocardiogram The 12-lead ECG will demonstrate an inferior wall or posterior wall infarction. If a RVMI is suspected recording of V4 R—V6 R is recommended to identify ST elevation in these leads (Spiers 2006). These lead are recorded by removing the V4-V6 leads from the left precordium and placing them in the identical place on the patient's right precordium. These leads give a highly specific and sensitive view of the right ventricle which is not afforded by the standard left sided ECG.

Nursing measures to manage right heart failure The goals of management for RVMI include reperfusion, optimization of ventricular preload using volume loading, inotropic stimulation, and maintenance of normal cardiac rhythm (Haji & Movahed 2000). Carter & Ellis (2005) offer a useful mnemonic guide to nursing management—*RRVVII*—reperfusion, rhythm, vital signs, volume, inotropes and intra-aortic balloon pump (IABP).

♦ *Reperfusion*—early coronary reperfusion by thrombolysis or primary coronary intervention is the mainstay of managing patients with STEMI.

♦ *Rhythm*—cardiac output can be enhanced by ensuring an appropriate heart rate and rhythm, regular monitoring is required.

♦ *Vital signs*—regular, continuous monitoring of heart rate, rhythm, respiratory rate, oxygen saturations and peripheral perfusion is essential.

♦ *Volume*—volume loading is not usually used in managing patients with acute STEMI. However, in RVMI volume loading (fluid challenge) is aimed at enhancing right ventricular contractility and is based on Starling's law of the heart, which states that within physiological limits the greater the degree of muscle stretch, the greater the amount of muscle contraction. Hence, volume loading with an isotonic solution such as sodium chloride will stretch the right ventricle and improve the right ventricular output. Volume loading will improve hypotension and the aim is to maintain the blood pressure at systolic 90 mmHg. It is advisable to monitor the patient carefully during volume loading as it may worsen any concomitant left ventricular failure.

♦ *Inotropic support*—if volume replacement therapy is not sufficient, it may be necessary to improve right ventricular contractility with an inotropic infusion such as dobutamine.

♦ *Intra-aortic balloon support*—finally, if cardiogenic shock develops an intra-aortic balloon pump may be utilized; this will improve coronary perfusion and reduce afterload (Carter & Ellis 2005). Patients receiving IABP support need to be managed in a high-dependency or coronary care unit.

Cardiogenic shock

Cardiogenic shock is the final result of failure of the compensatory mechanisms described above. Cardiogenic shock is a complex syndrome caused largely as the result of severe myocardial damage where more than 40% of the ventricular wall is infarcted (Julian *et al.* 2007). In some patients the cause is due to mechanical dysfunction such as ventricular septal defect or papillary muscle rupture. There is significantly reduced cardiac output and peripheral resistance insufficient to compensate for this.

Clinical presentation Cardiogenic shock usually presents rapidly and the presentation includes:

♦ tachycardia—heart rate >100 beats/min

♦ hypotension SBP <90 mmHg

♦ tachypnoea—respiratory rate >22 breaths/min

♦ peripheral vasoconstriction—cool, clammy, cyanosed extremities

♦ altered mental state—confusion

♦ oliguria—<0.5 mL/kg/h—leading to anuria

♦ intractable chest pain.

Management of cardiogenic shock Extreme vigilance is required in managing patients post-STEMI to identify the early features of cardiogenic shock. A falling blood pressure compromises coronary blood flow and further worsens myocardial ischaemia. Hypoxia, reduced blood flow, and anaerobic metabolism results in a spiralling cycle of events that further compromises cardiac function.

Despite advances in cardiology in the last two decades, patients in cardiogenic shock following a STEMI have a mortality rate of 50%. The use of intravenous dobutamine or dopamine to provide pharmacological inotropic support is useful, but should be used with caution as it will increase myocardial workload and exacerbate myocardial ischaemia.

Inotropic drugs Inotropic drugs are usually given by continuous intravenous infusion, preferably via a central line as any extravasations into local tissues can cause severe necrosis. Inotropic drugs include dopamine, dobutamine, and adrenaline. All three drugs have advantages and disadvantages in a patient with cardiogenic shock due to their complementary and opposing actions. All inotropes increase myocardial contractility, primarily by actions on the β-1 adrenergic receptors. Most inotropic drugs are also chronotropic and will thus increase the heart rate. Augmentation of stroke volume and heart rate will increase cardiac output but at the expense of myocardial oxygen demand.

Subsequently the choice of inotropic drugs depends on the clinical presentation and patient response. Dopamine may be given at a low dose of 2.5 mcg/kg/min; at this dose dopamine increases renal flow and urinary output (so called 'renal dopamine'). At higher doses—5 mcg/kg/min dopamine increases myocardial contractility but shows increased propensity to cause cardiac arrhythmias and vasoconstriction. Dobutamine at doses of 5 mcg/kg/min increases myocardial contractility, heart rate, and potential for cardiac arrhythmias. Low dose adrenaline (0.04–0.10 mcg/kg/min) may be useful as it causes vasodilation, hence reducing afterload and reducing cardiac workload. At higher doses, adrenaline causes strong arterial vasoconstriction and should be avoided in cardiogenic shock.

All patients receiving inotropic support via a central line require intensive monitoring and support and should generally be nursed in a high-dependency unit if possible. Continuous cardiac monitoring to identify potential ventricular and tachyarrhythmias and continuous blood pressure recordings are essential.

The intra-aortic balloon pump can provide temporary clinical improvement and is valuable as a bridge to support the patient before other interventions such as percutaneous coronary angioplasty for a blocked coronary artery or surgical intervention to correct mechanical dysfunction.

Nursing care of the patient with cardiogenic shock Nursing actions aim to monitor vital signs, detect deterioration, maintain tissue perfusion, and prevent further ischaemia.

The patient should be nursed in the semi-upright position and high flow oxygen should be administered; some patients may benefit from CPAP. Use of low-dose or even continuous diamorphine infusion will help reduce preload and also support the patient, who may be extremely anxious. Drug therapy should be reviewed as many of the commonly used drugs during acute myocardial infarction may exacerbate the hypotension and shock. In particular ACE inhibitors, β-blockers, and nitrates should be used with caution.

Continuous monitoring of heart rate, rhythm, blood pressure, and oxygen saturation is essential. Sphygmomanometer readings may be difficult to interpret and Dynamap recordings should be used. The patient and family will need expert, skilled nursing support as this situation is potentially fatal.

Clinical link 3.3 (see Appendix for answers)

You are caring for a 65-year-old female patient who is recovering from a STEMI suffered 4 days ago. Plans for discharge are well advanced and the patient is due to go home tomorrow. She has seen the cardiac rehabilitation team and has also discussed her discharge medications with the pharmacist.

It is 18:00 and you record a routine set of vital signs:
temperature: 36.4°C.
radial pulse: 95 beats/min irregular (recording at 06:00 was 65 beats/min regular).
blood pressure: 90/50 mmHg (recording at 06:00 was 120/70 mmHg).
respiratory rate: 26 breaths/min (recording at 06:00 was 14/min).
O_2 saturations: 90% on air.

You note that she is breathless on minimal exertion and you also note that she appears slightly cyanosed peripherally. Capillary refill is 3 s. She denies any chest pain.

♦ What would your next immediate actions be and why?

♦ What other investigations is the doctor likely to perform and why?

♦ What are the potential problems evolving in this situation?

Overview of types of shock

Shock is a syndrome characterized by hypoperfusion of body tissues. In order for blood flow to occur to the tissues and homeostasis to be maintained, the following three factors are necessary:

♦ an adequate amount of blood

♦ an ability of the heart to pump the blood

♦ blood vessels with good tone and ability to constrict and dilate in response to physiological changes.

Shock may be classified as hypovolaemic, cardiogenic, neurogenic, anaphylactic, and septic. Specific treatment and management of each type of shock is given in the specific chapters in this book. Clinical shock is a life-threatening condition requiring immediate attention.

Hypovolaemic shock (see Chapter 7)

This is the most common type of shock, resulting from any reduction in the volume within the vascular compartment. Causes include:

♦ excessive blood loss: haemorrhage (trauma, gastrointestinal bleeding, post-operative surgical causes)

♦ loss of body fluids other than blood: excessive diuresis (diabetic ketoacidosis), plasma loss from burns, fluid loss from excessive vomiting, or diarrhoea

♦ movement of fluid into another body space ('the third space'), for example bowel obstruction or peritonitis.

Clinically patients with hypovolaemic shock will present with the following:

♦ dizziness, disorientation, confusion

♦ anxiety

♦ hypotension

♦ tachycardia

♦ oliguria

♦ decreased oxygen saturation.

Cardiogenic shock (see Chapter 3)

Cardiogenic shock results from the inability of the heart to pump sufficient cardiac output to perfuse the cells of the body. Causes include:

♦ myocardial infarction (this is the commonest cause and as discussed above, is potentially fatal)

♦ cardiac tamponade (blood in the pericardial space caused by trauma, surgery, or malignancy)

♦ valvular heart disease in particular mitral regurgitation or papillary muscle rupture secondary to an acute myocardial infarction

♦ cardiac arrhythmias.

Clinically patients with cardiogenic shock will present with the following:

♦ hypotension

♦ tachycardia

♦ cardiac arrhythmias

♦ signs of heart failure (raised CVP, pulmonary oedema and breathlessness).

Neurogenic shock

Neurogenic shock is due to disruption of the sympathetic nerve activity which helps to maintain vasomotor tone. The autonomic nervous system is unable to maintain systemic vascular resistance and this results in massive dilation of the blood vessels. Causes include:

♦ spinal cord injury

♦ trauma or disease to the brain stem

♦ spinal anaesthesia.

The failure of the sympathetic nervous system results in the following features:

♦ massive vasodilation

♦ profound bradycardia

♦ hypotension.

Anaphylactic shock (see Chapter 13)

Anaphylactic shock results from a severe allergic reaction in which an antigen–antibody reaction has occurred. This results in bronchospasm, severe vasodilation, and increased permeability of the blood vessels. It is a medical emergency and requires urgent attention otherwise death can occur within minutes. There are a variety of causes, including:

♦ antibiotics

♦ vaccinations

♦ blood transfusions

♦ latex

♦ food (nuts, eggs and fruit are common culprits)

♦ insect bites.

The patient's symptoms will present very rapidly and the upper airway is particularly vulnerable. The following signs and symptoms may occur:

♦ airway compromise; hyperventilation, tachypnoea, hypoxia

♦ cardiovascular collapse; tachycardia, hypotension, oedema

♦ allergic reaction; urticaria, itching, burning, stinging of skin and mucous membranes

♦ extreme anxiety.

Septic shock (see Chapter 8)

Septic shock is a systemic response to a severe infection and is characterized by a response to the toxin resulting in profound vasodilation, increased microvascular permeability, and neutrophil activation. Conditions that predispose to septic shock include:

♦ the very old and the very young

♦ patients who are immuno-suppressed, receiving chemotherapy or steroids

♦ patients who have undergone gastrointestinal or urological surgery

♦ patients with hypertrophic or cancerous prostate glands (these patients are more likely to develop urinary tract infections and to have undergone urologic procedures).

Initially the patient with early septic shock will present with 'hot' shock due to the excessive vasodilation. There will be the following characteristics:

- tachycardia
- increased cardiac output
- peripheral vasodilation (skin flushing)
- increased renal output (polyuria)
- fever
- oedema formation.

End of chapter test

The following assessment will enable you to evaluate your theoretical knowledge of cardiovascular assessment and management as well as your ability to apply this theory to clinical practice. You should undertake the following assessment with an appropriately trained member of staff in clinical practice. If you are unable to answer any questions it may be helpful to revisit the section in this chapter.

Knowledge assessment

With the support of your mentor/supervisor from practice, work through the following prompts to explore your knowledge level about cardiovascular assessment, care, and management.

- Describe the anatomy and blood flow through the heart.
- Discuss the coronary artery circulation and the anatomical regions supplied by each coronary artery.
- Describe the normal waveforms on the ECG and discuss the normal amplitude and duration parameters.
- Explain the important aspects of taking a cardiac history and discuss commonly presenting symptoms of cardiac disease.
- Differentiate the various causes of chest pain.
- Critically analyse factors which contribute to the formation of atherosclerosis.
- Recognize commonly encountered arrhythmias (supraventricular tachycardia, atrial fibrillation. and third degree AV block) and discuss nursing and medical interventions.
- Define acute coronary syndromes and differentiate between the presentation of different types of acute coronary syndromes.
- Discuss why 'time is myocardium' and explain how processes are used to ensure timely treatment for patients with suspected acute coronary syndromes.
- Critically analyse your roles and responsibilities in managing a patient who requires thrombolysis.
- Discuss the underlying pathophysiology for left ventricular failure and explain how management strategies are used to treat patients with this condition.
- Differentiate the causes, presentation, and management of acute right heart failure from acute left heart failure.
- Discuss signs of impending cardiogenic shock and appropriate management.
- Differentiate types of shock, including; hypovolaemic, cardiogenic, anaphylactic, neurogenic, and septic shock.

Skills assessment

Under the guidance of your mentor/supervisor, undertake a cardiovascular assessment followed by appropriate interventions for any significant abnormality. Your mentor/supervisor will assess your ability and provide feedback based on the following skills:

+ Takes a cardiac history, including key points in relation to assessment of cardiac symptoms.
+ Conducts a comprehensive cardiovascular assessment and explains normal/abnormal findings related to the patient's symptoms and presentation.
+ Demonstrates an ability to perform 12-lead ECG, continuous cardiac monitoring, oxygen saturation monitoring, and other vital signs.
+ Identifies the need for and frequency of vital signs observation.
+ Facilitates the completion of relevant clinical investigations such as blood, urine, X-ray, and ECG tests and evaluates results.
+ Liaises with other members of the health care team as necessary, including nurse in charge, doctor, pharmacist, and healthcare assistant.
+ Recognizes the need for fast and appropriate response if cardiovascular function is deteriorating.
+ Reports any new or worsening chest pain and records appropriate assessments.
+ Reviews need for cardiovascular assessment and frequency of vital signs monitoring.
+ Informs patient/relative of any changes.
+ Demonstrates clinical reasoning and provides justification for all interventions for a patient with acute left or right heart failure.

References

ACC/AHA/ESC. (2006) Guidelines for the management of patients with ventricular arrhythmias and the prevention of sudden cardiac death—executive summary. *Eur. Heart J.* **27**, 2099–140.

Albarran, J.W. (2002) The language of chest pain. *Nurs. Times.* **98**, 38–40.

Albarran, J.W. (2007) Analysing the presentation of women with chest pain and other symptoms associated with coronary heart disease and myocardial infarction. In: Albarran, J. and Tagney, J. (eds) *Chest pain: Advanced assessment and management skills.* Blackwell Publishing, Oxford.

Anti-Platelet Trialists' Collaboration. (1994) Overview 1: prevention of death, myocardial infarction and stroke by prolonged anti-platelet therapy in various categories of patients. *BMJ.* **308**, 81–106.

Antman, E.M., Anbe D.T., Armstrong, P.W. *et al.* (2004) ACC.AHA guidelines for the management of patients with ST-elevation myocardial infarction: a report of the American College of Cardiology/American Heart Association Task Force on Practice Guidelines. Writing committee to review the 1999 guidelines for the management of patients with acute myocardial infarction. *J. Am. Coll. Cardiol.* **44**, 671–719.

Banner, D. (2008) The pathophysiology and management of atrial fibrillation. *Br. J. Cardiac Nurs.* **3**, 201–9.

Berne, M. and Levy, M.N. (2001) *Cardiovascular physiology*, 8th edn. Mosby, St Louis.

Boersma, E., Maas, A.C., and Simoons, M.L. (1996) Early thrombolytic treatment in acute myocardial infarction: reappraisal of the golden hour. *Lancet.* **348**, 771–75.

British Heart Foundation (2006) Coronary Heart Disease Statistics Database Annual Compendium. British Heart Foundation, London.

Carter, T. and Ellis, K. (2005) Right ventricular myocardial infarction. *Crit. Care Nurse.* **25**, 52–62.

Castle, N. (2006) Reperfusion therapy. *Emerg.* Nurse. **13**, 25–35.

Clinton, H. (2003) Haemodynamic monitoring in theatre. *Br. J. Anaesth. Recov. Nurs.* **4**, 10–16.

Collinson, P. (2006) Cardiac troponins T and I: Biochemical markers in diagnosing myocardial infarction. *Br. J. Cardiac Nurs.* **1**, 418–23.

Conover, M.B. (2003) *Understanding Electrocardiography*, 8th edn. Mosby, St Louis.

Department of Health (2000) *National Service Framework for Coronary Heart Disease*. Stationery Office, London.

Department of Health (2005) Arrhythmias and sudden cardiac death. In: *National Service Framework for Coronary Heart Disease*. Stationery Office, London.

Department of Health (2008) *National Infarction Angioplasty Project (NIAP): interim report*. Stationery Office, London.

Epstein, O., Perkin, G.D., Cookson, J., and de Bono, D.P. (2003) *Clinical Examination*, 3rd edn. Mosby, St Louis.

Fibrinolytic Therapy Trialists Collaborative Group. (1994) Indications for fibrinolytic therapy in suspected acute myocardial infarction: collaborative overview of early mortality and major morbidity results from all randomised trials of more than 1000 patients. *Lancet.* **343**, 311–22.

Fox, K.A.A. (2004) Management of acute coronary syndromes: an update. *Heart.* **90**, 698–706.

Fuster, V., Ryden, L.E., Cannom, D.S., *et al.* (2006) for the American College of Cardiology/American Heart Association Task Force on Practice Guidelines and the European Society of Cardiology Committee for Practice Guidelines. Guidelines for the management of patients with atrial fibrillation. *Circulation.* **114**, e257–354.

Goldberger, A.L. (2006) *Clinical Electrocardiography: A Simplified Approach*, 7th edn. Mosby, St Louis.

Grace Registry. Available at: http://www.outcomes.org/grace.

Greenfield, F. (2008) Continuous ST-segment monitoring using EASI vector-derived ECG in suspected ACS. *Br. J. Cardiac Nurs.* **3**, 343–48.

Haji, S.A. and Movahed, A. (2000) Right ventricular infarction—diagnosis and treatment. *Clin. Cardiol.* **23**, 473–82.

Julian, D.G., Campbell Cowan, J., and McLenachan, J.M. (2005) *Cardiology*. Elsevier, Edinburgh.

Katz, R. and Purcell, H. (2006) *Acute Coronary Syndromes*. Elsevier, Edinburgh.

Keeley, E.C., Boura, J.A., and Grines, C.L. (2003) Primary angioplasty versus intravenous thrombolytic therapy for acute myocardial infarction: a quantitative review of 23 randomised trials. *Lancet.* **361**, 13–20.

Kelly, J. (2007) Mending broken hearts: acute stress cardiomyopathy. *Br. J. Cardiac Nurs.* **2,** 525–31.

Khan, E. (2004) Clinical skills: the physiological basis and interpretation of the ECG. *Br. J. Cardiac Nurs.* **13**, 440–46.

Moye, S., Carney, M.F., Holstege, C., *et al.* (2005) The electrocardiogram in right ventricular myocardial infarction. *Am. J. Em. Med.* **23**, 793–99.

Nehyba, K. (2006) Continuous positive airway pressure ventilation part one: physiology and patient care. *Br. J. Cardiac Nurs.* **1**, 575–79.

Nehyba, K. (2007) Continuous positive airway pressure ventilation part two: indications and contraindications. *Br. J. Cardiac Nurs.* **2**, 18–24.

Newby, D.E. and Grubb, N.R. (2005) *Cardiology: An illustrated Colour Text*. Elsevier, Edinburgh.

NICE (2002) *The clinical effectiveness and cost effectiveness of drugs for early thrombolysis in the treatment of acute myocardial infarction*. National Institute for Health and Clinical Excellence, London.

NICE (2006) *Atrial fibrillation: National clinical guideline for management in primary and secondary care*. National Institute for Health and Clinical Excellence, London.

Nicholson, C. (2007) *Heart Failure: A Clinical Nursing Handbook*. John Wiley & Sons, Chichester.

Opie, L.H. and Gersch, B.J. (2004) *Drugs for the Heart*. 6th edn. WB Saunders, Philadelphia.

Owens, C.G., Agney, A., and Adgey, J. (2006) Electrocardiographic diagnosis of non-ST segment elevation acute coronary syndromes: current concepts for the physician. *J. Electrocardiol.* **39**, 271–4.

Pope, J., Aufderheide, T., Ruthazer, R. *et al.* (2000) Missed diagnoses of acute cardiac ischaemia in the emergency department. *New Eng. J. Med.* **342**, 1163–70.

Resuscitation Council (2005) Adult Advanced Life Support Guidelines. Resuscitation Council UK, London.

Silber, S., Albertsson, P., Aviles, F.F. *et al.* (2005) Guidelines for percutaneous coronary interventions The Task Force for Percutaneous Coronary Interventions of the European Society of Cardiology. *Eur. Heart J.* **26**, 804–47.

Spiers, C.M. (2003) Detecting failed thrombolysis in the accident and emergency department. *Accid. Emerg. Nurs.* **11**, 221–25.

Spiers, C. (2006) Using the ECG in the early detection of right ventricular myocardial infarction Br. *J. Cardiac Nurs.* **3**, 512–18.

Thygesen, K., Alpert, J.S., White, H.D (2007) (Joint ESC/AACF/AHA/WHF Task Force). Universal definition of myocardial infarction. *Eur. Heart J.* **28**, 2525–38.

Van de Werf, F.J., Antman, E.M., and Simoons M.L. (2002) Managing ST-elevation myocardial infarction. *Eur. Heart J. Suppl.* **4**, (SuppE) E15-E23.

Van de Werf, F., Ardissino, D., Betriu, A. *et al.* (2003) Management of acute myocardial infarction in patients presenting with ST-segment elevation: Task Force on the Management of Acute Myocardial Infarction of the European Society of Cardiology. *Eur. Heart J.* **24**, 28–66.

Wolff, A. and Cowan, C. (2009) 10 Steps before you refer for palpitations. *Br. J. Cardiol.* **16**, 182–86.

Woodrow, P. (2004) Reading electrocardiograms and recognising common dysrhythmias. In: Moore, T. and Woodrow, P. (eds) *High Dependency Nursing Care*. Routledge, London.

Yusuf, S., Hawken, S., Ounpui, S. *et al.* (2004) Effect of potentially modifiable risk factors associated with myocardial infarction in 53 countries (INTERHEART): case control study. *Lancet.* **364**, 937–52.

Chapter 4

Neurological care

Fiona Creed

Chapter contents

In order to understand how to assess and manage the patient with neurological conditions it is essential to have an understanding of the structure and function of the brain and how injury/illness can affect this. This chapter will examine:

+ normal physiology.
+ physiological changes following illness and injury
+ the physiology of raised intracranial pressure and cerebral oedema
+ immediate assessment of neurological function
+ formal neurological assessment (to include Glasgow Coma Scale)
+ nursing care of the patient with neurological injury, to include:

  • stroke
  • subarachnoid haemorrhage
  • mild brain injury
  • seizures.

Learning outcomes

This chapter will enable you to:

+ develop understanding of the normal structure and function of the nervous system
+ develop an understanding of changes during illness/injury
+ understand the significance of neurological assessment
+ examine the practice of neurological assessment
+ discuss the management of common neurological problems
+ understand common treatments for neurological illness
+ understand when the patient with deteriorating neurological function requires urgent medical attention
+ understand the impact of neurological problems on the patient and their carers
+ use a skills assessment tool to assess your clinical practice.

Introduction

The human brain is composed of billions of specialized cells (neurons). All the neurons a person has are present at birth. These specialist cells do not have mitotic capacity and are not replaceable. In cases of illness and injury it is therefore essential that care is delivered to prevent cell death and to preserve nervous system functioning. An adequate understanding of the nervous system's structures and functions is essential to ensure adequate assessment of this complex system, and timely and appropriate care delivery. This initial section aims to revise basic anatomy and physiology, and enable the reader to understand the potential consequences of injury to the brain and central nervous system.

Normal anatomy and physiology

The nervous system is divided into two main anatomically different parts:

+ the central nervous system, which includes structures and nerves within the cranium and spinal cord
+ the peripheral nervous system, consisting of nerves outside the brain and spinal cord and which is further subdivided into somatic and autonomic nervous systems.

The main focus of this chapter will be role of the central nervous system and the function of the brain. Reference will be made to the autonomic system in Chapters 2, 3, and 7. It may be beneficial to refer to a specific neurophysiology text if more detail is required.

The brain

The brain constitutes about 2% of total body weight. The average weight of a young adult brain is 1400 g, decreasing with age to approximately 1200 g. Simplistically, the brain is divided into three main areas: the cerebrum, the brain stem, and the cerebellum. Other subdivisions are sometimes used in clinical practice. Reference may be made to areas known as 'fossae', including anterior, middle, and posterior fossae areas. Because of the significant functions of the brain, adequate protection from injury is required. The brain is protected by the skull, the meninges, and the cerebral spinal fluid (CSF).

The skull

The purpose of the skull is to protect the most vulnerable parts of the brain. The skull provides a bony framework and consists of 8 bones of the cranium and 14 bones of the face. The bones of the skull join at various places (suture lines). At around the age of 14 the bones become fused and the brain is encapsulated in a closed box. This can cause problems if the brain swells as there is little capacity for swelling/oedema. The skull offers varying protection to the brain, but because of the irregular nature of the inner skull it can actually worsen injury, especially during traumatic injury.

The meninges

Immediately below the skull are the three layers of the meninges (see Figure 4.1). These cover both the brain and the spinal cord and are detailed below.

Dura mater

The dura mater is a double layered, white, inelastic membrane that lies beneath the bone. Folds of dura are also situated within the skull cavity to support and protect the brain. These folds of dura mater further divide areas of the brain. The most important of these is the tentorium cerebri. The area above the tentorium is supratentorial, the area below infratentorial.

Arachnoid membrane

The arachnoid membrane is an extremely thin and delicate layer that loosely encloses the brain. It is separated from the dura by the subdural space. CSF flows around the subarachnoid space.

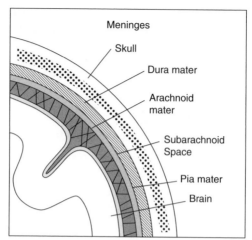

Figure 4.1 The meninges.

It contains a large number of blood vessels. The arachnoid membrane also contains pressure sensitive 'valves', or arachnoid villi, that allow reabsorption of CSF.

Pia mater

The pia mater is a mesh-like vascular membrane that covers the entire surface of the brain.

Spaces of the meninges

The meninges are not fused together and three important potential spaces occur:

- the extradural (epidural) space, between the periosteum and outer layer of dura
- the subdural space, between the inner layer of dura and the arachnoid membrane
- the subarachnoid space, between the arachnoid membrane and pia mater.

These potential spaces are of significance in clinical practice as they may become the focus of bleeding/haematoma formation following traumatic brain injury. They are also the focus for infection in bacterial/viral meningitis.

The cerebrum

The first major subdivision within the brain is the cerebrum. The cerebral cortex is often linked to higher functioning of the nervous system. The cerebrum is made up of two cerebral hemispheres, separated by the sulcus. The surface of the cerebral hemispheres has a wrinkled appearance (gyri) that substantially increases the surface area of the brain. Each hemisphere is covered by a cerebral cortex of gray matter that contains billions of neurons. Under the cerebral cortex is white matter that contains nerve fibres. The cerebrum is further divided into pairs of lobes. Historically, attempts have been made to match the functions of these lobes and therefore predict expected damage following injury and illness. The advent of functional scans has allowed for further classifications, but it is essential to stress that this work is not complete and more research is required. Examination of the lobes allows for understanding of the functions of each lobe and a degree of prediction of loss of function if the area sustains damage. The following section highlights some of the functions of the cerebrum and

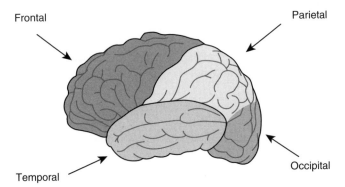

Figure 4.2 The cerebrum.

discusses some symptoms of lobe damage that may occur in the patient with neurological damage.

The cerebrum is divided into frontal, parietal, occipital, and temporal lobes (see Figure 4.2).

The frontal lobe

Major functions of the frontal lobe include:

♦ higher level cognitive functioning such as reasoning and concentration

♦ memory

♦ emotional states

♦ control of voluntary eye movement

♦ Speech (Broca's area)

♦ motor function.

Frontal damage can lead to some of the following:

♦ inability to solve problems

♦ personality changes

♦ disordered eye movement

♦ speech problems (expressive dysphasia)

♦ decreased memory.

The parietal lobe

Major functions of the parietal lobe include:

♦ analysis of gross aspects of sensation (touch, position, pressure etc)

♦ awareness of body

♦ orientation in space

♦ perception of body positioning.

Parietal damage can lead to:

♦ lack of conscious sensation on half of the body

♦ neglect of half of the body

+ disorders of spatial awareness
+ agnosia (difficulty in perceiving objects normally).

It should be noted that the frontal and parietal lobes work closely together to control motor/sensory function, since the sensory and motor cortex is located between these two lobes (central sulcus).

The temporal lobe

Major functions of the temporal lobe include:

+ primary auditory receptive area
+ speech (Wernicke's area)
+ memory
+ learning
+ intellect

Temporal lobe damage can lead to:

+ disorders in learning verbal information
+ memory loss
+ speech problems (receptive dysphasia).

The occipital lobe

Major functions of the occipital lobe include:

+ visual perception
+ visual reflexes
+ involuntary smooth eye movements.

Occipital lobe damage can lead to:

+ visual disturbances
+ alterations in visual reflexes.

Cerebral dominance

At birth, both cerebral hemispheres have an equal capacity for development. As the child grows, one cerebral hemisphere develops more rapidly in relation to the other one. In adulthood most adults will have one dominant hemisphere. Left cerebral dominance is found in approximately 90% of the population. It is generally held that the patient's speech centres are located in the dominant region of the brain, hence for the majority of the population the speech centre is in the left cerebral hemisphere. This can cause significant problems with the perception and articulation of speech if the dominant side of the brain is affected by injury.

Corpus callosum

Although studies suggest that the right and left cerebral hemispheres function independently, it is important to acknowledge that the areas are linked. The cerebral hemispheres are connected by the corpus callosum, a thick area of nerve fibres connecting one part of the hemisphere with its corresponding part on the other side. Because of this connection the two hemispheres are intricately linked. Studies in children with damage suggest that if one hemisphere is damaged the other can take over its role. This is not the case in adults and neurological damage may be more debilitating in adults as the capacity for compensation is limited.

Other structures within the cerebrum

Basal ganglia: control movement that involves both cognitive and motor processing.

Dicephalon: a major division of the cerebrum, divided into four regions, including:

- the thalamus, the last area where impulses are processed before ascending to the higher function areas of the cerebral cortex
- the epithalamus, which is thought to have a role in growth and development and in 'food-getting reflex'
- the hypothalamus, which controls the following: temperature regulation, water metabolism, pituitary secretions, excitatory/inhibitory functions of the autonomic nervous system, sleep/wakefulness cycles
- the subthalamus, which is similar in function to basal ganglia.

The brain stem

The brain stem is the second major subdivision of the brain. The brain stem has specific functions and contains the nuclei of several of the cranial nerves. It is made up of:

- the midbrain
- the pons
- the medulla.

Damage to the brain stem can be confirmed by a specific examination of cranial nerve function (this is commonly referred to as brain stem death testing, which involves testing of brain stem reflexes and an apnoea test, and is only conducted on ventilated patients in the intensive therapy unit (ITU) (Dawson & Shah 2005).

The midbrain

The midbrain's function is to act as a pathway for the cerebral hemispheres and lower brain. It is the centre for auditory and visual reflexes, and contains the nuclei of the occulomotor and trochlear cranial nerves.

The pons

The pons acts as a bridge between the midbrain and the medulla. A large number of tracts (nerve pathways) go through the pons, connecting higher cerebral regions with the lower levels of the nervous system. The pons also has some control over respiratory function, including the apneustic centre and the pneumotaxic centre.

The medulla oblongata

This part of the brain stem joins the spinal cord. It is level with the foramen magnum (a hole in the base of the skull where spinal cord and brain connect). The decussation of pyramids occurs here (this means that the motor fibres from the left side of the brain cross over to the right side of the body, enabling the left brain to control right body movement and vice versa). The medulla also contains the cardiac, respiratory, and vasomotor centres. The reflex centres for sneezing, coughing, vomiting, and hiccoughing are also here.

Special systems within the brain

Two other systems of clinical significance are the reticular activating system and the reticular formation.

The reticular activating system The reticular activating system (RAS) is a diffuse system that extends from lower brain to cerebral cortex. The RAS controls sleep/wake cycles, consciousness, and focused attention. Stimulation of the brain stem portion of the RAS results in wakefulness throughout the entire brain. The RAS is the physical basis of consciousness. Certain drugs can affect RAS. It is suppressed by alcohol and tranquillizers, and enhanced by some mood-altering drugs, e.g. LSD.

The reticular formation The reticular formation is a group of neurons originating within the brainstem that project towards the higher parts of the nervous system. It is involved in:

♦ sleep/waking cycles

♦ control of sensory information (either inhibit or allow sensory messages to pass)

♦ control of responsiveness.

The cerebellum

The cerebellum is the last major subdivision within the brain. It is located at the posterior fossa and is attached to the brain stem. The cerebellum has a large number of functions. These include control of fine motor movement, coordination of muscle groups, and maintenance of balance (through feedback loops). It is quickly affected by alcohol consumption and is often damaged in patients with a history of alcohol abuse. Damage to the cerebellum can lead to abnormal gaits and this is often seen in patients with a history of long-term alcohol abuse.

Blood supply to the brain

About 20% of oxygen consumption in the body occurs in the brain and this is used for glucose metabolism. The brain is totally dependent on glucose for its metabolism. A lack of oxygen, and hence glucose metabolism, for more than 5 min can cause irreversible brain damage.

The blood supply to the brain is via two pairs of arteries (the internal carotid and vertebral basilar arteries). These vessels join together to form the circle of Willis. In favourable instances the circle of Willis may allow an adequate blood supply to reach the brain even if one of the four component vessels has been cut off (see Figure 4.3).

The venous drainage is largely managed by two vascular channels, the dural sinuses. The dural sinuses empty into the jugular veins and then back to the heart.

There are several distinct characteristics of cerebral blood flow:

♦ Cerebral arteries are often thinner than other arteries of comparable size.

♦ The veins are also thinner and lack a muscle layer.

♦ The veins and sinuses have no valves.

♦ The venous return does not retrace arteries but has own course.

♦ The dural sinuses are unique to cerebral circulation.

The blood–brain barrier

In order for the brain to function normally, it must maintain its own stable environment. The blood–brain barrier is a term used to describe the tight network of cells and capillaries that prevent anything not required by the brain from entering. Substances that cross the blood–brain barrier easily include lipids, oxygen, carbon dioxide, water, and glucose. In clinical practice it is important to note that drugs, unless bound in lipids (e.g. propofol), do not cross the blood–brain

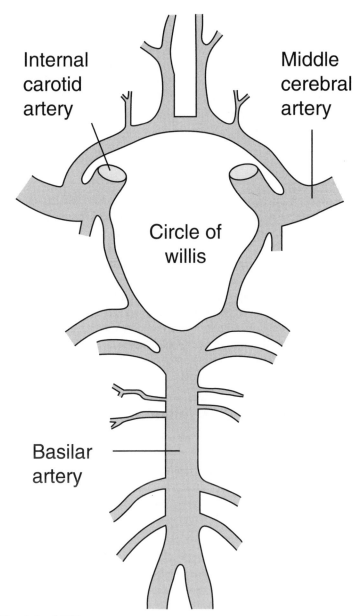

Figure 4.3 The circle of Willis.

barrier easily. This is of particular significance when considering antibiotics for cerebral infection.

Cerebral spinal fluid

It was highlighted earlier that cerebral spinal fluid (CSF) has a role in the protection of the brain by acting as a 'shock absorber', cushioning the brain from injury. It also has a significant role in the carriage of nutrients to the brain and is sometimes referred to as a 'third circulation'. CSF is composed of water, a small amount of protein, oxygen, and carbon dioxide. It also carries electrolytes (sodium, potassium, and chloride) and glucose (necessary for cerebral metabolism). CSF is produced in the choroid plexus, a small cauliflower-like structure within the ventricles of the brain. The choroid plexus produces about 25 mL of CSF per hour. This flows through the ventricular system and around the brain and spinal cord, where it is reabsorbed by pressure-sensitive arachnoid villi. Sometimes in neurological damage there can be problems with obstruction to flow or problems with reabsorption and this can lead to hydrocephalus.

The spinal cord

There is clearly a need for the messages from the brain to quickly reach receptor sites, and for messages from the peripheral nervous system to link to the central nervous system. This is the role of the spinal cord. As stated earlier, the spinal cord is part of the central nervous system. The spinal cord is continuous with the medulla oblongata; it runs from the upper borders of the atlas (first cervical vertebra C1) to the lower border of the first lumbar vertebra (L1). The spinal cord is protected from injury by the spinal column and the meninges. The spinal cord allows messages to travel from the peripheral nervous system to the brain and messages from the brain to get to the peripheral nervous system. It can on occasion act as an activating centre in its own right by receiving incoming sensory impulses and initiating outgoing motor signals. This is seen in reflex arcs and is an important consideration in neurological assessment (the practitioner needs to be sure that any motor response testing is a true test of motor function and not a spinal reflex; this will be discussed under neurological assessment).

Damage to the central nervous system

The nursing management of patients with any neurological condition requires an understanding of the pathophysiology of the disease process and complications that can arise as a result of these changes. This next section will consider the main pathophysiolocal consequences of disease/damage to the central nervous system. Additional detail, in relation to specific illness/disease processes, may be found later in the chapter under condition-related subheadings.

Cerebral metabolism

The brain is very dependent on blood flow to provide oxygen and nutrients to the neurons and remove the end products of metabolism. Damage will quickly occur to the neuron if it is deprived of oxygen or blood for a short period or if excessive carbon dioxide accumulates. Following damage, because of their inability to replicate, neurons die and are not replaced. If sufficient numbers of neurons are damaged the patient will exhibit significant loss of neurological function. A number of factors have been shown to influence the amount of blood the brain receives (cerebral blood flow). These are often described as extracerebral (outside the brain) or intracerebral (within the brain).

Extracerebral factors:

These are primarily related to the cardiovascular system and include changes in blood pressure, cardiac function, and viscosity of blood. Usually in adults, cerebral blood flow is held constant unless the mean arterial pressure (MAP) falls below 50–60 mmHg. Factors that may reduce cardiac function, e.g. atherosclerosis, advancing age, and cardiac dysfunction, will again only impact on cerebral blood flow if pressure is low. Cerebral blood flow is generally held constant by the ability of the brain to autoregulate its own blood flow all the time systemic pressure is sufficient. Blood viscosity changes may have an impact on flow and it is acknowledged that if the patient is anaemic, flow is increased (less resistance to flow) whereas polycythaemia may decrease flow (increased resistance to flow).

Intracerebral factors:

The primary intracerebral factors are cerebral vascular artery disease and increased intracranial pressure (ICP). Widespread cerebral vascular disease can cause increased cerebral vascular resistance and hence decrease flow. Raised intracranial pressure increases the pressure within the brain that the blood has to flow against, deceasing overall perfusion. Additional changes to blood flow will occur in relation to chemical changes within the brain (see Table 4.1).

In terms of blood flow to the brain, it is usually considered more appropriate to consider cerebral perfusion pressure. Cerebral perfusion pressure (CPP) is an estimate of the adequacy of cerebral circulation and the calculation is:

$$CPP = MAP - ICP$$

Normal CPP is 60–70 mmHg. It is not directly possible to measure this in a ward/high dependency unit environment, since the equation for CPP necessitates the measurement of ICP. In ward terms it is useful to monitor systemic blood pressure whilst considering any impact potential neurological damage may have on ICP.

Compensation

The brain is able, to an extent, to compensate for slight changes in ICP. According to the Monro–Kelly hypothesis, the skull is a rigid box filled to capacity with non-compressible contents: 80% brain, 10% CSF, and 10% blood. The volume of each of these should remain constant. If there is an increase in any of these then ICP will rise unless compensation occurs. Compensation within the skull is limited and is dependent on altering one of the contents, usually blood or CSF (since it is not possible to decrease amount of brain tissue). This can be done by:

♦ increasing CSF absorption
♦ decreasing CSF production
♦ shunting of CSF to the spinal column
♦ alterations in cerebral blood flow(vasoconstriction).

The ability to compensate is small and if not treated quickly the patient's ICP will rise and cause further problems with cerebral blood flow.

Table 4.1 Factors affecting cerebral blood flow

Chemical change	Net effect
Increased CO_2	Cerebral vasodilatation
Decreased CO_2	Cerebral vasoconstriction
Decreased oxygen	Vasodilatation
Increased H^+ concentration	Vasodilatation

Pathophysiology of cerebral ischaemia

Patients with neurological damage are usually affected by secondary injury that worsens the effect of their original condition/injury. The secondary injury is usually related to problems where metabolism of neurons exceeds blood flow, resulting in ischaemia. When the brain is deprived of oxygen (for whatever reason) a chain of events occurs called the ischaemic cascade. The end point of this cascade is neuronal dysfunction and then death. In the centre of the ischaemic area (referred to as the penumbra) are a number of minimally surviving cells. The lack of O_2 and CO_2 causes these cells to switch to anaerobic metabolism, with a resultant decrease in adenosine triphosphate (ATP) production. ATP is required to power neurotransmission. The process of anaerobic metabolism causes the release of an excitatory neurotransmitter glutamate, which has a neurotoxic effect and ultimately causes cell lysis and eventual neuronal death. The survival of the penumbra neurons is dependent on the re-establishment of effective cerebral circulation. If the cells of the penumbra die, the core of dead tissue increases and ultimately causes cerebral oedema and eventual death if not treated quickly. Nursing management needs to be effective to prevent further deterioration.

Nursing management of neurological conditions

Nursing management of this group of patients has some common features. Specific management will be detailed under specific subheadings. The main aim of treating patients with neurological injury is to prevent secondary damage and the cascade of problems that may lead to cerebral ischaemia and further neuronal death. It is vital that neuronal function is optimized to facilitate patient recovery and prevent further neurological deterioration. Care should be aimed at:

♦ accurate and timely neurological assessment

♦ management of symptoms to prevent secondary damage

♦ timely nursing/medical intervention.

Of these management tools, the most important is neurological assessment and this will be discussed in detail as it is a fundamental part of neurological care. Early diagnosis of problems will lead to timely treatment that may reduce the impact of damage. It is essential that all staff should understand how to perform neurological assessment correctly so that early changes can be identified and treated promptly. Timely escalation of the patient with neurological problems is vital.

Nursing assessment

Neurological assessment is carried out for a wide variety of reasons. The depth of neurological assessment varies between practitioners. Doctors will conduct a more in-depth neurological assessment that includes full neurological examination, assessment of cranial nerves, and motor/sensory function. In practice you may be asked to carry out a very simplistic assessment of neurological function (AVPU) or a more detailed assessment.

AVPU

AVPU is a very simplistic assessment that allows quick evaluation of conscious levels. It is not and should not replace a full neurological examination if the patient's condition requires this. It is a tool designed to be used in emergency situations to enable a very quick assessment of consciousness. It is ideal in the initial rapid ABCDE assessment of the acutely ill patient.

The AVPU scale is as follows:

♦ **A**lert

♦ responds to **V**oice

♦ responds to **P**ain

♦ **U**nconscious (Resuscitation Council 2006).

The AVPU scale is usually linked to a track-and-trigger scoring system and is used as part of the scoring system to detect acute deterioration (see Chapter 13). It may be necessary to conduct an in-depth neurological assessment following initial scoring.

There are a number of reasons to conduct an in-depth neurological assessment. These include:

♦ to establish a baseline of the patient's neurological function

♦ to determine whether the patient has a neurological condition

♦ to determine if the neurological condition is deteriorating

♦ to detect life-threatening situations and those that require immediate intervention

♦ to establish the impact of neurological illness on a patient (Shah, 1999).

Consciousness

The most significant indicator of neurological deterioration is changes in levels of consciousness. Consciousness is described as a state of general awareness of oneself and the environment (Hickey 2003). Consciousness is a dynamic state and levels of consciousness can change very rapidly. Consciousness is often described as having two parts:

♦ arousal or wakefulness: concerned with patients' appearance of wakefulness

♦ cognition: cerebral mental functions.

Physiologically there are a number of systems that contribute to arousal and consciousness: the reticular formation (a complex network of nerve fibres/tracts) and the reticular activating system (a series of interrelated neurons). It is essential that both of these components function to allow arousal from sleep and wakefulness, and focused attention. A number of factors may affect consciousness in the clinical environment and changes in levels of consciousness may be neurological in origin or be systemic/metabolic (see Table 4.2).

Subjective versus objective assessment

Various terms are used to describe alterations in consciousness. Theses include:

♦ fully conscious

♦ confused

♦ lethargic

♦ obtunded

Table 4.2 Factors affecting consciousness

Neurological causes	Systemic/metabolic causes
Traumatic brain injury	Hypoxia
Stroke	Hypoglycaemia
Subarachnoid haemorrhage	Hypercapnea
Tumours	Hypotension
Cerebral oedema	Hepatic failure
Cerebral abscesses	Drug induced
Brain stem infarction	Alcohol induced
Convulsions	Renal insufficiency/failure

+ stuporous

+ comatose.

Physicians may use these terms in clinical discussion about patients but there is no recognized definition of these terms and use of them can cause confusion and subjective interpretation and prevents the accurate conveying of the patient's condition between practitioners. In an attempt to provide clarity and decrease the subjective nature of neurological assessment the Glasgow Coma Scale (GCS) was introduced (Teasdale & Jennett 1974). Provided this tool is used correctly it has a number of advantages, including:

+ it provides standardized, consistent assessment of consciousness

+ it is reliable

+ it can be used by different observers and still provide consistent results

+ it should provide graphical data that is easy to evaluate

+ it is quick to use

+ it facilitates communication in the multidisciplinary team (Shah 1999).

It should be noted that the GCS was not designed to be used in isolation and it should be used alongside other tools, including pupil assessment, motor function assessment, and physiological measurements.

The Glasgow Coma Scale

There is evidence that the GCS is performed poorly in clinical practice (Addison & Crawford 1999). It is vital to understand how to perform an accurate GCS to effectively assess consciousness in practice. The GCS is subdivided into three main components:

+ eye-opening

+ verbal response

+ motor response.

It is important that each of these components is assessed appropriately to ensure the assessment is accurate.

Eye-opening Assessment of eye-opening demonstrates functioning arousal mechanisms (except in the case of persistent vegetative state where patients may have sleep/wake cycles but not be aware). Patients are scored from 1–4 dependent on their response:

spontaneously (4)

to speech (3)

to pain (2)

no response (1).

Spontaneously: The highest score is when the patient has their eyes open. If the patient's eyes are not open the level of simulation required to get the patient to open their eyes is recorded.

To Speech: If the patient's eyes are closed verbal stimulus should be attempted initially. The most effective verbal stimulus is to call the patient's name in a normal tone. Care should be taken if the patient has poor hearing or requires a hearing aid or has any neurological damage that may impede hearing, e.g. acoustic neuroma.

To pain: if the patient does not respond to speech it is necessary to apply a painful stimulus. There is significant controversy within the literature as to the most appropriate painful stimuli

(Dawson & Shah 2005). It is important to state that different painful stimuli can be used when testing eye-opening, these may not be appropriate when testing motor function. When testing eye-opening it may be appropriate to use peripheral stimulation, e.g. pen pressure to side of finger. This stimulation should not be used when testing motor function. It is also appropriate to consider central stimulation, for example:

+ trapezium squeeze (this is considered the 'gold standard' and is least likely to cause any damage)
+ supraorbital pressure (not recommended if patient has facial injury).

It is a nursing responsibility to decide the most appropriate painful stimuli, having assessed their patient. The level of stimuli should be documented in the nursing notes to facilitate standardization of assessment.

No response: It is important to note whether eye closure is due to swelling. In this incidence the nurse should document 'c' on the GCS chart. Eye-opening may also be impaired if the third cranial nerve (occulomotor) is damaged, a condition known as ptsosis.

Verbal response

This should follow eye-opening assessment and assesses whether a patient is aware of themselves and the environment. It tests whether speech is comprehended and whether the patient is able to articulate, therefore testing higher cerebral functioning (Jevon 2007). Patients should be asked questions relating to time place and person. Various responses may be seen (Moore & Woodrow 2004).

Orientated: The patient is able to state where they are, who they are, what month/year it is (never ask date!), and the season. A patient who is orientated scores 5.

Confused: This covers a range of responses and the same score applies to those patients who are mildly confused and those who are extremely confused. It is worth noting if your patient varies within this range, i.e. is becoming increasingly confused, as it is important to detect subtle changes of consciousness. Confused patients have the ability to talk in sentences but cannot accurately answer some questions. A patient who is confused scores 4.

Occasional words: The patient replies in words, but these may be said at random. Sometimes shouting and use of expletives may occur. This category scores 3.

Incomprehensible sounds: No understandable language. Grunts and groans may follow painful stimuli. This category scores 2.

No response: The patient is unable to speak. It is important here to acknowledge whether patient is unable to speak (e.g. recent tracheostomy, document 't') or whether the patient has dysphasia (document 'd' in most appropriate category). Patients who have damage to the Broca's area (frontal lobe) may well be able to understand what is said to them but may be unable to give a correct response. Patients who have damage to Wernicke's area (temporal lobe) are difficult to assess as they may not fully comprehend what you are asking them. If the patient makes no verbal response, for whatever reason, they should score 1.

Other considerations include a language barrier. It is often difficult to assess patients who speak little English or who speak different languages. Care should be taken when using family members as interpreters: it is important to stress the importance of the interpreter telling the nurse exactly what the patient says. Patients who have a history of language/hearing impediments and those patients with learning disabilities may be harder to assess and this should be taken into account when developing appropriate questions.

Motor response Motor response is testing a patient's ability to follow a command. This should always record the best arm response as the test of motor function is an assessment of upper limb movement. Legs should not be used as the responses are different. Any differences in motor response should not be documented here, merely the best response. Use of leg response may be testing spinal reflex and is not recommended (Hickey 2003).Useful tests include asking the patient to lift their arms, holding the thumb up or squeezing the fingers (note that it is essential if using the squeeze method that patients are instructed to 'squeeze and let go'). Patients with severe brain damage may demonstrate primitive reflexes. This is not a test of strength, so even mild movement in response to command is indicative of ability to respond. A central source of pain should always be used to eliminate the risk of a spinal reflex being documented inaccurately.

Obeys commands: Patients who are able to obey commands score 6.

Localizes to pain: There is purposeful movement to remove noxious stimuli. Shah (1999) and Moore & Woodrow (2004) both stress the need to apply central pain above the level of the chin, e.g. trapezium squeeze or supraorbital pressure. It is stressed that for true localization to occur, the patient should bring their hand up above the level of the chin (for this reason sternal rub is not recommended as it may be difficult to differentiate between true localization and flexion to pain). This category scores 5.

Flexion/withdrawal to pain: Different GCS tools use slightly different categories. Specialist neurological centres are likely to use the term 'flexion', more general hospitals may use term 'withdraw'. In this response patients flex their arm towards the source of pain but do not localize. This category scores 4.

Abnormal flexion: This represents severe damage to the nerve pathways. The patient will flex the arm at the elbow and rotate the wrist simultaneously in response to painful stimuli. This category scores 3.

Extension to pain: This also represents severe damage at brain stem level and indicates that messages are not able to extend to the cerebral hemispheres due to damage. Presence of extension usually indicates a poor prognosis. The patient will extend or straighten their arm at the elbow and may rotate the arm inwards. This category scores 2.

No response: This is an extremely poor sign, usually indicative of 'brain stem death'. It is important to rule out any spinal cord damage or the presence of muscle paralysis medication as both of these may affect the patient's ability to move their limbs.

Once the GCS is completed the nurse should graphically document these findings on a neurological assessment chart. It is important to note that when conveying information to other members of the team about the patient it is more useful to state where deficit is occurring (see Table 4.3).

Having completed the GCS the practitioner also needs to complete a pupil examination, assessment of motor function (to detect weaknesses), and physiological observations. These assessments are not part of the GCS but should be performed to give an overall impression of the patient's neurological status.

Table 4.3 Score divisions within the Glasgow Coma Scale

Normal Glasgow Coma Scale	Abnormal Glasgow Coma Scale (confused/sleepy)
E = 4	E = 3
V = 5	V = 4
M = 6	M = 6
Total = 15	Total = 13

E, eye-opening; V, verbal response; M, motor response.

Pupil responses

Normal pupil size ranges from 2 to 6 mm, and this can be influenced by the amount of light present — pupils will constrict in very light environments and dilate in darkened environments (Blows 2001). Pupil assessment is important and is the only cranial nerve assessment to be performed by ward staff. Cranial nerve iii (occulomotor) and to some extent cranial nerve ii (optic) are both tested. In health, the activation of a reflex arc will cause pupil constriction if a bright light is shone into the pupil. Additionally, the other pupil should produce a consensual reaction (i.e. constrict when a light is shone into the other pupil). The consensual reflex (indirect reaction) may be less than the reaction of the directly tested eye. The consensual reaction occurs as a result of the cranial nerve fibres crossing at the optic chiasma and the posterior part of the mid brain (Hickey 2003). Pupil abnormality is a late but important indicator of neurological deterioration and, taken in association with other neurological changes, is an indication of increasing ICP (Dawes *et al.* 2007). Cerebral oedema causes a partial herniation of the temporal lobe through the tentorium and places pressure on the occulomotor nerve, causing pupillary changes. Initially, pupil changes will be on the same side as the cerebral damage (ipsilateral changes), but as cerebral oedema worsens the other side will be affected and the patient will have contralateral changes. As the pressure increases on the cranial nerve the patient may present with the following progression of changes:

♦ pupil shape becomes ovoid

♦ pupil begins to dilate on affected side

♦ pupil fixes on affected side

♦ contra lateral changes occur.

The speed of these changes is dependent on the speed of the swelling and may happen very quickly in some patients.

Pupils should be examined for size, shape, and equality. The size documented on the chart should be the size of the pupil prior to direct light testing. It is worth noting that about 12–17% of the population have unequal pupils, with no underlying pathophysiology (Hickey 2003). However, in clinical practice abnormalities should be considered abnormal until proven otherwise.

Assessment of the pupil should follow the following stages (Shah 1999):

♦ looking at the size of the resting pupil of both eyes

♦ looking at the shape of the resting pupil of both eyes

♦ looking to see if both pupils are equal

♦ looking to see if both pupils react to light

♦ looking for a consensual reaction.

Pupil reaction should be recorded as + (brisk), − (negative), or sl (sluggish). Any changes to pupil shape and size should be quickly reported as urgent action/treatment may be required.

Assessment of motor function

The GCS is only required to assess best motor function and any differentiation in sides is not noted on that part of the assessment form. The motor function assessment is supplemental to the assessment of consciousness but provides additional information about the overall function of the nervous system. It is here where weaknesses and information on developing hemiparesis are recorded. An increasing weakness on one side may indicate further damage/swelling and is often a good indicator of further deterioration in subarachnoid haemorrhage patients and patients with

Table 4.4 Objective classification of motor function

Classification	Criteria
Normal power	Patient is able to match resistance applied by the observer, i.e. they are able to hold up the limb and resist moderate efforts to push limb down
Mild weakness	Patient is able to hold up limb against mild resistance but this may be overcome if resistance is increased slightly
Severe weakness	Patient is able to move limb but not against resistance
Flexion Extension No response	This is in response to central pain stimulus Pain should only be used if there is no spontaneous movement from the patient

traumatic brain injury. It is important to note that motor weakness is usually seen on the opposite side of the body to the damage. This is because the motor fibre tracts or pyramids swap sides at the medulla oblongata (decussation of pyramids), hence the right side of the brain controls the left side of the body below this level.

Motor function is assessed through the patient's ability to overcome weakness. There is a tendency for this to be a little subjective and it is recommended that specific criteria are used (see Table 4.4).

It is acceptable practice to note on this part of the assessment tool whether there is a difference between limbs and to plot this accordingly using L (left)/R (right) symbols. If motor response is the same a single dot will suffice.

Assessment of physiological status

It is important to record the patient's physiological status once the other parts of the neurological assessment are complete. There is a pattern of recognized changes in physiological measurements that may indicate that the patient's condition is deteriorating (Crawford & Guerro 2004). Again these are quite a late sign and it is probable that changes in levels of consciousness will have been noticed first.

As the patient's neurological condition deteriorates as a result of increasing ICP (see section on damage to the nervous system), changes in physiological measurements occur. These are referred to as the Cushing's triad and include the following.

Increased blood pressure There is an increase in blood pressure with a widening of the pulse pressure. The increasing blood pressure is the body's attempt to maintain cerebral perfusion as the ICP increases.

Bradycardia Bradycardia is caused by midbrain compression. As ICP increases, pressure is increased on the vagus nerve, which in turn causes a slowing of the heart rate.

Alterations to respiratory rate As the respiratory centres within the brain are compressed, the patient may show signs of respiratory alteration. In the initial stages there may be a decrease in respiration, but as ICP increases there is sometimes an increased respiratory rate. Abnormal patterns of respiration may be seen.

Temperature Temperature is not part of the Cushing's triad but damage to the hypothalamus due to oedema may result in pyrexia. Pyrexia can be of other origins and it is useful to exclude infection as cause of pyrexia.

Any indications that the patient is presenting with Cushing's triad signs (hypertension, brady-cardia, decreased respirations) should be reported promptly as they may indicate a potentially lethal rise in ICP.

Frequency of neurological observations

There is no real consensus about the frequency of neurological observations (Mooney & Comerford 2005). The only group of patients for whom there are specific guidelines are those with traumatic brain injury. The NICE guidelines (2007) highlight that the risk of intracranial complications is greatest in the first 6 h after injury. They state that observations should be recorded most frequently during this period. For this group of patients NICE (2007) base the frequency of observations on the initial GCS score. They state that GCS should be recorded half hourly until GCS has returned to 14. In those patients whose GCS is 15, observations should be recorded:

♦ half hourly for 2 h
♦ 1 hourly for 4 h
♦ 2 hourly thereafter.

It may be necessary to record the observations more frequently in unstable patients. It is also necessary to increase the frequency of observations if there is a decrease in the GCS (NICE 2007).

It is important that the practitioner uses the assessment tool with care. It is vital to note that no single change is more important than another and changes must be reported to enable timely and appropriate intervention. The practitioner should continue to use professional judgement if they feel the patient is deteriorating. NICE (2007) have issued some guidelines relating to changes that may require review. Although these are explicitly written for head-injured patients they are also applicable to other patients. NICE (2007) suggest urgent attention should be sought if:

♦ there is development of agitation or abnormal behaviour
♦ there is a sustained drop of 1 point in GCS (greater weight if this is related to motor function)
♦ there is any drop in the GCS of greater than 2 points, regardless of the time or GCS subscale
♦ there is development of new or increasing headache
♦ there are new or evolving neurological symptoms, e.g. pupil, limb, or facial movement asymmetry.

NICE (2007) also suggest that, in order to avoid interobserver reliability issues (and unnecessary referrals), a second member of staff who is competent to perform assessment should confirm deterioration immediately before informing the doctor. If this is not possible and there is

---

Clinical link 4.1 (see Appendix for answers)

A patient is admitted to your ward following a fall from a ladder. The GCS is initially 15 and you have been asked to observe this patient.
Consider the neurological observation (see Figure 4.4) of the patient and discuss:

♦ the frequency of observations
♦ the trigger for medical review
♦ the significance of drop in GCS and changes in motor function.

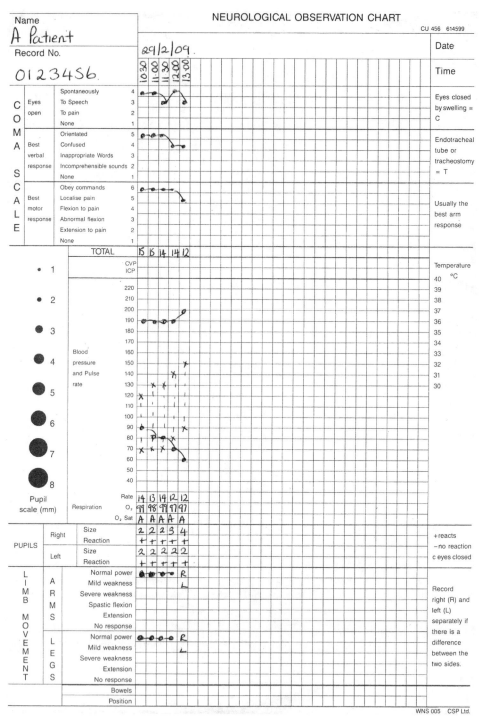

Figure 4.4 Neurological observation chart.

concern, medical contact without confirmation should occur. Rapid escalation of the deteriorating patient is vital and any cause for concern in relation to neurological deterioration should be reported to the medical staff immediately.

Common neurological disorders

Stroke

Care of the acute stroke patient

Around 150,000 people per year have a suspected transient ischaemic attack (TIA) or mild stroke and there is a 20% risk of stroke within the first 4 weeks after a TIA (Royal College of Physicians 2004). About two-thirds of these patients are nursed on a ward for all or some part of their hospital stay (Department of Health 2007). Recent Department of Health documents have stressed the need for a more urgent response to stroke and TIAs. Early assessment and intervention has been shown to halt the progression of stroke, limit neuronal death, and decrease morbidity (Rothwell 2007). It is suggested that those patients who receive care for strokes in an appropriate centre have better outcomes. The National Service Framework for older people (Standard 5) highlights that all people thought to have had a stroke should have:

+ access to appropriate diagnostic service
+ treatment by a specialist stroke team
+ access to multidisciplinary programme of prevention and rehabilitation.

The NICE guidelines (2008) make explicit recommendations for the admission of stroke patients to a specialist acute stroke unit where there is access to:

+ a separate ward area dedicated to stroke management
+ a specialist stroke multidisciplinary team
+ immediate computerized tomography (CT) scanning and imaging
+ continuous haemodynamic monitoring
+ thrombolytic therapy where indicated.

Pathophysiology of stroke

Ischaemic stroke Ischaemic stroke accounts for 85% of all strokes. This is further broken down into:

+ atherosclerotic cerebral vascular stroke: extra- and intracranial arteries are narrowed by arteriosclerotic changes; this is worsened by associated atheroma which can be the site for thrombus development. Around 40% of these patients will experience TIA before the stroke occurs (Hickey 2003).
+ small artery penetrating stroke (lucunar stroke): a lucune describes a small cavity that develops after the necrotic tissue from a deep infarct is removed. Although often small in size, the consequences can be devastating and are dependent on the area of injury.
+ cardiogenic embolic stroke: often caused by emboli from atrial fibrillation, valve disease, and other cardiac problems. Microemboli from the left side of the heart move, commonly through the carotid arteries. This often blocks the left middle cerebral artery as it is a relatively straight vessel and offers little resistance.
+ cryptogenic stroke: cause unknown
+ other causes: these include coagulopathies, vasospasm. and substance misuse.

All of these types of ischaemic stroke cause the same effect. Ischaemic stroke will lead to narrowing of the blood vessels, which causes ischaemia. If ischaemia is for a prolonged period of time this may lead to areas of infarction that will perpetuate the ischaemic cascade discussed earlier.

Haemorrhagic stroke Haemorrhagic stroke accounts for 15% of strokes. This is further subdivided into:

+ intracerebral stroke: bleeding into the brain caused by rupture of a small artery, often related to prolonged periods of poorly controlled hypertension
+ subarachnoid haemorrhage (SAH): bleeding into the subarachnoid space usually related to aneurysm (refer to section on SAH).

Haemorrhagic stroke leads to an immediate rise in ICP because blood from the bleeding artery causes an intracerebral haematoma that displaces brain tissue. Some degree of compensation may occur, but if the bleed is large enough then the associated ischaemic cascade discussed earlier will be triggered.

Patient presentation

This will vary according to the area of the brain involved and the severity of stroke. Signs and symptoms include (Dawson & Shah 2005):

+ reduced levels of consciousness
+ hemiparesis or hemiplegia
+ right or left hemianopias (loss of visual fields unilaterally)
+ deviation of head/eyes to one side (same side as stroke)
+ dysphasia
+ inattention to one side of the body(opposite side to stroke).

The Department of Health has launched an advertising campaign that aims to encourage people to recognize and respond to signs and symptoms of acute stroke. The campaign uses the FAST acronym to help identify changes:

Facial weakness

Arm weakness

Speech disturbance

Time to seek help

Treatment

Treatment is dependent on cause of the stroke and immediate CT to establish whether the stroke is ischaemic or haemorrhagic is essential, as the treatment is different and misdiagnosis could have disastrous consequences.

Ischaemic stroke Thrombolysis is an effective treatment but it must be administered within 3 h of the patient's onset of symptoms (this time window may change as evidence develops). If there is a delay in diagnosis then it is not appropriate, as it is unlikely to be effective (Department of Health 2007). It is thought that 1.9 million neurons are lost for each minute a stroke is untreated (Department of Health 2007). Conservative management is appropriate if thrombolysis is not indicated. Early anticoagulation therapy should be given. NICE (2008) recommend that aspirin is administered within 24 h of the onset of symptoms (unless there is a history of allergy), either orally or rectally.

Haemorrhagic stroke Management is symptom related. It may be necessary to remove the haematoma if it is large, and this would be performed in a specialist neurological centre. Protocols should be available for referral of appropriate patients (NICE 2008).

Thrombolytic therapy NICE (2008) highlights the significant improvement in outcome that thrombolytic therapy may have if given early, but it is not without risks and they report a 6% incidence of haemorrhage. The guidance makes the following recommendations:

♦ Thrombolytic therapy should be given in the first 3 h of symptom development.

♦ It should only be given if brain haemorrhage has been definitively excluded by imaging.

♦ Tissue plasminogen activator (t-PA) is the drug of choice and manufacturer's recommendations should be adhered to.

Thrombolytic therapy should only be administered:

♦ if staff are trained in delivery of the drug and understand potential complications

♦ in units that can provide care for level 1 and 2 patients (see Table 1.1 in Chapter 1)

♦ in units with immediate access to imaging, where staff are skilled at image interpretation.

Nursing care The immediate focus of nursing care of the patient following stroke involves many different factors (see Table 4.5). Long term stroke care and rehabilitation is significant but beyond the focus of this book.

Subarachnoid haemorrhage

Care of the patient following subarachnoid haemorrhage

Although technically a form of stroke, subarachnoid haemorrhage (SAH) is discussed separately as its treatment and management is different from other forms of stroke. SAH accounts for 5% of strokes. The incidence of SAH is 6–7 per 100,000 of the population (Van Gijn *et al.* 2007). Approximately half of those patients who have a SAH are under 55 years of age. The mortality rate, despite advances in treatment, remains high at about 50% (this includes the 10% of patients who die immediately post SAH). The morbidity rate is also high and approximately one-third of patients will be left with some degree of neurological dysfunction (Al Shahi 2006). Timely and effective diagnosis and treatment is vital.

Clinical link 4.2 (see Appendix for answers)

A 67-year-old man is admitted to your ward following diagnosis of stroke. He delayed seeking medical attention and therefore was not an appropriate candidate for thrombolytic therapy. He has suffered a left-sided stroke with a right sided weakness. His blood pressure is 187/112 and he has a prominent facial weakness of the left and is dribbling/spluttering. Consider the following:

♦ What are his potential nursing problems and associated management?

♦ What are your nursing priorities (and why)?

♦ What other members of the multidisciplinary team will need to review this patient's care?

Table 4.5 Nursing care of the patient following stroke

Potential problem	Nursing care
Ineffective airway due to deteriorating consciousness levels	• Careful positioning to maintain airway • Elevation of head of bed to 30° • Use of airway adjuncts; consider anaesthetic referral if Glasgow Coma Scale below 8 • Suctioning and oxygen as required
Potential deterioration of respiratory function	• Monitor respiratory rate • Provide supplemental oxygen if saturations below 95% (NICE 2008) • Appropriate respiratory assessment (see Chapter 2) • Physiotherapy
Risk of aspiration (see nutrition)	• A swallow screen should be carried out before anything is given orally. This should occur in first 24 h. Patients should remain nil by mouth until this. • Patients with swallow difficulties should have a swallow assessment by an appropriately trained specialist • Elevation of head of bed to 30°
Potential neurological deterioration	• Neurological assessment is paramount • Maintain venous return from brain by elevation of head of bed to 30° • Maintain patient's head in neutral alignment • Avoid activities that may increase intracranial pressure • Ensure analgesia if required
Hypertension	• Monitor blood pressure/pulse • Report significant changes immediately • Hypertension may only be treated if evidence of a hypertensive emergency (NICE 2008) • Blood pressure reduction to 185/110 mmHg should be considered if thombolysis indicated (NICE 2008)
Pyrexia	• Monitor temperature • Temperature may increase post stroke but important to eliminate infection as cause • Conservative management of pyrexia
Blood glucose instability	• High glucose levels will increase intracranial pressure • Maintenance of blood glucose within range of 4–11 mmol (NICE 2008) using intravenous insulin if necessary
Risk of dehydration	• Establish intravenous insertion • Fluid balance chart/24 h balance • Observe for signs of dehydration/fluid overload (see Chapter 7)
Nutrition	• Patients who are unable to swallow will require nasogastric feeding and referral to dietician • Patients should have nutritional assessment and assessed regularly for risk of malnutrition
Communication difficulties	• Assess type of deficit • Develop appropriate communication methods • Speech and language therapist assessment

Hickey (2003); Hinkle & McKenna Guanci (2007); Jones et al. (2007); NICE (2008).

Pathophysiology of subarachnoid haemorrhage

Approximately 85% of SAH are caused by ruptured cerebral aneurysms. An aneurysm is a weakness in the cerebral artery wall. Aneurysms normally occur at the bifurcations and branches of large arteries. Studies suggest that 85% occur in the anterior part of the circle of Willis, the remaining 15% in the posterior circulation. Although the exact cause of aneurysms is not fully understood, there are some common risks factors, including hypertension, smoking, and excessive alcohol intake. At the time of aneurysm rupture, arterial blood (under high pressure) is forced into the subarachnoid space. Tissues surrounding the aneurysm stop the initial bleeding and the coagulation process forms a plug, which seals off the initial bleed. The blood that has entered the subarachnoid space is irritant and sets up an inflammatory response that enhances cerebral oedema and causes later secondary damage. At the time of rupture, significant subarachnoid haemorrhage occurs, which rapidly increases ICP/decreases the level of cerebral perfusion and this may lead to a transient loss of consciousness (Hickey 2003).

Patient presentation

Signs and symptoms of SAH depend on the severity and region of the injury and include:

- sudden thunderclap headache 'the worst of my life'
- loss of consciousness/decreased level of consciousness
- motor dysfunction, e.g. hemiparesis/hemiplegia
- potential speech deficits
- signs of menigeal irritation, including:
  - neck stiffness
  - vomiting
  - back/neck pain
  - blurred vision
  - photophobia

Later symptoms include:

- increased cerebral oedema
- increased ICP
- pituitary dysfunction (electrolyte imbalance)
- delayed ischaemic neurological deficit (prevalence 30%).

Diagnosis of SAH

No single clinical feature is sufficiently reliable to make diagnosis, and it is usually made by a combination of the following:

- history and neurological examination
- CT scan/magnetic resonance imaging scan
- cerebral angiography
- lumbar puncture may be used with caution.

Treatment

Immediate treatment is dependent on the severity of SAH. A number of factors are used to determine this, including patient's age, comorbidity, and time from onset of aneurysm. Severity of SAH can also be classified in accordance with the World Federation of Neurological Surgeons

Table 4.6 WFNS scale

WFNS scale	Glasgow Coma Scale	Motor deficit
i	15	Absent
ii	14–13	Absent
iii	14–13	Present
iv	12–7	Present or absent
v	6–3	Present or absent

scale (WFNS, see Table 4.6), although other scales may be used (Cavanaugh & Gordon 2002). These help to determine how and when the aneurysm should be secured. The main aim is to prevent rebleeding, but it should be noted that securing the aneurysm is only part of the treatment process. Effective management post intervention is essential to prevent further complications.

Intervention for treatable aneurysms is either by:

♦ neurosurgical clipping: the goal of which is to prevent rebleeding by securing the neck of the aneurysm with a clip or

♦ endovascular occlusion using coils 'coiling', which involves packing the aneurysm with platinum coils to facilitate clotting within the aneurysm to prevent rebleeding.

Treatment is usually offered within first 72 h to suitable patients.

Immediate nursing care Patients who are suitable for aneurysm treatment should be promptly referred to a neuroscience centre for supportive treatment and prevention of complications. Initial ward management is aimed at observation and prevention of complications, e.g. rebleeding (approximately 15% of patients rebleed in the first day (Van Gijn *et al.* 2007), see Table 4.7).

Complications of SAH

These include:

♦ delayed neurological deficit (vasospasm)

♦ hydrocephalus

♦ further bleeds

♦ neurological deterioration

♦ development of permanent neurological deficit.

Once the patient receives appropriate intervention to secure the aneurysm, treatment may alter to focus on triple-H therapy (hypertension, hypervolaemia, haemodilution). This is usually provided in specialist neuroscience centres (Ogungbo *et al.* 2005).

Mild head injury

Care of the patient following mild head injury

Approximately 700,000 people attend emergency departments each year following traumatic head injury (NICE 2007). The most common causes of injury include falls, road traffic accidents, and assault. Of these patients:

♦ 90% are classified as minor or mild (GCS 13–15)

♦ 5% are moderate (GCS 9–12)

♦ 5% are serious (GCS 3–8).

Clinical link 4.3 (see Appendix for answers)

A 45-year-old lady is admitted to a medical assessment unit, awaiting transfer to a neuro-science unit. On admission her GCS is 15, her WFNS is 1. She is complaining of severe head ache and nausea. She has not eaten or drunk anything since admission and is feeling very thirsty. She is complaining of photophobia and neck stiffness. Her intravenous insertion has tissued and needs replacing.

♦ What are your nursing priorities (and why)?

The patient and her family are extremely anxious and she asks for more information. She demands to know when she will be transferred to the neurological centre and what treatment is best.

♦ How will you deal with this lady's anxiety?

♦ What information will you provide regarding transfer and subsequent treatment?

Patients with moderate/serious head injuries will normally receive specialist or ITU care. Of the 90% with mild head injury, some may be admitted to a ward for observation of their condition. NICE (2007) have identified those patients who should remain in hospital for observation or treatment. These include:

♦ patients with significant abnormalities on imaging (likely to be transferred to a neuroscience centre)

♦ patients whose GCS has not returned to 15, regardless of imaging results

♦ patients who fulfil the criteria for scanning (see Table 4.8), but cannot be scanned because of resourcing issues/insufficient cooperation for scanning

♦ continuing worrying signs (e.g. persistent vomiting, severe headache)

♦ other sources of concern (e.g. alcohol intoxication, other injuries, CSF leak).

Pathophysiology of head injury

The primary head injury is the injury that occurs at the time of the accident, causing damage to cell structure and function and potential cell death (Littlejohn *et al.* 2003). Injury can happen as a consequence of acceleration (when a moving object hits a stationary head, e.g. a blow from a blunt object) or deceleration (when the head hits a stationary object, e.g. a windscreen). In addition the patient's head may be subject to rotational forces causing stretching and shearing of the nerve fibre (Dawson & Shah 2005). Primary injury is irreversible and the damage cannot be repaired.

Secondary injury occurs as a response to damage from the primary injury. It includes factors such as cerebral oedema, ischaemia, and chemical changes as a result of trauma (Littlejohn *et al.* 2003). Nursing management is aimed at the prevention of secondary injury and is potentially reversible.

A careful history will be taken of the mechanism of injury as this will enable greater understanding of the likely injury. Injuries are further classified as either focal or diffuse.

Focal injury Focal injuries have an identifiable focus to the injury, which may be treated surgically. Classifications of focal injury include:

♦ contusions: bruising to the surface of the brain that may give rise to decreased consciousness and development of cerebral oedema

Table 4.7 Nursing care of the patient following subarchnoid haemorrhage

Potential problem	Nursing care
Potential neurological deterioration	• Frequent neurological observation • Assess and report any changes in Glasgow Coma Scale quickly, a change of just 1 point may be sign of complications • Report any changes in motor function/focal neurological deficits/cranial nerve deficits quickly • Monitor for complications of subarachnoid haemorrhage
Pain	• Assess location and severity of pain • Administer prescribed analgesia (this may be paracetamol and/or other opiate based analgesia, e.g. codeine) • Avoid overstimulation • Patient may prefer darkened room if photophobic • Reduction in activity • Psychological support • Administer antiemetic if nausea and vomiting associated with drugs or condition
Prevention of rebleeding 1	• Patient should be placed on complete bed rest • Anti-embolic stockings/intermittent pneumatic compression (e.g. flotron boots)
Prevention of rebleeding 2: blood pressure control	• Blood pressure should be carefully monitored as extreme hypertension will increase risk of rebleed • Blood pressure should be kept at systolic of >130 mmHg and <180 mmHg (Dawson & Shah 2005) • Antihypertensive drugs should be used with extreme caution • Hypotension should be promptly treated
Prevention of rebleeding 3: constipation	• Analgesia likely to cause constipation • Straining at stool increases likelihood of rebleed • Bowel management program with stool softeners is essential
Fluid balance/ maintenance of hydration	• Intravenous line mandatory • Give at least 3 L of fluid in 24 h • Insert indwelling catheter • Compensate for negative fluid balance and for high temperature • Electrolyte monitoring (at least daily) • Assess and treat severe emesis/prevent dehydration
Drug therapy	• Nimodipine is recommended for the prevention of delayed neurological deficit (shown to enhance collateral blood flow and improve long term outcome (Hickey 2003) • Phenytoin may be required if patient has had a seizure, not normally given as prophylaxis (Al Shahi et al. 2006)
Reduction in anxiety	• Assess patient for signs of anxiety • Endeavour to identify source of anxiety • Offer reassurance as appropriate • Keep patient and family informed of progress/treatment changes

♦ haemorrhage/haematoma formation, including:

• extradural haematoma: bleeding between the periosteum and dura mater

• subdural haematoma: bleeding between the dura mater and subarachnoid layer, often classified according to speed of onset into acute (immediate), subacute (between 48 h and 2 weeks), and chronic (after 2 weeks)

Table 4.8 NICE recommended criteria for CT scanning

Criteria for scanning

Glasgow Coma Scale less than 13 at any point since admission

Glasgow Coma Scale equal to 13 or 14 2 hours post injury

Suspected open or depressed fracture

Any sign of basal skull fracture

Post-traumatic seizure

Focal neurological deficit/amnesia for more than 30 min

More than one episode of vomiting (clinical judgement may be used)

Additional categories of patients requiring scanning

Patient aged over 65 years

Coagulopathy, including history of bleeding, clotting disorder, current treatment with warfarin

Dangerous mechanism of injury (e.g. fall from higher than 1 m)

NICE (2007).

- intracerebral haematomas: bleeding into the brain parenchyma rather than meninges, which is often related to further bleeding post-contusion injury.

These patients usually require transfer to a neuroscience centre for surgical treatment and evacuation of these injuries.

Diffuse injury Diffuse injuries are injuries that are widespread and have no particular focus. They are usually treated conservatively with appropriate medical management and include:

- concussion: occurs as a result of brain acceleration/deceleration injury. Concussion means 'to shake violently' and can follow trauma to the head. Patients may experience a loss of consciousness. CT scan is usually normal.
- acute axonal/diffuse injury: often follows road accidents and is caused by a mechanical shearing of the axons. Initial CT changes are minimal but often the patient is deeply unconscious. These patients often require specialist ITU nursing care.

Treatment of head injury

Treatment of head injury is dependent on the nature of the head injury.

Focal injuries The majority of patients with focal head injury will be transferred to a neuroscience centre for surgical intervention. If the bleed is minor, e.g. chronic small subdural haematoma, they may potentially be referred to a ward whilst awaiting an available bed.

Diffuse head injuries Patients with diffuse head injuries may be transferred to a neuroscience centre for conservative management. Those patients with severe diffuse head injury will probably require an ITU bed.

Most patients with minor head injury who fulfil the requirement of NICE guidelines for hospital admission will be admitted for general observation and only transferred to a neurological centre if their condition worsens/does not improve.

Nursing management

Nursing management of the patient with minor head injury largely revolves around accurate neurological assessment and immediate reporting and action on deteriorating neurological function. Other issues may be pertinent (see Table 4.9).

Table 4.9 Nursing care of the patient following head injury

Potential problem	Nursing care
Neurological deterioration 1	Neurological assessment to include GCS, pupil size and reactivity, limb movement, respiratory rate, heart rate, blood pressure, temperature, oxygen saturation
	The NICE guidelines suggest the frequency should be determined upon neurological deficit, therefore if GCS below 14, half hourly observations are required. If GCS returns to 15 then observations should be recorded half hourly for 2 h, hourly for 4 h, 2 hourly thereafter until discharge.
	Care should be taken to report any deterioration immediately. Doctors should be prepared to liaise with neurosurgical team if patient's condition deteriorates.
Neurological deterioration 2	The following criteria should be used as a guide for reporting any deterioration (NICE 2007): • there is development of agitation or abnormal behaviour • there is a sustained drop of 1 point in GCS (greater weight if this is related to motor function) • any drop in the GCS of greater than 2 points regardless of the time or GCS subscale • development of new or increasing headache • new or evolving neurological symptoms, e.g. pupil, limb, or facial movement asymmetry
Potential dehydration	Dehydration is damaging to the neurological patient so it is important to ensure adequate fluid intake. This may be oral fluids if tolerated or intravenous infusion. This is of particular importance if the patient appears to have been drinking alcohol because of the diuretic effects. Fluid balance should be recorded.
Headache	Patients may experience pain due to injury. It is important to offer adequate analgesia, but at the same time important to ensure that analgesia will not affect neurological assessment. Paracetamol and codeine are useful analgesia in the management of headache. Stronger opiates may make the patient drowsy and compound the difficulties with adequate assessment.
Maintaining a safe environment	It is important to ensure a safe environment is maintained at all times. Consideration should be given to: • location of patient's bed to enable close supervision • use of pillows and other protective equipment to protect patient from injury • close supervision at all times
Patient positioning	A quiet environment is useful especially if the patient has severe headache/photophobia
	Patient should not be nursed flat and kept at 30° to facilitate venous return
Treatment of other injuries	Other injuries should have been assessed and documented in the emergency department
	Observe for any other injuries and take appropriate action

GCS, Glasgow Coma Scale.

Neurological assessment and alcohol consumption

Increasingly nurses are caring for patients admitted with head injury following the consumption of alcohol (Iankova 2006). This can sometimes make neurological assessment difficult. When patients are admitted and smell strongly of alcohol, healthcare professionals may assume the changes in the patient's condition are related to alcohol rather than injury. Alcohol consumption may affect basic physiological and psychological processes and may result in difficulties in thinking rationally, slurring of speech, and irrational behaviour. These behaviours are also associated with head injury and neurological deterioration. NICE (2007) stress the importance of excluding any serious head injury that may be causing this behaviour. They stress the importance of avoiding ascribing changes in conscious level to alcohol and stress the need to treat all patients, irrespective of alcohol consumption, as potential head injury patients. Assessment should follow the NICE guidelines and under no circumstances should neurological assessment be discontinued in this vulnerable group of patients.

Managing discharge

Once fit for discharge the nurse should ensure the patient receives appropriate advice regarding potential further deterioration/long-term consequences of mild head injury. NICE (2007) recommend that the patient should be encouraged to seek medical attention if they:

+ become unconscious (999 call)
+ become confused
+ become sleepy
+ develop problems with speech
+ develop problems with balance
+ develop a weakness in one or both arms/legs
+ develop problems with eyesight
+ develop severe headache
+ are persistently vomiting
+ have a seizure
+ have clear fluid coming out of nose/ears

In addition the patient may require referral to an acquired brain injury nurse specialist if they develop symptoms of post-concussion disorders. These can be extremely debilitating and may include memory loss, lethargy, persistent headache, fatigue, depression, and personality changes.

Seizure

Care of the patient following seizure

Seizure is a term used to describe abnormal neural activity within the brain. It is usually a single event, characterized by an alteration in the level of brain function. A seizure can occur either as a 'one off occurrence' or on a chronic level, often being referred to as epilepsy. It is argued that this term should be used with caution, as the term epilepsy/epileptic can cause the patient to be stigmatized (Dawson & Shah 2005). Epilepsy is quite common in the UK, with estimated figures of occurrence in 4–10 per 1000 of the population (Bassett & Makin 2000).

Pathophysiology

In some cases the cause of the seizure may be unknown (idiopathic); given the right circumstances any patient may experience a seizure, e.g. electrical shock, metabolic imbalance, certain drugs (Hickey 2003). Seizures are, however, more common in certain groups of patients. This includes patients with:

+ head trauma
+ central nervous system infection

Clinical link 4.4 (see Appendix for answers)

Part 1

You are caring for a 24-year-old patient admitted with mild concussion after a fight in a night club. He has a severe headache and is feeling very nauseated; his breath smells strongly of alcohol. On admission his GCS is 13. He is quite sleepy, awakes to verbal command but is aggressive and agitated when awake. He is speaking in sentences and is able to respond to command. Physiological observations are normal and pupils a size 3 and reacting to light consensually. Consider how you will:

+ manage this patient's aggression
+ ensure neurological assessment is appropriate.

Part 2

One hour after admission you note that he is sleepier and is requiring painful stimuli to awaken him; he is less agitated and once awake is able to obey commands. His pupils are a size 3 but they are ovoid and a little sluggish in reacting to light. Consider the following:

+ What is his GCS now?
+ What other assessments will you do?
+ When will you report these changes?
+ What other actions may be required?

+ cerebral tumours
+ cerebral vascular disease.

Some situations can induce a seizure. These include:

+ alcohol intoxication
+ drug overdose
+ electrolyte imbalance
+ endocrine disorders
+ pregnancy.

Seizures are caused by an alteration in the membrane potential of the neuron that creates hypersensitivity in the neuron. The hypersensitive neuron has a lower threshold for firing and can fire excessively. The cell can begin to fire repeatedly, producing sustained neural activity that results in seizure activity. During the period of the seizure there is a dramatic increase in cellular metabolism, increasing the neurons' need for glucose, oxygen, and ATP. Cerebral blood flow will increase to meet the demands of the overactive neural cells. If the seizure continues for a long period, this excessive increase in metabolic requirements can lead to cellular exhaustion and cellular destruction. The goal of nursing intervention is to prevent cellular damage caused by excessive seizure activity.

Seizures can be classified using a number of tools, the most simplistic being the international classification of epileptic seizure (ICES). This classification system divides seizures into two major categories depending on clinical observation of the seizure and EEG activity. The terms 'petit mal' and 'grand mal' are outdated terms and should not be used in clinical practice.

Partial seizures In partial seizures, clinical observation and EEG changes indicate that seizure activity is limited to one part of the cerebral hemisphere. They may be subdivided further into simple or complex partial seizures depending on whether or not consciousness is lost.

♦ Simple partial seizures: consciousness is not lost and the effects of seizure activity will be dependent upon area of brain affected. The patient may have abnormal movement or jerking of limbs/twitching of facial muscles. In some patients sensation is changed and they may complain of feelings of numbness/tingling in an area. The patient will often be quite frightened and can often explain the effects of their seizure on them. Simple seizures may evolve into complex seizure activity.

♦ Complex partial seizures: consciousness is impaired/lost and the patient will not be aware of their surroundings. Patients may present with bizarre behaviour (automatisms) or absences, or may experience hallucinations and motor disturbances, e.g. fumbling, repeated rubbing, and semi-purposeful movement. They are not aware of their behaviour (Hickey 2003; Dawson & Shah 2005).

Both types of partial seizures may terminate on their own or develop into a generalized seizure.

Generalized seizures Generalized seizures reflect involvement of both cerebral hemispheres. There are motor (movement) changes in a generalized seizure. These are usually bilateral and the patient usually loses consciousness. The symptoms of a generalized seizure are affected by the area of brain affected and different manifestations may occur. The most common generalized seizure is the tonic/clonic seizure.

♦ *Tonic/clonic seizure.* The patient may or may not experience an aura (a warning that a seizure is starting). In the tonic phase the voluntary muscles contract, the body, legs, and arms stiffens and the patient falls to the ground if standing. The muscles of the jaw cause the mouth to close tightly (this may cause the patient to bite their tongue). The bladder and (rarely) bowel will empty, the pupils dilate and are unresponsive to light. The patient will stop breathing and may become pale/cyanosed. This period usually lasts 1 min (Hickey 2003). In the clonic phase the patient will begin to develop violent, rhythmic muscular contractions accompanied by strenuous breathing (hyperventilation).The eyes may roll and there is excessive salivation/frothing at the mouth. The clonic phase usually lasts for 30 s but may be longer. After the clonic phase the patient is usually unconscious for a period of time, their extremities may be limp, they will breathe quietly, and pupils may be unequal but should respond to light. After awakening there is usually a period of confusion and amnesia and the patient may be very drowsy and sleepy. A more worrying form of this type of seizure is status epilepticus.

♦ *Status epilepticus* is defined as serial seizures without recovery of consciousness between seizures (Bassett & Makin 2000). Status epilepticus usually presents as tonic clonic seizures but it should be remembered that partial seizures can also cause continuous seizure activity and should be suspected if the patient with partial seizures have sustained significant alterations in consciousness. Status epilepticus is a medical emergency as neuronal death will quickly ensue if seizure activity is not halted.

Nursing care

Nursing care of the patient having a partial seizure largely involves observation, protecting the patient from harm, and documentation of seizure on the seizure chart. Documentation of seizure activity should include detail about:

♦ levels/alteration of consciousness

♦ presentation of seizure

Table 4.10 Nursing management of a seizure

Potential problem	Nursing care
Prevention of injury	If patient falls to ground, ensure area is free from hazards or remove hazards, e.g. hospital furniture
	Remove any glasses or objects that may cause injury
	Loosen constricting clothing
	Do not attempt to force anything into mouth
	Do not restrain the patient
	Stay with the patient
	Maintain patient dignity
Observation of seizure	You will need to note and document the following: • any aura or warning • part of body where seizure activity began • spread of movement • type of movement • duration of time (tonic and clonic) • pupils • continence/incontinence • post-ictal state
Aftercare following seizure	ABC assessment (crash call if respiration does not return)
	Ensure patient placed in comfortable position/recovery position
	Move the patient to bed from floor when able
	Support for patient
	Allow rest
	Observe for repeated seizure activity
	Check compliance with medication/medication levels

Note: Seizure activity can be a side effect of under/over dose of phenytoin—levels should be monitored.

Table 4.11 Management of status epilepticus

Potential problem	Nursing care
Supporting airway, breathing, circulation	Position patient to maintain airway Insert airway if possible (not in tonic phase) Administer 100% oxygen/suction airway if able Refer to anaesthetist—ventilation may be required Establish intravenous access Monitor blood pressure if able Cardiac monitoring if able
Administer medication	Several drugs may be administered but these should be at hand and include: ♦ short-term management drugs, e.g. diazepam ♦ longer-acting drugs, e.g. phenytoin Assess for cause
Transfer of patient	Patient may require artificial ventilation/closer observation and may be moved to an ITU bed to allow this

ITU, intensive therapy unit.

Clinical link 4.5 (see Appendix for answers)

You are called to see a patient in a side room. The patient has been in hospital for several weeks following a stroke and his room is quite cluttered. On your arrival the student nurse reports that the patient has just collapsed on the floor and is now beginning to shake violently. He is blue in the face and is foaming at the mouth.

- What are your immediate actions?
- What will you need to observe in relation to his seizure?
- How can you protect this patient from injury?

After about 1 min the seizure appears to stop and then the patient starts shaking again. This is still continuing after 3 min.

- Discuss your initial actions.
- What help will you summon?
- What equipment/treatment may you need?
- How will you organize this patient's transfer to ITU?
- What will you need to consider prior to transfer?

- length of seizure
- patient's condition post seizure.

Care of the patient having a tonic/clonic seizure revolves around protecting the patient from injury during the seizure, monitoring seizure activity, and calling for help if required (see Table 4.10).

Management of status epilepticus Immediate medical attention is vital this may be using a medical emergency call or follow hospital policy, see Table 4.11.

The patient may require additional assessment/tests post scan especially if they have not experienced a seizure before. This may include CT scan, EEG tests, and referral to a neurologist. A detailed description and documentation of the events of the seizure may assist the medical staff with diagnosis of the seizure type.

End of chapter test

It is important that you understand both the theory related to neurological care and the practice of specific neurological skills in order to safely care for patients with neurological problems. In order to test your knowledge and apply this knowledge to clinical practice you should undertake the following assessment with an appropriately trained member of staff in clinical practice. If you are unable to answer any questions it may be helpful to revisit the section in this chapter.

Knowledge assessment

Work with your mentor/supervisor in practice and ask them to test your knowledge in relation to the following. Incorrect answers/lack of knowledge will require further revision/re-reading of this chapter.

- Discuss the normal divisions within the central nervous system.
- Discuss why it is important to prevent damage to the neurons.
- Discuss the ischaemic cascade that occurs as a result of neuronal damage.

+ Discuss the factors that can influence consciousness.
+ Analyse common causes of decreasing levels of consciousness.
+ Identify signs and symptoms of common neurological emergencies, e.g. SAH, CVA, meningitis, brain injury.
+ Discuss the use of quick assessment of neurological function (AVPU).
+ Discuss the need for formal objective neurological examination.
+ Discuss which patients require formal neurological assessment.
+ Identify which structures within the brain are tested by each stage of assessment.
+ Discuss how to accurately perform each stage of assessment.
+ Describe responses to each assessment.
+ Describe the difference between central and peripheral painful stimuli.
+ Discuss the significance of pupil response.
+ Discuss causes of pupil constriction/dilation.
+ Evaluate the advantages and disadvantages of using a neurological assessment tool.
+ Analyse the reliability and validity of neurological assessment tools.
+ Discuss indicators for further nursing/medical intervention.
+ Analyse treatment options for patients with deteriorating conscious levels.
+ Identify causes of seizure and discusses management.
+ Discuss common neurological tests, e.g. CT, magnetic resonance imaging, and lumbar puncture, highlighting their role in assisting with each procedure.
+ Discuss risk issues related to transfer of patients with decreasing levels of consciousness to CT and other areas.
+ Discuss signs of swallowing difficulty and appropriate management.

Skills assessment

Work with your mentor/supervisor in practice and ask them to assess your ability to care for patients with neurological injury using the following criteria, where appropriate. Note that you may not be able to demonstrate all these skills. Ask your mentor/supervisor to give you feedback on areas that you did well and areas that may require improving.

+ Identifies need and frequency of observation.
+ Identifies whether AVPU or GCS is appropriate tool.
+ AVPU: systematically makes quick neurological assessment and determines need for GCS testing.
+ Tests blood glucose if suspected cause of loss of consciousness.
+ GCS: systematically tests eye-opening, verbal response, and motor function using appropriate assessment.
+ Tests pupils, noting for reaction and consensual reactions.
+ Highlights any treatment/cause of change in pupil size.
+ Reports any new or worsening confusion.
+ Reports changes in consciousness.
+ Ensures patient safety and appropriate positioning if required.

- Summarizes neurological findings and initiates appropriate management as required.
- Liaises with multi disciplinary team.
- Informs patient/relative of any changes.
- Recognizes need for fast and appropriate response if conscious levels deteriorating.
- Demonstrates neurological assessment technique at handover if appropriate.
- Reviews need for neurological assessment and frequency of neurological assessment.

Adapted from the University of Brighton skills template, authors: Fiona Creed and Denise Hinge.

References

Addison, C. and Crawford, B. (1999) Not badly used just misunderstood. *Nurs. Times* **95**, 52–53.

Al Shahi, R. *et al.* (2006) Subarachnoid haemorrhage. *BMJ.* **333**, 235–39.

Bassett, C. and Makin, L. (2000) *Caring for the seriously ill patient*, Hodder Arnold, London.

Blows, W. (2001) *The Biological Basis of Nursing, Clinical Observations*. Routledge, London.

Cavanagh, S.J. and Gordon,V.L. (2002) Grading scales used in the management of subarachnoid haemorrhage: A critical review. *J. Neurosci. Nurs.* **34**, 288–94.

Crawford, B. and Guerro, D. (2004) Observations: neurological. In: Dougherty, L. & Lister, S. (eds) *The Royal Marsden Handbook of Clinical Nursing Procedures*, 6th edn. Blackwell Science, Oxford.

Dawes, E., Lloyd, H. and Durham, L. (2007) Monitoring and recording patients' neurological observations. *Nurs. Stand.* **22**(10), 40–6.

Dawson, D. and Shah, S. (2005) Neurological care. In: Shepperd, M. & Wright, M. (eds) *Principles and Practice of High Dependency Nursing*. Elsevier, London.

Department of Health (2007) *National Service Framework for Older People*.

Department of Health (2008) *National Stroke Strategy*. HMSO, London.

Hickey, J.V. (2003) *The Clinical Practice of Neurological and Neuroscience Nursing*, 5th edn. Lippincott, Philadelphia.

Hinkle, J.L. and McKenna Guanci, M. (2007) Acute ischaemic stroke. *J. Neurosci. Nurs.* **39**, 285–93.

Iankova, A. (2006) The Glasgow coma scale: clinical application in emergency departments. *Emerg. Nurse.* **14**, 30–34.

Jennett, G. and Bennett, B. (1974) Assessment of coma and impaired consciousness: a practical scale. *Lancet.* **2**, 81–4.

Jevon, P. (2007) *Treating the Critically Ill Patient*. Blackwell Publishing, Oxford.

Jones, S.P. *et al.* (2007) Physiological monitoring in acute stroke: a literature review. *J. Adv. Nursing.* **60**, 577–94.

Littlejohn, L., Bader,M. and March, K. (2003) Brain tissue oxygen monitoring in severe brain injury. *Crit. Care Nurs.* **23**, 17–27.

Mooney, G. and Comerford, D.M. (2003) Neurological observations. *Nurs. Times* **99**, 24–5.

Moore, T. and Woodrow, P. (2004) *High Dependency Nursing Care: Observation, Support and Practice*. Routledge, London.

NICE (2007) *Guidelines 2007 Head injury—Triage, Assessment, Investigation and Early Management of Head Injury in Infants, Children and Adults*. HMSO, London.

NICE (2008) *Stroke. National Clinical Guideline for Diagnosis and Initial Management of Acute Stroke and Transient Ischaemic Attack (TIA)*. HMSO, London.

Ogbungbo, B., Prakash, S., Ushewkunze, S., Etherson, K., and Sinar, J. (2005) Value of triple H therapy in a patient with an ischaemic penumbra following subarachnoid haemorrhage (a case study). *J. Neurosci. Nurs.* **37**, 326–33.

Resuscitation Council (2006) *Advanced Life Support*, 5th edn. Resuscitation Council, London.

Rothwell, P. (2007) Effect of urgent treatment of transient ischaemic attack and minor stroke on early recurrent stroke: a prospective population based sequential comparison. *Lancet.* **370**, 1432–42.

Royal College of Physicians (2004) *National Guidelines for Stroke*, 2nd edn. Royal College of Physicians, London.

Shah, S. (1999) Neurological assessment. *Nurs. Stand.* **13,** 49–56.

Van Gijn, J., Kerr, R., and Rinkel, G. (2007) Subarachnoid haemorrhage. *Lancet.* **369**, 306–15.

Chapter 5

Renal assessment and support

Cristina Osorio

Chapter contents

Assessing and supporting kidney function is an integral aspect of acute care. The purpose of this chapter is to examine:

♦ the anatomy and physiology of the kidney

♦ the pathophysiological changes of kidney function in acute care

♦ the assessment of kidney function

♦ the conservative management of the patient with reduced kidney function

♦ renal replacement therapies.

Learning outcomes

This chapter will enable you to:

♦ apply knowledge of the normal anatomy of the kidney to demonstrate understanding of pathological mechanisms which cause acute kidney injury (AKI)

♦ identify tools for the assessment of kidney function and understand the relevance of findings to define the extent of kidney failure

♦ select appropriate interventions to alleviate symptoms, control severity. and stop aggravation of AKI

♦ demonstrate knowledge of renal replacement therapies and when to start them, as well as a working knowledge of which choices are best for solute clearance, restoration of fluid and electrolyte homeostasis, or physiological stability

♦ discuss with insight the importance of multi-disciplinary work towards pro-active and effective resolution of AKI.

Introduction

The modernization of renal services in the UK, expressed within the National Service Framework (Department of Health 2004, 2005), called for a change in terms when talking about kidney failure, mostly driven by a desire for simplicity. Different expressions may be used to describe the same clinical reality and therefore it is important to clarify early on the terms to be used.

AKI refers to what was previously described and is still internationally accepted as acute renal failure (Bellomo *et al.* 2004). In many instances the word 'renal' is replaced with 'kidney', for example kidney failure and chronic kidney failure.

Acute care nurses require a thorough understanding of their patients' kidney function because of the risk for AKI, and when it is known that early and swift intervention will reduce it markedly (Stewart *et al.* 2009). Technological developments have improved patient outcome in many areas of health care, yet the associated invasive actions such as contrast and angiographic procedures, and the use of artificial devices have also increased the risk of kidney injury (Stevens *et al.* 2001). This chapter will review kidney anatomy and physiology followed by the nursing care involved in assessing and managing abnormal kidney function. The focus is on relevance and applicability to clinical practice and this will be aided by reference to clinical link activities.

An estimated 5–20% of critically ill patients experience AKI during the course of their illness. In addition, data from the Intensive Care National Audit Research Centre indicates that AKI accounts for almost 10% of all intensive care bed days (Rowan & Harrison 2007). Prevention of kidney injury, early intervention and suitable follow-up are therefore important aspects of patient care if these findings are to be improved. From the patient's perspective, survival is not the only outcome: life without dialysis or significant kidney disability is likely to be an equally desirable outcome.

At the end of this chapter there is a knowledge and skill assessment for professional development.

Applied anatomy and physiology of the kidney

People will normally have two functioning kidneys. Figure 5.1 indicates their location and anatomic size.

The primary functions of the kidney are:

♦ to filter and excrete metabolic waste products

♦ to sustain homeostasis of blood pH, electrolytes and body water.

Additional functions of the kidney are:

♦ regulation of blood pressure

♦ production of erythropoietin

♦ regulation of parathyroid activity.

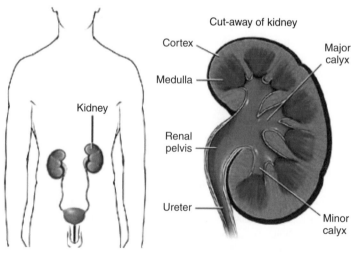

Figure 5.1 Location and macroscopic view of uro-kidney body system. Copied from: https://services. epnet.com/GetImage.aspx/getImage.aspx?ImageID=2454.

It is generally helpful to distinguish between the macroscopic and microscopic structures of kidney.

Macroscopic overview

The kidneys receive 20–25% of the cardiac output from the heart. This is equivalent to approximately 180 L/day, circulated via the renal arteries. An extensive vascular system delivers blood supply to every cell of the kidney, enabling quick and responsive filtration and homeostatic regulation.

The anatomic size and shape of each kidney is important in clinical investigations when ascertaining whether kidney injury is recent or silently ongoing. The simplest and quickest way to identify deviation from normal size and shape is to undertake a kidney ultrasound. Small kidneys are associated with chronic damage, often too advanced to enable diagnosis of underlying cause. The Renal Registry annual report (Ansell *et al.* 2008) identified that 25% of people in England and Wales receiving dialysis treatment did not know what caused their irreversible kidney failure because their kidneys had been too small to undergo diagnostic investigations. This indicates that by the time the first symptoms ensued, there was too much scar tissue and atrophy to identify a pathological mechanism.

In its 11 years of annual reporting, the Renal Registry has shown a small reduction in the number of late community referrals of patients with chronic kidney failure in England and Wales. Nevertheless the percentage of patients who present too late to have a primary diagnosis has remained relatively unchanged. This points towards the silent nature of chronic kidney failure but also the real possibility that patients admitted into hospital may already have kidney failure, unknown to them.

Possible causes, among others, of small kidneys are:

♦ undetected reflux nephropathy

♦ glomerulonephritis

♦ vascular atheroma.

Those who present clinically with symptoms of AKI and are found to have small kidneys on ultrasound visualization, can be considered to have had silent chronic kidney failure and are not likely to recover function. The therapeutic aim changes from recovery to halting progression. Success in preserving remaining kidney function relies on prompt identification of small kidneys as a significant risk factor for further kidney injury. The recently published report by the National Confidential Enquiry into Patient Outcome and Death (NCEPOD) Office specifically recommends 24-h access to kidney ultrasound facilities in all hospitals to improve early and pro-active identification of small kidneys in all UK hospitals (Stewart *et al.* 2009).

The signs and symptoms of chronic kidney failure are non-specific and numerous, making it easily confused with other possible differential diagnosis. Table 5.1 outlines signs and symptoms but very rarely would they present simultaneously.

Microscopic overview

The vascular network of arteries and arterioles of the kidney ends near the cortex, where just over 1.1 million nephrons are located. The nephron is a microscopic structure and the functional unit where the filtration and secretion functions of the kidney take place, culminating in the formation of urine, drained into the collecting duct. Figure 5.2 shows the anatomical structure in some detail.

Blood entering the glomerular capsule is filtered at a rate of 120–150 ml/min/1.73 m2 body surface, known as the glomerular filtration rate (GFR). Few substances or solutes remain unfiltered;

Table 5.1 Signs and symptoms of chronic kidney failure

Sodium and fluid retention:

- ◆ pitting oedema
- ◆ shortness of breath
- ◆ weight gain

Uraemia:

- ◆ sallow colour and uraemic breath
- ◆ nausea and vomiting, loss of appetite
- ◆ tiredness, lethargy and jerkiness
- ◆ lack of concentration, poor cognitive functioning
- ◆ disseminated itching

Endocrine alterations, causing:

- ◆ hypertension
- ◆ anaemia
- ◆ abnormal bone turnover

for example protein and red blood cells do not normally pass through the basement membrane. As the filtrate moves through the tubule, 99% of the water and glucose are re-absorbed into body circulation and several electrolytes are secreted, excreted, or actively transported through the tubular cells. Damage to the glomerular membrane or the tubular cells is likely to translate into the presence of protein and blood in urine. In acute care urinalysis is a simple, quick tool to detect early signs of kidney injury, both chronic and acute (Stevens *et al.* 2001).

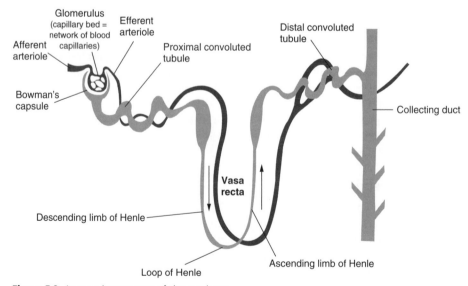

Figure 5.2 Anatomic structure of the nephron.

Kidney function, assessment, and investigations

Since 2006 and guided by the Renal National Service Frameworks (NSF), pathology laboratories in the UK now report routinely on the estimated GFR (e-GFR). This tool for the assessment of kidney function is most useful if the patient does not have acute sepsis, recent amputation, and is an adult. Above all it is most reliable to monitor chronic kidney failure or suspected acute-on-chronic kidney failure. It is less useful to monitor AKI because physiological changes are more immediate in the latter and need to be investigated through other means.

Estimation of e-GFR is currently based on the Modified Diet Renal Disease (MDRD) calculation formula, which has taken precedence over creatinine levels as a more reliable indicator of chronic kidney failure, especially when compared over time. Creatinine is a by-product of muscle activity and highly influenced by the individual's muscle body mass and drug intake. Creatinine is higher in those who take steroids and have high body muscle content, e.g. younger people, men, and individuals of black ethnicity. In those instances higher creatinine levels may not be indicative of reduced kidney function and it is more important to translate the serum creatinine level into an estimation of GFR. The MDRD formula is:

$$e - GFR = 186 \times (\text{serum creatinine})^{-1.154} \times (\text{age})^{-0.203} \times 0.742 \ (\text{if female})$$

The formula considers the person's measured serum creatinine and mathematically corrects for predictable variations associated with gender and age, making the result more accurate than serum creatinine alone. It is an approximate estimation and more complex formulas will make further corrections for other variables also known to influence GFR, for example body weight and ethnicity. However, more complex calculations are not practical for acute setting laboratories because it is unlikely that doctors and nurses will routinely enter the patient's weight and ethnicity on blood forms, whereas gender and age are easier to elicit from hospital computer records.

The MDRD formula for GFR estimation is a mathematical calculation validated by computer modelling from data on 1628 patients (Levey *et al.* 2006). There are other formulae widely recognized and validated to estimate GFR and the Cockcroft–Gault calculation is an example preferred by nephrologists (Renal Association 2007). However the MDRD formula above has been adopted nationally since 2006, as recommended by the Renal NSF, due to its simplicity, independent peer-reviewed reliability and ease of implementation (Department of Health 2004).

The e-GFR is helpful when chronic kidney failure is suspected, but serological changes are not noticeable until the e-GFR drops below 60 mL/min/1.73 m^2. People can tolerate loss of up to 70% loss of function without detriment to daily functioning, therefore great loss of kidney function may be present before there is any sign of it (Thomas 2004). Estimated GFR is also useful to enable monitoring and comparisons over time for individual patients in the absence of infections and acute illness. It is an unreliable calculation in AKI, including instances of sepsis, when the patient is catabolic and has disturbed muscle physiology affecting creatinine levels.

Kidney function is essential to human life. Kidney failure may be chronic over a long period of time or acute and related to specific conditions or recent events. Various investigations and detailed patient history will assist differential diagnosis. Patient history in particular is of great value when diagnosing AKI, especially for those admitted from the community with signs and symptoms. There may be environmental and patient-specific factors that only history-taking and good communication among health professionals will bring to the fore.

However nurses who work in hospitals–based acute settings are more likely to come across acute kidney injury as a complication rather than a reason for patient hospitalisation, in which case closer patient monitoring has greater prominence. Ongoing assessment and use of early-warning scores are recognized care-planning priorities for early detection and intervention (Department of Health 2000; NICE 2007).

Whilst glomerular damage affects the content of urine and is often a feature of chronic kidney injury, damage to the tubular structure affects urinary output more directly and is often implicated in AKI. However, tubular cells have the ability to regenerate and recover with therapeutic support, further highlighting the central role of the acute care nurse in assisting in the early detection and intervention of kidney injury.

As the kidney is an excretory organ, accumulation of related waste products in the bloodstream will give an indication of poor function. As mentioned earlier, creatinine has for many years been the preferred serum marker of kidney function.

To assess AKI, the preferred markers continue to be serum creatinine levels together with serum urea levels and urinary output. In acute care the first sign of abnormality may be reduced urinary output. This is known as oliguria, which is further defined as urinary output lower than 0.5 mL/kg body weight/h (Renal Association 2007).

In 2009 and following a UK-wide review of all cases of AKI, the NCEPOD revealed that 50% of patients admitted into hospitals received less than good care in the management of kidney injury (Stewart *et al.* 2009). There are several simple and inexpensive measures to significantly improve on this and they are alluded to throughout this chapter. This important report reflects on the negative impact of poor knowledge and communication together with organizational barriers and makes clear recommendations for immediate improvements. Physiological measurements of urinary output and serum electrolytes are already supported by early warning scores and outreach care (Department of Health 2000; NICE 2007). However NCEPOD found that 29% of the AKI cases reviewed had inadequacies in the management of their kidney injury, with lack of physiological monitoring a common feature. Worryingly for nurses, they found a proportion of patients with AKI whose urine had not been tested with a urinalysis reagent strip. This is a simple, inexpensive test that should be part of all hospital admissions, offering the opportunity to identify abnormalities immediately (Stewart *et al.* 2009).

Table 5.2 summarizes clinical investigations to determine kidney function and move towards a diagnosis.

Vital signs

Due to its regulatory role, the kidney has mechanisms to compensate physiologically for imbalance and it may take a while for abnormalities to be noted in the routine vital signs observations done by nurses and healthcare assistants.

The first abnormality to be noted is an increase in respiratory rate to compensate for metabolic acidosis. The kidney function is not sufficient to recycle and create new molecules of bicarbonate and therefore respiratory excretion of CO_2 increases in accordance with the Hasselbach formula for acid–base balance. Regular monitoring of respiratory rate will be an early indicator of deterioration, especially when trends can be identified over time.

Blood pressure is not likely to change until there are marked compensatory physiological changes. Hypovolaemia will usually translate into hypotension, and hypervolaemia into hypertension. However, by these extremes stages other physical signs are present on examination.

Chronic kidney failure

Health professionals in acute hospital settings need to remain alert to the possibility that patients may have renal failure unknown to them. Normally this will be of a chronic nature, progressing silently. Other clinical problems or the treatment given to the person may become the

Table 5.2 Renal investigations

Diagnostic investigation	How it is done	Utility
Kidney ultrasound	Sound waves are used to obtain visualization on screen of organs and surfaces of varying densities Gel is applied to the patient's skin and the probe moved round as images are observed on screen in real time This is a painless procedure that can be done anywhere: the machine can be taken to where the patient and an available technician are	Confirms size and presence of two kidneys It will give indication of cysts, if any Accumulations of fluid can be indicated but are less clearly defined
Urinalysis	A fresh urine sample is dipped with a suitable strip and readings taken in the given time, which will be up to 2 min	Leucocytes will indicate urinary infection, which can also be suspected from the presence of blood, protein, and nitrates. Where it is known the patient has acute renal failure, specific gravity can indicate acute tubular necrosis due to poor kidney perfusion
Urine creatinine/ protein ratio	Urine is collected any time of the day, but not the first void after waking up	Determine urinary loss of protein If more than 3 g/24 h, the patient has nephrotic syndrome
Urine pheresis and cytology	A fresh urine sample is spun and examined under the microscope.	Presence of Bence–Jones protein suggests chronic renal failure from amyloid disease
Kidney angiogram	Contrast substance is injected into the bloodstream and timed X-ray films taken of the kidneys	Stenosis and aneurysms will show up on the X-ray films, indicating problems in the blood circulating to the kidneys
Kidney biopsy	Under local anaesthesia and ultrasound guidance, a biopsy needle is pushed into the kidney to obtain a small number of nephrons for microscopic study	Damaged nephrons are inspected to determine causes Many glomerular and tubular pathologies can be diagnosed immediately

precipitating factors to what appears to be AKI, but is in fact an acute aggravation of underlying chronic kidney failure.

Routine reporting of e-GFR helps long-term monitoring of people who have reduced kidney function and assists care management plans, as outlined in Table 5.3.

Acute kidney injury in hospital settings

Acute kidney injury is characterized by rapid reduction in kidney excretory function due to a variety of causes. It is classically divided into pre-renal, renal, and post-renal causes. Table 5.4 shows a selection of common causes.

Healthcare professionals need to be particularly alert to the risk factors that can lead to AKI among inpatients. The NCEPOD report identified that 50% of patients with AKI received less than good care (Stewart *et al.* 2009).

Table 5.3 Stages of chronic kidney disease, internationally recognized and sanctioned by the UK Renal Association

Stage	Glomerular filtration rate*	Description	Treatment stage
1	90+	Normal kidney function but urine findings or structural abnormalities or genetic trait point to kidney disease	Observation, control of blood pressure
2	60–89	Mildly reduced kidney function and other findings (as for stage 1) point to kidney disease	Observation, control of blood pressure and risk factors
3A 3B	45–59 30–44	Moderately reduced kidney function	Observation, control of blood pressure and risk factors
4	15–29	Severely reduced kidney function	Planning for end-stage renal failure
5	<15 or on dialysis	Very severe, or end-stage kidney failure (sometimes called established renal failure)	Planning for renal replacement therapies, based on lifestyle

* All glomerular filtration rate values are normalized to an average surface area (size) of 1.73 m^2.

When the independent case reviewers looked at the post-admission AKI cases, in 43% of cases they identified an unacceptable delay in recognizing the condition. As a result they recommended that doctors and nurses be educated better to understand the risk, the necessary daily monitoring and investigations, as well as the actions that may deliver better outcomes in a timely way.

Pathophysiology of acute kidney injury

Acute kidney injury in the hospital setting is usually related to the admission problem or ongoing treatment and interventions. As examples, the patient may have been admitted for surgery or angiographic interventions and this alone places them at risk of kidney injury through hypovolaemia or drug nephrotoxicity. For inpatients, medication may have a nephrotoxic effect or the patient may contract sepsis or be unduly immobile, both of which also increase the risk of kidney injury (Nash *et al.* 2002).

In a responsive health service, it is helpful to the patient if nurses, doctors, and the care team remain alert to the risk of kidney injury and monitor physiological changes such as urinary output, changes in respiration rate, and blood pressure accordingly (NICE 2007). Acute kidney injury in the acute setting is most likely to affect the tubules in the nephron. There are two primary

Table 5.4 Pre-renal, renal and post-renal causes of acute kidney injury

Pre-renal	Renal	Post-renal
Hypovolaemia: ♦ vomiting and diarrhoea ♦ haemorrhage Reduced effective circulating volume: ♦ heart failure ♦ septic shock	Glomerular damage: ♦ glomerulonephritis ♦ vasculitis Tubular damage: ♦ acute tubular necrosis ♦ interstitial nephritis	Obstruction: ♦ calculi ♦ tumours

mechanisms of injury: acute tubular necrosis, which accounts for approximately 75% of acute renal failure, and interstitial nephritis (Renal Association 2007). Both pathological processes cause oliguria and anuria defined as urinary output less than 0.5 mL/kg/h.

Acute tubular necrosis

In acute tubular necrosis (ATN) the injury occurs within the tubular lumen, sometimes caused by nephrotoxic solutes in the glomerular filtrate, other times by reduced perfusion, as is the case in hypovolaemia and prolonged hypotension. It is known that a drop in mean arterial pressure (MAP) below 60 mmHg increases the risk of acute tubular necrosis.

ATN accounts for approximately 75% of the AKI episodes that occur in hospital, according to the Renal Association AKI guidelines compiled by Davenport and Stevens (2008). ATN may be the result of a direct insult to the tubular cells from drug metabolites and various other solutes, but it can also occur as a tubular response to pre-renal volume depletion.

Tubular cells receive nourishment and excrete some waste products directly on to the glomerular filtrate. Poor perfusion can starve them and lead to acute tubular ischaemia or acute tubular necrosis.

Interstitial nephritis

In interstitial nephritis the injury occurs in the interstitial space outside the tubular lumen, affecting normal tubular flow. The mechanism is different to acute tubular necrosis. Damage is caused by swelling of the space between the tubules, which constricts the tubular lumen. The accumulation of fluid may be caused by certain drugs, such as non-steroidal anti-inflammatory drugs. General causes of interstitial nephritis are:

♦ drug reactions, for example to vancomycin, especially if given too fast

♦ allergic processes, for example peanut allergy and wasp stings.

Acute kidney injury (AKI) and the nephrotic syndrome

According to the Renal Association (2007) the incidence of AKI in the community is around 1% and in hospital this increases greatly, to just over 7%. The nephrotic syndrome is a more likely cause of AKI, which starts in the community and later leads to hospital admission. Tubular cells remain intact in the early stages and serum urea and creatinine may be in normal range. The patient continues to urinate in amounts that appear normal but fluid retention escalates.

Physiologically the glomerular basement membrane becomes excessively permeable and vast amounts of serum albumin and protein are constantly lost in urine. The nephrotic syndrome is associated with inflammation of the glomerulus, otherwise known as glomerulonephritis (Thomas 2004). There may be an underlying condition or the result of a skin or throat streptococcal infection. Further investigation will clarify if the kidney injury is the result of an acute insult or a sign of acute exacerbation of a chronic condition. A kidney biopsy is the most informative investigation for patients presenting with nephrotic syndrome.

The process of kidney injury is reflected in extensive loss of protein in urine of greater that 3 g/24 h. This is confirmed by 24-h urine sample or a protein/creatinine ratio in a single-void (see Table 5.2 for details of the test).

Patient presentation The nephrotic syndrome patient develops low levels of serum protein—creatinine and urea often remain in acceptable range; albumin is less than 25 mmol/L, despite efforts to replace it by breaking down muscle protein. The presence of proteins in the blood and especially albumin is important to create oncotic pressure, which is a type of osmotic pressure that normally draws water from the body tissues into blood circulation. Loss of oncotic pressure changes the fluid distribution across body compartments, as explained in Chapter 7. The patient becomes fluid-depleted in the vascular space but fluid-overloaded in the interstitial space. Albumin and protein are lost in large amounts in the urine. This will be first suspected when performing urinalysis with a reagent strip that will react intensely to protein. The elements of the nephrotic syndrome are:

♦ hypotension

♦ pitting oedema and large amounts of fluid retention, to the point that mobility is difficult and weight rises sharply every day

♦ muscle breakdown and malnutrition

♦ clotting disturbances, with high risk of embolism.

Nursing management Whilst it is not life-threatening, the nephrotic syndrome creates a range of high-risk problems for the patient if not resolved. For the physician, the main priority is to identify and treat the cause of glomerular leakage of protein and to do that a kidney biopsy is needed.

To protect patient well-being, nursing care is directed to manage symptoms, monitor progress, and prevent clotting complications, such as deep-vein thrombosis and embolisms. Table 5.5 outlines a nursing care plan.

Once the cause of the nephrotic syndrome is known, the medical team will be able to formulate a treatment plan to address the underlying cause. As the glomeruli recover, so the protein loss in urine improves and the signs and symptoms recede.

In extreme cases where protein loss does not improve despite individualized treatment, kidney embolization may be required under angiographic guidance (Schwartz *et al.* 2006). This means a section of kidney will be lost but it is a justifiable step to prevent long-term complications of unstoppable urinary excretion of protein and hypoalbuminaemia.

Table 5.5 Nursing plan of care for nephrotic syndrome

Potential problem	Nursing care
Rapid malnutrition and oedema due to protein loss and low serum albumin	♦ Encourage food intake ♦ Explain to patient that appetite is impaired due to internal oedema to the stomach and bowel and advise to eat little and often ♦ Check weight daily ♦ Monitor blood pressure, which may be low; postural hypotension will indicate hypovolaemia due to lack of oncotic pressure from low serum protein levels, particularly albumin ♦ Monitor and document level of pitting oedema ♦ Take regular blood tests to monitor trend in serum albumin level ♦ Encourage light exercise to prevent rapid tissue deterioration and type 2 pressure ulcers
Embolisms caused by serum accumulation of lipoprotein as a by-product of muscle breakdown	♦ Measure, supply and help the patient wear anti-thromboembolism stockings ♦ Ask doctor to prescribe thrombus prevention sub-cutaneous heparin ♦ Observe for respiratory distress/chest tightness or deep leg pain—all possible sites for thrombus obstruction

Clinical link 5.1 (see Appendix for answers)

Consider this case. Mr T, 72-year old man, living alone and managing independently, had a fall on the street, landing on his coccyx. Next day he presented to hospital with back pain, which had started with his fall and gradually got worse. There were no detectable abnormalities on X-ray and the pain was thought to be musculoskeletal. The plan was to discharge once the analgesics were sufficiently effective. Mr T was not thriving in hospital, appeared unexpectedly bed bound despite physiotherapy collaboration and in day 2 of admission appeared disorientated, had a temperature of 37.5°C and was complaining of urinary urgency. At the same time his abdomen appeared distended and he reported diarrhoea.

Urine:
Leucocytes   Present ++
Protein   Present +++
Blood   Present ++
Ketones   Negative
Glucose   Negative

Blood results:
K^+ 2.9 mmol/L
Na^+ 139 mmol/L
Urea   45 mmol/L
Creatinine   400 µmmol/L
White blood cells 18.0×10^9/L
Haemoglobin   12.3 g/dL
Blood pressure   124/86 mmHg
Pulse   130 bpm
Respirations   24 rpm

Past medical history: Bowel cancer in remission for 5 years, hypertension, awaiting urology appointment for suspected prostate enlargement.

+ What would your priorities be for this patient? Justify your actions.

+ What interventions from the doctors would you anticipate?

+ What types of assessment and monitoring will you continually undertake?

+ Why would serum potassium be low and how can this be resolved?

+ What type of acute renal failure may be occurring here? Identify how it can be compensated.

Notes

+ Hypokalaemia is a rare presentation and hyperkalaemia is much more likely in AKI, but Mr T reports diarrhoea.

+ Refer to Table 5.6 for conservative nursing plan of care.

The patient experience of acute kidney injury

AKI usually has sudden onset and the patient may be too ill to realize and react to the inevitable worry. This will not be the case for relatives, who often report feeling powerless and fearful. Relatives and significant others require much reassurance and above all to be kept informed.

This is of great importance as they observe the rapid change to more invasive devices such as urinary catheterization, intravenous infusions, oxygen therapy, and stepping up of nursing monitoring.

Relatives and significant others also report concerns that the patient is becoming malnourished and is not eating. In fact there is evidence that aggressive parenteral nutrition is damaging to kidney recovery (Daugirdas *et al.* 2006). It is important to give reassurance that a short period of fasting is not deleterious and equally that a change in clinical condition is expected within days, therefore malnutrition is not likely to become a problem.

Conservative management of acute kidney injury

A series of published cases on AKI suggests that up to 30% of cases may be preventable, with a further percentage helped through simple interventions (Ho and Sheridan 2006; Boldt 2007; Landoni *et al.* 2007). In 2001 an international group of nephrologists and intensivists working together compiled *Risk/Injury/Failure/Loss/End-stage* (RIFLE), a classification system for AKI that has proved useful in clinical practice and has become increasingly popular. It gave prominence to the concept that AKI does not happen suddenly and that there is a build-up that, if identified early enough, can generate early and effective intervention. As experience continued to inform evidence, it soon appeared that renal replacement therapies were routinely introduced too late to deliver dual outcomes of survival and kidney recovery. As a result, in 2004, the Acute Kidney Injury Network adapted RIFLE by advocating that invasive treatment should be introduced earlier–at the stage of F for failure (Stevens *et al.* 2001; Bellomo *et al.* 2004) (Figure 5.3).

Whatever the gravity of acute renal failure experienced by the patient, there are two priorities for the healthcare team:

♦ to help the patient survive – mortality varies between 20 and 80% depending on co-morbidity and speed of diagnosis and treatment

♦ to rehabilitate kidney function for the long-term – although survival is an immediate priority, in reality dialysis and filtration therapies make it a realistic outcome. On the other hand, survival with irretrievable and disabling loss of kidney function offers poor prognosis and makes rehabilitation a significant priority.

Nursing management

In contemporary nursing care, management of AKI starts with prevention. Patients admitted for elective procedures and surgery should be routinely assessed for early abnormal signs with simple tools such as urinalysis and blood pressure measurement. Certain patient groups are at greater risk of silent chronic renal failure, for example those with diabetes, history of hypertension or heart failure, and the person aged over 50 years.

A simple and effective preventative measure to avoid pre- and post-operative hypovolaemia is proactive and effective management of patient fasting. The Royal Society of Anaesthetists collaborated with nurses and other health professionals to publish much-needed guidance on fasting for surgery in the UK (Royal College of Nursing 2005). The group's recommendations are upheld by the NHS and advocate clear fluids to be drunk up to 2 h pre-surgery. In reality, effective hydration by hospital inpatients continues to be a daily challenge aggravated by lack of clarity on times for procedures. Evidence is empirical and experiential; it is not uncommon for patients

	Non-oliguria	Oliguria	Intervention
Risk	Abrupt – 1-7 days, decrease (>25%) in GFR Or serum creatinine x 1.5. Sustained for more than 24 h	Decreased urine output relative to the fluid input. Urine output less than 0.5ml/kg/h for longer than 6 hours	
Injury	Adjusted creatinine or GFR decrease more than 50%, or serum creatinine x 2	Urine output less than 0.5ml/kg/h for longer than 12 hours	
Failure	Adjusted creatinine or GFR decrease >75%, serum creatinine x3 or serum creatinine >4mg% or 5mg/% when acute	Urine output less than 0.5ml/kg/h for longer than 24 hours and/or anuria for longer than 12 hours	ARF – earliest point for provision of RRT
Loss	Irreversible ARF or persistent ARF for more than 4 weeks	Irreversible ARF or persistent ARF for more than 4 weeks	
ESRF	ESRF for longer than 3 months	ESRF for longer than 3 months	

GFR (glomerular filtration rate), ARF (acute renal failure), ESRF (end stage renal failure), RRT (renal replacement therapy)

Figure 5.3 RIFLE classification of acute renal failure, including later revision by Acute Kidney Injury Network (AKIN 2004).

and nurses to report consecutive days of patient fasting in excess of 6 h for clear fluids, whilst waiting for different procedures or rescheduled surgery. It is interesting to note that there is much published evidence to indicate that hospital inpatients have a high risk of hypovolaemia and associated kidney injury. Although a variety of reasons may be explored, there is a lack of evidence and evaluation of levels of fluid intake by hospital inpatients.

Nurses are in a key position to ensure effective hydration and educate their patients to the advantages of following this simple action. Good hydration is a positive step to protect kidney function that can be improved greatly with patient involvement.

The effect of low water intake could be further aggravated by the administration of diuretic medication. Whilst this medication is suitable at home, it may aggravate dehydration in the hospital setting if fluid intake drops. Diuretic medication should be reviewed on a daily basis before symptoms of hypovalaemia may appear.

The same follows for medications known to have a nephrotoxic effect, such as metformin and angiotensin-converting enzyme inhibitors. Whilst the patient may continue to have a clinical need to take these medications, sustained hydration with intravenous fluids during operative procedures that use contrast substances is a simple intervention to help preserve good kidney perfusion.

In conclusion, the successful conservative management of AKI is a highly desirable goal. The role of acute care nurses in identifying patients at risk and implementing a set of simple but highly effective measures cannot be underestimated. Good communication with patients and other health professionals is an integral aspect of conservative management, for example reviewing the need for diuretic and nephrotoxic medication, clarifying fasting times, and evaluating and discussing response to fluid challenges (Scales & Pilsworth 2008). Table 5.6 summarizes the nursing plan of care for conservative management.

Table 5.6 Nursing plan of care for conservative management of acute kidney injury

Potential problem	Nursing care
AKI evidenced by oliguria. One of the first signs of AKI is reduced urinary output, less than 0.5 mL/kg body weight/h.	◆ Advocate and implement urinary catheterization for the purpose of accurate, hourly measurement of urinary output ◆ Maintain fluid balance chart ◆ Work closely with doctor to implement fluid challenge as soon as possible ◆ Take vital signs observations four times a day and look for changes in breathing and blood pressure ◆ Listen to chest sounds for crackles and observe for dyspnoea ◆ Observe for cyanosis and take oxygen saturation readings; if below 92%, review oxygen therapy
Infection risk indicated by the presence of invasive devices such as urinary catheter and central line	◆ Review need for urinary catheter daily and aim to remove on day 5 (Department of Health 2006) if possible ◆ Observe intravenous cannula daily for signs of infection, give it a phlebitis score once daily, shift, and resite after 72 h in-situ ◆ Use aseptic non-touch technique when opening the central line ◆ If central line is used for renal replacement therapies, do not use it for anything else—to remain a dedicated line ◆ Support good hygiene practice around the patient environment and with their person, including catheter cleansing ◆ Assess temperature fluctuations four times a day ◆ Encourage nutrition and hydration
Fluid imbalance aggravating AKI	◆ Encourage patient to keep up fluid intake and keep hydrated. Observe progress and investigate obstacles ◆ If there is a central line in place, take regular readings for central venous pressure ◆ If the patient appears dry, take lying and standing blood pressure; differential greater than 20 mmHg is indicative of dehydration, unless he/she takes medications likely to cause it ◆ If patient is hypotensive review diuretic and anti-hypertensive medication with medical staff
Lack of recovery from AKI	◆ Notify doctor urgently and contact outreach team if available in hospital (Department of Health 2000) ◆ Review nephrotoxicity of all medications and discuss with medical team ◆ Take urgent blood sample for urea and electrolytes ◆ Take ECG looking for hyperkalaemic changes—inverted T wave and shortened PR interval
Polyuria during recovery phase from AKI	◆ Polyuria is likely to take 2–3 days to normalize; in the meantime polyuria has to be managed ◆ Monitor hourly urine output and give variable fluid replacement therapy ◆ Educate the patient and reassure that polyuria is transitional, a sign that tubular cells are recovering and it is important to continue drinking and avoid dehydration

AKI, acute kidney injury.

Pulmonary oedema and its pathophysiology

Pulmonary oedema is a life-threatening and rapidly escalating condition associated with acute decompensated cardiac failure (see Chapter 3). Non-cardiogenic causes are also possible, such as in sudden fluid overload caused by rapid infusions, severe hypertension, and kidney disease.

Clinical link 5.2 (see Appendix for answers)

You are caring for Lydia, a patient 48 h post appendicectomy. Yesterday she had a pyrexia of 39.4°C and a peripheral blood culture sample was taken. The results yields MRSA septicaemia, and Lydia commenced intravenous vancomycin. Lydia is aged 57 and known to have congestive heart disease and takes ramipril and furosemide regularly. However, today her breathing is laboured, bubbly, and distressed. Lydia reports a sense that something terrible is about to happen. Her oxygen saturation is 85% on air, so you start her on oxygen therapy.

♦ What other immediate actions would you undertake and why?

♦ What other signs and symptoms would indicate pulmonary oedema?

♦ If pulmonary oedema was confirmed, how would you co-ordinate care of the patient including interaction with the nurse in charge and medical team?

There is a rapid accumulation of fluid within the interstitial and alveolar spaces in the lung, leading to dyspnoea and a patient-reported sense of 'drowning'. Initially fluid accumulates in the lower lobes and the patient breathes more easily sitting up.

Patient presentation

The patient presents with dyspnoea, cyanosis, and agitation. Peripheral oxygen saturation is reduced, respiration rate increases and becomes laboured. Blood pressure may be within normal range and the pulse is weak or pounding. There may be a cough, with or without production of pink, frothy sputum.

Given that kidney failure is a non-cardiogenic cause of pulmonary oedema, the possibility should be investigated by monitoring urinary output and serum levels of urea, creatinine, and electrolytes. Close monitoring of urinary output at hourly frequency is necessary to confirm AKI and this is made possible with the insertion of a urinary catheter.

A patient exhibiting pulmonary oedema, oliguria, and sepsis should have a urinary catheter in place as soon as possible to enable accurate measurement of urine output. This outweighs the infection risks associated with urinary catheterization (Department of Health 2007).

Fluid challenge and replacement

Fluid challenge is the practice of administering a large volume of intravenous fluids, possibly combined with diuretics. There is a long tradition of using this approach in an attempt to stimulate return to improved levels of kidney function. Its success is not guaranteed where the kidney function does not respond to the drugs. More recent randomized controlled trials are adding evidence that popular drugs used in acute renal failure such as furosemide and dopamine are ineffective or have benefits neutralized by its side effects and complications (Mehta *et al.* 2002; Ho & Sheridan 2006; Lauschke *et al.* 2006; Van der Voort *et al.* 2009). In the majority of cases, AKI can be resolved by adequate fluid challenge or replacement and the treatment of underlying medical conditions, such as sepsis and haemorrhage, as well as avoidance of nephrotoxic drugs.

There is currently no evidence to positively define a pharmacological strategy in the management of AKI. Loop diuretics such as furosemide have in the past proved very popular to convert oliguria to increase levels of urinary output. Equally, furosemide has been statistically linked to increased failure to recover renal function and higher mortality in anuric patients (Ho & Sheridan 2006). On the latter point it has been theorized that furosemide administration

Clinical link 5.3 (see Appendix for answers)

Following on from Clinical link 5.2, 12 h have passed. Her condition has deteriorated further but she is still able to sustain her own breathing. The chest X-ray shows upper lobe blood diversion, urinary output is a total of 200 mL in the last 12 h.

Vital signs:
Blood pressure   92/58 mmHg
Pulse   136 bpm
Respirations   32 rpm
Oxygen saturations   82%
Temperature   37.4°C

Recent blood results:
K^+ 6.9 mmol/L
Na^+ 139 mmol/L
Urea   45 mmol/L
Creatinine   450 μmmol/L
Bicarbonate   13 mEq/L

♦ What may be causing Lydia's problems?

♦ Why is potassium high?

♦ What will the medical team do next?

has neutral benefits and it is the delay in implementing renal replacement therapies whilst waiting for the drug to act that causes the increased risk, not the drug itself (Davenport & Stevens 2008).

Similarly popular over the years is the use of dopamine to promote vasodilation, improve renal blood flow and reduce cell oxygen consumption. A number of studies challenge that view and a more recent meta-analysis (Friedrich *et al.* 2005) showed no clinical benefits arising from the use of dopamine to aid recovery from AKI. Other studies have even suggested that dopamine has a detrimental effect when serious side effects are considered, such as cardiac arrhythmias, and myocardial and intestinal ischaemia (Lauschke *et al.* 2006).

Fenoldopam is a selective dopamine A-1 receptor agonist that decreases systemic vascular resistance, whilst increasing renal blood flow. So far, small clinical studies have proved inconclusive, but improved kidney function has been reported with fenoldopam, when using it in cases of severe hypertension (Landoni *et al.* 2007). There is a clear need for more substantial evidence from multicentre controlled trials in the search for effective pharmacological solutions.

Patient presentation

Patients with AKI will present the following problems:

♦ *Metabolic acidosis*, identifiable in elevated respiration rate and hyperkalaemia. Hyperkalaemia is the result of potassium displacement inside the cells in preference to the retention of hydrogen ions in an acidotic state.

♦ *Oliguria* or *anuria*, expressed as urinary output less than 0.5 mL/kg/h. Reduced fluid output may be accompanied by nausea and vomiting as physiological ways to avoid fluid overload. Uncompensated anuria is likely to result in pulmonary oedema.

+ *Uraemia* is an indicator of poor excretion of metabolic products. Accumulation of uraemic products causes the uraemic syndrome. Amidst its most serious consequences is the interference in the clotting cascade, with an extension of bleeding times, combined with gastrointestinal erosive effects. The risk of severe and uncontrolled haemorrhage is a threat to well-being.

Each problem, on its own and with sufficient gravity in presentation, is enough reason to commence renal replacement therapies (RRT). Patients with a degree of heart or respiratory failure suffer a quicker escalation of the above problems because their tolerance to compensatory hyperventilation and pulmonary oedema is lower.

The importance of nursing focus on prevention and early detection of reduced kidney function cannot be overemphasized, alongside the need to communicate effectively with the multidisciplinary team. When the clinical problems listed above are present and serious, acute kidney failure becomes life-threatening. Survival rate is reported in the region of 20–80% depending on co-morbidity. RRTs improve both survival and prognosis, but are resource-intensive, not readily available outside intensive care or renal units, and carry new risks associated with their invasive requirements.

All forms of RRT share the following new risks to the patient:

+ embolism, accidental puncture of a central vein, and septicaemia due to the need for a double-lumen central vascular catheter

+ loss of blood due to clotting in the RRT circuitry or excessive bleeding due to oversitivity to anticoagulant during therapy.

At the stage of needing RRT, failure to act rapidly worsens the patient's prognosis. Once a decision is made to instigate RRT, the physician has to choose the best option available at the time. That decision should be primarily guided by the clinical priority, which will be based around one of these parameters:

+ correction of metabolic acidosis to reduce the cardiac threat of hyperkalaemia

+ fluid removal across body compartments to correct pulmonary oedema

+ solute removal to improve uraemic syndrome.

Renal replacement therapies

RRTs have in common the purpose of replacing the homeostatic function of the kidney normally regulated by the production of urine. They have evolved greatly over the years and presently offer safe, effective means to support kidney function and maintain acceptable levels of fluid and electrolyte balance. Nevertheless, two important challenges arise. Firstly, preservation and recovery of kidney function, because a long-term outcome of life on dialysis would prove unacceptable to many surviving patients. Secondly, RRTs are costly and resource-intensive. If demand is greater than availability, a level of rationing will occur, raising ethical questions.

Despite a wide range of small studies comparing RRTs in the treatment of AKI, statistical adjustment renders the evidence-base inconclusive (Davenport & Stevens 2008). What is known with certainty in the nephrology world is that recurrent hypotensive episodes will cause further kidney injury and increase the likelihood of long-term dialysis as a patient outcome, therefore a choice of therapy that preserves haemodynamic stability as much as possible for the individual patients is the best option.

There are several choices to consider and Table 5.7 summarizes these.

RRT is linked to approximately 4.9% of admissions to intensive-care units. Patients with single-system failure or recovering well from other complications may, however, be able to transfer to

Table 5.7 Choices of renal replacement therapies, all of which require extra-corporeal blood circulation and anticoagulation

Therapy	Overview of therapy	Best suited to these patients	Advantages and shortfalls
Haemofiltration	A pump pushes patient blood through a filter and a closed circuit Plasmatic fluid is drained, depending on the flow pressure through the filter Treatment will continue for more than 8 h, and up to 24 h	Patients whose clinical priority is fluid removal Patients who need up to 15 L removed from their blood circulation in 24 h	Gradual fluid removal helps sustain blood pressure levels Equipment easier to set-up and cheaper than the other options Requires sustained anticoagulation for a long period
Haemodialysis	Same as above but therapy takes 2–4 h only Blood is exposed to purified water across a semi-permeable membrane, allowing for diffusion	Patients whose clinical priority is solute removal and correction of acidosis, with fluid removal no more than 3 L per session	Physiological shifts of solutes and fluid are rapid and effective Water treatment facilities and sophisticated dialysis machines are required Anticoagulation is needed but can be dispensed with if necessary
Haemodiafiltration	Same as above but therapy takes 6–8 h. In this option sterile water is used. Blood is exposed to it across a membrane as in haemodialysis, however water is also mixed with blood, usually in a pre-filter dilution regimen but can also be post-dilution.	Patients whose clinical priority is solute removal and large fluid removal Patients who need to achieve this and are severely hypotensive.	Good diffusion of larger molecules than any of the above, good for removal of body toxins produced in septicaemia Good fluid and solute removal with least hypotension risk Requires sterile water, which can be provided in large bags Sterile water requirement added to the limited availability of machines makes this is the most expensive therapy Anticoagulation is needed during therapy

level 2, high-dependency areas, of which there is a recognized lack in the UK (Department of Health 2000; NICE 2007; Davenport & Stevens 2008). The Department of Health (2000) defines level 2 patients as those needing highly dependent care, usually due to one organ failure. Managed in clinical areas with the right nursing skills and ratio, level 2 patients do not require an intensive-care bed. level 3 patients also require highly dependent care, but have multiorgan failure and need intensive-care accommodation and one-to-one specialist nursing.

The ideal model of care offers fluidity and collaborative critical care networks that are responsive to patient need in a timely fashion. Much of it relies on good communication and collaboration

> ## Clinical link 5.4 (see Appendix for answers)
>
> Following on from Clinical link 5.3, Lydia was prescribed 50 mL of 50% glucose mixed with 10 units of human insulin administered over 30 min. She was also given intravenous calcium gluconate 10%.
>
> A double lumen central line was inserted into the femoral vein and arrangements were made for Lydia to receive 6 h of haemodiafiltration.
>
> ♦ Why was Lydia prescribed the above drugs?
>
> The physician opted for haemodiafiltration as RRT. This decision was based on the need to remove both fluid and solutes.
>
> ♦ Why was haemodialysis not given instead, when the same outcome can be delivered?

between doctors and nurses in general hospital areas, renal and intensivist specialities (Stewart *et al.* 2009). If care remains patient-centred, professional boundaries and systems are less likely to drive their clinical outcome. More level 2 high-dependency areas would increase the flexibility to offer the patient RRT without having to take an intensive or renal unit bed. This would be an entirely appropriate way to manage the individual who has kidney failure but has not yet developed further complications.

Acute care nursing

Nurses have a unique role protecting patients from kidney injury, firstly by understanding that every individual with a health problem is at risk; hospital admission, and all that comes with it, enhances that risk. The tenets of *Essence of Care* (Department of Health 2001) outline evidence-based and effective standards of basic care that all patients have a right to expect from their health service. Upholding the benchmarks on nutrition, self-care, infection control, communication, and documentation will protect many patients from kidney injury.

Secondly, nurses in acute care settings need to understand that certain conditions combined with the invasive nature of surgery, strong medications or procedures, and the deteriorating health of their patients increase the risk of AKI with poorer prognosis. Early-warning scores widely introduced across the NHS include respiration rate and urinary output (NICE 2007). A rising early-warning score based on faster respiration and lower urinary output in the previous 6 h should be escalated for medical attention. In the meantime, seeking further information from the patient and obtaining additional clinical data would help a timely, differential diagnosis of AKI, for example:

♦ fluid intake

♦ urinalysis

♦ medication review

♦ urgent urea and electrolytes blood test

♦ electrocardiogram looking for rhythm changes related to potassium or calcium.

Lastly, acute care nurses need to understand that life without dialysis is an important outcome for any patient recovering from kidney injury. This desirable outcome relies on early intervention in the face of deteriorating kidney function. Effective intervention to avoid permanent kidney injury requires sound clinical judgement but also equipment and expertise that are not available in every hospital. It therefore important to build networks of care and support across NHS trust organizations; acute care nurses should be aware of how to access specialist advice at regional level. Renal services in the UK are organized centrally for each county. Usually there is a main unit located at an acute hospital where the expertise for the region is centralized. Although the main unit will have satellite units in other hospitals, these are often nurse-led. At various stages of the patient journey, interventions are simple, albeit effective and for that reason the value of expert advice at the end of the phone should not be under-estimated. Through networks of care and local contacts, acute care nurses can be aware of the location and services offered at their regional renal unit, for example access to renal pharmacy, dieticians, and counselling from nursing colleagues with expertise in renal care.

End of chapter test

The following assessment will enable you to evaluate your theoretical knowledge of acute renal failure and its management as well as your ability to apply this theory to clinical practice.

Knowledge assessment

With the support of your mentor/supervisor from practice, work through the following prompts to explore your knowledge level about assessment of kidney function and management of acute renal failure.

+ Describe the functions of the kidney and relate kidney failure to its main signs and symptoms.
+ Define acute and chronic renal failure.
+ Differentiate between acute, chronic, and acute-on-chronic renal failure, referring to respective patho-physiological processes.
+ Identify and explain how and why AKI becomes life-threatening.
+ Explain your role and responsibilities as a nurse in the active preservation of kidney function.
+ Recognize risk factors for kidney failure and critically discuss current methods to document information and communicate relevant findings.
+ Explain how blood tests, investigations, and observations contribute to an assessment of kidney function.
+ Critically relate fluid balance to the progression of AKI and planning of nursing care.
+ Critically analyse the impact of renal recovery and survival as two different treatment outcomes.
+ Contrast and analyse the advantages of and limitations of fluid challenge and renal replacement therapies.
+ Compare and contrast models for the organization of care across multi-disciplinary teams when patients experience kidney failure.
+ Choose a case from personal practice where the patient experienced AKI and explore what happened, what worked well, and what could have been different.

Skills assessment

Under the guidance of your mentor/supervisor, plan care for an individual in acute renal failure, followed by appropriate interventions and evaluation. Your mentor/supervisor will be able to assess your ability and provide feedback based on the following skills:

+ Conducts a patient history and physical assessment with a systems review to support a clinical judgement on their likelihood of developing AKI.

♦ Monitors patient's urinary output, fluid intake, vital signs, and blood test results and comment on how they interlink.

♦ Assesses all sources and amount of fluid intake and output from a patient undergoing fluid challenge and fluid replacement therapy.

♦ Facilitates the completion of relevant clinical investigations such as blood, urine, and radiology tests and evaluate results.

♦ Reviews current medications and intravenous therapy rationalizing impact on kidney function.

♦ Explains clinical reasoning and provide justification for all interventions in the patient's journey of AKI.

♦ Liaises with other members of the healthcare team as necessary to demonstrate an ability to support sustained, positive kidney function for hospital inpatients.

♦ Documents care plans, completed actions, and evaluation of actions as per local policy.

References

AKIN (2004) Available at: http://www.nature.com/ncpneph/journal/v2/n7/images/ncpneph0218-f1.jpg (accessed 27 October 2009).

Ansell, D. *et al.* (2008) *UK Renal Registry: The Eleventh Annual Report.* The Renal Association, London.

Bellomo. R., *et al.* and the ADQI workgroup (2004) Acute renal failure—definition, outcome measures, animal models, fluid therapy and information technology needs. The second international consensus conference of Acute Dialysis Quality Initiative (ADQI) Group. *Crit. Care.* **8**: R204–R212.

Boldt, J. (2007) The balanced concept of fluid resuscitation. *Br. J. Anaesth.* **9**, 312–15.

Davenport, A. and Stevens, P. (2008) Renal Association Guidelines: Acute Kidney Injury. Available at: http://www.renal.org/pages/pages/guidelines/current/arf.php (accessed 10 February 2009).

Daugirdas. J., Blake, P., and Ing T. (2006) *Handbook of Dialysis.* Little Brown, Philadelphia.

Department of Health (2000) *Comprehensive Critical Care—A Review of Adult Critical Care Services.* HMSO, London.

Department of Health (2001) *The Essence of Care: Patient-*focussed *benchmarking for health care practitioners.* HMSO, London.

Department of Health (2004) *The National Service Framework for Renal Services: Part One.* HMSO, London.

Department of Health (2005) *The National Service Framework for Renal Services: Part Two: Chronic Kidney Disease, Acute Renal Failure and End of Life Care.* HMSO, London.

Department of Health (2007) *Essential Steps to Clean, Safe Care.* Urinary Catheter Care. HMSO, London.

Department of Health (2007) Using High Impact Interventions: Using Care Bundles to Reduce Healthcare Associated Infection by Increasing Reliability and Safety. Available at: http://www.dh.gov.uk/en/Publichealth/Healthprotection/Healthcareacquiredinfection/Healthcareacquiredgeneralinformation/ThedeliveryprogrammetoreducehealthcareassociatedinfectionsHCAIincludingMRSA/index.htm (accessed 29 January 2009).

Friedrich, J.O., Adhikari, N., and Herridge M.S. (2005) Meta-analysis: low-dose dopamine increases urine output but does not prevent renal dysfunction or death. *Ann. Int. Med.* **142**, 510–24.

Ho, K.M. and Sheridan, D.J. (2006) Meta-analysis of frusemide to prevent or treat acute renal failure. *BMJ* **333**, 420–25.

Landoni, G., *et al.* (2007) Beneficial impact of fenoldapam in critically ill patients with or at risk for acute renal failure: a meta-analysis of randomised clinical trials. *Am. J. Kidney Disease.* **49**, 56–68.

Lauschke, A. *et al.* (2006) Low-dose dopamine worsens renal perfusion in patients with acute renal failure. *Kidney Int.* **69**, 1669–74.

Levey, A.S. *et al.* (2006) Using standardized serum creatinine values in the modification of renal diet in renal disease equation for estimating glomerular filtration rate. *Ann. Int. Med.* **145**, 247–54.

Mehta, R.L. *et al.* (2002) Diuretics, mortality, and non-recovery of renal function in acute renal failure. *JAMA.* **288**, 2547–53.

Nash, K., Hafeez, A., and Hou, S. (2002) Hospital-acquired renal insufficiency. *Am. J. Kidney Disease.* **39**, 930–6.

NICE (2007) *Acutely Ill Patients in Hospital: Recognition of and Response to Acute Illness in Adults in Hospital.* National Institute for Health and Clinical Excellence, London.

Renal Association (2007) *Treatment of Adults and Children with Renal Failure: Recommended Standards And Audit Measures*, 4th edn. Royal College of Physicians, London.

Rowan, K.M. and Harrison, D.A. (2007) Recognising and responding to acute illness in patients in hospital. *BMJ.* **335**, 1165–6.

Royal College of Nursing (2005) *Perioperative Fasting in Adults and Children.* Royal College of Nursing, London.

Scales K. and Pilsworth, J. (2008) The importance of fluid balance in clinical practice. *Nurs. Stand.* **22**, 50–7.

Schwartz, M.J. *et al.* (2006) Renal artery embolization: clinical indications and experience from over 100 cases. *BJU International.* **99**, 881–6.

Stevens, P.E. *et al.* (2001) Non-specialist management of acute renal failure. *Quart. J. Med.* **94**, 533–40.

Stewart, J. et al. (2009) *Adding Insult to Injury –a Report by the National Confidential Enquiry into Patient Outcome and Death.* National Confidential Enquiry into Patient Outcome and Death, London.

Thomas, N. (2004) *Advanced Renal Care.* Blackwell, Oxford.

Van der Voort, P. *et al.* (2009) Furosemide does not improve renal recovery after hemofiltration for acute renal failure in critically ill patients: a double blind randomised-controlled trial. *Crit. Care Med.* **37**, 533–8.

Further reading

Hegarty, J. *et al.* (2005) Severe acute renal failure: place of care, incidence and outcomes. *Quart. J. Med.* **98**, 661–6.

Chapter 6

Gastrointestinal tract

Kathy Martyn

Chapter contents

This chapter will provide an overview of the gastrointestinal (GI) system, and explore:

+ the normal anatomy and physiology of the GI tract
+ the normal anatomy and physiology of accessory organs (liver, gall bladder and pancreas)
+ the care and management of patients presenting with symptoms of the GI tract and associated organs
+ the nutritional support of the patient in the acute care setting, including enteral and parenteral nutrition.

Learning outcomes

This chapter will enable you to:

+ describe the normal anatomy and physiology of the GI tract
+ describe the stages of the swallowing reflex
+ describe the vomiting reflex
+ explain common symptoms associated with GI disorders using the relevant anatomy and physiology
+ understand the importance of nutritional support in the acutely ill patient.

Normal anatomy and physiology of the gastrointestinal tract

The GI tract is a hollow tube that runs from the mouth to the anus. Along its length it is modified according to its function. At the mouth, the buccal cavity, the main function is the mastication or chewing of food to form a bolus, which can then be swallowed into the oesophagus. The formation of a bolus requires the tongue, lips, cheeks, and teeth to be functioning. The teeth break the food into small segments and movement of the tongue and cheek mixes the food with saliva, salivary amylase, and lingual lipase. The amylase has a limited impact on the starch content of the food. Lingual lipase begins the digestion of fat, whilst the saliva, containing water, mucus, and electrolytes, dissolves molecules of flavour to be detected by taste receptors on the tongue and provides a lubricant to moisten the food for swallowing. During the chewing process the food is gradually moved to the back of the throat, the oropharynx, and a swallowing reflex is initiated.

Swallowing

Swallowing is a complex neurological response controlled by a swallowing centre in the brain and is in three distinct stages.

- The first stage is the formation of a bolus as described above.
- The second stage, the pharyngeal phase, is triggered as soon as the bolus reaches the tonsils and is automatic. During this phase the soft palate closes against the back wall of the throat, separating the oral cavity from the nasal cavity to prevent food or liquid from coming up through the nose. The vocal cords close, shutting access to the trachea to prevent food or liquid from being aspirated into the lungs. Next the throat muscles contract in a rhythmic, coordinated fashion to propel the bolus downwards towards the oesophagus. There is movement of the larynx and epiglottis to both protect the vocal cords and to ensure the bolus goes in the correct direction. Finally, the oesophageal sphincter relaxes and the bolus enters the oesophagus.
- The third and final phase occurs once the bolus is in the oesophagus, the oesophageal phase, and describes the active movement of the bolus through peristalsis. The bolus moves down the oesophagus, through the lower oesophageal sphincter, and into the stomach, when swallowing is complete.

Patients presenting with an altered swallow—dysphagia

The ability to swallow can be affected by many different conditions and situations. The most common in an acute care setting are related to altered neurological function due to trauma, illness, or general anaesthesia. Patients with a reduced level of consciousness will automatically have a reduced ability to swallow and this should be considered within the general management of the patient (see Chapter 4). Patients with altered cognitive functioning such as dementia may also have a swallow that is compromised, as they no longer respond to the triggers for the swallowing reflex or even recognize when to swallow.

Early recognition of the signs and symptoms (Box 6.1) associated with a reduced ability to swallow will help to prevent aspiration of gastric secretions or food and reduce the risk of aspirate pneumonia developing.

Box 6.1 Signs and symptoms of a dysphagia

- Difficulty in coordinating breathing with eating or drinking
- Wet 'gurgly' voice when speaking
- Frequent coughing
- Unexplained weight loss, altered diet or loss of appetite
- Dribbling of saliva from the mouth
- Recurrent chest infections
- Difficulty with chewing with prolonged meal times
- Aspiration of food or liquid
- Laboured breathing
- Difficulty in speaking

Adapted from SIGN 78 Managing patients with stroke; Identification and management of dysphagia (SIGN 2004).

The stomach and small intestine

The stomach acts as a reservoir, allowing food to be consumed in large amounts, and a mixer, mixing the food with mucus, hydrochloric acid (HCl), and gastric enzymes (pepsin and lipase). These enzymes play a limited role in the digestion of the fat and protein components of food, which are predominantly broken down by pancreatic and brush border enzymes. The main functions of the stomach are protection and denaturing (unfolding) of complex protein structures. Food often contains many microbes and during swallowing a large number of microbes will be swallowed. Parietal (also known as oxyntic) cells are stimulated by:

- acetylcholine, released by parasympathetic neurons
- gastrin, secreted by G cells
- histamine, secreted by mast cells.

Parietal cells secrete HCl into the lumen of the stomach, which reduces the bacterial load as the contents of the stomach fall to a pH of 1–3. This acid environment denatures proteins, making them more accessible to enzyme activity, and activates the enzyme pepsinogen.

The movement of food as it passes through the GI tract is due to rhythmic contractions, known as peristalsis, which are controlled by the vagus nerve through the parasympathetic divisions of the autonomic nervous system. The type of movement along the GI tract will reflect the function of that component. In the body of the stomach, peristalsis takes the form of waves of vigorous muscle contraction that mix the food with HCl, mucus, gastric lipase, and pepsin, until a thick paste called chyme is formed. It then pushes about 3 mL of chyme through the pyloric sphincter.

The rate at which chyme leaves the stomach, gastric emptying, depends on the composition and volume of food or liquid consumed. Water leaves the stomach quickly, whilst complex meals begin to leave after a lag time of between 20 and 30 min, 2–4 h after consumption. The greater the fat content of a meal, the slower gastric emptying is. This ensures that the small intestine is not overloaded with nutrients and maximizes the likelihood of nutrient absorption. The emptying time of liquids will also be slower if they contain fat or protein molecules. For an estimation of the time taken for gastric emptying see Figure 6.1.

Once the chyme has passed through the pyloric sphincter it is in the first part of the small intestines, the duodenum. The duodenum does not play an extensive role in digestion and absorption but allows the food remnants to be mixed with bile salts and pancreatic juices.

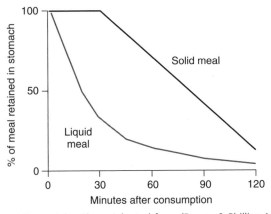

Figure 6.1 Estimated gastric emptying time. Adapted from (Degen & Phillips 1996).

The small intestine comprises the duodenum (25 cm), the jejunum (1 m), and ileum (2 m), and joins with the large intestine at the ileocaecal sphincter.

As the chyme enters the duodenum the presence of lipids (fatty acids) and peptides trigger the release of the hormone cholecystokinin that stimulates secretion of pancreatic juice and contraction of the wall of the gall bladder. In addition it:

♦ slows gastric emptying by promoting the pyloric sphincter to contract

♦ enhances satiety by acting on the hypothalamus

♦ maintains the normal growth of the pancreas and enhances the effect of secretin.

The presence of chyme triggers the release of the hormone secretin from S cells in the duodenum. In response to secretin the flow of pancreatic juices containing bicarbonate ions is increased, buffering the acidic chyme and inhibiting the secretion of gastric juices.

The structure of the small intestine is modified to increase its surface area by the presence of circular folds, villi and micro villi (the brush border), which enhance its absorptive function. The circular folds also ensure that the chyme spirals as it is moved through the small intestine by muscle contractions, known as the migratory motility complex (MMC).

The villi are finger-like projections that have a central lymphatic capillary (lacteal), arteriole, venule, and capillary network that is essential for nutrient absorption. These vessels are embedded in a connective tissue, lamina propria, which also contains mucosa-associated lymphoid tissue. This lymphoid tissue along with lymphatic nodules along the length of the GI tract (forming Peyer's patches) are an important component of the immune system, making the GI tract the largest immune organ in the body.

The outer layer of a villus is composed of several different cells:

♦ absorptive cells that have microvilli (the brush border) on their surface, which increases the surface area, and have brush border enzymes (see Table 6.1) inserted into their plasma membrane, allowing some enzymatic digestion to occur at the surface of the absorptive cells

♦ goblet cells that secrete mucus

♦ enteroendocrine cells that secrete secretin, cholecystokinin or glucose-dependent insulinotropic peptide

♦ paneth cells, which secrete lysozyme and are capable of phagocytosis.

The movement of chyme through the small intestine is through MMC, which begins as a slow wave at the lower portion of the stomach, reaching the end of the ileum in 90–120 min, before another wave begins. In this way chyme remains in the small intestine for 3–5 h. A second type of peristalsis, segmentation, is a localized contraction that mixes the chyme with the digestive juices and brings the particles of food into contact with the mucosa for absorption.

At the end of the ileum is a fold of mucous membrane called the ileocaecal sphincter or valve, which allows the remnants of food to enter into the large intestine. This valve has an important

Table 6.1 Brush border enzymes

Substrate	Enzyme	End product
Sucrose	Sucrase	Glucose and fructose
Lactose	Lactase	Glucose and galactose
Maltose	Maltase	Glucose
Dipeptides	Dipeptidases	Amino acids

regulatory function as it slows the flow from the ileum into the caecum. Distension and irritation to the caecum results in a reflex increase in the tone of the ileocaecal valve and inhibits ileal peristalsis.

Functions of the small intestine

The main function of the small intestine is the absorption of nutrients, water, and drugs through the mucosal membrane and into the hepatic portal vein or lymphatic system. (Table 6.2).

Absorption of nutrients and fluids Absorption of nutrients, amino acids, glucose, fructose and galactose, fatty acids, vitamins, minerals, and trace elements is through several distinct mechanisms, which may be compromised during periods of ill-health or due to specific disease processes. Some areas of the small intestine have precise roles in absorbing micronutrients. Vitamin B12 is only absorbed in the ileum because of the presence of intrinsic factor and

Table 6.2 The absorption of macronutrients

Food	Enzymes	Absorption
Carbohydrates found in foods such as bread, pasta, rice, fruit, and vegetables	Salivary amylase Pancreatic amylase Sucrase Maltase Lactase Galactase	Fructose is absorbed by facilitated diffusion, so there is no need for metabolic energy, but a specific carrier is required. Once inside the cell, fructose is phosphorylated and converted to glucose prior to entering the portal blood. Galactose and glucose are actively transported into the mucosal cell by a common transport protein. The energy for this active transport is provided by the electrochemical Na+ gradient. The glucose carrier has binding sites for Na+ and glucose. When both are bound, the protein translocates across the membrane.
Protein found in meat, fish, dairy products, fruit, vegetables, pulses, and grains	Pepsin Pancreatic peptidases	Dipeptides and tripeptides are transported across the brush border membrane. Amino acids are transported across the brush border plasma membrane into the intestinal mucosal cell by way of certain specific amino acid transport systems. There are three main sodium-dependent active transport systems for amino acids that occur in brush border membranes. The neutral brush border system transports most of the neutral amino acids, both hydrophobic and hydrophilic.
Fat found in all food groups, with most dietary fats coming from animal and dairy products	Gastric lipase Pancreatic lipase The absorption of fat requires bile salts to emulsify fat and aid formation of micelles	The fat digestion products, i.e. monoglycerides, fatty acids, cholesterol, and phospholipids, are present in the intestinal lumen in the form of micelles (aggregates). Micelle formation is aided by the presence of bile acids. These products are absorbed into the intestinal mucosal cell from these micelles. They enter the lacteals in the villi in the form of chylomicrons entering the blood stream at the vena cava. As the micelles travel down the small intestine they become more concentrated with cholesterol. Although the duodenum and jejunum are active in absorbing fatty components, most of the ingested fat is absorbed at the mid jejunum. Free fatty acids diffuse across the brush border membrane.

carrier proteins. Alterations in the length and surface area of the small intestine can compromise absorption of nutrients.

Common symptoms associated with malabsorption include:

+ osmotic diarrhoea (carbohydrate malabsorption)
+ steatorrhoea (fat malabsorption)
+ pernicious anaemia (vitamin B12 malabsorption)
+ iron deficiency anaemia (iron malabsorption).

Approximately 2000 mL of fluid are consumed each day, with a further 7000 mL of water made up from saliva, gastric secretions, bile, pancreatic juice, and intestinal secretions entering the lumen of the GI tract. Most of this volume is absorbed in the small intestine as part of the digestive processes, with only 1400 mL entering the colon. Inflammation of the mucosal membranes due to infection or disease will compromise this function, leading to diarrhoea (see section on altered bowel function). Excessive water and electrolytes loss can be seen in:

+ ulcerative colitis
+ Crohn's disease
+ gastroenteritis.

Protection In addition the GI tract is an integral part of the first line of defence immune mechanism, by limiting entry of ingested pathogens or toxins to the body. The acid environment of the stomach created by the release of HCl reduces the bacterial load of any food ingested. The structures of the lining of the small intestine do not normally come into direct contact with nutrients, potential pathogens, or allergens and as such the immune tissue are not stimulated. However, it is possible for individuals to develop intolerance to a nutrient if the functions of the GI tract are altered or an allergy to a specific nutrient, if the lining of the small intestines is compromised and the immune system is activated.

Lactose intolerance, caused by a failure to secrete the enzyme lactase, is found in as many as 30% of northern Europeans (Wilson 2005). Lactose intolerance will lead to crampy stomach pain, flatulence, bloating, and diarrhoea, as undigested lactose passes through the small intestine.

Food allergies can occur in people who are considered to be atopic, and may have other allergies such as hay fever, bee sting allergy, or seasonal rhinitis. Common food allergies include milk protein allergy, peanut allergy, and shellfish allergy. An allergy means that the immune system has been activated, most commonly leading to the production of the antibody IgE, which increases inflammation and risk of anaphylaxis. Patients who are known to have food allergies should be identified, as they may also be allergic to latex or iodine, both of which are commonly used in hospitals. Patients with food allergies may also be allergic to some medications, such as salicylic acid (aspirin).

Both food intolerances and food allergies can have implications for nutritional support (see section on nutritional support).

The large intestine

The large intestine is 1.5 m in length and is divided into the caecum, colon, rectum, and anus. The remnants from digestion and absorption are slowly moved along its length by peristalsis. In addition there is haustral churning. The haustra are a series of pouches formed by contraction of longitudinal bands, which when relaxed fill until distension triggers contraction, squeezing the contents into the next haustrum. As the contents move towards the transverse colon a strong peristaltic wave begins (mass propulsion), quickly driving the contents of the colon into the rectum. Once in the rectum, stretching of the rectal wall stimulates stretch receptors, initiating a defaecation reflex. After consuming food, a gastrocolic reflex is initiated in the colon, triggering mass peristalsis three to four times per day during or shortly after a meal.

The colon also contains a large population of commensal bacteria of as many as 10^{12} per cubic millilitre (mL^3) of colonic fluid. These bacteria are essential for maintaining the health of the colon but can easily be transmitted to other tissues and organs, causing infection (Table 6.3).

Functions of the large intestine

The functions of the large intestine include chemical digestion, absorption of water and the end products of fermentation, and faeces formation. Chyme, containing the remnants of digestion and non-digestible substances, enters the colon and is mixed with mucus. Unlike the small intestine, no enzymes are secreted. Instead, bacterial fermentation, from commensal bacteria, breaks down remaining carbohydrates, proteins, and fats. In the fermentation process methane is produced causing flatulence, which can cause distress to patients. In addition, short chain fatty acids (butyric acid and propionic acid) are produced, which are utilized by the cells of the colon as an energy substrate, maintaining colonic health, with the excess entering the bloodstream for use by other body tissues. In addition, bacteria decompose bilirubin to form stercobilin, the brown pigment associated with faeces.

The chyme will have been in the GI tract for as long as 10 h and during this time 90% of the water will have been reabsorbed along with nutrients in the small intestine. Of the remaining 0.5–1 L of water that enters the large intestine, up to 800 mL will be reabsorbed, making the large intestine an important organ for maintaining fluid balance.

The remaining faecal matter contains a mixture of inorganic salts, sloughed off epithelial cells, products of bacterial fermentation, unabsorbed digested materials, and the indigestible parts of food.

The liver and gall bladder

The liver is the major metabolic organ and, weighing almost 1.4 kg in adults, it occupies most of the right hypochondriac region. Almost completely covered by visceral peritoneum, it is divided into two principal lobes: a large right lobe and smaller left lobe. The lobes are made up of functional units called lobules, each containing hepatocytes, a central vein, highly permeable capillaries called sinusoids, and fixed phagocytes called Kupffer cells.

The hepatocytes secrete bile into small canals, the canaliculi, which empty into small bile ductules. These ductules finally emerge at the periphery of the lobules into the right and left hepatic duct, which unite to form the common hepatic duct. The common hepatic duct joins the cystic duct from the gall bladder to form the common bile duct. About 1 L of bile is secreted each day and it is made up of water, bile salts, cholesterol, lecithin, bile pigments, and several ions. Bile is the major way of excreting excess cholesterol and bilirubin from the haem component of phagocytosed red blood cells.

Table 6.3 Infections caused by bacteria found in the colon

Infection	Bacterium
Urinary tract infections	E coli, enterococci and Proteus species
Intra abdominal infections	Bacteriodes fragilis
Diarrhoea and vomiting	E. coli

The liver has two blood supplies. The hepatic artery supplies oxygenated blood for cell function and the hepatic portal vein supplies absorbed nutrients, drugs, microbes, and toxins from the GI tract. Products manufactured by the hepatocytes and nutrients are secreted into the blood via the central vein, which feeds into the hepatic vein. In this way the liver controls what enters the central circulation. Portal hypertension is a common complication of liver disease and can lead to a distended liver, ascites, and enlargement of the oesophageal varices.

Functions of the liver

The liver has many vital functions, which are discussed below.

Carbohydrate metabolism The liver is essential for maintaining a normal blood glucose level of between 4 and 6 mmol/L. When blood glucose is high the liver converts glucose to glycogen and triglyceride for storage. In this way, excess dietary carbohydrate can lead to excessive triglyceride production and weight gain (see Box 6.2). When blood glucose is low the liver can break down glycogen to glucose and convert certain amino acids and lactic acid to glucose. It can also convert other sugars such as galactose and fructose to glucose.

Lipid metabolism Hepatocytes can store some triglycerides and break down fatty acids to generate ATP. Importantly, the hepatocytes synthesize very low density lipoproteins (VLDL) and high density lipoproteins (HDL) to transport fatty acids, triglycerol, and cholesterol to and from the liver. Altered blood lipids are risk factors for coronary heart disease (Box 6.3). Cholesterol is synthesized by the liver. When cellular cholesterol stores are full excess is excreted in bile salts. Excessive excretion of cholesterol can lead to the formation of gall stones.

Protein metabolism Hepatocytes deaminate, removing $-NH_2$ from amino acids (Box 6.4), so that the amino acid can be used for ATP production or converted to carbohydrate or fats. The resulting ammonia, NH_3, is converted to urea, which can then be excreted in urine. Hepatocytes also synthesize most plasma proteins, including albumin, C-reactive protein, prothrombin, and fibrinogen.

Drugs and hormones The liver detoxifies substances such as alcohol and can excrete drugs such as penicillin and erythromycin. During metabolism of drugs the metabolites can be active or toxic, as in the case of paracetomol. The toxic metabolites then need to be detoxified in order to be excreted (Box 6.5). If the toxic metabolite exceeds the liver's capacity to detoxify it then damage to the hepatocytes can occur.

Box 6.2 Fatty liver disease

Patients at risk of fatty liver disease

Patients who are being artificially fed via a parenteral route are at risk of developing fatty liver disease, as triglyceride is synthesized and stored in the liver. Liver function tests are recommended twice weekly when patients are fed via a parenteral route (NICE 2006a).

Other patients at risk are those who are overweight and those who consume large quantities of alcohol, who may then develop liver cirrhosis.

Symptoms of fatty liver disease

♦ A third of patients have no symptoms.

♦ Liver is enlarged and may be tender.

Box 6.3 Management of coronary heart disease

The prescription of statins and fibrates influences liver synthesis and regulation of VLDL, HDL, triglycerol, and cholesterol, and they are used in the management of coronary heart disease. Patients may also be prescribed omega-3 fatty acids, which improve the synthesis of HDL molecules and contribute to an improved lipid profile. High concentrations of cholesterol in bile can lead to the formation of gall stones.

Excretion of bilirubin Bilirubin is the end product of haem metabolism. Initial bilirubin is unconjugated and insoluble in water. After uptake by hepatocytes the unconjugated bilirubin is conjugated, made water soluble, and excreted into the biliary tract for storage in the gall bladder. Alterations in the metabolism of bilirubin can lead to jaundice (Box 6.6).

Other functions of the liver

+ Synthesis of bile salts: bile salts act like biological soap and solubilize ingested fat and fat-soluble vitamins, facilitating their digestion and absorption.

+ Storage of glycogen and vitamins such as B12, A, D, E, K: in health, glycogen is stored in the liver and skeletal muscle. These stores are sufficient to provide glucose for approximately 24 h in the absence of dietary intake (see section on energy balance). Stores of vitamins in the liver ensure their availability when dietary intake is compromised.

+ Activation of vitamin D: fat-soluble vitamin D is essential for calcium metabolism. Biologically inactive once synthesized in the epidermis or ingested as part of the diet, it must be activated by the liver. Deficiency in vitamin D increases the risk of osteoporosis developing.

+ Phagocytosis of bacteria, aged red blood cells and white blood cells by Kupffer cells.

Gall bladder

The gall bladder is a store of bile. In the presence of cholecystokinin the gall bladder contracts and the hepatopancreatic sphincter (sphincter of Oddi) opens, allowing bile to enter the duodenum.

In some patients gall stones will form in the gall bladder. These can pass through the biliary tract, causing biliary colic (see section on abdominal pain).

Box 6.4 Essential amino acids

There are 20 amino acids which are found as constituents of proteins. These are essential for metabolism but not all have to be preformed in the diet because they can be made from other precursors in the liver. Only eight amino acids are considered to be essential. These are leucine, isoleucine, valine, phenylalanine, threonine, methinonine, tryptophan, and lysine. Consuming more amino acids in the diet than you need will increase the rate of excretion via urea or undigested in faecal matter. During acute illness the amino acid glutamine is considered to be conditionally essential.

In times of acute illness the rate of synthesis of plasma proteins such as prothrombin and fibrinogen will exceed the availability of amino acids, and prothrombin and fibrinogen levels will fall. This increases the risk of bleeding.

Box 6.5 Liver disease and drug metabolism

Liver disease can affect the way drugs are metabolized. This may:

♦ increase the availability of an active drug, increasing the risk of toxic effects

♦ decrease the availability of the active drug

♦ increase the time taken for a drug and its metabolites to be excreted, increasing the risk of toxic effects,

The pancreas

The pancreas is a gland that is about 15 cm long and 1 cm wide and lies posterior to the greater curvature of the stomach. It is divided into three regions: the head, the body, and the tail, and is usually connected to the duodenum by two ducts: the accessory duct and the hepatopancreatic duct.

The pancreas is both an exocrine and endocrine gland. The larger exocrine portion is made up of small clusters of glandular epithelial cells known as acini, which secrete up to 1.5 L of fluid containing a mixture of digestive enzymes, sodium bicarbonate, and some salts. These enzymes include pancreatic amylase, pancreatic lipase, ribonuclease, and deoxyribonuclease. In addition, trypein then activates the remaining inactive pancreatic enzymes, trypsinogen, chymotrypsinogen, procarboxypeptidase and proelastase, in the duodenum. These enzymes are inactive to prevent autodigestion of pancreatic cells. The aciner cells also produce a trypsin inhibitor should any active trypsin be produced. Once in the duodenum, the inactive trypsinogen comes into contact with a brush border enzyme, enterokinase, which splits the trypsinogen to active trypsin. Trypsin then activates the remaining inactive enzymes.

The remaining cells of the pancreas form islets called pancreatic islets (islets of Langerhan), which produce the hormones glucagon, insulin, somatostatin, and pancreatic polypeptide, which are secreted into the bloodstream. (see section on blood glucose regulation).

Nursing assessment of a patient with dysphagia Formal assessment of the swallow is normally completed by the speech and language team (SALT), but it is important that nurses complete a basic assessment if there is a change in the patient's condition, the patient complains of having

Box 6.6 Jaundice

Jaundice is a common symptom associated with disease of the liver, gall bladder, or head of the pancreas (blocking the hepatopancreatic duct). It can also occur if the red blood cells die too quickly—haemolytic anaemia.

Jaundice associated with the gall bladder or obstruction of the hepatopancreatic duct will be caused by the decreased excretion of conjugated (water soluble) bilirubin, and the stools will be pale and clay-like; the urine will be much darker. The patient may complain of generalized pruritis.

Jaundice associated with liver disease will lead to an increase in unconjugated bilirubin in the plasma. The stools will be pale and clay-like. The urine will not be as dark but the level of jaundice can be severe.

difficulty in swallowing, or there are concerns about a patient's ability to eat. The assessment is as follows:

- Check to see if dysphagia is due to airway obstruction.
- Observe for obstruction such as enlarged tonsils.
- Ensure patient has a clean, moist mouth and, if present, correctly fitting dentures. This will aid the formation of a bolus which will assist swallowing.
- Evaluate swallowing reflex by placing your fingers along the thyroid notch and instruct the patient to swallow. If you feel the larynx rise, the reflex is functioning. If uncertain, follow local protocol and refer to SALT for swallowing assessment.
- Ask patient to cough to assess the cough reflex.
- If certain that both the swallowing and cough reflex are present, assess the gag reflex. This can be achieved by touching the pharyngeal mucosa with a tongue depressor.
- Look at the face and listen to the speech for signs of muscle weakness. Does the patient have aphasia or dysarthria? Is the voice nasal, wet, hoarse, or breathy? Can the patient poke out their tongue?
- Ask whether solids or liquids are more difficult swallow.
- Ask whether the symptoms disappear after trying to swallow a few times. Is the swallow affected by the position in bed or chair?
- Is it painful to swallow?

Nursing management of a patient with dysphagia Dysphagia will not only compromise food and fluid intake, increasing the risk of malnutrition and dehydration, but will also increase the risk of oral infections and mouth discomfort, as the secretions remain in the oral cavity or are lost through the mouth. Oral infections increase the risk of infections in the heart and lungs, and the possibility of septicaemia and bacteraemia developing. The following steps should be taken:

- Ensure frequent oral hygiene is performed (Rawlins 2001; Jones 1998).
- Administer prescribed medication to reduce secretions.
- Use suctioning as required.
- Provide nutritional support (see section on nutritional support).

Clinical link 6.1 (see Appendix for answers)

Rosie Hubbard, 84, has been admitted into hospital following a right sided CVA. She is conscious and a CT scan has confirmed she has had a bleed. She has been seen by the physiotherapist who has confirmed that she can sit unaided. An intravenous infusion has been commenced; she is currently receiving 1 L of dextrose saline over 8 h. You notice she has difficulty in drinking.

- What would your priorities be for this patient?
- What actions will you take to ensure her nutritional and fluid needs are met?
- What signs might indicate that she has a problem with swallowing?

The patient with raised blood glucose

Patients who are acutely ill can have a raised blood glucose, and accurate monitoring and effective management is essential for positive health outcomes (Alm-Kruse *et al.* 2008).

In health, blood glucose is maintained between 4 and 6 mmol/L by the action of the pancreatic hormones, insulin and glucagon, and the function of the liver. Following a meal, blood glucose will rise and this will stimulate the release of insulin to promote the cellular uptake of glucose by the liver and skeletal muscle. This anabolic response enables excess glucose to be stored in the form of glycogen and tricyglycerol. During periods of starvation, such as during the night, blood glucose will begin to fall and glucagon is released. This catabolic response will stimulate the release of glucose from glycogen and fatty acids from the lipids. If starvation is prolonged then fatty acids from adipocytes and amino acids derived from skeletal muscle will be used by the liver to synthesize new glucose in a process known as gluconeogenesis.

Diabetes mellitus

Impaired regulation of blood glucose is commonly known as diabetes mellitus. In this condition insulin is either not produced or is not effective. Type 1 diabetes can occur at any age but is commonly first seen in younger people, whilst type 2 diabetes is associated with older people, although it can also occur in individuals who are obese. Without insulin the body is unable to regulate blood glucose levels and the glucose in the blood is not able to enter the cells.

Insulin therapy is increasingly used to lower blood glucose if this is persistently high when using oral hypoglycaemic therapy.

Acute illness and increased blood glucose

An increase in blood glucose can also be observed in acute illness, when dietary intake is often suppressed. This increase in blood glucose occurs due to:

♦ the presence of acute phase catabolic hormones (adrenalin and cortisol)
♦ the presence of circulating cytokines (chemicals), which increase glucose synthesis
♦ the development of insulin resistance (see section on energy balance).

Monitoring the blood glucose of an acutely ill patient is important, as uncontrolled blood glucose will lead to fluid and electrolyte imbalance (Alm-Kruse *et al.* 2008). It has been demonstrated that tight glycaemic control in patients following a myocardial infarction or stroke can reduce morbidity and mortality (McMullin *et al.* 2007). Research is now focusing on whether improved glycaemic control will have similar benefits in other acutely ill patients.

Patients with type 1 and type 2 diabetes can find their blood glucose is unstable and less easy to manage when they are acutely ill. It is important that they continue with their oral hypoglycaemics or insulin, even if they are not eating, and also that their blood glucose levels are closely monitored.

Fluid and electrolyte disturbances when blood glucose is raised

Within the kidneys, glucose is normally filtered via the glomeruli in the Bowman's capsule of the nephron and reabsorbed in the proximal convoluted tubule back into the bloodstream. If the blood glucose concentration is higher than 10 mmol/L, the capacity for reabsorption of glucose in the proximal convoluted tubule is exceeded and glucose remains in the lumen of the nephron.

The fluid in the lumen of the nephron is now more concentrated than the surrounding blood and water is 'trapped' due to the process of osmosis. The osmotic diuresis caused leads to a water loss in excess of sodium loss, increasing the sodium concentration of the blood. Hypernatraemia can occur.

The excretion of excess glucose in urine (glycosurea) by the nephrons is one way in which blood glucose is regulated.

As blood glucose increases, the concentration (osmolality) of blood increases and water is drawn from the cells into the circulatory system through the process of osmosis. This shift of fluid into the vascular system can create hyponatraemia as the blood is diluted. As the cells become dehydrated, antidiuretic hormone (ADH) is released from the posterior pituitary gland and the thirst centre is triggered. ADH binds to receptors at the distal convoluted tubule of the nephron and triggers the reabsorption of water. Monitoring fluids and electrolytes is essential in the management of patients with raised blood glucose (see Chapter 7).

In patients with hyperglycaemia it is important that the patient is monitored and that nurses recognize the point at which additional support is required. Monitoring should include the following:

- capillary blood test BM stix
- fluid balance charts
- conscious level using GCS.

All patients who are acutely ill can present with, or develop, raised blood glucose. For those who have type 1 or type 2 diabetes this can lead to the development of diabetic ketoacidosis or non-ketotic hyperosmolar states. These metabolic complications are potentially life-threatening and can lead to admission into the intensive care unit.

Diabetic ketoacidosis

The most common causes of diabetic ketoacidosis (DKA) are pneumonia, urinary tract infection, sinusitis, sepsis, and meningitis. In critically ill patients it can also be precipitated by trauma, myocardial infarction, surgery, pancreatitis, and failure to take insulin. The signs and symptoms of developing DKA include the following (Coursin *et al.* 2002):

- altered mental status
- deep and rapid breathing pattern—Kussmauls's respirations
- 'fruity' breath
- nausea and vomiting
- abdominal pain
- diffuse weakness
- hypothermia secondary to acidosis induced peripheral vasodilation.

The medical management of DKA will include aggressive fluid management using prescribed intravenous fluids:

- normal saline to lower the blood glucose (dilution effect), decrease the stress hormone levels associated with hypotension, and corrects the ketosis and acidosis
- hypotonic fluid (0.45% saline) to replenish intracellular losses in place of normal saline once intravascular volume has been restored.

Glucose and electrolyte imbalances are corrected by:

- insulin infusion using short-acting insulin to normalize blood glucose levels

- replacing potassium and phosphate as indicated by blood results
- 5% dextrose infusions to prevent hypoglycaemia.

The nursing role in the management of DKA is to provide continuing care of the airway, mouth care, personal hygiene, catheter care if *in situ*, and pressure area care. Also, to continue to monitor the haemodynamic status of the patient and to maintain accurate records of all fluids, insulin and electrolytes administered, to monitor urine output, and complete fluid balance charts.

Non-ketotic hyperosmolar states

Non-ketotic hyperosmolar states (NKHS) are more common in frail, elderly patients who suffer from type 2 diabetes and are unable to take adequate oral fluids. It can be precipitated by infection, medications such as diuretics, or during the perioperative period. Symptoms of NKHS developing include:

- confusion
- seizures
- focal deficits such as hemiplegia
- seizures.

In developing NKHS, patients will develop profound dehydration, hyperosmolarity and hyperglycaemia. Unlike DKA the breath is not 'fruity', as ketoacidosis does not develop. Instead, the poor tissue perfusion and dehydration leads to lactic acidosis. The dehydration, haemoconcentration, and hyperviscosity can result in the development of thrombi, which can adversely affect patient survival.

As with DKA, fluid replacement is the most important therapy and should commence with normal saline until the patient is no longer hypotensive and urine output has increased. Local policy will dictate whether insulin therapy is commenced, as there is some debate in the literature as to how this is managed (Coursin *et al.* 2002).

The nursing role, as with DKA, is to provide continuing care to ensure patient comfort during this episode and to monitor the haemodynamic status of the patient. The poor tissue perfusion as a result of the severe dehydration and the frail nature of the patients who develop HKNS will increase the risk of pressure sores developing, and attention to pressure areas is essential.

Hypoglycaemia

Although in most cases acutely ill patients have hyperglycaemia, hypoglycaemia can also occur. Hypoglycaemia is defined as a blood glucose <2.8 mmol/L (Coursin *et al.* 2002). The signs and symptoms associated with hypoglycaemia are neuroglycopenic:

- confusion
- irritability
- fatigue
- headache
- somnolence.

There are also adrenergic responses:

- anxiety
- restlessness
- diaphoresis

- tachycardia
- arrythmias
- hypertension
- chest pain.

In severe cases hypoglycaemia can lead to seizures, coma, and death. Recognizing the potential for hypoglycaemia should be considered in any patient who develops new neurological symptoms.

Hypoglycaemia can occur quickly in patients receiving exogenous insulin, have impaired gluconeogeneisis, or insufficient carbohydrate intakes. When patients are receiving artificial nutritional support, blood glucose levels should be routinely measured to avoid rebound hypoglycaemia developing if feeding is suddenly discontinued.

Alterations to gastrointestinal tract functioning

The nursing management of patients with altered GI tract function requires an understanding of how altered functioning impacts on the patients' wellbeing. In this section, common signs and symptoms associated with altered GI tract function will be explored in conjunction with the relevant disease processes.

The patient with nausea and vomiting

Nausea and vomiting are common symptoms experienced by patients and are a biological defence mechanism. Nausea is the sensation that the stomach 'wants' to empty and is associated with feeling hot, sweaty, and retching. Vomiting (emesis) is the forcible act of the stomach emptying.

Nausea and vomiting are very distressing to patients and can also lead to other complications, including:

- fluid and electrolyte imbalances
- bleeding
- aspiration pneumonia.

These complications can delay recovery and extend the patient's stay in hospital.

Nausea and vomiting are also common symptoms associated with specific treatments such as chemotherapy and radiotherapy, with as many as 25% of patients refusing chemotherapy treatments (Marin Caro *et al.* 2007) because of the discomfort they may feel. Recognizing the distress caused by nausea and vomiting, and alleviating the symptoms is important.

Vomiting (emesis) is multifactorial and can be caused by a range of stimuli, including medical interventions. In addition to poisoning and gastroenteritis, emetic stimuli include motion, surgery, GI tract obstruction, pregnancy, drugs, radiation, fear, and pain.

The vomiting reflex can be classified into three phases: nausea, retching, and vomiting.

Nausea is described as an unpleasant sensation that immediately proceeds vomiting. A cold sweat, pallor, salivation, a noticeable disinterest in the surroundings, loss of gastric tone, duodenal contractions, and the reflux of intestinal contents into the stomach often accompany nausea.

Retching follows nausea, and comprises laboured spasmodic respiratory movements against a closed glottis with contractions of the abdominal muscles, chest wall and diaphragm, without any expulsion of gastric contents. Retching can occur without vomiting but normally it generates the pressure gradient that leads to vomiting.

Vomiting is caused by the powerful sustained contraction of the abdominal and chest wall musculature, which is accompanied by the descent of the diaphragm and the opening of the gastric cardia. This is a reflex activity that is not under voluntary control. It results in the rapid and forceful evacuation of stomach contents up to and out of the mouth.

Neuronal pathways, transmitters, and receptors involved in nausea and vomiting

There are two types of receptors involved in nausea and vomiting:

- Mechanoreceptors are tension receptors that initiate emesis in response to distension and contraction, e.g. from bowel obstruction. They are located in the stomach, jejunum and ileum.
- Chemoreceptors respond to a variety of toxins in the intestinal lumina.

Once stimulated, nerve impulses are transmitted through common afferent neuronal pathways from the abdomen to the vomiting centre in the medulla, where the vomiting reflex is initiated. The vomiting centre controls the act of vomiting and instead of being a discrete site is a series of interrelated neural networks. Inputs include the vagal sensory pathways from the GI tract, neuronal pathways from the labyrinths, higher centres of the cortex, intracranial pressure receptors, and the chemoreceptor trigger zone (CTZ). The CTZ acts as an entry point for emetic stimuli and is in the area of the fourth ventricle known as the prostrema. It is outside the blood–brain barrier, and therefore responds to stimuli from either the cerebrospinal fluid (CSF) or the blood.

When activated, the vomiting centre induces vomiting via stimulation of the salivary and respiratory centres and the pharyngeal, GI, and abdominal muscles.

Schematically the major factors influencing nausea and vomiting can be illustrated as shown in Figure 6.2.

In the brain, a wide variety of receptor types and neurotransmitters are thought to have an impact on vomiting. The neurotransmitters include histamine, acetylcholine, dopamine,

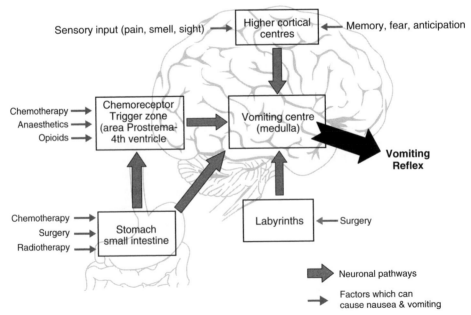

Figure 6.2 Factors influencing nausea and vomiting.

noradrenaline, adrenaline, 5-hydroxytryptamine (5HT), and Substance P. In support of their role in emesis, it has been shown that antagonists of receptors for each of these transmitters have anti-emetic effects.

The management of nausea and vomiting

The management of patients with nausea and vomiting should address a number of important issues:

- identification and elimination of the underlying cause if possible
- control of the symptoms if it is not possible to eliminate the underlying cause
- correction of electrolyte, fluid, or nutritional deficiencies.

It is important to care for the well-being and comfort of the patient, since poor management of this can lead to delayed recovery, poor clinical outcome, and aversion to future treatment.

Controlling symptoms: drug treatment of nausea and vomiting A wide range of drugs have been shown to have effects on nausea and vomiting. These include antihistamines, anticholinergics, dopamine receptor antagonists, 5-HT$_3$ receptor antagonists, cannabinoids, benzodiazepines, corticosteroids, and gastroprokinetic agents. Each of the drugs affects different receptors, and some act at a number of different sites. This determines their different clinical profiles.

The main classes of anti-emetic drugs commonly used are shown in Table 6.4, although it should be appreciated that many drugs have multiple mechanisms of action.

A multidrug approach to the treatment of different types of nausea and vomiting is often used in clinical practice, based on knowledge of the causes of the underlying nausea and vomiting and the sites of action of each of the available drugs (Figure 6.3).

Table 6.4 Prescribed anti-emetics

Class	Drug	Comments
Anti-cholinergic	Scopolamine (L-hyoscine)	
Anti-histamine	Cinnarizine	Useful for postoperative nausea and vomiting
	Cyclizine	Useful for motion sickness and nausea and vomiting associated with opiods
	Promethazine	
Dopamine antagonists	Metoclopramide	Useful for nausea associated with enteral tube feeding as prokinetic
	Domperidone	
	Haloperidol	Patients with suspected bowel obstruction should not be prescribed prokinetic drugs
Cannabinoid	Nabilone	
Corticosteroid	Dexamethasone	
Histamine analogue	Betahistine	
5HT$_3$-receptor antagonist	Granisetron	Useful for chemotherapy and radiotherapy-induced nausea and vomiting
	Ondansetron	

Based on data from British National Formulary (2008).

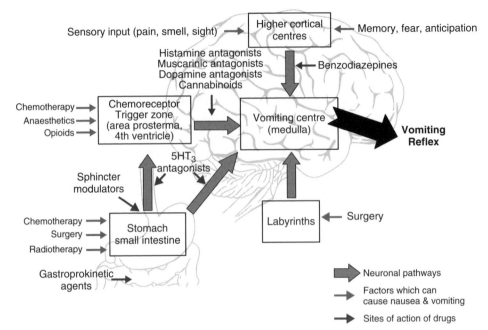

Figure 6.3 Drugs used to control nausea and vomiting and their sites of action.

⋆ **Nursing management of nausea and vomiting** Ensure antiemetic medication is given in a timely fashion to reduce the incidence of nausea and vomiting when patients undergo treatments that are known to induce nausea and vomiting. Because of the multifactorial nature of the stimulus to vomit, ensuring that prescribed medication is given will help to reduce the incidence of vomiting.

Measure and record all vomitus on a fluid chart and calculate fluid balance. The GI tract can secrete as much as 7 L of fluid into the lumen each day, which is normally reabsorbed as the gastric contents move from the stomach through to the colon. This fluid contains a mixture of HCl and electrolytes, predominantly sodium. Excessive vomiting can deplete the stomach of HCl, leading to a metabolic alkalosis. The loss of sodium and water will also lead to dehydration.

⋆ Offer regular mouth care. Vomiting is very unpleasant and will leave a bitter taste in the mouth. If nausea and vomiting is caused by obstruction in the small intestines it will contain bile, which can stain the mouth, and have an offensive smell depending on where the obstruction occurs (Jones 1998).

Vomiting and nausea associated with gastrointestinal tract obstruction Obstruction of the GI tract can be caused by many different factors, including position of a tumour and adhesions following previous GI surgery or inflammation (see section on GI tract obstruction).

Management of nausea and vomiting may include:

◆ insertion of nasogastric tube for drainage of stomach contents

◆ recording volume of vomit drained

◆ administration of prescribed anti-emetics (see Table 6.4).

Vomiting associated with enteral tube feeding (see section on nutrition) The most common factors that contribute to nausea and vomiting associated with enteral tube feeding are reduced gastric emptying, infection, and intolerance to the feed.

- When enteral tube feeding, ensure the patient is inclined at no less than 30°.
- Gastric motility can be enhanced through the use of prokinetic anti-emetics (see Table 6.4).
- Ensure hands are washed before preparing a feed and that feeding tube is changed every 24 h (NPSA 2005).
- Avoid use of milk-based feeds if patient is lactose intolerant. Alternative soya-based products are available after consultation with the dietetic department (see local protocol).

The patient with abdominal pain

Abdominal pain is one of the most common symptoms expressed by patients and can account for up to 50% of surgical emergencies (Jones *et al.* 2000; Smith & Lobo 2008). It can be triggered by many different stimuli, including indigestion. Acute and severe abdominal pain is almost always as a result of intra-abdominal disease.

As pain is experienced very differently by individuals it can be described in many different ways, and identifying where the pain comes from can be difficult (see Table 6.5).

Table 6.5 Abdominal pain

Pain description	Common causes
Pain after meals or on an empty stomach	Peptic ulcer
Pain can occur at night and may be relieved by antacids or food	
Pain is severe, lasting from 1 to 12 h	Biliary colic
Pain is sporadic and is located in the right epigastrum, the right upper quadrant and or right scapula	If the pain lasts longer than this it may be indicative of pancreatitis or cholecystitis. Following the episode of pain the patients feels generally well. If the common bile duct is obstructed this can also lead to fever (cholangitis) and jaundice.
Pain is often described as steady and radiating through to the back	Pancreatitis A patient can have several episodes and at its most severe can lead to shock. The patient may also suffer from nausea, vomiting, and weakness. Drinking alcohol can exacerbate the condition.
Waves of abdominal pain, often after eating	Iscahemic bowel disease can be caused by Crohn's disease, neoplasm, or volvulus. Patients who have a history of atherosclerosis have an increased risk of myocardial infarction, aortic abdominal aneurysm, and mesenteric ischaemia. The patient may also present with pyrexia, weight loss, nausea, vomiting, and fear of eating.
Severe left lower quadrant abdominal pain	Diverticular disease may lead to the development of peridiverticular abscess. Patient may also have a raised temperature. Diverticular disease is often asymptomatic.
Severe flank pain radiating to the groin	Renal colic, due to a stone passing through the uretur, may be accompanied by haematuria. Although not chronic it may be recurrent.
Recurring abdominal pain	In women, pelvic inflammatory disease or endometriosis may account for recurring abdominal pain. Patient is well between bouts of pain.

Based on data from Jones 2000.

Pathophysiology

Visceral pain Pain that originates from the internal abdominal organs is known as visceral pain and is innervated by the autonomic nerve fibres, which respond mainly to sensations of distension and muscular contraction, but not to cutting, tearing, or local irritation. This type of pain is carried by the sympathetic autonomic nerves and enters the spinal cord from T6 to L2. The parasympathetic system also carries pain sensation from the pelvic organs via S2, 3, and 4.

Visceral pain is often described as 'vague, dull, and nauseating'. The pain is often poorly localized, which means that the patient cannot always describe where it is due to the embryonic development of the tissue involved. In general:

+ pain in the upper abdomen is caused by distension or muscular contraction of the stomach, duodenum, liver, and pancreas structures
+ pain in the periumbicular region is caused by distension or muscle contraction of the small intestines, proximal colon, and appendix
+ lower abdominal pain is triggered by distension or muscular contraction of the distal colon and genital urinary tract.

Somatic pain In contrast to visceral pain, somatic pain comes from the parietal peritoneum, which is innervated by somatic nerves and responds to irritation from infectious, chemical, or other inflammatory processes. Somatic afferents supplying the abdominal wall enter the spinal cord between T5 and L2. Additionally, the undersurface of the diaphragm has innervation from the phrenic nerve (C3, 4, and 5). Thus, irritation of the diaphragm may refer pain to the shoulder.

Somatic pain is sharp and well localized.

Referred pain Some abdominal pain is known as referred pain as it is perceived some distance from its origin due to convergence of sensory neurons at the spinal cord. Common examples of referred pain include:

+ pain in the scapula due to biliary colic
+ pain in the groin due to renal colic
+ pain in the shoulder due to blood or infection irritating the diaphragm.

Other aspects of abdominal pain Abdominal pain can also be chronic in nature and reflect underlying disease processes or conditions. It can also be caused by conditions not associated with the abdomen, including (Stephenson 2008):

+ herpes zoster
+ alcoholic ketoacidosis
+ diabetic ketoacidosis
+ porphyria
+ sickle cell disease
+ myocardial infarction
+ pneumonia
+ pulmonary embolism
+ opiod withdrawal.

The main causes of abdominal pain are identified in Figure 6.4.

Abdominal Pain – Diffuse Pain: Peritonitis, leukaemia, early appendicitis, gastroenteritis, aneurysm, colitis, intestinal obstruction

Pain in Right Upper Quadrant – Cholycstitis, Hepatitis, Hepatic Abscess, Hepatomegaly, peptic Ulcer, Pancreatitis, Renal Pain, Myocardial infarction, pericarditis, Pneumonia

Pain in Left Upper Quadrant – Gastritis, Gastric Ulcer, Pancreatitis, Spleen; rupture, enlargement, infarction; aneurysm, Renal pain, Myocardial Infarction, Pneumonia, Aortic Aneurysm

Periumbilical – Intestinal obstruction, Acute pancreatitis, Early appendicitis, thrombosis, Aortic Aneuryms, Diverticulitis

Right Lower Quadrant – Diverticulitis, Intestinal Obstruction, Appendicitis, Leaking Aneurysm, Ectopic pregnancy, Ovarian cyst, Salpingitis, Endometriosis, Uretal calculi, Renal pain, Seminal vesiculitis, Cholcystitis, perforated ulcer, strangulated hernia

Left Lower Quadrant – Diverticulitis, Intestinal Obstruction, Appendicitis, Leaking aneurysm, Ectopic pregnancy, Ovarian cyst, Salpingitis, Endometriosis, Uretal calculi, Renal pain, Seminal vesiculitis, Strangulated hernia

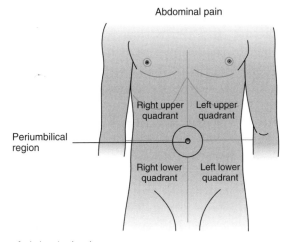

Abdominal pain

Periumbilical region

Right upper quadrant

Left upper quadrant

Right lower quadrant

Left lower quadrant

Figure 6.4 Causes of abdominal pain.

Nursing assessment of the patient with abdominal pain

The initial assessment of the patient with abdominal pain is important. In assessing the patient with abdominal pain, it is essential that complete physical history is obtained. Signs of anxiety, pale skin, and increased sweating (diaphoresis) can all be indicative of a serious problem.

Baseline observation, including blood pressure, pulse, state of consciousness, and altered peripheral perfusion, must all be recorded. Patients with abdominal pain may also present with concomitant symptoms such as nausea, vomiting, diarrhoea, constipation, jaundice, melaena, haematuria, haemetemesis, gastro-oesophageal reflux, mucus or blood in the stool, and weight loss.

Accurate recording of fluid loss, including consistency and odour, is important to aid diagnosis and to plan care (see Chapter 7).

Certain findings should be reported immediately:

♦ severe pain

♦ signs of shock (e.g. tachycardia, hypotension, diaphoresis, confusion)

♦ signs of peritonitis—see next section

♦ abdominal distension.

Distension of the abdomen can be caused by bowel obstruction and may indicate that peritonitis has developed. Patients who have had previous surgery are more at risk of obstruction due to adhesions (see section on obstruction). As the GI tract becomes obstructed, increased peristalsis occurs as the GI tract attempts to clear the blockage. This increased peristalsis can heard through a stethoscope, has a high-pitched sound and is known as borborygmi. If the obstruction is not cleared then peristalsis will stop and the patient will have a 'silent abdomen'. During this time the patient will be in severe pain, and may well be lying very still. As the GI tract close to the site of the obstruction will be inflamed and fluids will leak into the peritoneal cavity, leading to distension and peritonitis.

The patient with peritonitis

Peritonitis is inflammation of the peritoneal cavity. The most serious cause is perforation of the GI tract, which produces immediate chemical inflammation followed shortly by infection from intestinal organisms.

Peritonitis can also result from any abdominal condition that produces marked inflammation (Skipworth & Fearon 2008):

+ appendicitis, diverticulitis, strangulating intestinal obstruction, pancreatitis, pelvic inflammatory disease, mesenteric ischemia

+ intraperitoneal blood from any source (e.g. ruptured aneurysm, trauma, surgery, ectopic pregnancy)

+ barium, which causes severe peritonitis and should never be given to a patient with suspected GI tract perforation

+ peritoneo-systemic shunts, drains, and dialysis catheters in the peritoneal cavity, which all predispose a patient to infectious peritonitis, as does ascitic fluid (rarely, spontaneous bacterial peritonitis occurs, in which the peritoneal cavity is infected by blood-borne bacteria).

The most common symptom is pain, which may be localized or diffuse. Constipation is normally present unless a pelvic abscess develops, when the patient will present with diarrhoea. Peritonitis causes fluid shift into the peritoneal cavity and bowel, leading to severe dehydration and electrolyte disturbances. The immediate medical management will involve high flow oxygen, fluid resuscitation, analgesia, antibiotics, and positioning of a nasogastric tube to drain stomach contents to alleviate vomiting (Skipworth & Fearon 2008). In severe cases adult respiratory distress syndrome can develop rapidly. Kidney failure, liver failure, and disseminated intravascular coagulation can then follow. The patient's face becomes drawn into the mask-like appearance typical of hippocratic facies: a pinched expression of the face, with sunken eyes, concavity of cheeks and temples, and relaxed lips. This is often associated with impending death.

Nursing management of patients with abdominal pain

Assessment of pain is essential for effective pain management and the following questions may be useful. Careful questioning can provide essential information that will help in pain management (see Table 6.6). Using a simple pain scale to score the pain will enable the effectiveness of interventions to be monitored.

Management of symptoms Following a pain assessment it is important the pain is managed effectively.

Table 6.6 Questions related to abdominal pain assessment

Question	Potential responses	Indication
Where is the pain?		Location of the pain: visceral, somatic, referred.
What is the pain like?	Acute waves of sharp constricting pain that 'take the breath away'	Renal or biliary colic
	Waves of dull pain with vomiting	Intestinal obstruction
	Colicky pain that becomes steady	Appendicitis, strangulating intestinal obstruction, mesenteric ischaemia
	Sharp, constant pain, worsened by movement	Peritonitis
	Tearing pain	Dissecting aneurysm
	Dull ache	Appendicitis, diverticulitis, pyelonephritis
Have you had it before?	Yes	Suggests recurrent problems such as ulcer disease, gallstone colic, diverticulitis, or mittelschmerz
Was the onset sudden?	Sudden: 'like a light switching on'	Perforated ulcer, ruptured aneurysm, torsion of ovary or testis, renal stones
	Less sudden	Most other causes
How severe is the pain?	Severe pain	Kidney stone, peritonitis, pancreatitis
	Pain out of proportion to physical findings	Mesenteric ischaemia
Does the pain travel to any other part of the body?	Right scapula	Gall bladder pain
	Left shoulder region	Ruptured spleen, pancreatitis
	Pubis or vagina	Renal pain
	Back	Ruptured aortic aneurysm
What relieves the pain?	Antacids	Peptic ulcer disease
	Lying as quietly as possible	Peritonitis
What other symptoms occur with the pain?	Vomiting precedes pain and is followed by diarrhoea	Gastroenteritis
	Delayed vomiting, absent bowel movement and flatus	Acute intestinal obstruction
	Severe vomiting precedes intense epigastric, left chest, or shoulder pain	Emetic perforation of the intra abdominal oesophagus

- Pain caused by indigestion or trapped wind will respond to antacids and peppermint water.
- Severe pain will respond to opioid analgesia such as morphine 4–6 mg. Pain associated with renal colic will respond well to diclofenac. There is some concern that administering analgesia may mask other symptoms but there is no clinical evidence to support this (Smith 2008).
- Symptomatic control of nausea and vomiting using anti-emetics.

The patient with diarrhoea

Diarrhoea is characterized by the passage of frequent, watery stools, which may have an offensive odour. Normally it will last for 1–2 days but if it persists can lead to dehydration and electrolyte imbalances (see Chapter 7). Chronic diarrhoea can lead to weight loss and malnutrition. In serious cases diarrhoea is often accompanied with other symptoms, including fever, cramps, dyspepsia, and intestinal bleeding.

Diarrhoea can be caused by several different mechanisms: osmotic diarrhoea, motility, diarrhoea and secretory diarrhoea.

Osmotic diarrhoea can be caused by nutrient malabsorption as sugars such as glucose, fructose, lactose, and sorbitol draw water into the colon and increase faecal water content. This can occur as a result of lactose intolerance, excessive sorbitol consumption, excessive fructose consumption in the form of fruits, and high concentrated formulated feeds.

Motility darrhoea speeds up peristalsis and can accelerate entry of fluids into the colon. This can occur following gastric surgery and removal of the lower part of the ileuem and caecum, the ileoceacal valve.

Secretory diarrhoea is often caused by bacterial food poisoning or enteritis. In hospital infections, *Clostridium difficile* can be the major cause of diarrhoea. Patients suffering from inflammatory bowel disease (Crohn's, ulcerative colitis) may also suffer from chronic diarrhoea or acute episodes of diarrhoea during exacerbations of their condition.

Nurses' role in managing diarrhoea

During episodes of diarrhoea it is important that personal hygiene is maintained and the skin around the anal sphincter is protected from excoriation. Recording faecal loss is essential in order to maintain an accurate fluid balance chart and to ensure appropriate oral intake is maintained. In acute cases of diarrhoea, fluid loss can be excessive and intravenous rehydration will be required (see Chapter 7).

Treatment of diarrhoea is based on treating the underlying cause and, if food-related, omitting the dietary source. If the diarrhoea is caused by the administration of enteral feeds it is important that the feed is not stopped. Advice should be sought from the dietician, who may recommend that the rate of the feed is reduced or may prescribe fibre-containing feeds to increase the faecal bulk and reduce gastric transit time.

The patient with constipation

Many patients in hospital may complain of constipation. During acute illness, becoming constipated may exacerbate the management of other conditions as people strain to empty their bowels. In addition, constipation may exacerbate confusional states, especially in the elderly or, post operatively, as toxins from the colon enter the bloodstream.

Dietary management of constipation is focused on ensuring that adequate fluids and fibre-containing foods are consumed. In the management of the acutely ill patient, laxatives, suppositories, and enemas may be required as dietary intake is reduced (see Table 6.7).

The patient with intestinal obstruction

Mechanical obstruction is divided into obstruction of the small bowel (including the duodenum) (Box 6.7) and obstruction of the large bowel (Box 6.8). Obstruction may be partial or complete. About 85% of partial small-bowel obstructions resolve with non-operative treatment, whereas about 85% of complete small-bowel obstructions require operation. The most common causes of mechanical obstruction are adhesions, hernias, and tumours (Berg *et al.* 2002).

Table 6.7 Laxatives

Laxative type	Active ingredient	Method of action	Cautions
Fibre	Methylcellulose, psyllium	Increase stool weight and aid in formation of soft bulky stools	May increase flatulence. Psyllium may cause an allergic reaction
Emollient	Docusate sodium	Detergent action promotes mixing of water with stools	Limited effect
Osmotic laxative	Lactulose	Unabsorbed carbohydrate attracts water in large intestine	May cause flatulence and cramp
Saline laxatives (osmotic laxatives)	Magnesium hydroxide, sodium sulphate	Unabsorbed salt attracts and retains water in large intestine	May cause bloating and watery stools. Should be used with caution
Stimulant	Senna, bisacodyl, cascara, castor oil	Act as local irritants to colonic tissue; stimulates peristalsis and mucosal secretions	May alter fluid and electrolyte balance

Based on data from British National Formulary (2008).

Pathophysiology

In simple mechanical obstruction, blockage occurs without vascular compromise. Ingested fluid and food, digestive secretions, and gas accumulate above the obstruction. The proximal bowel distends and the distal segment collapses. The normal secretory and absorptive functions of the mucosa are depressed, and the bowel wall becomes oedematous and congested.

Strangulating obstruction is obstruction with compromised blood flow; it occurs in nearly 25% of patients with small-bowel obstruction. Venous obstruction occurs first, followed by arterial occlusion, resulting in rapid ischemia of the bowel wall. The ischemic bowel becomes oedematous and infarcts, leading to gangrene and perforation.

Box 6.7 Signs and symptoms associated with obstruction of the small intestine

- Abdominal cramps centred around the umbilicus or in the epigastrium.
- Vomiting.
- Complete obstruction—constipation or severe constipation (obstipation).
- Partial obstruction—diarrhoea.
- Severe, steady pain suggests that strangulation has occurred. In the absence of strangulation, the abdomen is not tender.
- Hyperactive, high-pitched peristalsis with rushes coinciding with cramps is typical.
- With infarction, the abdomen becomes tender and auscultation reveals a silent abdomen or minimal peristalsis.
- Shock and oliguria are serious signs that indicate either late simple obstruction or strangulation.

> **Box 6.8 Signs and symptoms associated with obstruction of the large intestine**
>
> ◆ Symptoms that develop more gradually than those caused by small-bowel obstruction.
> ◆ Increasing constipation leads to obstipation and abdominal distention.
> ◆ Vomiting may occur several hours after onset of other symptoms and may smell faecal-like but is not common.
> ◆ Lower abdominal cramps unproductive of faeces occur.
> ◆ Distended abdomen with loud borborygmi.
> ◆ Systemic symptoms are relatively mild, and fluid and electrolyte deficits are uncommon.

Nutrition and the acutely ill patient

During periods of acute illness the initial focus of care will be in maintaining the airway, breathing, and circulation, and managing the acute symptoms. Recognizing the importance of nutritional support at this time will help to avoid unnecessary complications and delayed recovery.

The key to nutritional management during the acute phase of an illness is ensuring that the patient is able to achieve energy balance, to minimize protein losses and to ensure fluid balance is maintained (Severino Brandi *et al.* 1997). In all patients, likely micronutrient and electrolyte needs must also be met and referral to a dietician at an early stage can minimize complications associated with micronutrient/electrolyte deficiency states developing (NICE 2006a). It is important that when planning nutritional support the patient is assessed, as both overfeeding and underfeeding can lead to complications.

Maintaining energy balance

In health it is important that the diet is balanced, with appropriate amounts of food, containing macro- and micronutrients consumed from each of the food groups. A healthy diet containing adequate amounts of starch, fat, and protein will supply adequate amounts of energy and ensure that energy stores in the form of glycogen in the liver and skeletal muscle, and as triglyceride in adipocytes, are maintained. If a wide range of foods from different food groups are consumed then stores of micronutrients and trace elements will also be maintained.

During acute illness the need for a balanced diet based on healthy eating is reduced, although if the illness is prolonged or if the patient is malnourished, dietary advice from the dieticians is essential to avoid micro- or macronutrient deficiency developing. Patients with poor dietary intake prior to their illness will have reduced reserves of energy and stores of micronutrients prior to admission into hospital and are therefore at greater risk of developing malnutrition in hospital. It is estimated that as many as one-third of patients will be malnourished on admission into hospital (Jebb 1994; Kondrup *et al.* 2002; Holmes 2007; Kubrak & Jensen 2007).

During periods of illness there is a natural reduction in dietary intake or loss of appetite as a result of the actual disease impacting on eating, digesting, and absorbing nutrients, or of the presence of circulating cytokines, which depress the appetite. The body's response to this is to mobilize stores of energy through hormonal and chemical signals: a stress response. Normal reserves of micronutrients and trace elements during this acute phase will be sufficient to meet the additional demands.

An optimum store of glycogen in the liver and skeletal muscle will provide glucose for approximately 24 h. These stores are mobilized by the action of glucagon, cortisol, and adrenaline. It is important in health and in ill-health that blood glucose is maintained at between 4 and 6 mmol/L and the utilization of glycogen can achieve this for a short period of time when no food is being consumed. Once the glycogen stores have been utilized there is a metabolic shift towards using stored lipids and functional proteins such as skeletal muscle. The release of fatty acids and amino acids into the bloodstream provide substrates for the liver to synthesize glucose. Hyperglycaemia as a result of the stress response, associated with acute illness, is not uncommon and must be managed (see section on raised blood glucose). Although lipids are more energy-dense than proteins, their use as an energy substrate is limited by the metabolic production of ketones and increased oxygen consumption. Unlike periods of starvation when there is conservation of body mass, during the acute phase of an illness there is continued use of both lipids and proteins. The continued loss of muscle mass can lead to complications such as respiratory infections, urinary tract infections, increased risk of pressure sores, and reduced mobility due to lethargy (Villet et al. 2005).

Protein requirements

In health the average adult requires approximately 0.75 g of protein per kilogram of body weight. This dietary intake of protein from a wide range of food sources is sufficient to ensure all essential amino acids are normally consumed. During acute illness, and where protein loss is exacerbated with complex wounds or high losses of exudates, protein intake can increase to as much as 2.0 g/kg body weight. Even when protein intakes are adequate, the continued catabolism of protein in the body due to metabolic stress can lead to a negative nitrogen balance.

Hypermetabolism and negative nitrogen balance

Metabolic stress causes hypermetabolism. This refers to the amount of energy needed to meet cellular requirements and occurs due to the release of chemicals known as cytokines and the hormones adrenaline and cortisol into the circulation. The extent of the hypermetabolism will reflect the nature of the disease or extent of trauma. Patients suffering from sepsis, head injuries, multiple fractures, malignant tumours, and burns can have a dramatically increased metabolic rate, which can exacerbate weight and lean tissue loss during the acute phase as energy and protein requirements are not met by dietary intake (Allan Palmer et al. 1996; Severino Brandi et al. 1997). In addition, the continued mobilization of amino acids from tissue proteins, hypercatabolism, and the depletion of essential amino acids causes a negative nitrogen balance as amino acids are utilized as a metabolic fuel. Negative nitrogen balance indicates the dietary protein intake (proteins contain nitrogen) is less than nitrogen loss. It is known that most patients who are acutely ill require nutritional support.

Calculating energy requirements

The Harris–Benedict equation is commonly used to estimate the basal energy expenditure and this is then multiplied by a stress factor to estimate the energy needs of the acutely ill patient (Box 6.9). Although this calculation is commonly performed by the dieticians in high dependency areas, it is helpful for nurses in a general clinical context when considering the energy requirements of patients who are acutely ill. Alternatively a more pragmatic approach is to multiply the patient's weight by a factor appropriate for the patient's condition or to use standard figures (Box 6.10).

Box 6.9 Estimating energy needs to support basal energy expenditure using the Harris–Benedict equation

Step 1 Calculate basal energy expenditure (BEE)

$$\text{Women BEE} = 655.1 + \left(9.563 \times \text{weight (kg)}\right)$$
$$+ \left[1.85 \times \text{height (cm)}\right) - \left(4.676 \times \text{age (years)}\right)$$
$$\text{Men BEE} = 66.5 + \left(13.75 \times \text{weight (kg)}\right)$$
$$+ \left(5.003 \times \text{height (cm)}\right) - \left(6.775 \times \text{age (years)}\right)$$

If patient is obese (BMI > 30) use adjusted weight in the equation.

$$\text{Adjusted weight} = \text{ideal body weight (IBW)}$$
$$+ \left(0.5 \times \left(\text{actual body weight} - \text{IBW}\right)\right)$$

Step 2 Multiply BEE by an appropriate stress factor

- Postoperative, no complications: 1.0
- Peritonitis: 1.05–1.25
- Cancer: 1.10–1.45
- Long bone fracture: 1.25–1.30
- Severe infection: 1.3–1.55
- Multiple trauma: 1.3–1.55
- Burns (over 40% body surface): 2.0

Adapted from (Johansen *et al.* 2004)

Nutritional screening and planning

It is generally considered that there is no gold standard for assessment of nutritional status and it is important that a range of data is gathered through nursing assessment, the use of nutritional screening tools, and biochemical markers (Brugler *et al.* 2005; Capra 2007). Nutritional screening to identify nutritional status and risk of malnutrition should be completed using a valid tool on all patients on admission into hospital (NICE 2006b). Several tools are available, with British Association of Enteral and Parenteral Nutrition (BAPEN) recommending the use of the Malnutrition Universal Screening Tool (MUST).

The MUST tool has been developed to provide a quick and reliable screening tool for use by nurses to establish the risk of malnutrition in hospital. It identifies three simple steps to identify

Box 6.10 Estimating energy and protein requirements for patients who are not severely ill or injured

Energy for a patient with sepsis: 25–30 kcal/kg body weight/day

Protein intake: 0.8–1.5 g/kg body weight/day

Adapted from NICE 2006b

Clinical link 6.2 (see Appendix for answers)

Eva, 84, has been admitted with a fracture of the left neck of femur and the left radius following a road traffic accident. She weighs 59 kg. She is 1.45 m tall.

◆ What actions will you take in order to plan the nutritional support for Eva during the acute phase of her illness?

After Eva returns from theatre she is confused and disorientated. She has had 3 units of packed cells whilst in theatre and there was an intravenous infusion of 1 L of normal saline running over 4 h. 24 h later she is still not eating or drinking well. No further intravenous fluids have been prescribed. She has a cannula in situ.

◆ What actions will you take to ensure that Eva's nutritional status is not compromised during this period?

nutritional risk (Table 6.8; Elia 2000; Weekes *et al.* 2004). Completion of this tool will enable appropriate referral to the dietetic department for additional nutritional support.

Biochemical markers, such as visceral proteins, total lymphocyte count, and nitrogen balance are also measured in the acutely ill patient. The measurement of visceral proteins such as albumin, immune complexes and total lymphocytes are associated with mortality and morbidity but not nutritional status (Kubrak & Jensen 2007).

NICE (2006b) recommend that nutrition support should be considered in people who are malnourished, as defined by any of the following:

◆ a BMI of less than 18.5 kg/m^2

◆ unintentional weight loss greater than 10% within the last 3–6 months

Table 6.8 MUST tool: Malnutrition Universal Screening Tool

Step	Scoring	
Step 1	BMI >20	Score = 0
	BMI 18.5–20	Score = 1
BMI < 18.5	Score = 2	Refer to BMI reckoner if needed
Step 2	In the past 3–6 months, has the patient experienced unplanned weight loss?	
	<5% loss	Score = 0
	5–10% loss	Score = 1
	>10% loss	Score = 2
	Refer to weight loss reckoner if needed	
Step 3	Is the patient acutely ill and:	
	has had no nutritional intake for more than 5 days?	
	is likely to have no nutritional intake for more than 5 days?	
	If the answer to either of these questions is 'yes', score = 2	
	If the answer to both of these questions is 'no', score = 0	
	Refer to guidance notes in ward nutrition folder	
Step 4	Overall score (Add the scores for Steps 1, 2 and 3)	

Adapted from BAPEN (Elie 2000).

- a BMI of less than 20 kg/m^2 and unintentional weight loss greater than 5% within the last 3–6 months.

Patients who have diseases where nutritional support is part of the clinical management will normally be referred to the dietetics department. This includes patients who have:

- diabetic ketoacidosis or non-ketotic hyperosmolar states
- liver failure
- pancreatitis
- renal failure
- inflammatory bowel disease—Crohn's disease
- burns.

If, after admission into hospital, a patient develops a condition that compromises their nutritional status, timely referral for nutritional support or advice is essential.

NICE (2006b) recommend that nutrition support should be considered in people at risk of malnutrition, as defined by any of the following:

- have eaten little or nothing for more than 5 days and/or are likely to eat little or nothing for the next 5 days or longer
- have a poor absorptive capacity, and/or have high nutrient loses, and/or have increased nutritional needs from causes such as catabolism.

Compromise of patient nutritional status

Factors that will compromise a patient's nutritional status whilst in hospital include the following.

Nil by mouth Prolonged periods spent 'nil by mouth' during diagnosis, investigations, or surgical procedures can compromise a patient's nutritional status. Any investigations and surgical interventions should be planned, and current guidance suggests that the periods when a patient is nil by mouth should be kept to a minimum (see Box 6.11). To avoid unnecessary delays with eating and drinking it is important that:

- a nutritional screen is completed and discussed with the multidisciplinary team in order for a nutritional plan to be devised that will indicate when eating and drinking will resume
- drinks and snacks are available in the clinical setting for when meals are missed

---

Box 6.11 Guidance for preoperative fasting in adults undergoing elective surgery: 'the 2 and 6 rule'

'2' intake of water up to 2 h before induction of anaesthesia

'6' a minimum preoperative fasting time of 6 h for food (solids, milk, and milk-containing drinks)

The anaesthetic team should consider further interventions for patients at higher risk of regurgitation and aspiration.

Postoperative resumption of oral intake in healthy adults

Patients should be encouraged to drink when ready, providing there are no complications.
Adapted from (RCN 2005)

- if investigations or operations are delayed, nurses and clinicians assess whether fluids and/or food can be given.
- if a patient is nil by mouth for more than 24 h, the dietetic team is informed and nurses and clinicians discuss whether alternative routes for providing nutritional support are required and complete a nutritional plan.

Other factors Various other factors can compromise patient nutritional status:

- uncontrolled vomiting or nausea—see section on nausea and vomiting
- uncontrolled faecal loss—see section on diarrhoea
- confusion and disorientation associated with infection, dehydration, or post anaesthesia
- uncontrolled pain—see section on abdominal pain
- increased breathlessness
- prolonged infection
- multiple pathology.

Nutritional support

In the acutely ill patient, nutritional support focuses on the patient's needs for energy, protein and fluids. It is important when managing the care of the patient that food intake as well as fluid intake is monitored and recorded. In all patients, likely micronutrient and electrolyte needs must also be met.

To help meet the increased energy and protein needs patients must be offered small, easily digested, energy dense foods. At this early stage it is less important that fruits and vegetables are consumed although as the patient's condition improves they should be included within the diet. Oral supplements in the form of formulated feeds are of use as they are nutritionally complete. However, if they are not well tolerated or disliked then using milk-based drinks is recommended. Studies have suggested that supplements can improve patient outcomes (Russell 2007; Stratton & Elia 2007).

For patients unable to meet their nutritional needs through an oral diet, nutritional support using an artificial route should be considered. The most common route for short-term feeding (less than 3 weeks) is with enteral feeding tubes via the nasogastric or orogastric route (Holmes 2004; Braga *et al.* 2006).

Enteral feeding

If the GI tract is functioning but the patient is unable to meet their nutritional needs with oral intake, then feeding using a fine-bore feeding tube is required. The decision to place a fine-bore feeding tube should be made if the patient (NICE 2006b):

- is malnourished or at risk of malnutrition
- has inadequate or unsafe oral intake
- has a functioning, accessible GI tract.

Enteral feeding should not be considered if the patient has a non-functioning GI tract due to:

- hypovolaemia, which leads to poor cardiac output and reduced perfusion of the GI tract
- peritonitis.

Enteral feeding can also be used to supplement oral intakes.

The position of all feeding tubes should be ascertained after placement using pH graded paper or X-ray (NPSA 2005) (Box 6.12). Local protocols should address the clinical criteria that permit

> ### Box 6.12 Checking the position of an enteral fine bore feeding tube
>
> Aspirate stomach contents using a 20 mL syringe. Test on pH graded paper. The pH should be less than or equal to 5.5.
>
> Note position of markers on tube and compare with those recorded on insertion.
> X-ray.

enteral tube feeding. These criteria should include how to proceed when the ability to make repeat checks of the tube position is limited by the inability to aspirate the tube or the checking of pH is invalid because of gastric acid suppression due to proton pump inhibitors and histamine-2 receptor antagonists (Marshall & West 2006).

Following insertion of a feeding tube it is important that its position is checked prior to feeding; that the tube is flushed before and after administration of a feed with clear water, and that where possible medications are not administered via the tube (NPSA 2005). Blockage of feeding tubes by incorrect administration of medications or a failure to flush the tube can delay provision of nutritional support, exacerbating the risk of malnutrition.

The formula feed will be prescribed by a dietician and should be administered and recorded to ensure nutritional support is maintained. Feeds can be administered in a bolus or a continuous mode using a pump. Normally nasogastric feeding is delivered continuously over 16–24 h. If the patient is prescribed insulin then 24-h feeding is recommended (NICE 2006b).

Parenteral nutrition

Nutritional support in acute care settings is predominantly through oral or enteral feeding. NICE (2006a) recommend that parenteral nutrition is considered in people who are malnourished or at risk of malnutrition due to:

+ inadequate or unsafe oral/enteral nutritional intake

+ a non-functioning, inaccessible, or perforated GI tract.

Parenteral feeds are complete feeds containing amino acids, fatty acids, and glucose. It is essential that prior to commencing feeding a full nutritional assessment is completed to ensure that micronutrient and macronutrient needs are met.

The parenteral route can be through dedicated, peripherally inserted central lines or a dedicated, centrally placed central venous catheter. Administering of parenteral nutrition via a

> ### Clinical link 6.3 (see Appendix for answers)
>
> George is 38 years old and has had multiple fractures following a road traffic accident. He is on traction and is immobile. Prior to his injury he ate a normal diet. A nasogastric tube has been inserted and a lactose-free standard formula feed has been prescribed. He is prescribed 2200 mL/24 h.
>
> + Critically discuss the actions will you take prior to commencing the feed.
>
> Eight hours later George complains of feeling sick and nauseous.
>
> + What actions will you take?

peripheral venous catheter should be considered for patients who will need nutritional support for less than 14 days. If parenteral nutrition is required for greater than 30 days then a tunnelled central venous catheter should be considered (NICE 2006b).

Nursing management of parenteral nutrition In addition to monitoring the haemodynamic status and fluids and maintaining patient comfort, strict asepsis must be maintained to avoid infections. Parenteral nutrition can cause alterations to biochemistry and fluid balance due to the increased osmolar load (see Chapter 7). The patient should be monitored for:

♦ hyperglycaemia

♦ liver dysfunction

♦ refeeding syndrome.

Refeeding problems

Severely malnourished patients or those that have had little or no food intake prior to their illness may suffer from complications associated with refeeding due to over-rapid or unbalanced nutrition (Braga *et al.* 2006).

Refeeding syndrome During starvation there are adaptive reductions in cellular activity and organ function accompanied by micronutrient, mineral, and electrolyte deficiencies. These include:

♦ whole-body depletion of intracellular potassium, magnesium, and phosphate

♦ increased intracellular and whole-body sodium and water

♦ low insulin levels and partial switch from carbohydrate metabolism to ketone metabolism to meet energy demand

♦ impaired cardiac and renal reserve with a decreased ability to excrete excess salt and water.

Refeeding the malnourished patient will lead to an increase in demand for electrolytes and micronutrients, whilst there is a shift of sodium and water into the extracellular compartment. This fluid and electrolyte imbalance can lead to life-threatening clinical and biochemical abnormalities, including (NICE 2006b):

♦ hypokaleamia

♦ hypophosphataemia

♦ hyperglycaemia

♦ hypomagnesaemia

♦ hypocalcaemia

♦ cardiac failure, pulmonary oedema, and arrhythmias

♦ acute circulatory overload or circulatory fluid depletion.

Patients at risk of developing refeeding syndrome include:

♦ those who have had very little to eat for >5 days

♦ those with a BMI of more than 16 kg/m^2

♦ those who have had unintentional weight loss of >15% within the previous 6 months

♦ those with low levels of potassium, phosphate, or magnesium prior to any feeding.

When feeding patients who meet any of the above criteria it is recommended that feeding is commenced at 50% of requirements for the first 2 days, before increasing to meet full needs if biochemical (see Chapter 10) and clinical assessment reveal no refeeding problems. Caution should also be taken when feeding patients if they have a history of alcohol abuse or are prescribed some drugs, including insulin, chemotherapy drugs, antacids, and diuretics (Kreymann *et al.* 2006).

Wernicke–Korsakoff syndrome Wernicke–Korsakoff syndrome is commonly associated with patients who, due to alcohol abuse or chronic vomiting, become depleted in thiamine. Thiamine is important for carbohydrate metabolism and as refeeding commences, the cells switch to carbohydrate metabolism and thiamine demand increases. The syndrome is associated with acute neurological disturbances, including:

- apathy and disorientation
- nystagmus, ophthalmoplegia, or other eye movement disorders
- ataxia
- severe impairment of short-term memory, often with confabulation.

Management of patients with refeeding problems Patients who are at high risk of refeeding syndrome should be commenced feeding at low levels of energy and protein but with additional thiamine and other B group vitamins, along with balanced multivitamins and trace elements.

Patients at risk of Wernicke–Korsakoff syndrome need high doses of daily thiamine and other vitamins intravenously for 3 days, e.g. Pabrinex® 1+2 once per day plus oral thiamine (NICE 2006b).

Nutritional support of patients with disorders of the gastrointestinal tract

Patients admitted with acute illnesses that affect the GI tract should be referred to the dietician for full assessment and nutritional management. The nurse's role is to ensure that:

- food and fluid intakes are monitored and recorded
- all feeds prescribed are administered and recorded
- all prescribed vitamin, mineral, and electrolyte supplements are administered and recorded
- nutritional status is monitored.

Nutritional support following gastric surgery

Many patients will undergo gastric surgery. Cancer remains the most common reason for gastric surgery, although it can be advocated in the treatment of peptic ulcers resistant to drug therapy and morbid obesity. In the surgical procedure, either all (total gastrectomy) or part (partial gastrectomy) of the stomach is removed and attached to the small intestine.

Following a gastrectomy the patient will normally be nil by mouth and once oral intake has resumed the dietary restrictions will depend on the size of the remaining stomach.

Nutritional support includes the following (Rolfes *et al.* 2006):

- small, frequent meals, eating slowly and chewing food thoroughly
- low fat foods
- avoiding milk and milk-based foods that are high in lactose
- foods high in complex carbohydrates

- avoidance of sweets and simple sugars as they can increase osmolarity and increase transit time
- limit liquids to those consumed at meal times, as liquids can increase transit time, and avoiding drinking fluids within 45 min before or after meals
- lying down for 30 min following a meal to help slow down gastric emptying.

The surgery not only reduces the size of the stomach but also influences food tolerance, due to increased transit time and risk of 'dumping syndrome'.

Dumping syndrome

Following gastrectomy or gastric bypass surgery, patients can suffer from 'dumping syndrome', which refers to a group of symptoms associated with increased transit time. Normally the pyloric sphincter controls the rate of chyme leaving the stomach into the duodenum. If the pyloric sphincter is removed or bypassed this control is lost and the patient can suffer from unpleasant side effects. Early symptoms occur within 30 min of consuming food and include:

- nausea
- vomiting
- rapid heart beat
- abdominal cramping
- diarrhoea.

These symptoms are normally due to the increased transit time, rapid shift of fluids from the blood plasma to the intestines and increased peristalsis. Several hours later, late symptoms can occur, associated with hypoglycaemia caused by an exaggerated release of insulin in response to the sudden increased in absorbed carbohydrate. These symptoms include:

- anxiety
- confusion
- headache
- palpitations
- sweating
- feeling faint.

Nutritional support of the patient with liver disease

Fatty liver disease The usual management will require the elimination of factors that contribute to the disease process.

- Patients who consume large amounts of alcohol would benefit from reducing alcohol intake.
- Patients with elevated blood lipids require lipid management through diet (reduction in obesity) or medication (statins/fibrates). Rapid weight-loss should, however, be discouraged (Schütz *et al.* 2004).

Cirrhosis Patients with cirrhosis can have great difficulties in consuming sufficient nutrients to prevent malnutrition. Ascites and GI symptoms such as nausea, vomiting, and fatigue can reduce food intake. Sodium restriction due to fluid overload can make many foods unpalatable. Nutritional management needs to include the following considerations.

Individualized nutritional plan. The diet should not restrict protein or fat, and advice as to how to increase energy intake may be required. This includes snacks between meals, oral supplementation, and use of high-energy supplements.

Sodium and fluids may be restricted in order to manage ascites. Helping patients to replace salt with herbs and other spices will help food to remain palatable. If diuretics are used potassium levels also need to be monitored.

Multivitamin supplements are recommended. If steatorrhea is present then fat-soluble vitamins can be provided in water-soluble forms.

Hyperglycaemia may occur due to insulin resistance and this may need to be managed with insulin.

Protein intakes need to remain high, between 1.2 and 1.5 g/kg/day to maintain nitrogen balance.

Nutritional support of the patient with pancreatitis

Acute pancreatitis is often as a consequence of gall stones or excessive alcohol use. Patients often have severe abdominal; pain, nausea, and vomiting with abdominal distension. Elevated serum levels of amylase and lipase can help to confirm diagnosis. In the acute phase of the illness, oral fluids and food are often withheld until the pain and tenderness has subsided. In some cases recovery is rapid and a low-fat oral diet can begin within 3–7 days of disease onset. In more severe cases an elemental diet via a fine bore jejunal tube can provide sufficient nutrients (Boulton-Jones *et al.* 2004). An elemental feed contains predigested formulated nutrients, amino acids, fatty acids, and glucose, which do not require pancreatic enzymes for digestion. Patients with severe disease or those who present with preexisting signs of malnutrition need nutritional support. Parenteral nutrition is often commenced in order to provide adequate nutrients whilst resting the bowel, although there is evidence to support the use of enteral nutrition.

Malabsorption results from a lack of pancreatic enzymes. If faecal fat is in excess of 10 g/day, pancreatic enzyme should be considered to facilitate nutrient digestion. Supplementation with fat-soluble vitamins is also important. In managing the nutritional support the following should be considered:

+ protein and energy requirements are often high due to catabolic and hypermetabolic responses
+ fat has a stimulating effect on the pancreas and low-fat diets may be better tolerated by the patient
+ pancreatic enzyme replacement may be required to correct steatorrhoea.

Nutritional support of the patient with malabsorption

Malabsorption can be caused by a wide range of conditions that affect the length of the small intestine or its ability to absorb nutrients. Common symptoms associated with malabsorption include:

+ diarrhoea
+ steatorrhea
+ malnutrition.

Patients at risk of malabsorption include those with Crohn's disease, ulcerative colitis, and short bowel syndrome. It is estimated that as many as 75% patients with Crohn's disease are malnourished in hospital. Malabsorption causes both vitamin and mineral deficiency, weight loss, and hypoalbuminia. Many patients with malabsorption will be anaemic, secondary to iron, folate, or vitamin B12 deficiency. In general patients with inflammatory bowel disease should have enteral nutrition with formulated feeds to compensate for the chronic malnutrition they may suffer. If absorbtive capacity is severely reduced parenteral nutrition may be required (see section on parenteral nutrition) (Crocella *et al.* 2008).

Following extensive small intestinal resection, patients may suffer from 'short bowel syndrome,' where less than 100 cm of small intestine remains. Resections of the distal ileum may affect vitamin B12 and bile acid absorption. This can result in diarrhoea and steatorrhea and the patient need to have a fat restricted diet. Referral to the dietetic department is essential for nutritional management. If the colon is present this will enable the absorption of short-chain fatty acids, which accelerate water and sodium absorption.

Following resection there is a gradual adaptation of the remaining intestines, improving the absorptive capacity. Many patients who need parenteral nutritional support immediately following resection can adapt to relying on oral or enteral nutrition after a period of time.

The nursing management will include referral to the dietetic department, ensuring nutritional support is provided, continuation of haemodynamic monitoring and maintaining an accurate fluid chart.

End of chapter test

The following assessment will enable you to evaluate your theoretical knowledge of GI assessment and management as well as your ability to apply this theory to clinical practice. You should undertake the following assessment with an appropriately trained member of staff in clinical practice. If you are unable to answer any questions it may be helpful to revisit the section in this chapter.

Knowledge assessment

With the support of your mentor/supervisor from practice, work through the following prompts to explore your knowledge level about the GI system and nutritional support.

♦ Describe the structure and function of the GI tract.
♦ Discuss the role of the liver and pancreas as accessory organs of digestion.
♦ Describe the three stages of the swallowing reflex.
♦ Discuss the impact diet has on gastric emptying.
♦ Discuss the factors that stimulate nausea and vomiting.
♦ Describe the components of pancreatic secretions and their involvement in digestion of nutrients.
♦ Describe the role of bile salts in the digestion of fats.
♦ Describe the structure of the villus.
♦ Name the brush border enzymes and the substrates they act on.
♦ Critically discuss the importance of fluid balance in relation to the function of the small intestine.
♦ Describe the difference between somatic and visceral pain.
♦ Explain why patients with disorders of the GI tract may have 'referred pain'.
♦ Explain why malabsorption of carbohydrate may contribute to diarrhoea developing.

- Describe why the stomach and the ileum are important for the absorption of vitamin B12.
- Explain the aetiology of jaundice and what physical findings you might observe.
- Explain the difference between DKA and HNKS.
- Explain why acutely ill patients develop hypermetabolism.
- Explain why blood glucose can increase when you are acutely ill.
- Explain why insulin therapy may be required in the acutely ill patient.
- Critically discuss how hypermetabolism and starvation differ.
- How would you calculate energy demand in an acutely ill patient.
- Discuss what criteria you would use to decide whether a patient requires nutritional support.
- Explain why the position of enteral feeding tubes should only be checked using two methods.
- Critically discuss the impact of proton pump inhibitors on checking the position of enteral feeding tubes.
- Critically discuss refeeding syndrome.

Skills assessment

Under the guidance of your mentor/supervisor, undertake a nutritional screen, pain assessment, and swallowing assessment followed by appropriate interventions for any significant abnormality. Your mentor/supervisor will be able to assess your ability and provide feedback based on the following skills:

- Conducts a full patient history with a systems review considering key points that are relevant for a nutritional assessment.
- Demonstrates the use of a nutritional screening tool to identify the risk of malnutrition.
- Identifies what physical observations would raise concern about a patient's ability to swallow.
- Identifies what actions should be taken if a patient if a patient is 'nil by mouth' for more than 6 h.
- Completes a nutritional plan for a patient who requires enteral nutrition.
- Demonstrates ability to commence enteral feeding safely.
- Reviews current medications and intravenous therapy, rationalizing impact on pain and nausea.
- Interprets all subjective and objective findings from the nutritional screening tool, rationalizes possible causes for these abnormalities, and plans appropriate actions.
- Explains clinical reasoning and provides justification for all interventions of the nutritional management plan.
- Interprets all subjective and objective findings from the pain assessment, rationalizes possible causes for these abnormalities, and plans appropriate actions.
- Explains clinical reasoning and provides justification for all interventions of the pain management plan.
- Liaises with other members of the healthcare team as necessary, including nurse in charge, doctor, dietician, pharmacist, physiotherapist, and healthcare assistant.
- Demonstrates an ability to follow infection control guidelines while undertaking enteral feeding.

♦ Documents the nutrition management plan, completed actions, and evaluation of actions as per local policy.

References

Allan Palmer, T.E., Griffiths R.D., and Jones, C. (1996) Effect of parenteral glutamine on muscle in the very severely Ill. *Nutrition.* **12**, 316–20.

Alm-Kruse, K., Bull, E., and Laake, J. (2008) Nurse-led implementation of an insulin-infusion protocol in a general intensive care unit: improved glycaemic control with increased costs and risk of hypoglycaemia signals need for algorithm revision. *BMC Nurs.* **7**, 1.

Berg, D.F., *et al.* (2002) Acute surgical emergencies in inflammatory bowel disease. *Am. J. Surg.* **184**, 45–51.

British National Formulary (2008) Available at: http://www.bnf.org/bnf/ (accessed August 2008).

Boulton-Jones, J.R., *et al.* (2004) Experience of post-pyloric feeding in seriously ill patients in clinical practice. *Clin. Nutr.* **23**, 35–41.

Braga, J.M. *et al.* (2006) Implementation of dietitian recommendations for enteral nutrition results in improved outcomes. *J. Am. Dietetic Assoc.* **106**, 281–4.

Brugler, L. *et al.* (2005) A simplified nutrition screen for hospitalized patients using readily available laboratory and patient information. *Nutrition.* **21**, 650–8.

Capra, S. (2007) Nutrition assessment or nutrition screening—How much information is enough to make a diagnosis of malnutrition in acute care?. *Nutrition.* **23**, 356–7.

Coursin, D.B., Coursin D.B., and Unger B. (2002) Endocrine complications in intensive care unit patients. *Seminars in Anesthesia, Perioperative Medicine and Pain.* **21**, 59–74.

Crocella, L., Rocca, R., Daperno, M., Migliardi, M., and Pera, A. (2008) Bowel malabsorption. *Immuno*-analyse & *Biologie Spécialisée.* **23**, 224–9.

Degen. L.P. and Phillips, S.F. (1996) Variability of gastrointestinal transit in healthy women and men. *Gut.* **39**, 299.

Elia, M. (2000) Guidelines for the detection and management of malnutrition. BAPEN, Maidenhead.

Holmes, S. (2004) Enteral feeding and percutaneous endoscopic gastrostomy (nutrition focus). *Nurs. Stand.* **18**, 41–3.

Holmes, S. (2007) The effects of undernutrition in hospitalised patients (Clinical report). *Nurs. Stand.* **22**, 35–8.

McWhirter, J.P. and Pennington, C.R. (1994) Incidence and recognition of malnutrition in hospital. *Clin. Nutr.* **13**, 267–8.

Johansen, N. *et al.* (2004) Effect of nutritional support on clinical outcome in patients at nutritional risk. *Clin. Nutr.* **23**, 539–50.

Jones, A., Turner, K., and Handa, A. (2000) Surgical emergencies:acute abdominal pain. *Student BMJ.* **8**, 56–7.

Jones, C. (1998) The importance of oral hygiene in nutritonal support. *Br. J. Nurs.* **7**, 74–83.

Kondrup, J., *et al.* (2002) Incidence of nutritional risk and causes of inadequate nutritional care in hospitals. *Clin. Nutr.* **21**, 461–8.

Kreymann, K.G., *et al.* (2006) ESPEN Guidelines on enteral nutrition: intensive care. *Clin. Nutr.* **25**, 210–23.

Kubrak, C. and Jensen, L. (2007) Malnutrition in acute care patients: a narrative review. *Int. J. Nurs. Stud.* **44**, 1036–54.

Marin Caro, M.M., Laviano, A., and Pichard. C. (2007) Nutritional intervention and quality of life in adult oncology patients. *Clin. Nutr.* **26**, 289–301.

Marshall, A.P. and West, S.H. (2006) Enteral feeding in the critically ill: are nursing practices contributing to hypocaloric feeding? *Intensive Crit. Care Nurs.* **22**, 95–105.

McMullin, J. *et al.* (2007) Lowering of glucose in critical care: a randomized pilot trial. *J. Crit. Care.* **22**, 112–8.

NICE (2006a) *Nutrition Support in Adults*. NICE, London.

NICE (2006b) *Nutrition support for adults oral nutrition support, enteral tube feeding and parenteral nutrition*. NICE, London.

National Patient Safety Agency (2005) *Advice to the NHS on Reducing Harm Caused by the Misplacement of Nasogastric Feeding Tubes*. (Online). National Patient Safety Agency. Available at: http://www.nrls.npsa.nhs.uk/resources/?entryid45=59794 (accessed 1 August 2008).

Rawlins, C.A, Ward, J., and Truman, I.W. (2001) Effective mouth care for seriously ill patients. *Prof. Nurse*. **16**, 1025–8.

Royal College of Nursing (2005) Perioperative fasting in adults and children. Royal College of Nursing, London.

Rolfes, S.R., Pinna, K., and Whitney, E. (2006) *Understanding Normal and Clinical Nutrition*, 7th edn. Thomson Learning, London.

Russell, C.A. (2007) The impact of malnutrition on healthcare costs and economic considerations for the use of oral nutritional supplements. *Clin. Nutr. Suppl.* **2**, 25–32.

Schütz, T., *et al.* (2004) Clinical practice of nutrition in acute liver failure—a European survey. *Clin. Nutr.* **23**, 975–82.

Severino Brandi, L., Bertolini, R., and Calafà, M. (1997) Indirect calorimetry in critically ill patients: clinical applications and practical advice. *Nutrition.* **13**, 349–58.

SIGN (2004) *Management of patients with stroke: identification and management of dysphagia*. SIGN, Edinburgh.

Skipworth, R.J.E. and Fearon, K.C.H. (2008) Acute abdomen: peritonitis. *Surgery (Oxford).* **26**, 98–101.

Smith, J.K. and Lobo, D.N. (2008) Investigation of the acute abdomen. *Surgery (Oxford).* **26**, 91–97.

Stephenson, M. (2008) Non-surgical causes of abdominal pain. *Student BMS.* **16**, 246–47.

Stratton, R.J. and Elia, M. (2007) A review of reviews: A new look at the evidence for oral nutritional supplements in clinical practice. *Clin. Nutr. Suppl.* **2**, 5–23.

Villet, S., *et al.* (2005) Negative impact of hypocaloric feeding and energy balance on clinical outcome in ICU patients. *Clin. Nutr.* **24**, 502–9.

Weekes, E.C., Elia, M., and Emery, P.W. (2004) The development, validation and reliability of a nutrition screening tool based on the recommendations of the British Association for Parenteral and Enteral Nutrition (BAPEN). *Clin. Nutr.* **23**, 1104–12.

Wilson, J. (2005) Milk intolerance: lactose intolerance and cow's milk protein allergy. *Newborn Infant Nurs. Rev.* **5**, 203–7.

Chapter 7

Fluid assessment and associated treatment

Heather Baid

Chapter contents

Evaluating a patient's fluid status is an integral aspect of any nursing assessment because an abnormally high or low fluid balance significantly influences the cardiovascular, respiratory, renal, and metabolic systems. The purpose of this chapter is to examine:

- the anatomy and physiology of fluid balance
- pathophysiological changes of fluid balance in acute care
- assessment of fluid status
- management of the patient with fluid excess
- management of the patient with fluid deficit
- administration of intravenous fluids and blood products.

Learning outcomes

This chapter will enable you to:

- describe the normal anatomy of fluids in the body, including the intravascular, interstitial, and intercellular fluid compartments
- explain the physiology of how the body maintains normal fluid homeostasis
- identify causes for an abnormal fluid balance with acute care patients
- explain how the body responds and compensates for an abnormal fluid balance
- discuss how normovolaemia can be maintained with acute care patients, including measures to prevent an abnormal fluid balance
- explore a systematic approach to assessing a patient's fluid status
- critically analyse normal and abnormal findings of a fluid assessment
- evaluate the nursing management of a patient with fluid excess and fluid deficit
- differentiate between crystalloid, colloids, and blood products
- discuss the nursing responsibilities for intravenous therapy.

Introduction

Water is the most abundant substance in the body, contributing to 55–60% of total body weight. Because there are continual losses of water as part of normal physiological function, an intake of water is required to achieve an equal net fluid balance. Acute care nurses require a thorough understanding of their patients' fluid status because of the risk for altered fluid balance with acute illness. This chapter will review the anatomy and physiology of fluid followed by the nursing care involved in assessing and managing an abnormal fluid balance.

Normal anatomy and physiology

Water in the body can be identified according to where the fluid rests. The majority is located inside the cells, with the remaining found in extracellular areas. Of this extracellular fluid (ECF), 80% is interstitial with the remaining 20% found in the intravascular space as plasma. If one area has an increase or decrease in total water content, fluid will shift across to maintain the normal distribution of two-thirds intracellular fluid (ICF) and one-third ECF. Fluid homeostasis is then maintained with a constant ratio of water across these three fluid compartments (see Figure 7.1).

There are a variety of physiological pressures preventing fluid from leaking out of its designated area otherwise the normal distribution of water between the intracellular, interstitial, and intravascular spaces would be lost. These pressures include *osmotic pressure*, *hydrostatic pressure*, and *oncotic pressure*.

Osmotic pressure pulls water across a semi-permeable membrane towards an area of greater solute concentration. As there is a higher amount of sodium in the ECF, sodium creates an osmotic pressure in the extracellular compartment. Similarly, potassium contributes to the osmotic pressure that maintains fluid within the cells.

Hydrostatic pressure is the pressure a fluid places onto the wall of a vessel and acts as a 'pushing force' because it pushes water out of the blood vessels into the interstitial space. Oncotic pressure keeps fluid inside vessels from the presence of large plasma proteins and is therefore a 'pulling force' pulling fluids into the blood from the interstitium. If the hydrostatic pressure is greater than the oncotic pressure, fluid leaves the intravascular space, resulting in a higher interstitial volume. Similarly, if the oncotic pressure rises more than the hydrostatic pressure, there is an increased movement of fluid into the intravascular space.

This interplay between hydrostatic and oncotic pressure occurs naturally in the body within the capillaries where at the arteriole side, hydrostatic pressure is greater than oncotic pressure, allowing fluid to move into the interstitial space. As the blood flows through the capillary, the amount of water in the blood then decreases by the time the fluid reaches the venule end. Large molecules such as albumin are not able to cross the capillary membrane with the escaping water, leading to an increase in oncotic pressure that pulls fluid back into the capillary. The end result is equilibrium because of the overall net balance of water remaining equal as the hydrostatic and oncotic pressures counterbalance each other (see Figure 7.2).

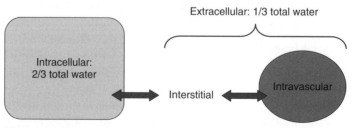

Figure 7.1 Fluid homeostasis.

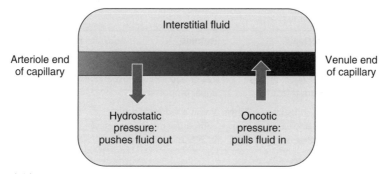

Figure 7.2 Fluid pressures.

There are further extracellular areas in the body where fluid is found in addition to those previously mentioned, such as fluid in the cerebral spinal space, pleural cavity, peritoneum, joints, and eyes. These are known as *transcellular fluids* but are not normally altered by significant daily losses or gains.

Normally, the amount of water gained during a day equals the amount of water lost, leaving the body with a net fluid balance of zero. Eating and drinking comprises the majority of water intake, with a small amount of water also produced through metabolic processes. In addition to the obvious water lost as urine, there are also insensible losses through the skin, lungs, and gastrointestinal (GI) tract. See Table 7.1 for a breakdown of water gain and water loss for an average adult (Tortora & Derrickson 2009).

Pathophysiology

Fluid deficit

A shortage of fluid in the intravascular and interstitial compartments occurs when there is a reduced amount of water and/or sodium due to abnormal losses, an inability to replace normal losses, or a combination of both. If there is an equal proportion of water and sodium lost, the extracellular fluid remains isotonic. Water then redistributes between the intra- and extracellular spaces, resulting in an overall reduction in each compartment. If mostly water is lost, the extracellular fluid becomes hypertonic, drawing water in from the ICF and causing *cellular dehydration*. Intravascular volume may initially improve from the fluid shift but will eventually drop if the

Table 7.1 Water gain and water loss

Water gain		Water loss	
Oral fluids	1600 mL	Urine	1500 mL
Oral food	700 mL	Skin	600 mL
Metabolic water	200 mL	Lungs	300 mL
	2500 mL	GI tract	100 mL
			2500 mL

GI, gastrointestinal.

Table 7.2 Fluid deficit

	Hypertonic	**Isotonic**	**Hypotonic**
Serum sodium level	>145 mmol/L	135–45 mmol/L	<135 mmol/L
Cause	More water than sodium is lost	Water and sodium lost in equal proportions	More sodium than water is lost
Effect	Fluid shifts from ICF into ECF—increased cellular dehydration	Volume reduced in all compartments (equal deficit in ECF and ICF)	Fluid shifts from ECF into ICF—increased hypovolaemia

ECF, extracellular fluid; ICF, intracellular fluid.

water loss continues. If there is predominantly a reduction in serum sodium, the subsequent hypotonicity of the extracellular fluid encourages water to shift into the cells, leaving the extracellular space volume depleted (see Table 7.2).

Reduced fluid in the intravascular space is clinically significant because a normal blood volume (*normovolaemia*) is essential for adequate tissue perfusion, transport of substances throughout the body, and functioning of all body systems. *Hypovolaemia* refers to an ineffective volume of circulating blood because of actual fluid loss or from fluid shifting out of the intravascular space to another compartment.

Hypovolaemia typically takes place when there is a reduction in total extracellular volume (intravascular + interstitial). However, there can be hypovolaemia with normal or increased extracellular volume if the amount of interstitial fluid is high while the intravascular volume is low. The total amount of water in the patient appears to be increased with a positive daily fluid balance but the abnormal fluid distribution leaves the vascular space relatively dry. In essence, there is a large amount of fluid in the body but it is in the wrong place to be effective. An example of this would be a low serum albumin causing fluid to leak out of the blood vessels to become oedema. The total amount of extracellular fluid remains high because of the excess fluid in the interstitial space, although the patient remains hypovolaemic because of the low intravascular volume.

When fluid builds up in the interstitium or another potential space that is not normally filled with fluid, it is referred to as *third-space fluid*. This fluid is physiologically useless and in large amounts causes hypovolaemia as fluid shifts out of the vasculature into the third-space area (Holcomb 2008). See Table 7.3 for causes of hypovolaemia with decreased interstitial volume compared with hypovolaemia with increased/normal interstitial volume.

Third-space areas:

♦ interstitium (peripheral/pulmonary oedema)

♦ peritoneum (ascites)

♦ pleural space (effusion)

♦ ileus (fluid accumulates within obstructed intestine).

Fluid deficit response

There are a variety of compensation mechanisms that take place in response to hypovolaemia to prevent detrimental effects from a low blood volume. Baroreceptors detect the reduction in pressure from the low volume and send a message to the central nervous system. The sympathetic nervous system is then stimulated, which increases the heart rate and force of myocardial contraction and causes vasoconstriction.

Table 7.3 Hypovolaemia

Hypovolaemia with decreased interstitial volume	Hypovolaemia with increased/normal interstitial volume
Fluid loss: • gastrointestinal—diarrhoea, vomiting, nasogastric suction • skin—sweating, burns, wounds • haemorrhage	Increased hydrostatic pressure: • chronic heart failure (increased hydrostatic pressure in veins) • liver failure (increased hydrostatic pressure in portal system)
Reduced intake of sodium and water: • poor oral intake of food and water • nil by mouth without intravenous replacement of sodium and water	Decreased colloid osmotic pressure: • low albumin Increased capillary permeability: • sepsis, shock, burns, trauma
Impaired retention of sodium and water: • diuretics • renal sodium wasting • adrenal insufficiency • osmotic diuresis	Impaired lymphatic drainage

The kidneys also sense a decreased glomerular filtration rate and activate the renin–angiotensin–aldosterone system. This begins when hypotension causes the kidneys to produce renin, which acts on circulating angiotensinogen to produce angiotensin I. Angiotensin-converting enzyme then transforms angiotensin I into angiotensin II and the following is a summary of the effects of angiotensin II:

• vasoconstriction

• increased reabsorption of sodium, chloride, and water in the proximal convoluted tubule

• adrenal cortex stimulated to release aldosterone that enhances sodium and water reabsorption in collecting ducts

• thirst sensation.

An increase in plasma osmolarity stimulates the pituitary gland to release antidiuretic hormone (ADH), also known as vasopressin. ADH enhances water reabsorption in the collecting ducts that concentrates the urine and increases the amount of water in the blood.

The goal of these compensation mechanisms is to have a net result of improving cardiac output and tissue perfusion that were compromised from the reduction in circulating blood volume. If hypovolaemia continues to the point where the compensation mechanisms fail, *hypovolaemic shock* develops (see Chapter 3). Inadequate tissue perfusion then impairs the ability of the cells to conduct aerobic metabolism, leading to anaerobic metabolism. If left untreated, the anaerobic metabolism will eventually result in acidosis, cardiac depression, intravascular coagulation, increased capillary permeability, and release of toxins.

Fluid excess

An overall gain in extracellular fluid results in increased water in the vascular and interstitial spaces. *Hypervolaemia*, commonly called 'fluid overload', occurs when there is a high amount of circulating blood volume which may be due to:

• increased retention of sodium and water

• heart failure

- liver failure
- nephrotic syndrome
- excessive administration of glucocorticosteroids
- SIADH (syndrome of inappropriate ADH)

♦ reduced excretion of sodium and water

- renal failure

♦ iatrogenic excessive administration of intravenous therapy

- crystalloid/colloid infusions
- blood transfusion
- total parenteral nutrition

♦ fluid shifting from interstitial space into the blood

- redistribution of oedema
- excessive administration of hypertonic solutions.

Although there are a variety of causes of hypervolaemia, a frequent reason seen in acute care is heart failure. Whether there is chronic heart failure present or a new acute cardiac problem causing the heart as a muscle to fail, blood is not ejected properly from the ventricles and becomes congested in the pulmonary and systemic regions (see Chapter 3).

A further consideration is the underlying processes involved with chronic heart failure. One of the normal compensation mechanisms for chronic heart failure is to increase the total blood volume, which allows for a greater stretch of ventricle wall thereby improving the force of contraction for each beat (Starling's law). However, hypervolaemia develops over time from the overall rise in blood volume and leads to fluid leaking out of the vascular space into the interstitial space. As the heart continues to fail, blood also starts to back up, causing pulmonary oedema with left ventricular failure and peripheral oedema with right ventricular failure.

Renal failure is another type of organ dysfunction resulting in hypervolaemia. Clearly, if there is fluid intake through drinking or an intravenous infusion but the kidneys are not excreting adequate amounts of sodium and water, then the total blood volume will continue to rise. See Chapter 5 for an extensive overview of renal failure.

An intravenous infusion may be necessary for a patient who is not taking in oral fluids, has recently had surgery, or requires total parenteral nutrition. Regardless of the type of crystalloid or colloid fluid being delivered, if the infusion rate or total amount of fluid being delivered is excessive, iatrogenic hypervolaemia may result. This occurs when the heart and kidneys are not able to keep up with their roles in maintaining normal homeostasis during the intravenous infusion.

Similarly, a blood transfusion will cause hypervolaemia if the resulting blood volume is increased to a level where the heart has difficulty pumping effectively or the kidneys do not draw off enough fluid to maintain a normal quantity of plasma. Patients with heart failure are particularly at risk for hypervolaemia from a blood transfusion, which is why they are often prescribed a diuretic to achieve a higher haemoglobin level while removing excess intravenous fluid (see Table 7.4).

Intracellular fluid excess

bundance of ICF develops when the extracellular fluid is hypotonic because the subsequent tic gradient pulls water out of the extracellular space into the cells. As the cells become ed with water, they lose their ability to function normally and tissues begin to swell. The brain

Table 7.4 Fluid excess

	Hypertonic	**Isotonic**	**Hypotonic**
Serum sodium level	>145 mmol/L	135–45 mmol/L	<135 mmol/L
Cause	Excessive sodium intake (rare)	Water and sodium gained in equal proportions	Excessive water intake, hyponatraemia
Effect	Fluid shifts from ICF into ECF	Volume increased in all compartments	Fluid shifts from ECF into ICF

ECF, extracellular fluid; ICF, intracellular fluid.

is particularly sensitive to swelling because the skull constricts the ability of the brain to expand. ICF excess due to *water intoxication* or *hyponatraemia* is life threatening when the central nervous system is affected and may present with changes to level of consciousness, seizures, or other abnormal neurological signs. Attempts to correct a low sodium level should be made slowly to prevent rapid fluid shifts and subsequent damage to the brain tissue that can occur if the hyponatraemia is resolved too quickly.

Fluid excess response

The body compensates for excessive water and solutes in the body by increasing their excretion in the urine. The regulation of renal sodium in the kidney is influenced by angiotensin II, aldosterone, and atrial natriuretic peptide. An increase in blood volume stimulates these hormones to reduce the reabsorption of sodium and water in the kidney tubules. As more sodium is then lost in the urine, water follows through the process of osmosis. In addition, the decreased osmolarity with a diluted high volume blood causes less ADH to be secreted, with a net result of further water loss in the urine. See Chapter 5 for a detailed explanation of the renal system's involvement in maintaining body water balance.

If these compensation mechanisms are insufficient because of underlying renal dysfunction or the high volume of intravascular fluid is simply too much for the kidneys to keep up with, there is a potential for cardiogenic shock to occur (see Chapter 3). Failure of the heart can therefore both cause hypervolaemia and result from a high volume of intravascular fluid. As the intravascular volume progressively increases, the excess fluid will redistribute, leaking out into other compartments (intracellular, interstitial, and other third-space areas) (see Figure 7.3).

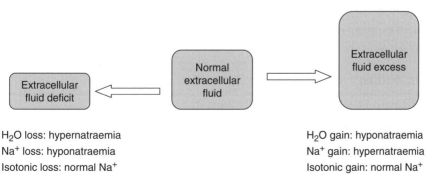

H_2O loss: hypernatraemia
Na^+ loss: hyponatraemia
Isotonic loss: normal Na^+

H_2O gain: hyponatraemia
Na^+ gain: hypernatraemia
Isotonic gain: normal Na^+

Figure 7.3 Influence of sodium on fluid shifts.

Prevention of altered fluid balance

As with any health problem, prevention of an altered fluid balance is an essential aspect of acute care nursing. Close monitoring and ongoing assessment of the patient will detect early changes seen with fluid excess or a fluid deficit. If a patient is nil by mouth, a crystalloid infusion will be necessary to maintain adequate amounts of fluid and electrolytes in the body. An intravenous infusion or nasogastric feeding may also be necessary if a patient is taking some oral food and fluid but not in adequate amounts. Patients at risk for a negative fluid balance but who can drink should have oral fluids encouraged. Equally, fluid restriction may be required for patients at risk for hypervolaemia. Close attention should be given to those patients who are particularly at risk of developing an abnormal fluid status.

Risk factors for fluid imbalance

Elderly

- ◆ Decreased skeletal muscle mass/increased adipose tissue = reduced total water.
- ◆ Decreased renal and cardiovascular function.
- ◆ Decreased mobility and cognition may impair drinking.
- ◆ Decreased thirst mechanism.
- ◆ Decreased skin elasticity prevents skin turgor from indicating hydration status.

Acute illness

- ◆ Surgery (nil by mouth pre-/postoperative, peri-operative fluid losses, bleeding).
- ◆ Nausea and vomiting.
- ◆ Diarrhoea.
- ◆ Nasogastric suction/drainage.
- ◆ Fever.
- ◆ Excessive sweating.
- ◆ Shock (septic, hypovolemic, cardiogenic, anaphylactic, neurogenic).

Chronic illness

- ◆ Impaired bodily functioning from illnesses affecting body systems.
- ◆ Renal insufficiency.
- ◆ Malnutrition influencing electrolytes and albumin.
- ◆ Reduced appetite and desire to drink water.
- ◆ Depression.

Infants/children

- ◆ Water 80% of total body weight with 40% in extracellular fluid.
- ◆ Kidneys immature.
- ◆ Acute changes within fluid status develops quickly.
- ◆ Body surface to water ratio is high—greater insensible water losses.
- ◆ Larger GI tract surface area.

Fluid optimization of surgical patients

Goal-directed therapy utilizes invasive monitoring to guide intravenous fluid delivery and has been shown to improve mortality and morbidity of surgical patients when used in the pre-operative and peri-operative period (Levett *et al.* 2002). Postoperative goal-directed therapy is also associated with reduced complications and hospital length of stay by ensuring an effective circulating blood volume for adequate tissue perfusion (Pearse *et al.* 2005). Although nursing care in acute and high dependency areas may not include the advanced cardiovascular monitoring necessary for goal-directed therapy, the principles of this approach to fluid management can be applied by nurses while sending a patient to surgery and continue once the patient returns to the ward/high dependency area. Close attention to fluid assessment and administration of intravenous infusions will ensure that the effective circulating blood volume is sufficient and prevent subsequent complications from occurring. Fluid optimization is particularly important for surgical patients because they may be nil by mouth for some time, there are large losses during surgery, and the normal physiological response in the immediate postoperative period is to have an increased cardiac output and blood flow to the tissues (Boyd 2005).

Patient assessment

Assessing fluid status benefits from a holistic approach incorporating a history and physical examination of all body systems because water is an integral aspect of each system's normal functioning. A comprehensive fluid assessment utilizing a systematic structure will consider whether the following signs and symptoms with normovolaemia are present.

Renal

- Clear yellow urine >0.5 mL/kg/h.
- Passing urine without pain or difficulty.

Respiratory

- Respirations regular and easy without shortness of breath.
- Oxygen saturations and respiration rate within normal values.
- Clear breath sounds.
- No cough.

Cardiovascular

- Peripheries pink, warm, and without oedema.
- Capillary refill <2 s.
- Mucous membranes pink and moist.
- Pedal pulses palpable.
- Heart rate, blood pressure, central venous pressure (CVP), and jugular venous pressure (JVP) within normal values.

Gastrointestinal

- Eating and drinking with normal appetite, thirst, and swallowing.

+ Normal bowel functioning.
+ Abdomen flat and soft (no evidence of ascites or internal bleeding).

Skin

+ Normal turgor (ability of skin to snap back to normal position when pinched).
+ Normal moisture (no sweating but not excessively dry).
+ Intact without wounds or drains.

Neurological

+ Alert and oriented to person, place, and time.
+ Normal strength and sensation to arms and legs.

Central venous pressure

The central venous pressure is frequently referred to as 'CVP' in practice and is a measurement of the pressure at the tip of a central venous catheter. Typically, this is assessed using a catheter placed in the internal jugular vein or subclavian vein where the catheter tip rests in the superior vena cava near the right atrium. A catheter inserted into the femoral vein can be used as long as the CVP is not interpreted as an absolute number and the trend of measurements followed instead with an understanding that the actual CVP reading may be inaccurate.

There is an assumption that the pressure in the vena cava where the end of the central venous catheter sits is the same as the pressure in the right atrium because of the close proximity. In addition, when the tricuspid valve opens, the pressure in the right atrium correlates to the pressure in the right ventricle, assuming there is a normal functioning tricuspid valve. The CVP measurement can thus be used as an indication of the pressure in the right ventricle. As volume and pressure are directly proportional to each other, the CVP as a pressure reading is then interpreted as the 'volume' status of the right side of the heart. A high CVP suggests a high blood volume and a low CVP suggests a low amount of circulating blood.

As well as hypervolaemia, other factors contributing to an increased CVP include decreased cardiac output (low heart rate or ventricular failure causing blood to back up into veins), venous constriction (activation of sympathetic system or vasoconstricting medications), and increased intrathoracic pressure such as through the Valsalva manoeuvre (compression of vena cava). These last two factors influence the CVP from primarily a change in venous compliance rather than venous blood volume although it is the relationship between CVP and blood volume that is most commonly relevant in clinical practice.

With intravascular fluid deficit, the response of the CVP to a fluid challenge is more clinically significant than the actual CVP number. The traditional approach is to assess whether a rise in CVP following the rapid intravenous infusion of 250–500 mL of fluid is sustained for at least 10 min otherwise it is likely there is hypovolaemia and a need for further intravenous fluid replacement. However, a recent systematic review by Marik *et al.* (2008) reveals that research has demonstrated a very poor correlation between CVP and blood volume and showed CVP monitoring as unreliable for predicting a haemodynamic response to fluid challenges. For this reason, some clinicians choose not to base decisions about fluid management on CVP measurements. Vincent & Weil (2006) recommend a modified approach to fluid challenges by using CVP as a safety limit and planning goals to be achieved from other clinical end points (e.g. blood pressure, heart rate, urine output, and skin perfusion).

If CVP is to be used as part of the ongoing patient assessment, the measurement can be obtained manually with a manometer or electronically with a transducer. Both systems require 'zeroing' to atmosphere pressure at the level of the right atrium and the most accurate reading will be found with the patient in the supine position. The level of the right atrium can be estimated at the phlebostatic axis (4th intercostal space, mid-axillary line) although the sternal notch is also utilized as a levelling point. Either landmark can be used as long as all colleagues are consistent in order for the measurement and trends to be following the same baseline. The range for a normal CVP reading is 2–8 mmHg or 5–10 cm H_2O.

Jugular venous pressure

The jugular venous pressure (JVP) can also be assessed externally without any invasive monitoring by identifying the level of venous distension in the neck. The JVP should be less than 4 cm above the sternum if the patient is lying supine and head of bed elevated to 45. A high JVP greater than 4 cm with the patient in this position or a visible JVP while the patient is fully upright could be caused by hypervolaemia, right ventricular failure, constrictive pericarditis, tricuspid stenosis, or superior vena cava obstruction. A low or absent JVP may indicate hypovolaemia, although the JVP can be difficult to find in many patients with normovolaemia, meaning it has limited use in assessing for intravascular dehydration.

The key land marking area for the JVP is in the triangular region between the two heads of the sternocleidomastoid muscle and has the following distinguishing features that differ from an arterial pulse:

♦ flickering, multiphasic pattern (two waves in the JVP for each cardiac cycle)

♦ non-palpable (should not have a palpable pulse like the carotid artery)

♦ variation with movement (JVP should decrease if the patient sits up)

♦ variation with respiration (JVP decreases with deep inspiration).

JVP is also referred to as jugular venous pulsation, jugular venous pulse, and jugular venous distension.

Patient weight

Weight is a significant aspect of a fluid assessment because it can indicate whether a patient is experiencing a deficit or excess of fluid. As with any objective number, the actual value of weight as a once-off reading does not contribute much to assessment findings. The trend of the weight as rising or falling is more clinically significant than the number itself because it can suggest whether total body fluid has been gained or lost. Typically, a change in 1 kg of body weight equates to 1 L of water. In acute care, the patient's pre-hospital weight should be recorded if available in order for clinicians to interpret daily weight within the context of a baseline number.

Although trends in a patient's weight may be useful for some clinical situations, caution should be taken while interpreting changes in weight because this may not be an accurate indicator of intravascular fluid volume. For example, if there is an increase in third-space fluid through the accumulation of peripheral oedema, the rise in the patient's weight could be viewed as fluid overload, although the effective circulating blood volume may be low.

Fluid balance

Calculating a net fluid balance is a crucial aspect of patient assessment in acute care to determine whether fluid input equals fluid output which occurs with normal hydration (Scales & Pilsworth 2008). A positive fluid balance indicates excessive water intake or a reduction in water excretion, which will lead to hypervolaemia if sustained. Conversely, hypovolaemia and cellular dehydration will eventually develop if a negative fluid balance continues from poor intake or increased fluid loss. However, it is always important to assess the trend of a daily fluid balance rather than interpret one number in isolation in case the high/low balance is an attempt to compensate for previous abnormality. A fluid balance chart is thus aided by a cumulative balance, which allows the nurse to incorporate daily calculations into a net balance from a wider range of time.

If a patient displays an alteration in fluid balance or has any type of organ dysfunction (particularly renal and cardiac), nurses should use clinical judgement to determine the frequency of fluid measurements and fluid balance calculation ranging from hourly to daily. While adding up the fluid balance, the following factors are included:

- ◆ fluid intake
  - oral fluids
  - intravenous infusions
  - intravenous medications
  - nasogastric feeding
- ◆ measurable fluid losses
  - urine
  - nasogastric
  - illeostomy/colostomy
  - drains.

Fluid input through the oral, nasogastric, or intravenous routes is easily identified and therefore monitored with precision of the actual amount. Fluid from urine, nasogastric suction, stomas, and drains can be collected, meaning this type of output can be accurately recorded. Other fluid losses cannot be readily captured into a container, making it more difficult to determine the exact volume. Examples of such fluid would be large amounts of diarrhoea, vomiting, and bleeding (internal or external). In these cases, an estimation of the fluid loss can be recorded but, more importantly, a critical evaluation of the fluid balance should be made taking into account other assessment findings and the direction of the cumulative fluid balance.

These assessment findings include other signs and symptoms of an alteration in fluid status that will help to confirm or refute whether an abnormal fluid balance number requires intervention. A fluid balance will never be truly accurate because of the inability to measure water loss from the skin, respiratory tract, and GI system although metabolic water production is thought to even out the deficit created from these insensible losses (Tortora & Derrickson 2009). Other questions to consider when evaluating fluid balance are whether the patient was already experiencing an abnormal fluid status before coming to acute care and if there are further immeasurable factors (e.g. losses during surgery or from a fever). As with all numerical observations, it is not a 'correct' fluid balance that is valuable to know. Rather, it is the relevance of the number as a trend and how it relates to the overall clinical picture that makes a fluid balance significant.

Because of the importance of early recognition of an abnormality in fluid status, the NICE (2007) recommends urine output to be included in physiological track and trigger systems. The aim is to utilize urine output as an early warning sign for acute illness along with other core assessment findings (see Chapter 11). The National Patient Safety Agency (2007) also promotes monitoring urine output and fluid balance regularly because of previous reports of serious incidents where fluid assessments have been neglected.

A summary of abnormal patient assessment findings is found in Table 7.5.

Clinical investigations

There are a variety of laboratory tests that may be of use while undertaking a comprehensive fluid assessment including:

- urine
  - specific gravity
  - sodium
  - osmolarity
- blood
  - urea
  - creatinine
  - sodium
  - chloride
  - potassium
  - haematocrit
  - haemoglobin
  - osmolarity
  - pH—arterial blood gas
  - Lactate.

Table 7.5 Fluid assessment findings

	Fluid deficit	Fluid excess
Skin	Dry, decreased turgor	Moist, shiny, oedematous
Tongue	Dry, coated	Moist
Skin	Dry, decreased turgor	Moist, shiny, oedematous
Tongue	Dry, coated	Moist
Thirst	Increased	May not be significant
Pulse	Rapid, thready	Rapid
Blood pressure	Low Orthostatic hypotension	High (unless cardiogenic shock develops)
Respirations	Increased rate	Increased rate, short of breath, productive cough (frothy)
Weight	Loss	Gain
JVP/CVP	Low	Elevated
Peripheries	Cool, pale, capillary refill >2 s	Warm, pink
Urine output	Reduced (except with conditions causing polyuria, e.g. DKA)	Normal/increased
Breath sounds	Clear	Fine inspiratory crackles

JVP, jugular venous pressure; CVP, central venous pressure; DKA, diabetic ketoacidosis.

Table 7.6 Urine investigations

Urine test	Normal range	Fluid deficit	Fluid excess
Specific gravity	1.020–1.030 g/mL	High	Low
Sodium	50–200 mmol/24 h	Low/high	Low/high
Osmolarity	300–1200 mOsm/L	High	Low

In addition, if fluid overload is suspected, a chest X-ray will aid in the medical diagnosis of pulmonary oedema. See Chapter 10 for further information on laboratory diagnostic tests and Tables 7.6 and 7.7 for a summary of typical findings from urine and blood tests with fluid deficit and fluid excess.

Nursing management

The goal of managing a patient with any alteration in fluid balance is to restore the intracellular and extracellular compartments back to their normal amounts of fluid and electrolytes. If there is an excess in fluid or electrolytes, nursing care will focus on restricting and promoting further excretion of both. If there are deficits, a plan will be made for replacing fluid and electrolytes as appropriate for intracellular or extracellular losses. Depending on the patient assessment findings, other components in the blood such as haemoglobin, platelets, and plasma proteins may also be replaced.

Fluid excess

The care of a patient with symptomatic hypervolaemia involves reducing the amount of circulating blood volume and taking measures to ensure normal functioning of the cardiovascular, respiratory, and renal systems. Sodium and water restriction will decrease the amount of water coming into the body. Diuretics will help to increase water loss in the urine, with common examples summarized in Table 7.8.

Evaluating the impact of a diuretic should include assessing whether it has increased urine output and resolved the hypervolaemia. Side effects of the medication such as the loss of electrolytes should also be observed. In particular, potassium levels need to be closely monitored and replaced as necessary. The diuresis should not go so far as to cause hypovolaemia therefore a comprehensive fluid assessment is necessary to establish the fluid status of the patient after administration of the diuretic. Included in this assessment will be a physical examination, which will inform the nurse if the signs and symptoms of fluid excess remain (e.g. tachypnoea and shortness of breath from pulmonary oedema).

Table 7.7 Blood investigations

Blood test	Normal range	Fluid deficit	Fluid excess
Urea	<7.5 mmol/L	High	Low
Sodium	135–145 mmol/L	Isotonic: normal Hypotonic: low Hypertonic: high	Isotonic: normal Hypotonic: low Hypertonic: high
Haematocrit	Male: 0.42–0.52 Female: 0.36–0.48	High	Normal/low
Osmolarity	280–300 mOsm/L	Isotonic: normal Hypotonic: low Hypertonic: high	Isotonic: normal Hypotonic: low Hypertonic: high

Table 7.8 Diuretics

Classification	Action in body	Examples
Loop diuretics	Inhibit water reabsorption from ascending limb of the loop of Henlé	Furosemide Bumetanide
Thiazides and related diuretics	Inhibit sodium reabosrption at beginning of the distal convoluted tubule	Bendroflumethiazide Metolazone
Potassium sparing diuretics	Aldosterone antagonist	Spironolactone

Diuretic medications depend on the kidneys responding to the medication, meaning hypervolaemia will continue if renal failure prevents an increase in urine production despite administering diuretic therapy. Ongoing hypervolaemia that is resistant to diuretics and compromising cardiorespiratory function will eventually need dialysis to remove excess intravascular fluid.

If a patient displays obvious signs of fluid excess, it is important to determine from the patient assessment where this abundance of fluid is located. If there is a surplus in the interstitial space, peripheral and pulmonary oedema becomes evident. As previously discussed, however, oedema does not necessarily mean there is hypervolaemia present if the amount of circulating blood volume is low despite the large amount of water in the interstitial space. The fluid status specific to the intravascular space can be evaluated using the CVP or JVP reading. With a normal or low intravascular volume, care should be taken while managing oedema because diuretics will also draw off fluid from the circulating blood volume, potentially leaving the patient with clinically significant hypovolaemia.

Fluid deficit

When the patient assessment findings indicate a fluid deficit, nursing care will aim to restore the normal fluid and electrolyte status. If a patient is able to drink, oral fluids can be encouraged, which obviously increases the water intake into the body. Oral intake of water will only suffice with mild volume loss; an intravenous infusion is necessary if the deficit is severe or the patient is unable to drink adequate amounts of water.

Intravenous infusions are used to replace fluid and electrolytes in the body following three basic principles:

+ replace abnormal losses
+ maintain and prevent further loss
+ repair acid–base and electrolyte imbalances.

The type of intravenous solution needed will depend on the severity of fluid deficit, fluid compartment affected, serum electrolyte levels (particularly sodium), and serum osmolarity.

Crystalloids

Crystalloids are clear solutions made up of water and electrolytes that are small molecules. As water and electrolytes are able to cross the semi-permeable membrane between the fluid compartments, both the fluid and the solute from this type of solution will shift among the intracellular and extracellular spaces depending on the concentration of the solution. If the crystalloid is isotonic, the fluid stays in the extracellular compartment and hypotonic solutions distribute through both intracellular and extracellular areas. Hypertonic intravenous crystalloids are not generally used on the acute ward because of the high risk of causing cellular dehydration and lack of evidence to support their use in acute care, although current research indicates that they may have a role with pre-hospital trauma patients (Hashiguchi *et al.* 2007) and post-traumatic cerebral oedema (Catrambone *et al.* 2008). See Tables 7.9 and 7.10 for a comparison of hypertonic, isotonic, and hypotonic crystalloid solutions.

Combined water and sodium loss

Isotonic dehydration where water and sodium are lost in the same proportion is the most common type of fluid deficit. This results in a depletion of fluid in both the intracellular and the extracellular compartments. An *isotonic intravenous infusion* is then needed as the replacement solution such as normal saline (0.9% NaCl). Isotonic solutions remain mostly in the extracellular areas with very little entering the cells because it contains the same concentration of dissolved substances as plasma. Although the main goal in delivering an isotonic infusion is to correct hypovolaemia, the infused fluid is distributed throughout the extracellular space. In fact, the majority of the water from the isotonic solution (70%) ends up in the interstitial space with only 30% left in the circulating blood volume (see Figure 7.4).

A sodium lactate solution (Lactated Ringer's or Hartmann's) is not only isotonic but also designed to be more physiologically equivalent to plasma with 111 mmol/L of chloride. Because normal saline has 150 mmol/L of chloride, it can contribute to hyperchloremic metabolic acidosis, although debate remains as to whether this is clinically significant or not (Boldt 2007). Other ingredients in a sodium lactate solution besides sodium and chloride are potassium, calcium, and lactate. The lactate is converted into bicarbonate by the liver, which helps to prevent a subsequent acidosis from developing. As normal liver functioning is required for this to occur, sodium lactate solutions should be avoided with patients who have liver failure.

> Avoid a sodium lactate solution with liver failure

Primarily water loss

If there has been more water lost relative to sodium loss, the extracellular fluid becomes hypertonic, which then draws water in from the cells, creating a fluid deficit in the intracellular compartment. Initially, this creates an increase of water in the extracellular area. With continual water loss, however, the extracellular spaces eventually become depleted of fluid as well because there is not enough water shifting in from the cells to maintain a normal blood volume. The end result is a lack of fluid in both the intracellular and the extracellular spaces and hypertonic blood (high sodium level). Ultimately, the cellular dehydration and depletion in blood volume requires replacement of free water to correct the underpinning fluid deficit. In this instance, a *hypotonic intravenous infusion* (e.g. 5% glucose or 0.45% NaCl) will distribute water evenly throughout the intracellular and the extracellular areas and help to correct the blood's hypertonicity (see Figure 7.5).

Pure water cannot be administered as an intravenous infusion because the osmotic gradient it creates pulls water in from the red blood cells until they burst (haemolysis). Although 5% glucose is technically isotonic as it exists in the bag, once administered the glucose is quickly metabolized, leaving the remaining water from the solution without causing haemolysis. This means that 5%

Table 7.9 Crystalloid solutions

Hypertonic	Isotonic	Hypotonic
3% NaCl	0.9% NaCl	0.45% NaCl
7.5% NaCl	Lactated Ringer's	5% glucose (once given)
	Hartmann's	4% glucose in 0.18% NaCl

Table 7.10 Crystalloid solutions

0.9% NaCl	4% glucose in 0.18% NaCl	5% glucose	Hartmann's
1 L water	1 L water	1 L water	1 L water
150 mmol Na$^+$	30 mmol Na$^+$	50 g glucose	131 mmol Na$^+$
150 mmol Cl$^-$	30 mmol Cl$^-$		111 mmol Cl$^-$
	40 g glucose		2 mmol Ca^{2+}
			5 mmol K$^+$
			29 mmol lactate

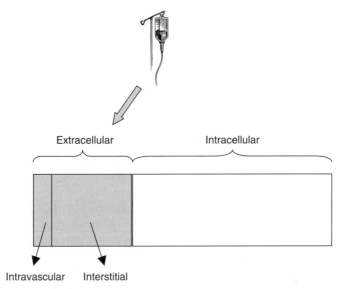

Figure 7.4 Isotonic crystalloid.

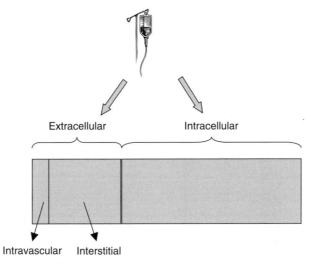

Figure 7.5 Hypotonic crystalloids.

glucose essentially functions as a hypotonic solution. As 5% glucose increases interstitial and intracellular water, it should be avoided with any patient who has a high intracranial pressure to avoid swelling of the cells and interstitial space in the brain.

Primarily sodium loss

A loss of more sodium than water creates the opposite problem, with hypotonic blood and fluid moving from the extracellular space to the intracellular space. This type of fluid deficit is relatively uncommon and can be caused by diuretics, salt-wasting renal disease, or when isotonic dehydration is replaced with a hypotonic intravenous solution. Normal saline (0.9% NaCl) is the preferred solution to provide replacement for the salt loss.

Colloids

Colloids contain macromolecules that normally stay within the plasma for a number of days because they are too large to pass through the vascular endothelial membrane and are metabolized slowly. The increased oncotic pressure from these added substances encourages the water to remain inside the intravascular space as well as draw off further fluid from the interstitium (see Figure 7.6). Compared with crystalloids then, colloids have an enhanced ability to expand plasma volume because much of the water from crystalloids ends up distributed across the extracellular area rather than remaining strictly in the plasma.

As a result, a smaller volume of colloid fluid needs to be infused and there is reduced peripheral and pulmonary oedema. The colloid will leak out of the plasma to cause oedema if the capillary endothelium is not intact such as with sepsis, acute respiratory distress syndrome, or blunt trauma. Other disadvantages are the potential for coagulopathy and anaphylaxis although both are quite rare (British National Formulary 2008). With large doses, some colloids cause pruitus and impair renal function particularly with septic patients where 'leaky capillaries' allow the macromolecules to settle in the skin and kidneys.

The crystalloid vs. colloid debate continues on with no consensus yet reached as to whether either one is preferential solution for intravenous fluid replacement. Colloids are more expensive

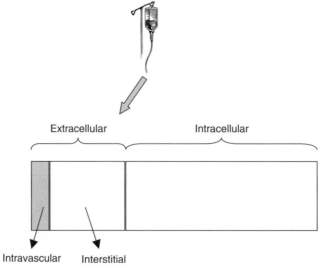

Figure 7.6 Colloids.

Table 7.11 Colloids

	Molecular weight (kDa)	Na$^+$ (mmol/L)	Cl$^-$ (mmol/L)
Gelofusine®–gelatine	30	154	120
Hetastarch–starch	450	154	154
Pentastarch–starch	200	154	154
Albumin 4.5%	70	150	120

and have not been shown to reduce mortality in critically ill patients (Finfer *et al.* 2004; Perel & Roberts 2007). However, it is difficult to make generalizations about fluid replacement because of individual variables with each patient and a theoretical role for both crystalloids and colloids depending on the type of fluid deficit (Marino 2007). Regardless of the conflicting literature, synthetic colloids continue to be popular in clinical practice such as those containing gelatine or etherfied starch. As of yet, there is no evidence that one colloid is more effective or safer than any other type of colloid (Bunn *et al.* 2008). See Table 7.11 for a comparison of colloids commonly used in acute care.

Blood products

Transfusing blood products is only indicated when there are specific deficiencies within the blood requiring replacement. Packed red blood cells are transfused for low haemoglobin or when patients are actively bleeding. If there is no evidence of haemorrhage or cardiovascular disease and vital signs are stable, the goal will be to achieve a haemoglobin level between 70 and 90 g/L. If cardiovascular disease is present, a stable patient who is not bleeding should receive packed red blood cells until the haemoglobin level is 90 to 100 g/L (McClelland 2007).

In order to ensure the right patient receives the right transfusion of blood products in the right manner, the correct administration procedure must be followed according to local polices. This is important to ensure the blood product infused is compatible with the patient's blood type. In addition, there are differences in how various blood products are stored and administered, which can be guided by protocols and clinical guidelines as well as from the UK Blood Transfusion and Tissue Transplantation Services (2008). See Table 7.12 for details about the indication, storage, shelf life, and transfusion time of different types of blood products.

Intravenous therapy

In addition to crystalloids, colloids, and blood products, other indications for intravenous therapy include administration of medications, electrolytes, and total parenteral nutrition. Intravenous therapy can be delivered peripherally in a small vein or centrally if a central venous catheter has been inserted into a larger vein (e.g. internal jugular, subclavian, or femoral). The most common type of central catheter used in acute care is a short-term non-tunnelled catheter, although some patients may come into hospital with a long-term tunnelled catheter such as a Hickman, Groshong, or Port-a-cath. Increasingly used is the peripherally inserted central catheter, which has a reduced risk of infection because the insertion site is farther away from the central cardiovascular system.

Regardless of the type of fluid or catheter being used, there are core principles of intravenous therapy that are necessary for all nurses to follow, including use of non-touch aseptic technique throughout preparation and administration, ongoing assessment of the intravenous site, which

Table 7.12 Blood products

	Packed red blood cells
Indication	Low haemoglobin from anaemia, bleeding
Storage	Blood fridge at 4°C
Shelf life	35 days
Transfusion time	Administer quickly if bleeding, otherwise over 2–3 h using caution with heart failure and a maximum of 4 h/bag
	Fresh frozen plasma
Indication	Clotting disorders
Storage	Blood fridge at 4°C once thawed
Shelf life	2 years at −30°C
Transfusion time	Administer as soon as possible 10–20 mL/kg/h
	Platelets
Indication	Very low platelet count
Storage	22 C—never refrigerate
Shelf life	5 days
Transfusion time	Administer as soon as possible over 30–60 min

should be free of complications and covered with a clear, intact dressing, and removal of intravenous cannula if it is no longer necessary.

Potential hazards of intravenous therapy

+ Infection—localalized, systemic.
+ Phlebitis—mechanical, chemical, infective.
+ Infiltration.
+ Extravasation.
+ Particulate contamination.
+ Embolism—air, clot, foreign body.
+ Fluid overload.
+ Anaphylaxis.
+ Speedshock.
+ Sharps injury.

Infection control measures are of particular importance while caring for a patient with intravenous access, especially those with a central venous catheter or with total parenteral nutrition. The Department of Health's (2007) Saving Lives Campaign emphasizes a standardized, evidence-based approach to reducing the incidence of catheter-related bloodstream infection. This includes the central venous catheter care bundle (High Impact Intervention 1) and peripheral intravenous cannula care bundle (High Impact Intervention 2), both of which provide guidance on actions for insertion and ongoing care.

To reduce the risk of incidents with medical devices used for intravenous therapy (pumps and syringe drivers), the National Patient Safety Agency (2004) recommends simplifying the range of devices that are available, monitoring systems centrally to allow for maximum use of equipment, and ensuring all staff have the necessary knowledge and skill to safely use the devices.

Table 7.13 Diabetic ketoacidosis and hyperglycaemic hyperosmolar syndrome

	Diabetic ketoacidosis	Hyperglycaemic hyperosmolar syndrome
Presentation	90% occur in known diabetes	Often initial
Frequency	Common	Uncommon
Usual type of diabetes	Type I	Type II
Precipitant	>1/3 due to infection	More severe illness, e.g. myocardial infarction, sepsis
Blood glucose	Often >16 mmol/L	Often >35 mmol/L
Serum osmolarity	Usually <350 mmol/L	Usually >350 mmol/L
Fluid deficit	5–8 L	8–12 L
Ketoacidosis	Present—ketones in urine, acidosis	Absent
Prodrome	Short time frame	Long time frame
Mortality rate	5–10%	40–60%
Peak age range	20–29 years	57–70 years

Common fluid disorders

Fluid deficit: severe hyperglycaemia

Diabetic ketoacidosis (DKA) and hyperglycaemic hyperosmolar syndrome (HHS) are both metabolic emergencies that can develop with diabetic patients. Although they appear to be very similar conditions, there are some differences, as outlined in Table 7.13.

Related pathophysiology

With DKA, there is a triad of:

1) hyperglycaemia

2) ketonaemia

3) acidosis.

The high blood sugar is caused by a lack of effective insulin from an infection, missed insulin injection, stress, trauma, or because the patient is a new diabetic. Ketogenesis occurs as fatty acids are used for energy instead of glucose that cannot be utilized without insulin. Ketone bodies are produced as a result, which acidifies the blood, bringing about a metabolic acidosis and increases the serum osmolarity.

In addition, the large glucose molecules enhance the high osmolarity even further, which draws water out of the cells creating intracellular dehydration. As the glucose molecules build up in the blood, they begin to spill over into the urine. Water follows in an osmotic diuresis, which also brings about intravascular volume depletion. The end result is a patient who has a severe fluid deficit in all fluid compartments.

There are absent ketones with HHS but the hyperglycaemia, hyperosmolarity, and fluid deficit are even greater, which leads to a high mortality with this particular clinical situation.

Patient presentation

The assessment findings of DKA and HHS are indicative of intracellular and intravascular fluid deficit:

- hypotension

- low CVP/JVP
- tachycardia
- thready pulse
- decreased skin turgor
- dry, coated tongue
- thirst
- pale, cool peripheries
- capillary refill >2 s.

With DKA and HHS there will also be polyuria (compared with other types of fluid deficit that tend to have a decreased urine output) due to the osmotic diuresis. Kussmaul's breathing is deep and laboured, which is an attempt to blow off more carbon dioxide to improve the acidosis. A patient with DKA will also have fruity smelling breath from ketones produced and results in ketoacidosis. Nausea, vomiting, and abdominal pain may also be present. Even if the serum potassium level is normal or high, this is from potassium shifting out of the cells and there will be an overall deficit of total body potassium. Once the insulin therapy is commenced, the potassium level will begin to drop dramatically without replacement indicating the need to closely monitor potassium.

Nursing management

The care of the patient with DKA/HHS focuses on intravenous therapy, including crystalloids, potassium, and insulin. If large amounts of potassium are needed, continual ECG monitoring and central venous access will be needed. The goal of the insulin is to lower the blood sugar slowly otherwise a sudden drop can create cerebral oedema. The insulin infusion is kept until ketoacidosis and osmolality resolve (10% glucose may be needed to maintain blood glucose). A systematic approach to managing DKA/HHS is provided by De Beer et al. (2008) and summarized in Figure 7.7.

For nursing care associated with DKA see Table 7.14.

Fluid deficit: haemorrhage

A patient who is actively bleeding will eventually begin to show signs of hypovolaemia because of the decreased effective circulating blood volume. Obvious signs of bleeding may be apparent when the skin integrity is broken, a patient has recently come back from surgery with an open wound/drains, or when blood is found in fluids being drained from the body such as urine from

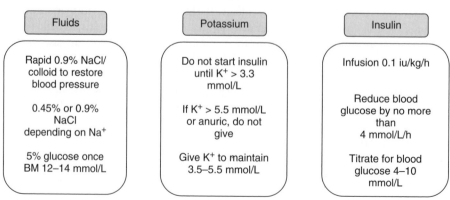

Figure 7.7 Management of DKA/HHS.

Table 7.14 Nursing care of hypovolaemia from diabetic ketoacidosis

Potential problem	Nursing care
Blood glucose instability	Monitor blood glucose hourly until stable
	Administer insulin infusion as prescribed and titrate to reduce a high blood glucose by no more than 4 mmol/L/h
	Continue to monitor blood glucose and provide glucose as needed to prevent hypoglycaemia
Hypotension	Monitor blood pressure regularly
	Monitor continuous heart rate
	Monitor central venous pressure
	Provide intravenous fluids to ensure an adequate blood pressure and central venous pressure
Fluid deficit	Establish intravenous therapy and administer crystalloid and colloid as prescribed
	Fluid balance chart
	24-h balance
	Monitor clinical signs and symptoms of fluid deficit/excess
Abnormal serum potassium	Monitor K^+ level hourly
	If K^+ <3.5 mmol/L, administer intravenous K^+ until at least 3.5 mmol/L
	If potassium <3.5 mmol/L, hold insulin infusion until potassium level >3.5 mmol/L
	Hold intravenous potassium if >5.5 mmol/L or anuric
	Continuous ECG monitoring
Altered level of consciousness	Monitor Glasgow Coma Scale regularly
	Assess ability to maintain airway
	Assess breathing and oxygenation saturations providing oxygen therapy as necessary to maintain saturations >92%
	Report any change in level of consciousness to medical team
Polyuria	Monitor urine output
	Fluid balance chart
	Monitor glucose in urine
Acidosis	Assess serum pH via with arterial blood gas until stable
	Monitor ketones in urine
	Maintain insulin infusion until ketones and acidosis resolved
	Monitor lactate
Nausea and vomiting	Monitor nausea and vomiting providing anti-emetic as necessary
	Record emesis loss in fluid balance

a foley catheter or pleural fluid from a chest tube. Internal haemorrhage should also be considered, which may not be visually seen on inspection but suspected from the patient's history.

Potential causes of internal bleeding include:

- gastrointestinal bleeding (e.g. varices, ulcer, cancer)
- ruptured abdominal aortic aneurysm or other blood vessels
- trauma
- fractures

Clinical link 7.1 (see Appendix for answers)

A 28-year-old type I diabetic has been admitted to hospital with diabetic ketoacidosis. He presented to A&E following a 3-day history of nausea, vomiting, and polyuria. In A&E, two peripheral intravenous lines were inserted and infusions of normal saline and insulin started prior to transferring to the high dependency unit.

Your initial assessment reveals a blood pressure of 85/50 mmHg, heart rate 130 beats/min, respirations 38 breaths/min (fruity smelling), temperature 38.3 C, and O₂ saturations 97%. The patient is awake and oriented to person, place, and time although appears restless and states he feels very tired and unwell. Mucous membranes are dry and he complains of severe thirst. The hands and feet are cool with a capillary refill of 4 s.

Results from investigations done 30 min previously in A&E include:

Arterial blood gas:

pH   7.14
HCO₃   6 mmol/L
PCO₂   17 mmHg/2.27 kPa
PO₂   82 mmHg/10.9 kPa
Lactate   3.0 mmol/L

Urine:

Ketones   Present
Glucose   Present

◆ What would your priorities be for this patient? Justify your actions.

◆ What interventions from the doctors would you anticipate?

◆ What types of assessment and monitoring will you continually undertake?

◆ Why would the lactate be elevated and how can this be resolved?

◆ Identify possible causes for this episode of DKA and how the clinical picture fits the diagnostic criteria for DKA.

◆ What type of shock is occurring? Rationalize your answer.

◆ brain haemorrhage
◆ ectopic pregnancy
◆ clotting disorder
◆ retroperitoneal bleeding.

Pathophysiology

Up to 10–15% of total blood volume can be lost without clinical significance because of the body's compensation mechanisms to maintain adequate tissue perfusion. This involves normal hypovolae- mia responses such as peripheral vasoconstriction, increase in heart rate, increase in cardiac output, secretion of ADH, and activation of the renin–angiotensin–aldosterone system. In addition, the liver acts as a reservoir (it holds up to 15% of the total blood volume at any given time) and is able to release blood during an incident of haemorrhage to improve the amount of blood in circulation.

As the amount of blood loss increases, so does the compensation, which then becomes evident in the patient assessment findings. Even further bleeding will overwhelm the body, causing the failure of the compensation mechanisms and leading to severe complications or death if left untreated.

Patient presentation

The American College of Surgeons Committee on Trauma (2004) has classified blood loss according to a severity scale:

- Class I (<5% blood volume): no changes to vital signs
- Class II (15–30% blood volume): tachycardia, narrow pulse pressure, pale, cool, respiratory rate 20–30 breaths/min
- Class III (30–40% blood volume): tachycardia, narrow pulse pressure, hypotension, capillary refill >3 s, cold, clammy, respiratory rate >30 breaths/min, oliguria, anxiety, confusion
- Class IV (>40% blood volume): compensation mechanisms fail with severe tachycardia and hypotension, respiratory rate >35 breaths/min, anuria, altered mental status.

This scale highlights how blood pressure may remain normal despite a moderate amount of blood loss. Obvious abnormality in the strength of peripheral pulses, systolic blood pressure, and mental status are thought to be late clinical signs of central hypovolaemia (Ryan *et al.* 2008). Tachycardia in the supine position may also be absent until quite severe blood loss (Marino 2007).

Although haemoglobin level is useful to measure in the patient with haemorrhage, it is expressed as a concentration, meaning that the total blood volume influences the numerical result. In an actively bleeding patient, it takes time for the fluid compartments to adjust to the decrease in intravascular volume therefore the haemoglobin level as a concentration may be misleading (Gutierrez *et al.* 2004). Crystalloid or colloid infusions dilute the blood, which further complicates the interpretation of a haemoglobin level after the initial fluid resuscitation. Transfusing one unit of packed red blood cells typically increases a haemoglobin level by 1 g/dL in the absence of bleeding although if the haemorrhaging remains, it is difficult to assess the exact effect of a transfusion on the blood volume through the haemoglobin level. Haemoglobin or haematocrit (percentage of red blood cells in the blood) are useful investigations to measure in the patient with blood loss but the values must be considered within the context of when the haemorrhage occurred as well as the types and amount of fluid replacement used.

Clinical link 7.2 (see Appendix for answers)

You are caring for a patient who returned from surgery 4 h ago from a right hemicolectomy. Initially, the vital signs were stable, pain was well controlled with an epidural, abdominal dressing was dry and intact, and there was minimal drainage from the nasogastric tube and abdominal drain. While doing a routine set of vital signs, you notice that the patient appears anxious, has cool peripheries, is tachycardic (115 beats/min), hypotensive (80/45), and has a high respiratory rate (25 breaths/min).

- What would be your next immediate actions and why?
- What other signs and symptoms would indicate post-operative bleeding is occurring?
- If active bleeding was ruled out, what other reasons could be causing these abnormalities?
- If active bleeding was confirmed, how would you coordinate care of the patient, including interaction with the nurse in charge and surgical team?

Nursing management

If a patient was previously bleeding or appears to be having continual blood loss, care should focus on identifying the source and liaising with the medical and the surgical teams for interventions that will stop the haemorrhage. In the meantime, ongoing assessment of vital signs, physical assessment signs of hypovolaemia, and blood results (haemoglobin, haematocrit, and lactate) will provide information for establishing trends and allow an estimation of whether the bleeding is resolving or getting worse (see Table 7.15).

Table 7.15 Nursing care of hypovolaemia from blood loss

Potential problem	Nursing care
External bleeding	Monitor for evidence of external bleeding from skin, wounds, drains, intravenous sites, or body orifices (eyes, nose, ears, tracheostomy, anus, urethral, vaginal)
	Report increase in bleeding to doctor
	Apply pressure if possible to site of bleeding
	Document estimated amount of bleeding on fluid balance
	Monitor vital signs and Hb regularly
Internal bleeding	Consider patient history while assessing for possible internal bleeding
	Monitor bodily fluids for signs of bleeding (urine, stool, sputum, gastrointestinal drainage/emesis)
	Assess abdomen: inspection, palpation, percussion, auscultation
	Liaise with doctor about further investigations (ultrasound, CT scan, X-ray)
	Document bodily fluids with signs of blood on fluid balance
	Monitor vital signs and Hb regularly
Decreased Hb and oxygen carrying capacity	Monitor haemoglobin level until stable
	Transfuse packed red blood cells as prescribed
	Consider the impact of intravenous infusions (crystalloid, colloid, and packed red blood cells) on haemoglobin level
	Monitor for signs of poor oxygenation (shortness of breath, cyanosis, low PaO_2, high lactate)
	Administer oxygen therapy as needed to maintain O_2 saturation >92%
	O_2 saturation may be normal (i.e. Hb molecules fully saturated) but total amount of Hb low from blood loss making it difficult to use O_2 saturation as clinical sign of oxygenation
Hypotension	Monitor blood pressure regularly
	Administer intravenous fluids as prescribed
Tachycardia	Monitor heart rate regularly
	Monitor ECG
	Monitor electrolytes
Impaired tissue perfusion	Assess peripheral pulses and capillary refill regularly
	Assess skin colour, warmth, movement, and sensation regularly
	Monitor lactate

Table 7.15 Nursing care of hypovolaemia from blood loss *(Continued)*

Potential problem	Nursing care
Altered level of consciousness	Monitor Glasgow Coma Scale regularly
	Assess ability to maintain airway
	Assess breathing and oxygenation saturations providing oxygen therapy as necessary to maintain saturations >92%
	Report any change in level of consciousness to medical team
Fluid deficit	Establish intravenous therapy and administer crystalloid, colloid, and blood products as prescribed
	Fluid balance chart
	24-h balance
	Monitor clinical signs and symptoms of fluid deficit/excess
Acute renal failure	Monitor urine output regularly
	Report to doctor if urine output drops below 0.5 mL/kg/h
	Monitor urea, creatinine, and electrolytes
	Administer intravenous therapy as prescribed to maintain adequate blood pressure and CVP
Reaction to blood transfusion	Monitor vital signs as per local protocol for administration of blood products
	Assess for signs and symptoms of acute or delayed reaction, post transfusion purpura, and acute lung injury
	If reaction suspected, stop transfusion and report to doctor and blood bank as per local protocol

CVP, central venous pressure.

Fluid deficit: vomiting and diarrhoea

A patient who is experiencing vomiting or diarrhoea has the potential to lose a significant amount of fluid as well as electrolytes. Without replacement, a negative fluid deficit will occur, placing the patient at risk of hypovolaemia.

Pathophysiology

Large amounts of GI fluid can be lost from the body through nasogastric drainage/suction, vomiting, and diarrhoea. In addition to the water loss, this also depletes the patient of hydrogen ions, sodium, chloride, and potassium. Gastric secretions contain very little magnesium, although prolonged vomiting for a number of weeks can result in hypomagnesaemia. As a result of the acidic nature of gastric fluid, continual loss eventually leads to metabolic alkalosis. The loss of bicarbonate from the lower GI tract contributes to the development of metabolic acidosis. There are numerous causes for both vomiting and diarrhoea, including infection, side effects from medication, and GI illness (see Chapter 6).

Patient presentation

A patient losing excessive amounts of GI fluid from vomiting or diarrhoea will display clinical signs and symptoms of volume depletion if the fluid deficit is severe enough:

- hypotension
- low CVP/JVP

Clinical link 7.3 (see Appendix for answers)

An 80-year-old male patient was originally admitted to hospital 10 days ago due to confusion, reduced mobility, and the inability of his wife as the main care giver to cope with caring for him. He is now experiencing yellow, watery stools, which are increasing in frequency and amount. Although he had been eating and drinking well up until 2 days ago with encouragement and assistance, today he has only agreed to minimal oral intake. At 15:30, you realize he has not had any urinary output since the beginning of your shift at 7:30 and there was no fluid balance chart recorded for the previous day. The patient is not catheterized and when you question him whether he needs a urinal, his answer is vague and not appropriate.

- Identify all the potential causes for fluid and electrolyte deficit with this patient.
- How would you manage the diarrhoea?
- How would you manage improving the fluid input?
- What investigations and treatments does this patient appear to need?

- tachycardia
- thready pulse
- decreased skin turgor
- dry, coated tongue
- thirst
- pale, cool peripheries
- capillary refill > 2 s.

As a result of the loss of electrolytes, hydrogen ions, or bicarbonate, the patient is also at risk of:

- hyponatraemia
- hypocholeremia
- hypokalaemia
- hypomagnesenaemia
- metabolic acidosis or alkalosis.

For nursing care associated with vomiting and diarrhoea see Table 7.16.

Fluid excess: liver failure

Patients with liver failure may have normal or decreased fluid in the intravascular space but an abundance of total body fluid because of the fluid leaking out into the interstitum. As a result, peripheral oedema and ascites develop.

Pathophysiology

The liver has a number of different functions, including synthesizing albumin, which is a large plasma protein. Because of its size, albumin creates an oncotic pressure that helps to maintain fluid within the intravascular space. With liver failure, the ability to produce albumin

Table 7.16 Nursing care of hypovolaemia from diarrhoea

Potential problem	Nursing care
Hypotension	Monitor blood pressure regularly
	Administer intravenous fluids as prescribed
Electrolyte imbalance	Monitor sodium, chloride, potassium, and magnesium and replace as prescribed
	ECG monitoring
Metabolic acidosis/alkalosis	Monitor blood pH if acid-base imbalance is severe
	Treat underlying cause of metabolic acid–base imbalance
Altered level of consciousness	Monitor Glasgow Coma Scale regularly
	Assess ability to maintain airway
	Assess breathing and oxygenation saturations providing oxygen therapy as necessary to maintain saturations >92%
	Report any change in level of consciousness to medical team
Impaired tissue perfusion	Assess peripheral pulses and capillary refill regularly
	Assess skin colour, warmth, movement, and sensation regularly
	Monitor lactate
Acute renal failure	Monitor urine output regularly
	Report to doctor if urine output drops below 0.5 mL/kg/h
	Monitor urea, creatinine, and electrolytes
	Administer intravenous therapy as prescribed to maintain adequate blood pressure and CVP
Fluid deficit	Establish intravenous therapy and administer crystalloid, colloid, and blood products as prescribed
	Fluid balance chart
	24-h balance
	Monitor clinical signs and symptoms of fluid deficit/excess
Tachycardia	Monitor heart rate regularly
	Monitor ECG
	Monitor electrolytes
Large amounts nasogastric drainage/vomiting	Monitor amount and type of gastric fluid and document on fluid balance chart
	Administer anti-emetics as prescribed
	Treat underlying cause of excessive nasogastric drainage/vomiting
Diarrhoea	Monitor amount and type of diarrhoea and document on fluid balance chart
	Send stool specimen for culture and sensitivity
	Strict infection control measures to prevent cross-contamination with other patients
	Close attention to skin care—washing after diarrhoea with protective spray/cream to keep skin intact

CVP, central venous pressure.

is impaired, which decreases the oncotic pressure and allows water to redistribute to the interstitial area.

A further influence on fluid status for patients with liver failure is the ascites that develops as fluid collects in the peritoneal cavity. The underlying contributing factors for ascites include sphlanchnic vasodilation, arterial hypotension, increased cardiac output, and decreased vascular

---

Clinical link 7.4 (see Appendix for answers)

You are caring for a 55-year-old female patient with chronic liver disease. She has been admitted to an acute ward because of severe ascites and suspected infection of unknown cause as of yet (temperature 38.3°C and white blood cells 16×10^9/L). On your initial assessment you note peripheral oedema up to her knees bilaterally and her breathing appears laboured at 25 breaths/min. Paracentesis was performed by the doctor, which drained off 6 L of clear yellow fluid. An albumin infusion was then prescribed, which you administer.

♦ Explain why hypotension due to hypovolaemia may occur with this patient, who has both peripheral oedema and ascites.

♦ What impact does the excessive fluid in the peritoneal space have on other body systems?

♦ Why was an albumin infusion prescribed?

---

resistance. The subsequent decrease in intravascular volume leads to impaired renal function and sodium/water retention. As water is retained proportionally more than the sodium, the patient then presents with dilutional hyponatraemia.

Patient presentation

Depending on a patient's albumin and retention of sodium and water, the intravascular volume may appear to be normal, low, or high as indicated by the CVP/JVP. The interstitial space will reveal fluid excess with the following clinical signs and symptoms:

♦ peripheral oedema

♦ ascites—round abdomen, central tympany with lateral dullness on both sides of the abdomen, fluid wave/shifting dullness tests, confirmation by ultrasound/CT scan

♦ pulmonary oedema—fine crackles to lower lung fields bilaterally, coughing up pink frothy sputum, shortness of breath

♦ increase in weight.

For nursing care associated with liver failure and fluid management see Table 7.17.

Fluid excess: iatrogenic intravenous infusion overload

Any patient with an intravenous infusion has the potential to receive an excessive total amount of fluid or to have the infusion administered too quickly for the cardiovascular system to cope with. The use of a pump ensures the exact amount of fluid at the prescribed rate which decreases the chance of overloading the patient with fluid while providing an intravenous infusion. This is particularly important for patients with heart failure or renal failure who are already at risk for hypervolaemia.

Pathophysiology

With fluid being delivered directly into the intravascular space, there will be an increase in the circulating blood volume. Whether it is a crystalloid, colloid, blood product, total parenteral nutrition or medication, intravenous therapy can potentially deliver too much fluid, resulting in water leaking out to the interstitium. Normally, this would be prevented because the liver expands ⟩ help manage the increased level of circulating blood volume and the kidneys produce more 'ne. However, when there is far too much fluid for the compensation mechanisms to cope with 'he function of the heart and kidneys are impaired, iatrogenic hypervolaemia would develop.

Table 7.17 Nursing care of hypovolaemia from liver disease

Potential problem	Nursing care
Hypotension	Monitor blood pressure regularly
	Administer intravenous fluids as prescribed
Electrolyte imbalance	Monitor sodium, chloride, potassium, and magnesium and replace as prescribed
Altered level of consciousness	Monitor Glasgow Coma Scale regularly
	Report any change in level of consciousness to medical team
Acute renal failure	Monitor urine output regularly
	Report to doctor if urine output drops below 0.5 mL/kg/h
	Monitor urea, creatinine, and electrolytes
Fluid excess	Fluid balance chart
	24-h balance
	Monitor clinical signs and symptoms of fluid imbalance
Ascites	Assess abdomen for evidence of ascites
	Assist doctor with ascites treatment documenting amount of any fluid drained off in fluid balance chart
	Sodium and water restriction
	Administer diuretics as prescribed
	Monitor for signs and symptoms of infection
Peripheral oedema	Assess arms and legs for oedema noting where oedema ends
	Administer diuretics as prescribed
Impaired respiratory function	Assess ability to maintain airway
	Assess breathing and oxygenation saturations
	Administer oxygen therapy as needed to maintain O_2 saturation >92%
	Monitor work of breathing and chest expansion as influenced from ascites
Liver failure	Monitor liver function tests and clotting factors
	Assess for signs and symptoms of liver disease (e.g. jaundice)

Clinical link 7.5 (see Appendix for answers)

A 75-year-old male patient (70 kg) has been receiving a normal saline infusion at 125 mL/h. The patient is currently nil by mouth because a previous stroke has left him with dysphagia and he continually pulls out the nasogastric tubes that were providing him with enteral nutrition. A PEG tube insertion has been scheduled for 2 days' time.

You noticed at 12:00 that the urine output has been 25 mL/h for the past 2 h and the fluid balance has become increasingly positive. The previous day's fluid balance was 3 L positive which included 1000 mL colloid given overnight when the urine output had decreased. Although he does not have a central line to measure the CVP, you were able to see an elevated JVP. The respiratory rate has increased from 16 to 28 breaths/min and the O_2 saturations are now 90% on room air, which were previously 98% this morning.

- What other signs and symptoms would indicate to you that this patient has become hypervolaemic?
- What would be your immediate actions and why?
- What medical investigations would help to confirm whether the patient has hypervolaemia?
- Provide an explanation for why the patient has a reduced urine output despite having an increase in total blood volume.

Table 7.18 Nursing care of hypervolaemia from iatrogenic fluid overload

Potential problem	Nursing care
Hypervolaemia	Monitor CVP/JVP Assess patient for clinical signs and symptoms of fluid excess Stop/limit intravenous infusions as discussed with doctor
Fluid excess	Fluid balance chart 24-h balance Monitor clinical signs and symptoms of fluid imbalance
Pulmonary oedema	Monitor respirator rate, O_2 saturations, cough, work of breathing, and chest expansion Administer oxygen therapy as needed to maintain O_2 saturation >92% Liaise with doctor regarding need for chest X-ray Administer diuretics as prescribed Sit patient up to improve work of breathing
Peripheral oedema	Assess arms and legs for oedema noting where oedema ends Administer diuretics as prescribed
Heart failure	Monitor for signs and symptoms of reduced cardiac output Monitor blood pressure and heart rate regularly Monitor urine output and renal function

CVP, central venous pressure; JVP, jugular venous pressure.

This is clinically significant when oedema not only develops in the peripheries but also begins to form pulmonary oedema, which impairs gas exchange in the lungs.

Patient presentation

Intravascular fluid excess from an intravenous infusion may present with the following:

+ peripheral oedema
+ pulmonary oedema: shortness of breath, increased respiratory rate, decreased O2 saturations, bilateral fine inspiratory crackles, pink frothy sputum
+ raised CVP/JVP
+ increased urine output (diluted) if renal function normal
+ decreased urine output with renal/cardiac function abnormal
+ signs and symptoms of heart failure.

For nursing care associated with iatrogenic fluid overload see Table 7.18.

End of chapter test

The following assessment will enable you to evaluate your theoretical knowledge of fluid assessment and management as well as your ability to apply this theory to clinical practice.

Knowledge assessment

With the support of your mentor/supervisor from practice, work through the following prompts to explore your knowledge level about fluid assessment and management.

+ Describe the fluid compartments in the body and how fluid homeostasis is maintained.
+ Differentiate between osmotic pressure, hydrostatic pressure, and oncotic pressure.

+ Identify all sources for water gain and water loss in the body.

+ Define normovolaemia, hypovolaemia, and hypervolaemia.

+ Define hypertonic, isotonic, and hypotonic.

+ Explain the role of sodium in maintaining fluid homeostasis.

+ Identify third-space areas and define the term third-space fluid.

+ Explain how there can be hypovolaemia even with an increased amount of total water in the body.

+ Critically analyse causes of fluid deficit along with the body's compensation mechanisms.

+ Define hypovolaemic shock.

+ Critically analyse causes of fluid excess along with the body's compensation mechanisms.

+ Explain your role and responsibilities as a nurse in preventing an altered fluid balance.

+ Recognize risk factors for fluid imbalance.

+ Define fluid optimization and describe its role in acute care.

+ Critically analyse the clinical presentation of fluid deficit and fluid excess.

+ Explain how blood tests, urine investigations, and chest X-ray contribute to a fluid assessment.

+ Differentiate between types of diuretics, including actions on the body, indications, contraindications, and side effects.

+ Compare and contrast crystalloids with colloids, including benefits, limitations, indications for use, contraindications, and side effects for each.

+ Discuss different types of crystalloids, including isotonic, hypotonic, and hypertonic solutions.

+ Discuss different types of colloid infusions, including those containing gelatine, starch, and albumin.

+ Critically analyse your role and responsibilities in transfusing blood products.

+ Discuss different types of blood products, including packed red blood cells, fresh frozen plasma, and platelets.

+ Differentiate between peripheral and central venous access.

+ Critically analyse potential hazards of intravenous therapy.

+ Explain the relevance of the Saving Lives Campaign for intravenous therapy, identifying all relevant high impact interventions.

+ Describe how fluid assessment and management are documented where you work.

+ Discuss the role of urine output in contributing to an early warning sign score.

+ Identify the three key features of DKA and explain how fluids are managed with a patient presenting with diabetic ketoacidois or HHS.

+ Recognize possible causes of internal bleeding and how you would act if you suspected a patient was experiencing internal bleeding.

+ Critically analyse the progression of blood loss as it becomes more severe.

+ Discuss how vomiting and diarrhoea influence fluids and eletrolytes in the body.

+ Explain how an alteration in fluid balance occurs with liver failure.

+ Explain how an alteration in fluid balance occurs with acute and chronic heart failure.

Skills assessment

Under the guidance of your mentor/supervisor, undertake a full fluid assessment followed by appropriate interventions for any significant abnormality. Your mentor/supervisor will be able to assess your ability and provide feedback based on the following skills:

+ Conducts a full patient history with a systems review, considering key points that are relevant for a fluid assessment.

+ Demonstrates a comprehensive physical assessment and explain normal/abnormal findings related to the patient's fluid status from the renal, respiratory, cardiovascular, GI, skin, and neurological systems.

+ Weighs the patient and explains the clinical significance of the actual number as well as any trends.

+ Assesses all sources and amount of fluid intake and output from the patient.

+ Calculates the current net fluid balance and explains the clinical significance of the actual number as well as any trends.

+ Facilitates the completion of relevant clinical investigations such as blood, urine, and X-ray tests and evaluate results.

+ Reviews current medications and intravenous therapy, rationalizing their impact on fluid status.

+ Interprets all subjective and objective findings from the fluid assessment, identifies significant abnormalities, rationalizes possible causes for these abnormalities, and plans appropriate actions.

+ Explains the clinical reasoning and provides justification for all interventions of the fluid management plan.

+ Liaises with other members of the healthcare team as necessary, including the nurse in charge, doctor, pharmacist, physiotherapist, and healthcare assistant.

+ Demonstrates an ability to follow infection control guidelines while undertaking intravenous therapy, including the management of the intravenous access and intravenous fluid.

+ Documents a fluid management plan, completed actions, and evaluation of actions as per local policy.

+ Incorporates fluid assessment findings into an early warning sign score as appropriate.

References

American College of Surgeons Committee on Trauma (2004) *Advanced Trauma Life Support for Doctors: Student Course Manual.* American College of Surgeons, Chicago.

Boldt, J. (2007) The balanced concept of fluid resuscitation. *Br. J. Anaes.* **99**(3), 312–5.

Boyd, O. (2005) Optimisation of the high-risk surgical patient—the use of 'goal-directed' therapy. In: *Recent Advances in Surgery*, Taylor, I. and Johnson, C. (eds). Royal Society of Medicine Press, London.

British National Formulary (2008) *British National Formulary.* BMJ Publishing Group, London.

Bunn, F., Trivedi, D., and Ashraf, A. (2008) Colloid solutions for fluid resuscitation. *Cochrane Database of Systematic Reviews.* Issue 4. Art. No.: CD001319. DOI: 10.1002/14651858.CD001319.pub2.

Catrambone, J.E., He, W., Prestigiacomo, C.J. *et al.* (2008) The use of hypertonic saline in the treatment of post-traumatic cerebral edema: a review. *Eur. J. Trauma Emer. Surg.* **34**(4), 397–409.

De Beer, K., Sindhu, M., Thacker, M. *et al.* (2008) Diabetic ketoacidosis and hyperglycaemic hyperosmolar syndrome—clinical guidelines. *Nurs. Crit. Care.* **13**(1), 5–11.

Department of Health (2007) Using High Impact Interventions: Using Care Bundles to Reduce Healthcare Associated Infection by Increasing Reliability and Safety (online). Available at: http://www.dh.gov.uk/en/Publichealth/Healthprotection/Healthcareacquiredinfection/Healthcareacquiredgeneralinformation/ThedeliveryprogrammetoreducehealthcareassociatedinfectionsHCAIincludingMRSA/index.htm (accessed 03 Aug 2009).

Finfer, S., Bellomo, R., Boyce, N., *et al.* (2004) A comparison of albumin and saline for fluid resuscitation in the intensive care unit. *New Engl. J. Med.* **350**, 2247–56.

Gutierrez, G., Reines, H.D., and Wulf-Gutierrez, M.E. (2004) Clinical review: hemorrhagic shock. *Crit. Care.* **8**, 373–81.

Hashiguchi, N., Lum, L., Romeril, E., *et al.* (2007) Hypertonic saline resuscitation: efficacy may require early treatment in severely injured patients. *J. Trauma* **62**(2), 299–306.

Holcomb, S.S. (2008) Third-spacing: when body fluids shift. *Nursing* **38**(7), 50–3.

Levett, D.Z.H., Grocott, M.P.W., and Mythen, M.G. (2002) The effects of fluid optimization on outcome following major surgery. *Transfusion Alternatives Transfusion Med.* **4**(3), 74–9.

Marik, P.E., Baram, M., and Vahid, B. (2008) Does central venous pressure predict fluid responsiveness? A systematic review of the literature and the tale of seven mares. *Chest* **134**(1), 172–8.

Marino, P.L. (2007) *The ICU Book*. 3rd edn. Lippincott Williams & Wilkins, Philadelphia.

McClelland, D.B.L. (2007) *Handbook of Transfusion Medicine*, 4th edn. The Stationery Office, Norwich.

NICE (2007) *Acutely Ill Patients in Hospital: Recognition of and Response to Acute Illness in Adults in Hospital*. National Institute for Health and Clinical Excellence, London.

National Patient Safety Agency (2004) *Improving Infusion Device Safety* (Online). Available at: http://www.npsa.nhs.uk/nrls/alerts-and-directives/notices/infusion-device/ (accessed 03 Aug 2009).

National Patient Safety Agency (2007) *Safer Care for the Acutely Ill Patient: Learning from Serious Incidents*. (Online). Available at: http://www.npsa.nhs.uk/nrls/alerts-and-directives/directives-guidance/acutely-ill-patient/ (accessed 03 Aug 2009).

Pearse, R., Dawson, D., Fawcett, J. *et al.* (2005) Early goal-directed therapy after major surgery reduces complications and duration of hospital stay. A randomised, controlled trial. *Crit. Care* **9**, R687–93.

Perel, P. and Roberts, I. (2007) Colloids versus crystalloids for fluid resuscitation in critically ill patients. *Cochrane Database of Systematic Reviews* 2007, Issue 3. Art. No.: CD000567. DOI: 10.1002/14651858.CD000567.pub3.

Ryan, K.L., Batchinsky, A., McManus, J.G. *et al.* (2008) Changes in pulse character and mental status are late responses to central hypovolaemia. *Prehospital Emergency Care* **12**(2), 192–8.

Scales, K. and Pilsworth, J. (2008) The importance of fluid balance in clinical practice. *Nurs. Stand.* **22**(47), 50–7.

Tortora, G.J. and Derrickson, B.H. (2009) *Principles of Anatomy and Physiology: Maintenance and Continuity of the Human Body*, 12th edn. John Wiley & Sons, Hoboken.

UK Blood Transfusion and Tissue Transplantation Services (2008) *UK Blood Transfusion and Tissue Transplantation Services*. (Online). Available at: http://www.transfusionguidelines.org.uk/index.aspx (accessed 03 Aug 2009).

Vincent, J.L. and Weil, M.H. (2006) Fluid challenge revisited. *Crit. Care Med.* **35**(2), 1333–7.

Bibliography

Beattie, S. and Metules, T. (2007) Bedside emergency: haemorrhage. Third in a four-part series. *RN* **70**(8), 30–5.

Chapelhow, C. and Crouch, S. (2007) Applying numeracy skills in clinical practice: fluid balance. *Nurs. Stand.* **21**(27), 49–56, 58, 60.

Chernecky, C.C. (2006) *Fluids and Electrolytes*, 2nd edn. Saunders Elsevier, St Louis.

Cotter G, Metra, M. and Milo-Cotter, O., *et al.* (2008) Fluid overload in acute heart failure—re-distribution and other mechanisms beyond fluid accumulation. *Eur. J. Heart Failure* **10**(2), 165–9.

David, K. (2007) IV fluids: do you know what's hanging and why? *RN* **70**(10), 35–40.

Davidson, J., Griffin, R. and Higgs, S. (2007) Introducing a clinical pathway in fluid management. *Preview J. Perioperative Pract.* **17**(6), 248–50, 255–6.

Garcia Levia, J., Martinez Salgado, J., Estradas, J., *et al.* (2007) Pathophysiology of ascites and dilutional hyponatremia: contemporary use of aquaretic agents. *Ann. Hepatol.* **6**(4), 214–21.

Garretson, S. and Malberti, S. (2007) Understanding hypovolaemic, cardiogenic and septic shock. *Nurs. Stand.* **21**(50), 46–55, 58, 60.

Le Fever Kee, J., Paulanka, B.J., and Purnell, L. (2004) *Handbook of Fluids, Electrolytes and Acid-base Imbalances*, 2nd edn. Thomson Delmar Learning, Clifton.

Moore, T. and Woodrow, P. (2004) *High Dependency Nursing Care: Observation, Intervention and Support.* Routledge, London.

Naughton, C. (2006) Central venous pressure monitoring: a practical guide. *Br. J. Cardiac Nurs.* **1**(3), 110–16.

Noble, K.A. (2008) Fluid and electrolyte imbalance: a bridge over troubled water. *J. Perianaesthesia Nurs.* **23**(4), 267–72.

Reilly, R.F. and Perazella, M.A. (2007) *Acid–base, Fluids, and Electrolytes.* McGraw-Hill Medical, New York.

Royal College of Nursing (2003) *Standards for Infusion Therapy.* (Online). Available at: http://www.rcn.org.uk/publications/pdf/standardsinfusiontherapy.pdf (accessed 03 Aug 2009).

Sheppard, M. and Wright, M. (2005) *Principles and Practice of High Dependency Nursing.* 2nd ed,. Elsevier, London.

Spaniol, J.R., Knight, A.R., Zebley, J.L. *et al.* (2007) *J. Trauma Nurs.* **14**(3), 152–62.

Sumnall, R. (2007) Fluid management and diuretic therapy in acute renal failure. *Nurs. Crit. Care* **12**(1), 27–33.

Wagih, M.I. and Arthurs, G. (2008) Central venous pressure. *Care Crit. Ill* **24**(3), 53–7.

Weinstein, S. and Lawrence Plumer, A. (2006) *Plumer's Principles and Practice of Intravenous Therapy.* 8th edn. Lippincott Williams & Wilkins, Philadelphia.

Woo, A., Sutton, H., and Stephens, R. (2007) An introduction to fluid therapy. *J Hosp. Med.* **68**(4), M62–4.

Chapter 8

Assessment and care of the septic patient

Kevin Barrett

Chapter contents

In order to understand how to assess and manage the patient with sepsis it is essential to have an understanding of the pathophysiology of an infective process that has resulted in a global, rather than localized, inflammatory response by the patient. This chapter will examine:

- physiological changes following widespread inflammation
- physiological changes to the cardiovascular system in particular
- definitions of sepsis, severe sepsis, and septic shock
- assessment of sepsis
- nursing care of the patient with sepsis to include:
  - care bundles and their rationale
  - nursing management of the septic patient
- infection control.

Learning outcomes

This chapter will enable you to:

- consolidate your understanding of the normal inflammatory response
- develop an understanding of changes to this response during sepsis
- understand the significance of early and repeated assessment in patients with suspected sepsis
- examine the practice of assessment in septic patients
- discuss the management of patients with sepsis
- understand when the patient with worsening symptoms requires an escalation of support
- understand the impact of sepsis on the patient and society
- use the clinical assessment framework to guide your practice.

Introduction

Sepsis is a complication of infection and is a leading cause of death and critical illness worldwide—and one that is increasing in its occurrence (Townsend *et al.* 2005). Infection is caused by microbes—most often bacteria—invading the tissues, which results in a localized inflammatory response from the immune system. Sepsis, or septicaemia as it used to be called, is the body's *systemic*, rather than localized, inflammatory reaction to infection (Llewellyn & Cohen, 2007). It is recognized that an understanding of what sepsis is and why it is such a dangerous condition is poor in nurses (Robson *et al.* 2006) and doctors (Poeze *et al.* 2004) alike and that education about the condition is often inadequate for medical staff (Cohen 2007). It is also realized that the general public need help in understanding the condition (International Sepsis Forum 2003). This widespread lack of awareness about sepsis alone constitutes a barrier in recognizing when these patients are becoming very unwell and require an escalation of interventions to try and avoid the very serious, often fatal, consequences of the condition—whether the patient begins to deteriorate at home or in hospital.

Epidemiology: 'the world's oldest killer'

The epidemiology of sepsis, which is the study of the spread of the condition throughout popula-tions, is helpful to look at because its incidence is so pervasive and yet is underestimated by healthcare professionals (Surviving Sepsis Campaign 2007). Worldwide, there are over 18 million cases of sepsis each year—which is equivalent to the combined populations of Ireland, Norway, Denmark, and Finland. Every day some 1,400 people die of sepsis (Townsend *et al.* 2005). Although the focus of this chapter is on ward-based patients, it is worth realizing that once patients with sepsis are transferred to an intensive therapy unit (ITU) setting, where they can best be supported, even then 35% of these patients will not survive and 47% of patients admitted to ITU with sepsis will die at some point in their hospital stay (Padkin *et al.* 2003). This is an extremely high mortality rate.

In the UK, the estimated annual figure for deaths from sepsis is in the region of 37,000: a higher mortality than lung cancer and also higher than the *combined* figures for bowel and breast cancer (Daniels 2007). Globally, the incidence of sepsis has risen by 329% over the past 20 years (Surviving Sepsis Campaign, 2007), and the most recent figures for this country show the number of deaths from sepsis is increasing, too (Harrison *et al.* 2006).

This escalating trend—estimated at a 1.5% increase per year (Angus *et al.* 2001)—is thought to be due to an increasingly older population becoming ill with a greater co-morbidity; older, more poorly patients are simply not able to fight infection and become overwhelmed by it. In addition, the therapies used in hospitals are often invasive and any breach in a patient's anatomical barriers to infection will increase their vulnerability to opportunistic infection (Daniels 2007a; Vila & Martinez, 2007). Widespread use of antibiotics has resulted in many strains of micro-organisms developing resistance to antibiotic therapy and thus are immune from the mainstay of treatment for infection (Dolan, 2003); consequently, the infection becomes much more difficult to contain and suppress.

Sepsis also places a huge financial strain on healthcare budgets around the globe—European estimates are for 7.6 billion Euros per year and the UK estimate is £1.5 billion per year (Daniels 2007), with the cost in the USA being over $1.6 billion (Townsend *et al.* 2005). Much of the high expenditure results from this patient group requiring very intensive nursing care; the nurse to patient ratio for very dependent patient groups is high, often one-to one (Galley & O'Riordan 2003).

The surviving sepsis campaign

Appreciating the vast scale of sepsis worldwide, as well as the unacceptably high mortalities involved, an initiative to form the Surviving Sepsis Campaign, endorsed by many of the major critical care societies in North America and Europe, was put into effect in 2002. The initial mandate of the campaign was to reduce mortality by 25% by 2009 (Surviving Sepsis Campaign 2007a). The means by which this is to be accomplished is through a six-point strategy:

♦ Awareness: increasing the awareness of healthcare workers, government agencies that fund health care as well as the general public of the dangers of sepsis.

♦ Diagnosis: improving early and accurate diagnosis of sepsis, partly by providing a consensus definition of sepsis that is relevant worldwide.

♦ Treatment: disseminating a range of treatment options and urging their timely intervention. Since 2004 there have been internationally accepted guidelines for the bedside management of sepsis (Dellinger, *et al.* 2004), including the early stages of sepsis, which nurses will be managing on the wards.

♦ Education: providing support and information to all professionals who manage patients with sepsis, including interventions and standards of care.

♦ Counselling: providing a framework for improving and accelerating access to post-ITU care and counselling for patients who have had sepsis.

♦ Referral: recognize the need for clear referral guidelines adopted by all countries through the development of global guidelines.

All of the above six points are relevant for ward nurses and all points are addressed in this chapter.

Sepsis, severe sepsis, and septic shock

Because sepsis can manifest in varying degrees of severity, leading, in the worst instances, to a state of shock and collapse of multiple organ systems, there are terms to define the progression of the illness that aim to define the scale of the damage that sepsis is causing to the patient. The terms used are sepsis, severe sepsis, and septic shock, which we should have a look at and consider— they are terms which have remained unclear for some professionals (Alberti & Brun-Buisson 2003) and which have now had definitions agreed upon (Dellinger *et al.* 2008) (see Tables 8.1 and 8.2). Essentially, sepsis is the presence of an infection together with the systemic signs and symptoms of infection (Dellinger *et al.* 2008).

One term that is used in close association with sepsis is 'SIRS', which is worth explaining. When a patient exhibits the systemic signs and symptoms of infection, but does not have a documented infection, the term systemic inflammatory response syndrome (SIRS) is used. This could be caused by any event provoking inflammation in multiple sites throughout the body simultaneously; examples being burns, pancreatitis, or trauma (Hinds & Watson 2005). These patients will exhibit broadly similar clinical signs to sepsis.

One of the difficulties in recognizing sepsis in its early stages is that the patient will complain of very general symptoms that might be attributable to any number of causes. Also, although there

Table 8.1 Definition of key terms (Dellinger et al. 2008)

Sepsis	Infection plus systemic manifestations of infection
Severe sepsis	Sepsis plus sepsis-induced organ dysfunction/tissue hypoperfusion. This sepsis-induced hypotension is defined as a systolic pressure of less than 90 mmHg or a systolic decrease of over 40 mmHg. Tissue hypoperfusion is evidenced by elevated lactate or oliguria*
Septic shock	Sepsis-induced hypotension persisting despite adequate fluid resuscitation.

* Both of the terms 'lactate' and 'oliguria' are considered later in the chapter.

Table 8.2 Signs and symptoms of infection (Robson & Daniels 2008)

Temperature	>38.3 or<36 C
Heart rate	>90 beats/min
Respiratory rate	>20 breaths/min
White cells	<4 or >12 g/L
Mental status	Acutely altered
Blood sugar	Hyperglycaemic (> 6.6 mmol/L)unless diabetic

are a variety of signs that the patient is developing sepsis, none of them alone are definitive of a septic patient. They also do not allow for any sense of the 'staging' or progression of the condition, nor of prognosis (Levy *et al.* 2003); it is difficult to predict how poorly someone is becoming in early sepsis. These signs and symptoms are detailed in Table 8.3.

It is easy to see how the development of sepsis might remain unsuspected in a patient with one or two of the above signs or symptoms. What is needed is an enhanced ability to suspect sepsis earlier, catch its development, and provide an escalation of support for the patient as quickly as possible. One way of doing this is to consider which patients might be at an increased risk of sepsis. When a change in temperature or an unexplained tachycardia is noted, for example, in these patients, it is imperative to monitor them closely and alert the shift leader or outreach team about their condition quickly. Patients who are at a high risk of developing sepsis are those who:

♦ are very young (premature babies, for instance) or who are very elderly

♦ have an already compromised immune system from taking immune suppressant drugs for auto-immune disorders or chemotherapy for cancer

♦ have addictions to drugs or alcohol

♦ have deep tissue wounds: for example from burns or trauma

Table 8.3 Signs and symptoms of early sepsis (International Sepsis Forum 2003)

Temperature	High—can be with rigours: this is especially associated with early sepsis but not always found OR can be low—especially in very young or elderly
Breathing	High respiratory rate, possibly with shortness of breath. Purulent sputum if associated with a chest infection
Heart rate	Tachycardia
Urine output	Low urine output (oliguria) or may be painful or foul smelling urine if associated with urinary tract infection
Abdominal symptoms	Pain if associated with abdominal infections or surgery
Central nervous system symptoms	Headache if associated with CNS infection (eg: meningitis)
Skin signs	Warm to touch and/or possible skin rash OR can be cool to touch
General weakness	'Fluey' symptoms
White cell count	Can be raised OR can be abnormally low
Microbiology report	Positive to bacteria or other organisms in biological fluids: blood, urine, sputum, etc.

+ have indwelling intravenous lines or catheters

+ are more prone to develop sepsis because of their genetic makeup (International Sepsis Forum 2003).

The first three groups are those with weak (or immature) immune systems and the next two groups are those who have been made vulnerable to invasion from micro-organisms. It is helpful to bear these two points in mind when caring for patients who cause concern in terms of changes in their routine observations or who begin to complain of feeling generally unwell. Each of the signs and symptoms will be reviewed throughout the course of the chapter; however, to appreciate why a 'systemic' or 'global' response to infection is so problematical, it is important to review what the body's normal or expected response would be.

The immune system: layers of defence

For an infective agent, be it a bacteria, fungus, or virus, to establish itself within our physiological systems—or 'colonize' them—it must initially bypass the body's many surface barriers. An infection occurs once our immune system cannot defend against colonizing micro-organisms and they begin to damage tissue (Kozier *et al.* 2008). The surface barriers constitute the first in a series of defences against the outside world. An intact skin surface with a slightly acid pH provides an effective obstacle, as there is no easy way through the skin and the pH is unsuitable for many organisms to inhabit. As the skin is keratinized and thus waterproofed, water-soluble organisms are kept at bay. A number of organisms do manage to colonize the skin surfaces but because the epidermal layers are constantly shedding, the colonies of micro-organisms are shed too.

In general, good personal hygiene means that the areas that are most likely to become colonized, such as the mouth, perineum, and hands, are kept clean and do not allow colonization to develop. The body cavities that are exposed to the outside world such as the respiratory, digestive, and uro-genital tracts secrete enzyme-laden fluids that are either directly antimicrobial or are lined with mucous that obstruct the pathogen from attaching to and colonizing those areas (Delves & Roitt 2000). The gastrointestinal (GI) tract uses extreme changes in pH to kill foreign bodies. As long as this first line of defence stays undamaged and intact, patients are protected from most invading organisms. Later in the chapter the frequently encountered breaks to the integrity of these surface barriers found in ward patients and the significance of these breaks in relation to sepsis will be considered.

However, once a foreign body does penetrate these defences, there are two further levels of protection—the innate responses and the acquired or adaptive reactions (Rote & Trask 2006). The innate system, although including the surface barriers, also consists of cellular and molecular components as well as the inflammatory response. Cells that employ phagocytosis—that is, they ingest other cells—circulate in the blood, lymph, and interstitial fluids as well as inhabit tissues: macrophages and neutrophils, for example. They engulf particles that are recognized as foreign and destroy them with powerful enzymes.

Macrophages are cells that can also release powerful inflammatory mediators, which are responsible for much of the classical inflammatory reaction: localized production of heat, redness, swelling, and pain. The inflammatory response is central to and definitive of the second line of defence, and it is the inflammatory response—when it becomes widespread rather than contained—that causes many of the problems encountered in sepsis. This is examined in the next section.

The molecular element of the innate immune system is the collection of 'chemical messengers' that control the inflammatory and clotting responses and help contain them just to the area that is affected. One of the key points here is that the inflammatory reaction is carefully controlled and manifests only in a limited area. These reactions occur in relation to *any* invading organism or breach in the first line of defence—they all form part of what is termed non-specific immunity; that is, they respond in the same way to any provoking agent and are not specific to purely that agent.

The third line of defence is the adaptive immune system, the behaviour of antigen-specific B- and T-cells that bind to antigen. Antigen is what the immune system interacts with and which helps it to recognize self- and non-self molecules (Hannigan 2000). B-cells secrete immunoglobulins; antibodies which are antigen specific and which kill that antigen. T-cells assist B-cells making these antibodies (Chapel *et al.* 2006). A key point here is that these defences are *specific* to individually identified molecules and are thus called our specific immunity.

The inflammatory response and sepsis

It is the second line of our immune system—and in particular the inflammatory reaction—that is responsible for the exaggerated physiological response and the complications that we see in sepsis. Inflammation is a rapid and coordinated reply to cellular injury (Trask *et al.* 2006), characterized by the classic findings of redness, heat, swelling, and pain as well as loss of function. Blood tests will reveal a concentration of leucocytes—white blood cells (Levick 2003). As much of the problem with sepsis is caused by inflammatory changes, this process is reviewed in-depth below.

When tissue is damaged or becomes contaminated with invading organisms, cells that are scouting for foreign bodies—mast cells and macrophages—are activated. Mast cells located in the interstitium around the affected area will degranulate—that is, release a number of chemical messengers into the bloodstream. These chemicals will both attract white blood cells—primarily neutrophils, which are the most abundant white cell type—to the area to help fight the infection and also influence the permeability the cells making up the lining of the capillary wall, the endothelium. They will also cause vasodilation, widening of the blood vessel, to increase blood flow to that localized area, increasing the supply of the oxygen, white cells, and nutrients needed to combat the infection.

Macrophages will be also be among the first components of the innate response to encounter the invading organism. They will release numerous cellular messengers called cytokines to alert other parts of the immune system of the invasion and they, too, attract neutrophils to the site of infection. Cytokines will also instruct bone marrow cells to produce more neutrophils (Helbert 2006)—they are sometimes referred to as the hormones of the immune system. Not all of the messengers involved are cytokines so the term inflammatory mediators can be used to address all of the different 'families' of chemicals released during inflammation.

The role of the endothelium

The inflammatory response is carefully orchestrated and something that plays a remarkable part in the coordination of events is the endothelium itself. As a single layer of cells, the capillary endothelium acts as a semi-permeable barrier between the bloodstream and the interstitium (Levick 2003). Nevertheless, the endothelium is an extremely dynamic membrane:

+ It controls exchange of proteins, hormones, minerals, and immunoglobins between the blood and the tissues.

+ It secretes numerous substances that help control the degree of contraction of the muscle wall in the blood vessels, affecting blood flow and pressure.

+ It secretes substances to encourage and also inhibit clotting processes and ensures that clotting is contained locally.

+ It responds to the mediators that are released in inflammation by becoming more permeable or 'leaky' (Levick 2003).

It is not so important to remember the names of the various substances that are involved in the behaviour of the endothelial cells, but it is necessary to appreciate that once the endothelium is subject to widespread damage, as with sepsis, all of the above controls are lost.

The role that the permeability of the endothelium plays in the normal inflammatory reaction is absolutely central (Playfair & Chain 2005). For example, when neutrophils arrive at the site of inflammation, they will need to be allowed passage through the blood vessel wall to the affected tissue. The neutrophils are normally too large to squeeze through the tiny junctions between the individual cells of the capillary wall. This particular process, called diapedisis, is managed by cytokine influence on the integrity of the endothelium (Male 2003), making the endothelium 'porous' enough for the neutrophils to migrate out of the vascular space. Here the white cells can begin the process of ingesting and destroying foreign particles; it is the concentration of white cells and bacterial debris that is largely responsible for the colour of pus (Actor 2007). This increase in permeability results in the collection of white cells found in inflamed tissue and also for the escape of plasma fluid that causes inflammatory swelling.

This rather complex sounding series of events can be simplified through the flow chart representation shown in Figure 8.1.

The cardinal signs of inflammation are:

♦ redness (erythema): caused by vasodilation and the increased blood flow to the affected area

♦ heat: also caused by vasodilation and increased blood flow as well as the increased metabolic activity at the area

♦ swelling: caused by the collection of plasma exudate

♦ pain: caused by some inflammatory mediators (noticeably one called bradykinin) (Levick 2003)

♦ loss of function: caused by the localized swelling and the effects of pain

♦ leucocytosis (concentration of white cells): facilitated by the permeability of the endothelium.

Tissue injury or infection

Mast cell and macrophage activation: release of inflammatory mediators

- Attraction of neutrophils, to fight infection
- Increase to the permeability of the vessel wall, to allow neutrophils across to affected tissues
- Vasodilation to increase blood flow and supply of oxygen and nutrients

Formation of exudate

Figure 8.1 Inflammatory reaction.

These inflammatory processes are controlled in what is called a positive feedback loop. In the presence of an alien organism, an increase in macrophage activity and cytokine populations signal the need for a further increase of macrophage activity and release of even more cytokines, which, in turn, results in an even further increase and so on. These processes, by virtue of being influenced by positive feedback, are very powerful and fast acting; they need to be in order to respond to infection and contain it locally (Sompayrac 2003). When the infection becomes spread throughout the body—as with sepsis—these same powerful responses are activated *everywhere*, which results in a massive over-reaction and the body's response becomes uncontrolled and dysfunctional. The term 'systemic inflammatory response syndrome' is easier to appreciate in this light. The overwhelming inflammatory response acting globally on the epithelium actually damages it—it is not particularly the infection that is causing the damage but the patient's response to it-their own inflammatory process (Marini 2007). Sometimes sepsis is therefore termed a type of hypersensitivity reaction (type V hypersensitivity) (Hannigan 2000). The widespread leakiness across the endothelium throughout the body results in significant losses of circulating plasma volume—causing hypovolaemia and hypotension—and also in widespread oedema. These are frequent findings in severe sepsis.

The increased presence of neutrophils (their production in the bone marrow having been stimulated by cytokines) contributes to a rise in the total number of white cells in the blood generally and this becomes a marker for infection. In general, the white cell count (WCC) is between 3.7 and 9.5 × 10^9/L (Blann 2006). A WCC above these limits is indicative of an infective process.

The flooding of inflammatory mediators into the bloodstream typifies the acute-phase response to infection in which core temperature is increased and certain proteins in the plasma become activated (Helbert 2006). These are key findings in most patients who have sepsis; the development of a temperature is an especially important one to be vigilant about. The increase in temperature—pyrexia—is caused by the hypothalamus' reaction to the presence of specific cytokines. The autonomic nervous system then 're-sets' the body's core temperature in an attempt to make the body's internal environment hostile to the replication of invading organisms. The acute-phase proteins will be monitored by the medical team in patients suspected of having a systemic infection; the most commonly measured of these proteins is called C-reactive protein (CRP).

One further blood test may be for the erythrocyte sedimentation rate (ESR). This test is also suggestive of infection if the value is prolonged. The ESR indicates that cells are taking longer to 'settle' or 'sediment' in a sample of blood than expected. This, in turn, indicates that the blood has become more viscous or sticky. The viscosity is the result of an increased presence of released cytokines and activated plasma proteins secondary to infection. CRP is a more sensitive test for infection and inflammatory processes than ESR and more likely to be done (Higgins 2007).

The infective agents that are associated with sepsis can be bacteria, viruses, fungi, and some parasites (Morton *et al.* 2004). Predominantly, it is bacteria that are the causative agents and particularly the 'Gram negative' bacteria. Gram negative simply describes the fact that these bacteria do not retain a stain—called the 'Gram stain'—which is applied in the laboratory to differentiate bacteria. Gram negative bacteria contain molecules called 'endotoxins' that are responsible for much of the cardiovascular dysfunction seen in septic patients (Parrillo 2001). Endotoxins are a component of the gram negative bacterial cell wall and directly injure the endothelial lining of capillary vessels; endotoxin will cause vasodilatation, inappropriately activate the coagulation cascade, and depress the myocardium (Barnett & Cosslett 1998). Gram positive bacteria also result in similar compromises, although through different mechanisms (Dolan 2003).

One group of patients that require particular vigilance in terms of the development of severe sepsis and shock are neutropenic patients. Neutropenic patients are unable to mount a normal response to infection because their white cell population is very low. By definition the WCC will be less than $4 \times 10^9/L$ (Kitchen *et al.* 2007), but it can be much lower than this. Neutropenia may be congenital or, more likely, acquired due to infections, autoimmune disorders or due to chemotherapeutic regimens in cancer treatment, for example (Murphy *et al.* 2005). Neutrophils have a very short lifespan and the stem cells that produce them in bone marrow must divide very rapidly to maintain circulating levels in the bloodstream (Kindt *et al.* 2007)—for this reason drugs that target rapidly reproducing cells (such as tumour cells) will effect neutrophils levels, too. Neutropenia is commonly found in patients undergoing chemotherapy or radiation therapies for cancer (Kitchen *et al.* 2007).

Neutrophils help contain infection and without them infection can spread unhindered and become systemic quickly (Nairn & Helbert 2007). An infection in the lungs, for example, will not result in localized symptoms and pus formation, but will spread rapidly into the blood. The macrophage activity is still intact, however, so cytokine release will still produce a temperature and shivering responses. Sometimes this is the only warning sign in neutropenic patients that an infection is present and in these patients sepsis may develop quickly. It may be that patients simply report feeling generally poorly, which is not uncommon in chemotherapy or radiation therapy patients. If a temperature is noted in a neutropenic patient, intravenous antibiotics are indicated and should be given immediately—within 1 h of the pyrexia being noted—in order to combat the bacteria and the effects of its endotoxin. If a tachycardia and hypotension are noted in the patient, it signifies that severe sepsis and shock are already developing and these patients need an urgent medical review and urgent fluid resuscitation.

Review point 1

+ Sepsis is infection with a systemic, rather than localized, inflammatory response.
+ Sepsis can lead to shock states with a very high mortality.
+ The prevalence of sepsis is very high but this is underestimated by healthcare professionals. The Surviving Sepsis Campaign aims to raise awareness of sepsis and provides treatment guidelines.
+ The inflammatory response is influenced and moderated by the endothelium. When the endothelium is damaged in a widespread fashion this moderation is lost and inflammation becomes a global event.
+ Neutropenic patients cannot mount a normal white cell response and infection may become systemic quickly. These patients may only show a temperature or vaguely complain of feeling unwell. Time is of the essence in these patients, particularly in terms of having a medical review and intravenous antibiotics being administered.

Clinical link 8.1 (see Appendix for answers)

+ Septic shock is sometimes referred to as 'distributive' shock. Why do you think this is?
+ The hypovolaemia found in sepsis is sometimes referred to as 'relative' hypovolaemia. Why do you think this is?

Pathophysiology: the cardiovascular system

Sepsis will affect every system in the body to some degree, partly because the infective agent is blood-borne and thus is spread everywhere, but also because the effects upon the cardiovascular system, responsible for blood pressure and oxygen delivery to all cells, is so profoundly and immediately affected. The cardiovascular manifestations of sepsis are essentially vasodilatation, maldistribution of blood flow (due to clotting abnormalities) and myocardial depression (Bridges & Dukes 2005). The main cardiovascular response to sepsis is vasodilation—the relaxing of the smooth muscle wall inside the blood vessels which leads to a looser, wider vessel. The vasodilation is caused by the release of a substance called nitrous oxide, which the endothelial cells release in response either to changes in blood flow or in response to cytokines (Levick 2003). Vasodilation is responsible for many physical assessment findings in the septic patient.

The main consequence of vasodilatation is that of hypotension—inadequate blood pressure to supply the tissues and cells with nutrients and, in particular, oxygen. Hypotension, if it is left unnoticed and untreated will affect every body system simply because they all rely upon the cardiovascular system to deliver oxygen and remove waste products. The worst case scenario in terms of hypotension is shock. Shock can be defined as circulatory insufficiency (Franklin & Darovic 2002); the cardiovascular system cannot meet the metabolic demands of the cells and they begin to dysfunction. This leads, if unsuccessfully treated, to multiple organ failure—because all cells are affected—and death. One of the end-stage consequences of septic shock is multi-organ dysfunction syndrome (MODS) (Gordon 1999), each cell type is affected in its own way by the disease processes and one failing system will compound the effects of the others.

In order to appreciate exactly why hypotension occurs in these patients it is helpful to quickly review how blood pressure is maintained in health—see also Chapter 3. The cardiac cycle is the sequence of events that the heart undergoes throughout one heart beat (McCance 2006). The heart pumps blood through the pulmonary and systemic vasculature by generating enough pressure to propel the blood that has drained into the ventricles—the 'stroke volume'—forward. This is called the systolic pressure and is produced by forceful contraction. The heart then relaxes and allows the next stroke volume to drain into the ventricles—this stage of the cycle is termed diastole. Clearly, the previous stroke volume will stop its forward movement as the propelling force from the heart comes to rest—as in diastole. There must be some other influences that support both the forward movement of blood and also the pressure that the blood is under in order for it to reach the tissues far from the heart at a pressure high enough to perfuse those tissues. These other influences are the behaviour of the blood vessels—there are cardiac and vascular components to blood pressure, hence the term 'cardiovascular'.

When the arterial vessels receive the stroke volume under high systolic pressure, they distend to accommodate the bolus of blood. They are able to do this because of the elastic nature of their walls—they have a layer of smooth muscle and elastic tissue, called the 'tunica media', which provides the ability to stretch. Whilst the heart stops contracting, the vessel wall can recoil from their stretched position, further squeezing the blood onward and this provides some continuity of forward propulsion for the blood. The most important factor, however, in preserving the blood pressure throughout the cardiac cycle is the tension that the blood vessel wall is kept under. This accounts for the pressure of blood in the vessels during the period that the heart is resting and filling—diastolic pressure. This is the pressure that the heart has to overcome to provide the next stroke volume and is termed the systemic vascular resistance (SVR) (Darovic 2002). SVR is maintained by a number of factors, although primarily through the sympathetic nervous system (SNS). The SNS innervates the smooth muscle wall of the vessels and sustains a level of contraction, or tone, to ensure that the lumen—or internal diameter of the vessel—is within a range of functional limits. The cardiac cycle is approximately two-third diastole and one-third systole, and thus the vessel wall tone contribution to maintaining blood pressure is very significant.

With a wider lumen in the blood vessels, it is increasingly harder for the heart to maintain the blood pressure at its normal value. An analogy here would be of a hose pipe with a narrow lumen—perhaps because a thumb has been partly placed over the opening—providing a good pressure of water. Compare that with the pressure of water from the hose when the thumb is removed, the pressure drops because the lumen is wider. When the blood vessel lumen widens, the diastolic component or SVR is lost. In response to the decreased SVR, the heart rate increases to compensate for the loss in diastolic pressure and tachycardia is a classic finding in patients in early stages of sepsis. The bounding, tachycardic heart beat is indicative of the cardiovascular system adjusting for vasodilation and the patient is said to be in a 'hyperdynamic' state. At this stage of sepsis the patient has a high cardiac output but only a normal or adequate blood pressure (Darovic 2002).This hyperdynamism can only be maintained for a limited amount of time. After a while the patient's physiological reserve becomes exhausted and the blood pressure becomes 'de-compensated' and falls to inadequate levels. At this point the pulse will feel 'thready' or weak. This is when shock is likely to develop very quickly. One of the reasons that patients with sepsis will be moved to a critical care unit is that their blood pressure and cardiac output can be monitored very closely and supported with powerful drugs, such as inotropes, which are considered in Chapter 3.

Vasodilatation is also responsible for, or contributes to, some of the other frequently encountered assessment findings in the patient with sepsis. These include the heat of their skin—surface temperature, their flushed appearance, and widespread peripheral oedema—although this is most markedly noticeable in patients in the latter stages of sepsis; hopefully these patients have already been re-located to the high dependency unit (HDU) or ITU by this point. The flushed appearance and, in part, increased skin temperature are due to the inappropriate dilation of peripheral vessels close to the skin, bringing an increased flow of blood close to the skin surface. Some of the surface temperature changes will be due to the re-setting of the internal thermostat mentioned earlier. Physiologically, the formation of oedema is more complex.

Oedema formation

In health, a constant balance of the 'escape' and return of plasma from the intravascular space into the interstitial space and back to the intravascular space is maintained. Fresh plasma fluid bathes the cells and so helps to deliver dissolved oxygen, electrolytes, and nutrients directly to respiring cells. The homeostatic mechanisms that regulate this circulation prevent any build up of fluid in the interstitium which would interrupt the supply, for example, of fresh oxygen and the removal of waste gas. As oedema can be global and very exaggerated in septic patients and because it can cause a number of secondary complications requiring nursing care, it is helpful to review how oedema occurs in sepsis.

Typically, blood arrives at the capillary beds from arterioles at a perfusing pressure of approximately 32 mmHg. This perfusing pressure is enough to push a small yet constant volume of the plasma—complete with all of its dissolved contents—through the microscopic junctions that exist between the single cell layer of the capillary vessels. The volume able to leave the vascular space is regulated by the perfusing pressure and the size of the cell junctions and the integrity of the vessel wall—there are only a certain number of tiny outlets for the fluid. It is also regulated by a force exerted by molecules in the capillary blood called colloid molecules; these are large molecules that are too big to squeeze through the cell junctions—red and white blood cells and proteins, for example—and create what is known as colloid or oncotic pressure. Oncotic pressure, approximately 20 mmHg in the capillaries—serves to hold most of the plasma fluid in the vascular space. It exercises a holding force on the fluid which can only escape its influence if the perfusing pressure is greater. At the arteriolar end of the capillary bed, the perfusing pressure (32 mmHg) *is* greater and plasma leaves the vascular space and becomes part of the interstitial fluid.

Once the fresh plasma has bathed the cells it will be depleted of fresh oxygen, nutrients, etc. and also will have picked up the waste products of the cells' metabolism—noticeably, carbon dioxide gas. This exchange will be due to concentration gradients of the various substances between the cell and the interstitial fluid. Unless the interstitial fluid is able to 'drain' itself back into the vascular space, there will be an accumulation of waste products and an interruption of the concentration gradients. This drainage happens because of the constant oncotic pressure in the capillary vessels provided by the presence of the large molecules: in a healthy, intact capillary vessel the large colloid molecules cannot escape through the vessel wall and this guarantees a consistent oncotic pressure along the length of the vessel. The perfusing pressure, however, decreases along the length of the capillary from the arterioles (32 mmHg) to venules (12 mmHg) (Figure 8.2).

Note now that the colloid pressure (20 mmHg) exceeds the perfusing pressure at the venous end (12 mmHg). At this point the interstitial fluid can be drawn back into the vascular space, through the same epithelial wall junctions, because the 'pulling', colloid influence of all of the large molecules now exerts a stronger influence than the 'pushing' perfusing pressure. In this way there is a constant flow of fluid into and out of the interstitium. Any residual fluid that might collect is drained by lymphatic vessels and then drained back into the bloodstream.

Sepsis disrupts this mechanism predominantly through compromising the integrity of the vessel walls. Endotoxin injures the endothelium directly and excessive cytokine activity causes the capillary junctions to become inappropriately permeable: sepsis has 'over-induced' the inflammatory response, causing it to 'over react' (Figure 8.3).

The combined effect is to let not only far too much fluid into the interstitium, but also to allow some of the colloid molecules—especially the smaller proteins—to enter the interstitial space and thus ruin the oncotic balance responsible for draining fluid back into the circulation. Too much

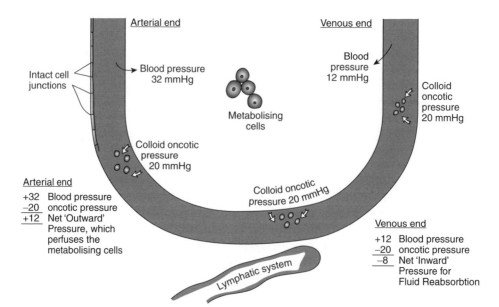

Figure 8.2 Normal tissue perfusion and drainage.

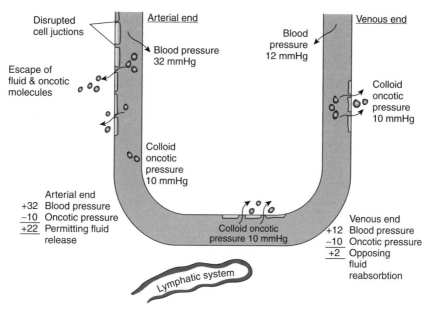

Figure 8.3 Formation of oedema.

fluid into the interstitium and not enough out results in the oedema that develops in more advanced cases of sepsis and also in the patients who have returned from ITU settings after having survived sepsis. Oedema can be incapacitating for patients because it may lead to blisters and rashes and cause restrictive, swollen joints and swelling of, or effusions around, vital organs (Levick 2003). The oedema experienced by patients who have had severe sepsis will have been profound and as well as its debilitating physical effects on the patient themselves it may have had a disturbing effect on relatives as the swelling of the soft facial tissue such as eyelids and lips can render people unrecognizable.

Secondary to hypotension and poor perfusion will be hypoxia of the tissues. When cells are in an oxygen-poor environment they begin to respire anaerobically, a by-product of which is lactate. Lactate is acidic and when it builds up in the tissues it has a toxic effect on cells. We have all experienced a miniature version of lactic acidosis when we develop a 'stitch' from running too fast for too long. Lactate levels in health are low—normal values are 0.5–2 mmol/L (Higgins 2007)—and raised levels signify that tissues are being under-perfused, hence lactate has become a frequently monitored blood value at the bedside. Other clinical signs of poor perfusion are acutely diminished mental status, a slow capillary refill time when a nail bed is pressed, and cool and/or mottled skin (Guardiola *et al.* 2007).

Another of the key features of cardiovascular compromise in sepsis is the effect upon the body's clotting mechanisms. In sepsis the epithelium has a prominent role in the derangement of clotting controls—coagulopathy (Levi & van der Poll 2004). Damage to the epithelium from excessive cytokine activity or endotoxin from Gram negative bacteria will activate the extrinsic pathway of the clotting cascade (Bridges & Dukes 2005). As a result of the extensive nature of the injury to the endothelium in sepsis, the clotting cascade will be activated in numerous sites, resulting in microthrombi, which occlude vessels supplying vital organs and tissue beds. This contributes to the development of organ failure that is seen in severe sepsis and septic shock (Rutherford 1996). The indiscriminate nature of thrombus formation throughout the body results in the profound depletion of clotting factors and this leads, in turn, to uncontrolled bleeding or 'oozing' of blood from any puncture sites such as intravenous access or the patient's gums or invisibly as internal bleeds from ulceration points, for instance. As the clotting processes are widespread rather than locally contained and because the thrombus is formed inside blood vessels, the condition is termed disseminated intravascular coagulopathy (DIC). DIC is largely responsible for the maldistribution of blood during severe sepsis. When the occlusion of vessels is combined with poor perfusing pressure due to vasodilation and loss of circulating fluid due to oedema formation, the effects are catastrophic and patients develop refractory shock—shock which is unresponsive to fluid resuscitation and drugs—and MODS, which has no means of treatment as, to date, there is no way to support respiration at the cellular level (Papathanassoglou *et al.* 2008).

The last of the three main cardiovascular compromises is myocardial depression, which is commonly met in severe sepsis (Guardiola *et al.* 2007). This is caused directly by some inflammatory mediators—in fact, one is named myocardial depressant factor. The result upon the heart is a reduced contractility so that even when fluid is given to resuscitate the blood pressure, the heart fails to respond adequately (Taiberg *et al.* 2005). This reduced contractility affects the ability to generate sufficient systolic pressure—this is dangerous for the septic patient as they also have a loss of circulating volume in the form of oedema and a reduced diastolic pressure due to vasodilation. All three situations together wreak havoc with the body's ability to supply enough oxygen to cells, which is why shock states develop so frequently in sepsis and why mortality is so high. The important point is to suspect its development and act quickly with the other multidisciplinary team (MDT) members to support the patient early—this is how septic patients are most likely to survive.

Review point 2

♦ Global endothelial dysfunction results in profound cardiovascular compromise, which in turn will affect all body systems.

♦ Sepsis causes vasodilation due to endothelial damage and massive inflammatory mediator release, resulting in hypotension from compromise of the diastolic function.

♦ At a time when increased oxygen is needed, the myocardium becomes 'depressed', resulting in hypotension from compromises of the systolic function.

♦ Widespread oedema, caused by global endothelial permeability changes, is a common finding in severe sepsis that effectively renders the patient hypotensive.

♦ Sepsis, through damaging the endothelium, can initiate the clotting cascade globally. This can result in multiple microthrombi that occlude vessels, resulting in poor perfusion of vital organs that can lead to their failure.

♦ Lactate is an indicator of tissue hypoxia and shock.

Sepsis thus affects the cardiovascular system in a profound way, but all systems are affected. The respiratory system is a major indicator of physiological changes in sepsis. The increased metabolic demand for oxygen and increase in production of carbon dioxide will result in a higher respiratory rate (tachypnoea), which in one study was found in 89% of patients who developed severe sepsis (Carter 2007). Tachypnoea is viewed as being the most sensitive of the basic observations in terms of patient deterioration (Ahern & Philpott 2002). Other signs of the patient struggling with respiratory function are use of accessory muscles which include the abdomen, shoulder girdle, and facial muscles. If the infection has come from the respiratory system, which is likely as in Europe, 50–60% of severe sepsis cases are from pneumonia (Daniels 2007b), there may be other signs of respiratory distress such as coughing, painful breathing, low saturation levels, or purulent sputum. Sputum samples should be sent for microbiological culture and sensitivity testing (MC&S).

The renal system relies on a perfusing pressure to filter blood plasma at the glomerulus to begin to form urine (Huether 2006). Without this pressure urine production falls or ceases altogether. Urine output is a good indicator of the perfusion of the kidneys (and thus all other vital organs) and so it is important for us to have a clear indication of the patient's renal function. The minimum that a normal urine output amounts to is 0.5 mL/kg, so in a person weighing 80 kg, 40 mL per hour is expected—anything less is termed oliguria. The complete absence of urine output, which is a serious indication of renal failure, is called anuria.

It is important to recognize if a patient is becoming oliguric before they become anuric; once organ failure is evidenced the patient is in severe sepsis and beginning the decline into the awful morbidity and mortality associated with it. To this end an hourly urine output is helpful as it alerts to possibly small but consistent changes in kidney function and a catheter can facilitate these observations. However, catheters are also a frequent source of hospital-acquired infection (Department of Health 2006) and, indeed, sepsis. Needless to say, strict asepsis is always imperative in catheter insertion (Department of Health 2006).

If the original infection has come from the urinary tract, the patient may complain of discomfort when passing urine and the urine itself may well be cloudy, discoloured and foul smelling. A urine-analysis dip stick test can identify the presence of leucocytes or nitrites—both indicators of bacterial presence. Any abnormal findings from this simple and quick test need to be followed up or referred on to the senior nurses or medical team. In the case of a positive result for bacterial presence a urine sample needs to be sent for MC&S; urinary tract infections (UTI) make up 7–10% of infective sources for sepsis (Daniels 2007b).Other markers of renal function will be gleaned from biochemistry results such as urea and creatinine levels and are discussed in Chapter 5.

The other significant source of infection in sepsis is the GI tract; 25% are from abdominal sources (Daniels 2007b). Abdominal pain would be an obvious cause for concern as would a distended abdomen—this may be caused by collections of gas or fluid. These collections, in turn, are due to poor perfusion of the gut causing an 'ileus' or immobile intestine, which allow fluids to collect rather than be absorbed or transported. One interesting point in relation to the GI tract is that it will allow much of its own blood supply to be diverted to the other vital organs in hypovolaemic or shock states. If the shock state is not resolved quickly, the GI tract begins to suffer the consequences of poor perfusion.

Immediate response: the 'sepsis six'

It has been known for some time that delayed identification and response to serious illness like sepsis results in poorer care for the patient, which will impact on their morbidity and mortality (McQuillan et al. 1998). It is also well known that recognition and therapeutic support given early—or in the 'golden hours' of illness—provide the most benefit for patients (Rivers et al. 2001). There are elements of evidence-based care that all patients should receive, but which are subject to variability—sometimes they are not put into effect in the same way (Adair & Kernohan 2008). To uniformize care into best practice everywhere, these elements are sometimes grouped into 'care bundles', and there are two care bundles for sepsis: one for the first 6 h and one for the first 24 h (Daniels 2007c). Care bundles are number six in the Department of Health top ten high impact changes, aiming to improve patient care (NHS Modernisation Agency 2004), and implementation of the 6-h bundle has already been shown to improve survival (Gao et al. 2005). In order to have their positive impact on patient care *all* components of the bundle must be carried out.

Clinical link 8.2 (see Appendix for answers)

One way of defining different stages of sepsis is to call early sepsis 'hot' sepsis and later sepsis can be called 'cold' sepsis. Why do you think this is?

In order to improve implementation of these two sepsis care bundles in the UK, an educational programme entitled 'Survive Sepsis' (see 'Resources' section, below) has been initiated aimed at junior doctors and ward staff. It recognizes that initiation of early management steps outside of designated critical care areas is an essential part of providing the best care for patients who are ill with sepsis. Some elements of the 24-h bundle and the early goal-directed approaches do require specialist environments with specially trained staff and equipment. Nonetheless, there are six points of care that can be delivered quickly by ward nurses within the first hour of recognizing deterioration from sepsis and have a major impact on whether the patient survives or not (Survive Sepsis 2007). These are called the 'sepsis six' and are outlined below.

1) 100% oxygen: Metabolic demand for oxygen throughout the body is hugely increased by sepsis and it is essential to at least ensure the *supply* of oxygen is maximized; as discussed earlier in the chapter delivery uptake at cellular level may be impaired. The best way of delivering maximum oxygen will be via a non-rebreathe mask (Robson & Daniels 2008). The patient will also benefit from an arterial blood gas sample being taken, so a member of the medical team will need to be involved for this. High-flow oxygen will be drying to the patient's upper respiratory tract mucosa so a humidified delivery system should be offered. The patient should not be left alone at this stage—reassurance is particularly important and their observations may need repeating frequently—especially for those with advanced chronic obstructive pulmonary disease whose respiratory drive may be reduced because of the high oxygen concentration (Robson & Daniels 2008). It is also important for the mask to be kept on—if a patient is becoming hypoxic and confused they will often try and remove the mask.

2) Blood cultures: It is imperative to identify the infecting organism and blood cultures must be taken before administration of antibiotics. At least two sets should be drawn: one percutaneously, from a peripheral vein, and one from each intravascular device if in for more than 24 h. Consideration should be given to other samples, including sputum, urine, cerebrospinal fluid, and pus. Strict asepsis whilst obtaining the samples is vital (Kleinpell 2005). Contamination of blood results could be as high as 10% and leads to 'false positive' results suggesting infection where there is none (Department of Health 2007). Typically, results are ready within 48 h and all members of the team should be involved in actively seeking the results.

3) Intravenous antibiotics: The early administration of broad-spectrum antibiotics is associated with significant reductions in mortality (Survive Sepsis 2007). Prescriptions should be reviewed once positive blood cultures are obtained to ensure that the identified organism is being targeted in as specific a fashion as possible.

4) Intravenous fluids: Patients with sepsis often require early, rapid fluid resuscitation to optimize tissue perfusion and limit subsequent shock and multiorgan dysfunction—see also Chapter 7. Fluid resuscitation is replacing some of the circulating volume that has been 'lost' because of capillary leak and oedema. Crystalloid or colloid fluids may be used. It is suggested that fluid is administered in bolus volumes of 20 mL/kg (Survive Sepsis 2007); alternatively it may also simply be infused as a given volume immediately or as infusion of the fluid at a given millilitre per hour rate. Failure to respond to fluid therapy indicates a need for invasive monitoring and early goal-directed therapy. A successful response would be indicated by a rise in blood pressure and central venous pressure—where that is being measured—and these

improvements would be maintained without the need for further fluid. Patients who we must observe especially closely here are those with a history of heart failure,—left ventricular failure in particular—because of the ease with which they can become fluid overloaded and begin to develop pulmonary oedema. Patients in renal failure must also be cautiously monitored during fluid resuscitation.

5) Lactate and haemoglobin levels: Tissue perfusion is compromised in sepsis and when cells are in a hypoxic environment they respire anaerobically resulting in lactate production. Lactate therefore provides an indication of the adequacy of tissue perfusion. Normal values are 0.5–2 mmol/L (Higgins 2007) and values above 4 mmol/L are diagnostic of shock, irrespective of the blood pressure and specify that more invasive support such as the early goal-directed therapies be started (Robson & Daniels 2008). Lactate is important in the recognition of severe sepsis and carries some prognostic value. Serial measurements may demonstrate response or lack of response to resuscitation. If the fluid resuscitation is raising blood pressure and improving perfusion, the cells can begin to respire aerobically once again and stop producing the lactate. Lactate can be measured using a blood gas analyser or hand-held device. Failing this, a sample may be sent to the laboratory.

Haemoglobin is the molecule in red blood cells which transports oxygen, so a low haemoglobin will result in a reduced capacity of the blood to transport oxygen. Because in sepsis the metabolic demands for oxygen are increased, poor ability to transport and deliver oxygen can result in tissue and organ failure. The haemoglobin must be measured early and transfusion arranged if found to be less than 7 g/dL. Too much haemoglobin increases the blood's viscosity (thickness) and may actually impair perfusion as it is now too thick to pass easily through the tiny capillary vessels, many of which may be 'shut down' due to peripheral vasoconstriction.

6) Measure and improve urine output: This often requires insertion of a urinary catheter where not already in place; some patients are still able to urinate spontaneously but ideally urine output should be measured hourly to notice when it begins to fall. Urine output is a direct measure of blood flow to the kidneys and therefore an easily observable measure of cardiac output for most people. A low cardiac output will mean poor blood supply to all organs, not just the kidneys. Early recognition of a low urine output, and taking steps to improve it, will help to reduce the likelihood of acute renal failure (ARF) developing. ARF in combination with severe sepsis carries a mortality rate of between 50 and 70% (Survive Sepsis 2007).

A helpful, preliminary step may be to ensure that the patient has a patent intravenous access for the intravenous therapies mentioned above. It may be prudent to ensure two cannulae are in place so that antibiotics and fluid can run concurrently. Are the cannulae patent? Is it a large enough lumen to run fluid in quickly, if needed? Check for signs of phlebitis at any existing cannula site and the need to change it, as this can be a precursor to infection and even sepsis in itself. These checks for phlebitis can be extended to other catheters, central venous lines for instance, and a check on how long they have been in situ is also valuable. If a central line is in place and asymptomatic then ensuring that the ports are all patent and available for infusions, in keeping with local policy, is sensible.

The other essential point is that specialist help is available to commence any additional interventions—such as the early goal-directed therapies. Certainly, the critical care outreach team will be involved in the care of this patient and a referral to the HDU will need to have been made. This is because the continuing care for these patients does generally require specialist facilities. One area of support that can be provided for ward-based patients is blood glucose monitoring: in sepsis the cells' ability to take up the glucose they need is impaired and there is a resultant hyperglycaemia. It may be that an intravenous insulin regime needs to be initiated to control high glucose levels as good glycaemic control is associated with better survival levels (Dellinger et al. 2008).

Referral

It has been acknowledged that some acutely ill patients have received 'suboptimal' care in hospitals, leading to their condition worsening unnecessarily (McQuillan *et al.* 1998). Errors in the early management of these patients include failure of organization within the MDT, lack of knowledge on the part of some individual practitioners, failure to appreciate the clinical urgency of the situation, lack of supervision, and failure to seek senior advice (McQuillan *et al.* 1998). Since that time a series of government documents have extolled the need for track and trigger systems to be in place for patients who are deteriorating in hospitals (Audit Commission 1999; Department of Health 2000, 2005). These are addressed in Chapter 11. The same documents articulated the need for critical care outreach services so that critical care be understood as a service rather than a place, such as an HDU (Department of Health 2000). These issues are addressed in Chapter 12. Essentially, there should be a means of identifying patients who are beginning to deteriorate and to refer them on to designated teams of practitioners who can help to supervise their care, the patient at risk team (PART) and medical emergency team (MET) are examples.

There have been two more recent publications that address the concerns that still remain about the safety of care in some instances (National Patient Safety Agency 2007), which provide guidelines for the identification of patients who are deteriorating (or at risk of doing so) and the responses that ought now to be in place for them (NICE 2007). Both of these seminal documents state that often patient deterioration can be preceded by hours or even days of physiological changes that go unrecognized. This is especially likely with the patient who is developing sepsis because the signs and symptoms of *early* sepsis are so generic and non-specific and there is concern, therefore, that the presentation of sepsis is attributed to other conditions (Poeze *et al.* 2004). Nonetheless, in the same way that nurses have contributed to the dramatic fall in mortality from acute myocardial infarction—from 30% in the 1960s to 8% nowadays (Vincent *et al.* 2002), nurses now have a role in the management of sepsis, especially in its early recognition (Robson 2004; Dawson 2002). Nurses must be willing to initiate an escalation of concern and therapeutic support for patients suspected of developing sepsis and to be proactive in their care provision, particularly for critically unwell patients such as those with sepsis (Department of Health 2001).

There are issues, however, involved in what is seemingly a simple process of referral. Studies to date in the utilization of care bundles and early recognition of sepsis outside of critical care, for instance, have shown that there is a need for improvement (Simmonds *et al.* 2008). Some of the obstacles recorded to successful referral have been vague handover of information or incomplete recordings of the observation charts (Carter 2007). Moreover, the recording of basic observations such as respiratory rate and fluid balance are known to be inconsistent. One study identified 55% of patients as not having had their respiratory rate done for 8 h and 22% having incomplete fluid balance charts (Chellel *et al.* 2002). Of particular concern here is that these were patients who were deemed to require closer support and observation than 'typical' ward patients (Chellel *et al.* 2002). The cause for these omissions was considered to be inadequate staffing and workload, but it is known that basic physiological observations are delegated to healthcare assistants in many instances and that a reliance on automated machinery to take blood pressures, for example, is commonplace (Wheatley 2006). This removes us as nurses from core physical assessment findings that we would be exposed to if we were doing them—noticing that a pulse was weak by feeling it rather than reading it from a display or feeling that an arm was very cool whilst taking a blood pressure, for example. As we meet more patients being cared for on wards that are especially unwell or prone to deterioration, the role of our physical assessment abilities is vital and these skills are needed by all nurses (West 2006), particularly to enable proactive and responsive care for these patients (Department of Health 2001).

These issues cannot be viewed in too simplistic a manner, however. Reports from ward nurses looking after critically ill patients identify that there are not only educational issues that still need to be met (Cutler 2002), but that assertiveness in professional relationships appears to be a key skill—and one that often comes with experience—in terms of ensuring that a patient is reviewed (Cox *et al.* 2006). Early feedback from outreach nurses suggested that the decisions about whether to refer a patient on for help or not were in need of investigation (McArthur-Rouse 2001) and more recently the concerns about calling the medical team inappropriately has been voiced, as well as a need for emotional support in terms of dealing with unstable patients in a ward setting and dealing with inter-professional issues (Cox *et al.* 2006).

Counselling and support

A critical illness, in its entirety, can be viewed as a continuum (Rattray & Crocker 2007) and ward nurses are in a position to be with the patient at the start and the end of their stay in hospital. Care needs for those patients who have survived sepsis need further consideration.

Typically, patients with severe sepsis will be cared for in an ITU. For many patients and their families, leaving the perceived security of a critical care unit to anywhere else in the hospital can be anxiety provoking (Streater *et al.* 2001). Caring for patients after a stay in ITU is addressed specifically in Chapter 15, but we should think about the counselling and support required by patients having survived a septic episode as it is a component of the Surviving Sepsis Campaign. Patients and their loved ones begin to try and make sense of what will have been a near-death experience in what has been described as a 'quest for meaning' (Storli *et al.* 2008): nurses have a role in helping to facilitate this quest.

It is well recognized that patients experience a range of debilitating effects after a critical illness (Cuthbertson *et al.* 2005) and follow-up afterwards is now a recognized component of critical care; the Department of Health in a review of critical care services (Department of Health 2000) recommended the provision of dedicated follow-up services and, in a subsequent report (Department of Health 2005), stipulated that hospitals should develop patient-centred rehabilitation services to optimize the recovery of patients discharged from critical care units. Furthermore, integration with primary care services after patients are discharged from hospital needs to be developed (Department of Health 2005). NICE guidelines are being compiled presently to make recommendations for good practice in these areas of care (NICE 2008) and a model along the lines of the rehabilitation programme provided for cardiac patients has been proposed (Rattray & Crocker 2007).

Much of the data about the need for follow up after surviving a critical illness is generic to intensive care rather than sepsis *per se*. However, extrapolation from the numbers of all intensive care admissions that are due to sepsis, 27% (Harrison *et al.* 2006), suggests that these data does apply very pointedly to the experience of patients who have survived sepsis.

Problems encountered after a serious illness requiring intensive care, such as sepsis, include physical, psychological, emotional, and cognitive dysfunction (Rattray & Crocker 2007). Patients report profound disorientation and disruption to their factual memory (Magerey & McCutcheon 2005), which exhibits a strong link to post-traumatic stress disorder (PTSD) (Ringdal *et al.* 2006). As PTSD has, potentially, a long-term effect on the patient—quite possibly over several years—caring strategies in the post-ITU stage are now being emphasized to try and prevent or ameliorate some of this distress (Corrigan *et al.* 2007). Strahan & Brown (2005) have compiled some practical recommendations for care for patients at this phase of their recovery:

♦ Nursing interventions should aim at maximizing patient control and help towards reducing anxiety levels—this will entail inclusion of the patient in possible choices available for medical or nursing care and explanations of all that is being done.

- Patients should be encouraged to re-adopt their 'normal' sleep pattern.
- Education regarding rehabilitation and diet is essential—physiotherapy and dietician input is important here.
- Families should be more involved in care and the rehabilitation process.
- Opportunity should be offered to discuss memories and nightmares, both real and hallucinatory. This is potentially time consuming for nurses on a busy ward but needs to be accommodated—it may also be that specially trained personnel such as hospital counsellors are best suited to this.

The need for patient information, explanation, and reassurance is real. One significant difference between critical care environments and wards is the staffing ratio, and patients and relatives should be assured that although staff may not be constantly at the bedside, they are available and approachable (adapted from Strahan & Brown et al. 2005: 169).

Patients' own accounts tell us that demonstrations of caring and attempts to allay worries and fears through explanation and reassurance were the most valued nursing skill (Hofhuis et al. 2008).The importance of reassuring behaviours during a time of great vulnerability is reiterated when patients revisit their experiences of critical illness. One study has recently compared patients' recall after 3 and 12 months and found that after 12 months highlights of the entire trajectory of their illness were of security and caring from staff (Lof et al. 2008).

However, many patients—up to 40% (Crocker 2003)—will experience a degree of amnesia in relation to their illness, which is felt as a loss of control over their experience and an obstacle to re-orientating to normal life (Combe 2005). Various approaches have been presented in an attempt to help with re-orientation, including diaries of the period of critical illness, although doing this retrospectively was found to be very time-consuming (Combe 2005). Certainly, a multidisciplinary approach for support is needed. The injurious effects of sepsis on the musculoskeletal system require physiotherapy expertise to regain function (Crocker 2003) and as many of the issues that patients will face at home cannot be assessed in hospital, occupational therapy input is vital in terms of successful follow-up care after hospital discharge (Crocker 2003).

This multidisciplinary approach is an important overview to keep when patients return to the ward. Relevant referrals are essential; perhaps to the occupational therapy department, the chaplaincy service, or other forms of spiritual support. It is possible that the mental health team might be an appropriate resource or a hospital counsellor would be able to offer practical input for the patient or family members. These referrals are within the remit of nurses to consider and put forward as practical, helpful options. As they can entail the addressing of sensitive issues, it is advisable to broach matters privately with the patient first. Some resources for patients or relatives that can be particularly meaningful are those that share the experiences of other patients, one online example being Dipex.org (see Resources Section, below); there may be support groups active locally, too.

It is also appreciated that the turmoil that relatives experience during a family member's critical illness can leave them very drained, physically and psychologically (Johansson et al. 2004). It is also highly likely that the care of the patient at home will involve family members, and to this end it may be appropriate to engage with social services to offer them support. As before, this referral needs to be done after consultation with the family members themselves. Early research has concluded that the relatives need support and counselling before they are discharged home as well as during recovery at home (Johansson et al. 2004). An important 'reality check' for relatives to be aware of is that psycho-social recovery from this kind of extreme illness often lags behind a recovery of physical functioning (Gardner & Sibthorpe 2002). This point is now becoming the focus of intensive care follow up and calls for research to be directed at supporting emotional outcome for patients are now being made (Rattray & Hull 2008).

It is known too, that a personal and financial burden can exist for family carers and that often they do not access health service input once home (Chaboyer 2006). The implications are that relatives need to be prepared and even encouraged to request support at home (Johnson *et al.* 2001), especially given the potentially multifaceted needs of a patient who has experienced a complex illness such as sepsis. The community nursing team will benefit from a very thorough handover of the history of the patient's stay in hospital and of any referrals that have been put in place.

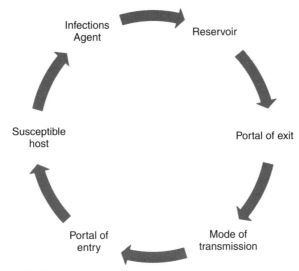

Figure 8.4 The chain of infection.

Sepsis prevention: infection control

The single most important element in preventing sepsis is infection prevention and control practice. Critically ill patients are at a pronounced risk of developing infection—17% of methicillin-resistant *Staphylococcus aureus* (MRSA) bacteraemias are found in patients who are already critically ill (Department of Health 2006 a). The overarching concept used to understand the spread of infection—and therefore how to combat it—is the 'chain of infection' (Figure 8.4).

Infectious agents are typically bacteria, but may also be viruses or fungi or parasites. The reservoir refers to the source of the infective agent—typically other people, but can also be animals, plants, food, water, dust, and dirt or faeces. The portal of exit is the initial outlet into the 'outside world'. There are multiple modes of transmission for infection, but they may be summarized as being direct, indirect, or airborne (Kozier, *et al.* 2008). Direct transmission is the immediate communication of the infective cause from one peron to another, for example coughing or touching. Indirect transmission involves an intermediary to transfer the infective agent, either a 'vehicle' or a 'vector'. A vehicle can be any object that carries the infective agent, so food, bedrails, soiled gloves or contaminated blood products used for transfusion all count as vehicles. The list is almost inexhaustible. A vector is an animal or insect that transmits the infection. Airborne transmission entails droplets of contaminated matter being sprayed into the environment by the infected person through coughing, sneezing, laughing, or talking, for example. It is also possible for dust laden with the spores of the infective agent to become airborne (Kozier *et al.* 2008). If any of the links in the chain are broken, then infection is not transmitted.

Clinical link 8.3 (see Appendix for answers)

List what you consider constitute the infection control aspects for each of the six links in the chain of infection.

Every year at least 300,000 patients in this country develop a healthcare acquired infection (HCAI); it is estimated that around one in ten patients pick up an infection during their stay in a UK hospital. A HCAI is any infection that has been acquired as a result of a patient's contact with the health service—it also applies to us as healthcare workers if we acquire an infection (Department of Health 2008). These infections can often be difficult to treat and they can complicate illnesses, cause distress to patients and their family, and in some cases may even be fatal (HCAI Research Network 2008). If a patient develops a HCAI, besides complicating their illness it may extend their stay in hospital, thereby leading to a loss of earnings for them and increased costs to the health service; a £1 billion per year cost is the current projection (National Patient Safety Agency 2008).

On average, patients with an HCAI have been found to be around seven times more likely to die in hospital than uninfected patients. It is estimated that as many as 5,000 patients die each year in the UK as a direct result of HCAI and it is one of the factors in another 15,000 deaths (HCAI Research Network 2008). It is estimated that up to 30% of these deaths are avoidable (National Audit Office 2004), and to counteract these disturbing trends a number of initiatives have been put in place that aim to address common causes of HCAI. Several high impact interventions (HII) have been identified to promote best practice for all patients who require common interventions (Department of Health 2007a). There is now a Code of Practice for Prevention and Control of Healthcare Associated infections (Department of Health 2008) that all individual practitioners and organizations are legally expected to adhere to. A number of risk elements have been recognized as being of central importance in terms of containing infection (Department of Health 2006b):

+ hand washing
+ use of personal protective equipment
+ aseptic technique
+ safe disposal of sharps.

These 'universal precautions' form the foundation of providing 'clean, safe, care' (Department of Health 2007a) and relate particularly to the most basic level of infection control practice. Hand washing is the single most effective measure to reduce HCAI (Pittet et al. 2006); it is also cheap and easy to perform when there is easy access to alcohol-based hand rub (Sax et al. 2007). As healthcare staff are in constant bedside contact with patients, nurses have the greatest potential to spread infection (National Patient Safety Agency 2008). It is at the point of care delivery—the patient's immediate environment wherein nurse-to-patient contact occurs—that good hand hygiene is crucial (National Patient Safety Agency 2008). To clearly identify the times at which we must clean our hands the World Health Organization has promoted the 'five moments' for hand hygiene (World Health Organization 2008), which are:

+ before patient contact—to protect patients from germs that we can all carry on our hands
+ before an aseptic task—to prevent micro-organisms, including the patient's own, from entering sterile tissues and spaces of their body
+ after body fluid exposure risk—to protect *yourself* from micro-organisms from the patient
+ after patient contact—to prevent the spread of patient's germs to the environment or to yourself

◆ after contact with patient surroundings—to prevent the spread of germs to the environment or to yourself.

Personal protective equipment (PPE) forms part of the universal precautions to prevent the spread of infection (Kozier *et al.* 2008):

◆ Gloves protect the nurse's hands from whatever may come into contact with them and reduce the transmission of harmful micro-organisms between the patient and the nurse and the environment.

◆ Aprons and gowns are disposable single-use items that help maintain uniform cleanliness. Sterile gowns may be used for more involved nursing activity such as changing extensive dressings; these gowns can then be re-sterilized and re-used.

◆ Eye wear—either splash guard masks or protective goggles to protect against droplet transmission and also 'splattering' of bodily fluids that could be contaminated.

◆ Face masks—for nursing those patients infected with germs that have an airborne route of transmission. Examples here would be tuberculosis, severe acute respiratory syndrome, and pandemic flu.

The choice and use of PPE is dependent on the assessment of the risk of transmission of micro-organisms to the patient or nurse and the risk of contamination of the nurse's clothing and skin by patients' body fluids (Pratt *et al.* 2007).

Aseptic technique is required in all clinical procedures where the patient is exposed to the potential introduction of micro-organisms into their sterile tissue. Aseptic technique is especially important for patients who are immune compromised but also for all patients with breaks in the integrity of their physical barriers to infection. There have been difficulties in assuring aseptic technique, partly because hygiene procedures have been highly variable across the NHS (Department of Health 2007b). To address this concern the use of aseptic non-touch technique (ANTT) is now being championed as the approach of choice across the NHS (ANTT™ 2008). ANTT is a Department of Health endorsed best practice aseptic technique developed on an evidence-based framework, and is now being advocated across the NHS and abroad (ANTT™ 2008). It provides an effective and standardized method for maintaining asepsis that has been seen to help cut infection dramatically (Department of Health 2007b).

One approach to infection control that is beyond the universal precautions is the notion of isolation. By isolating a vulnerable patient they can be better protected from infection than they would be when exposed to an environment with many other people (Smith *et al.* 2008). The ability to do this is dependent on the availability of single rooms. Needless to say, the psychosocial needs of the patients then become paramount as they are not only literally isolated from others, but also potentially stigmatized by the need for them to be isolated. The need for isolation itself can be either because they have a virulent infection that requires everyone else to be protected from (barrier nursing) or because they need extra protection from infective agents (reverse barrier nursing).

Using a care bundle approach, seven areas of care provision have been highlighted as being key areas for reducing HCAIs:

◆ central venous catheter care

◆ peripheral intravenous cannula care

◆ renal dialysis catheter care

◆ preventing surgical site infections

◆ care bundle for ventilated patients (or those with tracheostomies)

- urinary catheter care
- reducing the risk from *Clostridium difficile*.

Take a moment to consider the relevance of the above seven areas for patients at risk of sepsis. The dialysed and mechanically ventilated patients are special groups of patients, but general ward staff do meet the other situations frequently—they are areas that infection control practice ought to be guided by the HII care bundles. By using the care bundle approach nursing practice can combine the best evidence for a procedure with a measuring tool for its implementation for all patients and strategies to improve the process through which patients receive this care (Department of Health 2007c).

Urinary catheters are the most common source of an HCAI (Doughty & Lister 2008), amounting to 19.6% of all hospital acquired infections (Department of Health 2007d). One point of consideration, which applies to all invasive lines, is to assess its need; does one need to be inserted or, if already *in situ*, is it still needed or can it be removed? The vulnerable points, in terms of infection control, are the joints between the catheter components and the contact between the catheter and the patient. Poor technique whilst obtaining urine specimens or changing/emptying the collection bag are also common means for cross-infection (Doughty & Lister 2008). Strict asepsis must be employed whilst inserting the catheter—60% of healthcare acquired UTI are associated with catheter insertion (Department of Health 2007d), and the same precautions used whilst sampling from the catheter are needed.

Central venous catheters, or 'central lines' are seen frequently in critically ill patients (Theaker 2005) and have a strong association with bloodstream infections—over 40% of blood-borne infections in England are associated with a central line (Department of Health 2007d). Besides the need for universal precautions whilst interacting with patients' central lines, vigilance with security, cleanliness, and adherence to local policies must be observed (Department of Health 2007e).

Another commonly found invasive technique is the use of peripheral cannulae. Although vital in many therapies, these cannulae can introduce either the patient's own skin flora or contaminants from the injection port into the bloodstream (Department of Health 2007f). As with central lines, peripheral cannula should be observed at least daily for signs of inflammation and the dressing over the cannula must be transparent to allow this (Department of Health 2007f).

The high incidence of infections acquired through invasive equipment is followed by those involving surgical wounds—national studies have shown that over 14% of all HCAIs are from wound sites (Department of Health 2007g). The care bundle employed for wound care targets pre- and peri-operative elements, with the maintenance of a temperature above 36 C and blood sugars below 11 mmol/L provided as evidence-based support for wound healing. The decolonization of existing MRSA forms the foundation of pre-operative care. MRSA has been acknowledged as a primary agent in HCAI and, particularly, bacteraemia (Department of Health 2007h); guidelines for its control and prevention are now agreed across the UK (Coia *et al.* 2006).

Infection control practice is clearly evidence based and as the evidence base accumulates so best practice is being disseminated. Responsibility for adhering to these ways of working to protect patients remains with each of us individually. In many instances the infection control practices involve simple manoeuvres, yet are ones that have profound effects if they are forgotten or poorly practiced. This is also true of the simple practices of taking basic physiological observations and being alert to the possible signs of a patient deteriorating, as with those in our care that may be developing early sepsis.

Review of assessment practice

Below is a list of the main factors to consider in assessing a patient with sepsis or suspected sepsis. You can use this as a revision of the points discussed throughout the chapter and to prepare for

Clinical link 8.4 (see Appendix for answers)

John Earle-Grey is 78 years old and weighs 90 kg. He was admitted to hospital with abdominal pain, which was found to be due to a duodenal ulcer and treated with a laparotomy for a repair of the ulcer. He is now day 5 post operative and has been on your ward since this morning. He is receiving 1 L of 0.9% sodium chloride (normal saline) over 6 h via peripheral cannula, but has no appetite. He reports feeling 'queasy' and his temperature is 37.5 C. His urine output is being measured by his urinary catheter and over the past 4 h has only been 40 mL per hour. The past three blood pressure (BP) recordings and heart rate taken by the HCA are:

♦ BP = 120/80, heart rate = 85 bpm at 08.00 am, respiratory rate 18, temperature 37.0°

♦ BP = 110/66, heart rate = 98 bpm at 12.30 pm, respiratory rate 22, temperature 38.0°

♦ BP = 110/ 56, heart rate = 120 bpm at 14.30 pm, respiratory rate 24, temperature 38.5°

The last set of results have worried the healthcare assistant and you have been asked to review him as you start your shift.

♦ Which risk factors for developing sepsis does John have?

♦ What suggests to you that John is possibly developing sepsis? How advanced is this development?

♦ What possible sources for the infective agent might there be that are identified in the scenario?

♦ What other possible causes of infection might you follow up on?

♦ Which of John's recent laboratory results will the surgical team be particularly interested in, in relation to your findings?

♦ What would your course of action be in response to your findings for John?

the skills assessment. The assumption here is that you have only a sphygmomanometer and watch as equipment, even though you may well have access to other tools such as pulse oximetry, and are therefore employing a 'look, listen, and feel' approach to your assessment.

♦ Risk factors
  • Is the patient very elderly?
  • Do they have an already compromised immune system from taking immune suppressant drugs for auto-immune disorders or chemotherapy for cancer?
  • Do they have addictions to drugs or alcohol?
  • Do they have deep tissue wounds, for example from burns or trauma, or have had invasive surgery?
  • Do they have indwelling intravenous lines or catheters?

♦ Patient history
  • Do they have an identified infection (or have they had a recent infection)?
  • Do they have a past medical history that includes sepsis?

♦ Patient complaining of:
  • coughing phlegm, which is new for them
  • discomfort passing urine, or discoloured, malodorous urine

- dizziness
- vague responses when interacted with
- feeling unwell—non-specific or 'fluey' symptoms'

♦ Skin, hot to touch due to:
- vasodilatation carrying blood (and therefore) metabolic heat to peripheries
- viral/bacterial pathogens increasing metabolic/inflammatory response from cells
- hypothalamus 're-setting' the internal thermostat

♦ Blood pressure, hypotensive due to:
- vasodilatation—this is seen in the diastolic blood pressure
- myocardial depressant effect of sepsis—this is seen in the systolic blood pressure

♦ Pulse
- Fast—tachycardic
- In early sepsis this will feel to be a 'bounding' pulse
- Compensation for relative hypovolaemia/distributive shock
- In later or decompensated sepsis and shock the pulse will be felt to be thready (due to hypovolaemia)
- Difficult to find due to oedema

♦ Pallor:
- flushed (more noticeable with Caucasians) due to vasodilatation—more blood at periphery

or
- mottled, due to patchy maldisribution of blood and poorly perfused capillary beds

or
- pale, due to poor perfusion globally secondary to low cardiac output/oxygen delivery

also
- impeded oxygen delivery due to oedema
- poor capillary refill

♦ Brain

Acutely altered/low GCS due to:
- hypoperfusion
- endotoxin

Pupils—constricted—shock state.
Dull, responses obtunded—shock state

♦ Kidneys
- oliguric (poor urine output): less than 0.5 mL/kg/h

♦ Abdomen
- Possibly distended, hard, uncomfortable/painful
- Bowel sounds possibly absent due to ischaemia, poor GI tract perfusion, 'auto transfusion' of gut to other vital organs
- Ileus—poor motility secondary to hypoperfusion.

End of chapter assessment

The following assessment will enable you to evaluate your theoretical knowledge of sepsis and its management as well as your ability to apply this theory to clinical practice.

Knowledge assessment

With the support of your mentor/supervisor from practice, work through the following prompts to explore your knowledge level about sepsis and its management.

+ Demonstrate an understanding of the difference between SIRS, sepsis, severe sepsis, and septic shock.
+ Broadly discuss the role of the inflammatory reaction and sepsis.
+ Be able to identify common origins of sepsis, including hospital acquired.
+ Explain the broad differences in patient presentation between 'early' and 'late' sepsis.
+ Explain the rationale behind lactate readings.
+ Be aware of essential management responses of the 'sepsis six' and their underpinning rationale.
+ Discuss the notion of 'care bundles'.
+ Discuss the nurse's role with microbiology samples for septic patients.
+ Describe the clinical syndrome DIC and why it is related to septicaemia.
+ Understand the local policy for taking blood cultures.
+ Identify local, national, and international strategies to address sepsis.
+ Be aware of support resources available to relatives.
+ Be aware of support resources and research available to nurses.

Skills assessment

Under the guidance of your mentor/supervisor, undertake a full assessment of a patient for signs and symptoms of sepsis followed by appropriate interventions for any significant abnormality. Your mentor/supervisor will be able to assess your ability and provide feedback based on the following skills:

+ Conducts a full patient history with a systems review considering key points that are relevant for a patient with sepsis or suspected sepsis.
+ Demonstrates a comprehensive physical assessment and explain the physiological underpinnings normal/abnormal findings from the respiratory, cardiovascular, renal, GI, skin, and neurological systems.
+ Findings are related to the data already charted and trends in potential deterioration or compensation identified.
+ The likely source and course of sepsis for the patient are discussed.
+ Microbiological and biochemical laboratory results are related to the patient's condition.
+ Intravenous access and all invasive lines are checked for date and necessity. Line sites are assessed for signs of inflammation or infection.
+ Demonstrates an ability to follow infection control guidelines while undertaking intravenous therapy, including the management of the intravenous access and intravenous fluid.
+ Any potentially diagnostic samples are taken and documented.

- Any outstanding and relevant laboratory results are pursued and relevant personnel informed.
- Any vulnerability to further infection is identified in terms of threats of infection and the patient's own physiological reserve.
- If an early warning observations chart is in use, the patient is scored.
- Any indication from the observations gathered that member of the MDT or the MET/PART/ Outreach teams need to be informed is acted upon. Shift leader for the ward is also notified.
- Ensures an estimation of when these personnel are able to review the patient is provided and follow this up if necessary.
- Documents all interventions and referrals, including times as per local policy.
- Care for that shift is prioritized on the basis of the clinical picture gathered.
- All universal precautions are adhered to whilst clinically interacting with the patient.

Resources

The international homepage for the Surviving Sepsis Campaign. http://www.survivingsepsis.org/.

UK-based resource for healthcare professionals and the general public about sepsis. The official training programme of the Surviving Sepsis Campaign. http://www.survivesepsis.org

The DiPEX project is supported by the NHS and seeks to describe the patient experience using semi-structured interviews. The experiences of people who have experienced critical illness are available on the site. The site has been well evaluated recently by broadsheet newspapers as a favourite, trusted site for patients. http://www.dipex.com/DesktopDefault.aspx

Intensive Care After Care Network—for professionals and lay people alike. Requires a simple, free, registration. http://www.i-canuk.com/default.aspx.

Homepage of the NHS 'clean, safe care programme'; providing tools and information to help reduce HAIs. http://www.clean-safe-care.nhs.uk. Incorporating the NHS 'saving lives' campaign. You can access the high impact intervention guidance from: http://www.clean-safe-care.nhs.uk/public/default.aspx?level=2 &load=Tools&NodeID=181.

Homepage of the National resource for infection Control. NRIC is a project developed by healthcare professionals, aimed at being a single-access point to existing resources within infection control for both Infection Control and all other healthcare staff. http://www.nric.org.uk.

Infection Prevention Society, incorporating the Infection Control Nurses Association website: UK based. http://www.ips.uk.net.

Homepage of the Hospital infection Society. The HIS exists to foster the advancement of knowledge and education of all those who have an interest in the important field of hospital infection. http://www.his.org.uk.

Homepage of the National Patient Safety Agency. The NPSA leads and contributes to improved, safe patient care by informing, supporting, and influencing the health sector. http://www.npsa.nhs.uk.

Homepage of Aseptic Non Touch Technique (ANTTTM). Resources and education on ANTT. http://www.antt.co.uk/Site/Welcome.html.

References

Actor, J.K. (2007) *Elsevier's Integrated Immunology*. Mosby Elsevier, Philadelphia.

Adair, K. and Kernohan, A. (2008) Care bundles. *Student. BMJ* **1**(51), 17. Available at: http://student.bmj.com/issues/08/02/editorials/051.php (accessed 01.10.2008).

Ahern, J. and Philpott, P. (2002) Assessing acutely ill patients on general wards. *Nurs. Stand.* **16**(47), 47–54.

Alberti, C. and Brun-Buisson C. (2003) Epidemiology of infection and sepsis: A review. *Adv. Sepsis.* **3**(2), 45–55.

Angus, D.C., Linde-Zwirble, W.T., Lidicker, J. *et al.* (2001) Epidemiology of severe sepsis in the United States: analysis of incidence, outcome and association of costs of care. *Crit. Care Med.* **29**(7), 1303–10.

ANTT™ (2008) What is ANTT? (Online) Available at: http://www.antt.co.uk/Site/What_is_ANTT.html (accessed 22.10.2008).

Audit Commission (1999) *Critical to Success. The Place of Efficient and Effective Critical Care Services Within the Acute Hospital.* Audit Commission, London.

Barnett, M.I. and Cosslett, A.G. (1998) Endotoxin—a clinical challenge. *Br. J. Int. Care May/June*, 78–87.

Blann, A. (2006) *Routine Blood Results Explained.* M&K Update, Keswick.

Bridges, E.J. and Dukes, S. (2005) Cardiovascular aspects of septic shock. Pathophysiology, monitoring and treatment. *Crit. Care Nurse.* **25**(2), 14–40.

Carter, C. (2007) Implementing the severe sepsis care bundles outside the ICU by outreach. *Nurs. Crit. Care.* **12**(5), 225–30.

Chaboyer, W. (2006) Intensive care and beyond: Improving transitional experiences for critically ill patients and their families. *Int. Crit. Care Nurs.* **22**(4), 187–93.

Chapel, H., Haeney, M., Misbah, S., and Snowden, N. (2006) *Essentials of Clinical Immunology.* 5th edn. Blackwell, Oxford.

Chellel, A., Fraser, J., and Fender, V. (2002) Nursing observations on ward patients at risk of critical illness. *Nurs.* Times **99**(46), 36–9.

Cohen, J. (2007) Better Teaching About Sepsis: Why? Who? When? What? (online) Available at: http://www.sepsisforum.org/Paris/S38%20COHEN%20-%20Better%20Teaching.pdf (accessed: 05.09.2008).

Coia, J.E., Duckworth, G.J., Edwards, D.I. et al. (2006) for the Joint Working Party of the British Antimicrobial Chemotherapy, Hospital Infection Society and the Infection Control Nurses' Association. Guidelines for the control and prevention of meticillin resistant Staphylococcus aureus (MRSA) in hospital facilities. *J. Hosp. Inf.* **63**(S), S1–44. (online) Available at: http://www.his.org.uk/_db/_documents/MRSA_Guidelines_PDF.pdf (accessed 20.10.2008).

Combe, D. (2005) The use of patient diaries in an intensive care unit. *Nurs. Crit. Care.* **10**(1), 31–4.

Corrigan, I., Samuelson, K.A.M., Fridlund, B *et al.* (2007) The meaning of posttraumatic stress—reactions following critical illness or injury and intensive care treatment. *Int. Crit. Care Nurs.* **23**(4), 206–15.

Cox, H., James, J., and Hunt, J. (2006) The experience of trained nurses caring for critically ill patients in a general ward setting. *Int. Crit. Care Nurs.* **22**(5), 283–93.

Crocker, C. (2003) A multidisciplinary follow-up clinic after patients' discharge from ITU. *Br. J. Nurs.* **12**(15), 910–14.

Cuthbertson, B., Scott, J., Strachen, M. *et al.* (2005) Quality of life before and after intensive care. *Anaesthesia.* **60**(4), 332–9.

Cutler, L.R. (2002) From ward-based critical care to educational curriculum 1: A literature review. *Int Crit. Care Nurs.* **18**(3), 162–70.

Daniels, R. (2007) Incidence, mortality and economic burden of sepsis. (online) Available at: http://www.library.nhs.uk/Emergency/ViewResource.aspx?resID=269230&tabID=290 (accessed 12.08.2008).

Daniels, R. (2007a) Pathophysiology of sepsis. (online) Available at: http://www.library.nhs.uk/Emergency/ViewResource.aspx?resID=269238&tabID=290 (accessed 12.08.2008).

Daniels, R. (2007b) Defining sepsis, severe sepsis and septic shock. (online) Available at: http://www.library.nhs.uk/Emergency/ViewResource.aspx?resID=269236&tabID=290 (accessed 12.08.2008).

Daniels, R. (2007c) Severe sepsis care bundles. (online) Available at: http://www.library.nhs.uk/Emergency/ViewResource.aspx?resID=269247&tabID=290 (accessed 12.08.2008).

Darovic, G.O. (2002) Pulmonary artery pressure monitoring. In: Darovic, G.O. *Haemodynamic Monitoring. Invasive and Non-invasive Clinical Application.* Saunders, Philadelphia.

Dawson, D. (2002) Sepsis recognition—a greater role for nursing? *Int. Crit. Care Nurs.* **18**(3), 135–7.

Dellinger, R.P., Carlet, J.M., Mansur, H. *et al.* (2004) Surviving Sepsis Campaign guidelines for management of severe sepsis and septic shock. *Int. Care Med.* **30**, 536–55.

Dellinger, R.P, Levy, M.M., Carlet, J.M. *et al.* (2008) Surviving sepsis campaign: International guidelines for management of severe sepsis and septic shock: 2008. *Crit. Care Med.* **36**(1), 296–327.

Delves, P.J. and Roitt, I.M. (2000) Advances in immunology: The immune system (first of two parts). *N. Engl. J. Med.* **343**(1), 37–49.

Department of Health (2000) *Comprehensive Critical Care. A Review of Adult Critical Care Services.* Department of Health, London.

Department of Health (2001) *The Nursing Contribution to the Provision of Comprehensive Critical care for Adults. A Strategic Programme of Action.* Department of Health, London.

Department of Health (2005) *Quality Critical Care. Beyond 'Comprehensive Critical Care': A Report by the Stakeholder Forum.* Department of Health, London.

Department of Health (2006) *Essential Steps to Clean, Safe Care. Urinary catheter care.* Department of Health, London.

Department of Health (2006a) *Infection Prevention and Control in Adult Critical Care. Reducing the Risk of Infection through Best Practice.* Department of Health, London.

Department of Health (2006b) *Essential Steps to Clean, Safe Care. Preventing the Spread of Infection.* Department of Health, London.

Department of Health (2007) *Taking Blood Cultures. A Summary of Best Practice.* Department of Health, London.

Department of Health (2007a) *Saving Lives: Reducing Infection, Delivering Clean and Safe Care.* Department of Health, London.

Department of Health (2007b) Using High Impact Interventions. Department of Health, London. (online) Available at: http://www.dh.gov.uk/en/Aboutus/MinistersandDepartmentLeaders/ChiefMedicalOfficer/AboutTheChiefMedicalOfficerCMO/CMOAtLarge/DH_4102099 (accessed 22.10.2008).

Department of Health (2007c) *Using High Impact Interventions.* Department of Health, London.

Department of Health (2007d) *Saving Lives: Reducing Infection, Delivering Clean and Safe Care. High Impact Intervention No 6. Urinary Catheter Care Bundle.* Department of Health, London.

Department of Health (2007e) *Saving Lives: Reducing Infection, Delivering Clean and Safe Care. High Impact Intervention No 1. Central Venous Catheter Care Bundle.* Department of Health, London.

Department of Health (2007f) *Saving Lives: Reducing Infection, Delivering Clean and Safe Care. High Impact Intervention No 2. Peripheral Intravenous Cannula Care Bundle.* Department of Health, London.

Department of Health (2007g) *Saving Lives: Reducing Infection, Delivering Clean and Safe Care. High Impact Intervention No 4. Care Bundle to Prevent Surgical Site Infection.* Department of Health, London.

Department of Health (2007h) *Essential Steps to Clean, Safe Care. Working Together to Reduce Healthcare Acquired Infection (HCAI)(Including Meticillin Resistant Staphylococcus aureus (MRSA)). A Strategy for Local Health Economies.* Department of Health, London.

Department of Health (2008) *The Health Care Act 2006: Code of Practice for the Prevention and Control of Healthcare Acquired Infections.* Department of Health, London.

Dolan, S. (2003) Severe sepsis—a major challenge for critical care. *Int. Crit. Care Nurs.* **19**, 63–7.

Doughty, L. and Lister, S. (2008) *The Royal Marsden Hospital Manual of Clinical nursing Procedures.* Student edition. 7th edn. Wiley-Blackwell, Chichester.

Franklin, C. and Darovic, G.O. (2002) Monitoring the patient in shock. In: Darovic, G.O. *Haemodynamic Monitoring. Invasive and Non-invasive Clinical Application.* Saunders, Philadelphia.

Galley, J. and O'Riordan, B. (2003) *Guidance for Nurse Staffing in Critical Care.* Royal College of Nurses, London.

Gao, F., Melody,T., Daniels, D.F. et al. (2005) The impact of compliance with 6-hour and 24-hour sepsis bundles on hospital mortality in patients with severe sepsis: A prospective observational study. *Crit. Care.* **9**(60), R764–70. (online) Available at: http://ccforum.com/content/9/6/R764 (accessed 02.10.2008).

Gardner, A. and Sibthorpe, B. (2002) When will he get back to normal? Survival and functional status after intensive care therapy. *Int. Crit. Care Nurs.* **18**(3), 138–45.

Gordon, L. (1999) The sepsis continuum from systemic inflammatory response syndrome to multiple organ dysfunction syndrome. *Nurs. Crit. Care.* **4**(5), 238–44.

Guardiola, J.J., Saad, M., and J. Yu (2007) Cardiovascular monitoring in severe sepsis and septic shock. In: Rello, J., Killef, M., Diaz, E., and Rodriguez, A. (eds) *Infectious Diseases in Critical Care*, 2nd edn. Springer, Berlin.

Hannigan, B.M. (2000) *Immunology*. Arnold, London.

Harrison, D.A., Welch, C.A., and Eddlestone, J.A. (2006) The epidemiology of severe sepsis in England, Wales and Northern Ireland, 1996–2004: Secondary analysis of a high quality clinical database, the ICNARC Case Mix Programme Database. *Critical Care.* **10** (online) Available at http://ccforum.com/content/10/2/R42 (accessed 01.07.2008).

Health Care Acquired Infections Research Network (2008) The effects of HCAI on patients. (online) Available at: http://www.hcainetwork.org/about%20hcai.htm (accessed 15.10.08).

Helbert, M. (2006) *Flesh and Bones of Immunology*. Mosby Elsevier, Edinburgh.

Higgins, C. (2007) *Understanding Laboratory Investigations*. Blackwell Science, Oxford.

Hinds, C.J. and Watson, J.D. (2005) Intensive care medicine. In: Kumar, P. and Clark, M. *Clinical Medicine*, 6th edn. Elsevier Saunders, Edinburgh.

Hofhuis, J.G.M., Spronk, P.E., van Stel, H.F. *et al.* (2008) Experiences of critically ill patients in the ICU. *Int. Crit. Care Nurs.* **24**(5), 300–13.

Huether, S.E. (2006) Structure and function of the renal and urologic systems. In: McCance, K.L. and Huether, S.E. (eds) Pathophysiology. *The Biologic Basis for Disease in Adults and Children*. Elsevier Mosby, St Louis.

International Sepsis Forum (2003) *Promoting a Better understanding of Sepsis*. Second Edition (online) Available at: http://www.sepsisforum.org/whitebook.htm (accessed: 19.08.2008).

Johansson, I., Fridlund, B., and Hildingh, C. (2004) Coping strategies of relatives when an adult next-of-kin is recovering at home following a critical illness. *Int. Crit. Care Nurs.* **20**(5), 281–91.

Johnson, P., Chaboyer, W., Foster, M. *et al.* (2001) Caregivers of ICU patients discharged home: What burden do they face? *Int. Crit. Care Nurs.* **17**(4), 219–27.

Kindt, T.J, Goldsby, R.A., and Osborne, B.A. (2007) *Immunology*. 6th edn. W.H.Freeman and Company, New York.

Kitchen, G., Griffin, J. Arif, S. *et al.* (2007) *Crash Course: Immunology and Haematolgy*. 3rd edn. Mosby Elsevier, Edinburgh.

Kleinpell, R.M. (2005) Implementing the guidelines: Implications for nursing care. *Adv. Sepsis.* **4**(2), 61–3.

Kozier, B., Erb, G., Berman, A. *et al.* (2008) Fundamentals of nursing. *Concepts, Process and Practice*. Pearson, Harlow.

Levi, M. and van der Poll, T. (2004) The central role of the endothelium in the crosstalk between coagulation and inflammation in sepsis. *Adv. Sepsis.* **3**(3), 91–7.

Levick, J.R. (2003) *An Introduction to Cardiovascular Physiology*. 4th edn. Hodder Arnold, London.

Levy, M.M., Fink, M.P., Marshall, J.C. *et al.* (2003) 2001 SCCM/ESICM/ACCP/ATS/SIS International Sepsis Definitions Conference. *Int. Care Med.* **29**, 530–8.

Llewellyn, M. and Cohen, J. (2007) Septic shock. In: Rello, J., Killef, M.,Diaz, E., and Rodriguez, A. (eds) *Infectious Diseases in Critical Care*. 2nd edn. Springer, Berlin.

Lof, L., Berggren, L., and Ahlstrom, G. (2008) ICU patients' recall of emotional reactions in the trajectory from falling critically ill to hospital discharge: Follow ups after 3 and 12 months. *Int. Crit. Care Nurs.* **24**(2), 108–21.

Magerey, J.M. and McCutcheon, H.H. (2005) 'Fishing with the dead'—recall of memories from the ICU. *Int. Crit. Care Nurs.* **21**(6), 344–54.

Marini, P.L. (2007) *The ICU Book*. 3rd edn. Lippincott, Williams and Wilkins, Philadelphia.

Male, D. (2003) *Infectious Disease: Immunology*. Open University Press, Milton Keynes.

McArthur-Rouse, F. (2001) Critical care outreach services and early warning scoring systems: A review of the literature. *J. Adv. Nurs.* **36**(5), 696–704.

McCance, K.L. (2006) Structure and function of the cardiovascular and lymphatic systems. In: McCance, K.L. and Huether, S.E. (eds) *Pathophysiology. The Biologic Basis for Disease in Adults and Children*. Elsevier Mosby, St Louis.

McQuillan, P., Pilkington, S., Allen A. *et al*. (1998) Confidential enquiry into quality of care before admission to intensive care. *BMJ*. (316), 1853–8.

Morton, P.G, Fontaine, D, Hudak, C.M., and Gallo, B.M. (2004) *Critical Care Nursing. A Holistic Approach*. 8th edn. Lippincott, Williams and Wilkins, Philadelphia.

Murphy, M.F., Wainscoat, J., and Colvin, B.T. (2005) Haematological disease. In: Kumar, P. and Clark, M. (eds) *Clinical Medicine*. 6th edn. Elsevier Saunders, Edinburgh.

Nairn, R. and Helbert, M. (2007) *Immunology for Medical Students*. 2nd edn. Mosby Elsevier, Philadelphia.

National Audit Office (2004) *Improving Patient Care by Reducing the Risk of Hospital Acquired Infection: A Progress Report*. The Stationary Office, London.

National Health Service Modernisation Agency (2004) *10 High Impact Changes for Service Improvement and Delivery*. Department of Health, London.

National Patient Safety Agency (2007) *Safer Care for the Acutely Ill Patient: Learning From Serious Incidents*. National Patient Safety Agency, London.

National Patient Safety Agency (2008) *Cleanyourhands Campaign*. (online) Available at: http://www.npsa. nhs.uk/cleanyourhands/the-campaign/background/ (accessed 20.10.2008).

NICE (2007) Acutely ill patients in hospital. Recognition of and Response to Acute Illness in Adults in Hospital. National Institute for Health and Clinical Excellence, London.

NICE (2008) *Critical Illness Rehabilitation* Final Scope. National Institute for Health and Clinical Excellence, London. (online) Available at: http://www.nice.org.uk/nicemedia/pdf/ CriticalRehabFinalScope0708.pdf (accessed 02.10.2008).

Padkin, A., Goldfrad, C., Brady, A.R. *et al*. (2003) Epidemiology of severe sepsis occurring in the first 24 hours in intensive care units in England, Wales and Northern Ireland. *Crit. Care Med*. **31**(9), 2332–8.

Papathanassoglou, E.D.E., Bozas, E., and Giannakopulou, M.D. (2008) Multiple organ dysfunction syndrome pathogenesis and care: a complex systems' theory perspective. *Nurs. Crit. Care* **13**(5), 249–59.

Parrillo, J.E. (2001) The heart and vasculature in sepsis and septic shock. In: Galley, H.F. (ed.) *Cardiology in Critical Illness*. BMJ Books, London.

Pittet, D., Allegranzi, B., Sax, H. *et al*. (2006) Evidence based model for hand transmission during patient care and the role of improved practices. *Lancet*. **6**, 641–52.

Playfair, J.H.L. and B.M. Chain (2005) *Immunology at a Glance*. Blackwell, Malden.

Poeze, M., Ramsay, G., Gerlag, H. et al. (2004) An international sepsis survey: A study of doctors' knowledge and perception of sepsis. *Crit. Care*. **8**(6), R409–13. (online) Available at: http://ccforum.com/content/8/6/R409 (accessed 08.10.2008).

Pratt, R.J., Pellowe, C.M, Wilson, J.A. *et al*. (2007) epic2: National evidence-based guidelines for preventing healthcare associated infections in NHS hospitals in England. *J. Hosp. Inf.* **65S**, S1–64.

Rattray, J. and Crocker, C. (2007) The intensive care follow-up clinic: current provision and future direction?. *Nurs. Crit. Care*. **12** (1), 1–3.

Rattray, J.E. and Hull, A.M. (2008) Emotional outcome after intensive care: Literature review. *J. Adv. Nurs*. **64**(1), 2–13.

Ringdal, M., Johansen, L., and Lundberg, D. (2006) Delusional memories form the intensive care unit—experienced by patients with physical trauma. *Int. Crit. Care Nurs*. **22**(6), 346–54.

Rivers, E., Nguyen, B., Ressler, S. *et al*. (2001) Early goal-directed therapy in sepsis and septic shock. *N. Engl. J. Med*. **345**(19), 1368–77.

Robson, W.P. (2004) From A&E to ICU: How nurses can support the Surviving Sepsis Campaign. *Int. Crit. Care Nurs*. **20**, 113–5.

Robson,W., Beavis,S., and Spittle, N. (2006) An audit of ward nurses' knowledge of sepsis. *Nurs. Crit. Care* **12**(2), 86–92.

Robson, W. and Daniels, R. (2008) The sepsis six: Helping patients survive sepsis. *Br. J. Nurs.* **17**(1), 16–21.

Rote, N. and Trask, B.C. (2006) Adaptive immunity. In: McCance, K.L. and Huether, S.E. (eds) *Pathophysiology. The Biologic Basis for Disease in Adults and Children.* Elsevier Mosby, St. Louis.

Rutherford, I.A. (1996) Haemostasis and disseminated intravascular coagulation. *Int. Crit. Care Nurs.* **12**(3), 161–7.

Sax, H., Allegranzi, B., Uckay, I. *et al.* (2007) 'My five moments for hand hygiene': A user-centred design approach to understand, train, monitor and report hand hygiene. *J. Hosp. Inf.* **67**(1), 9–21.

Simmonds, M., Hutchinson, A., Chikhani, M. *et al.* (2008) Surviving sepsis beyond intensive care: A retrospective cohort study of compliance with the international guidelines. *J. Int. Care Soc.* **9**(2), 124–7.

Smith, S.F., Duell, D.J., and Martin, B.C. (2008) *Clinical Nursing Skills. Basic to Advanced Skills.* 7th edn. Pearson, Upper Saddle River.

Sompayrac, L. (2003) *How The Immune System Works.* Blackwell, Oxford.

Storli, S.L., Anders, L., and Asplund, K. (2008) A journey in quest of meaning: A hermeneutic-phenomenological study on living with memories from intensive care. *Nurs. Crit. Care* **13**(2), 86–96.

Strahan, E.H.E. and Brown, R.J. (2005) A qualitative study of the experiences of patients following transfer from intensive care. *Int. Crit. Care Nurs.* **21**(3), 160–71.

Streater, C., Golledge, J., Sutherland, H. *et al.* (2001) The relocation experiences of relatives leaving a neurosciences critical care unit: A phenomenological study. *Nurs. Crit. Care* **6**(4), 163–70.

Surviving Sepsis Campaign (2007) Survive Sepsis: The official training programme of the surviving sepsis campaign. (online) Available at: http://www.survivesepsis.org/attachments/11902833672252.ppt (accessed 01.08.2008).

Surviving Sepsis Campaign (2007a) Action Demanded on World's Oldest Killer. (online) Available at: http://www.survivingsepsis.org/background/worldsoldestkiller (accessed 01.08.2008).

Surviving Sepsis Campaign (2007b) Barcelona Declaration. Problems and issues associated with sepsis treatment. (online) Available at: http://www.survivingsepsis.org/background/barcelona_declaration (accessed 01.08.2008).

Survive Sepsis (2007) The Sepsis Six. (online) Available at: http://www.survivesepsis.org/content.php?name=surviving.php (accessed 01.08.2008).

Taiberg, L., Wong, J., and Kumar, A. (2005) Myocardial depression in sepsis and septic shock. *Adv. Sepsis* **4**(3), 82–94.

Theaker, C. (2005) Infection control issues in central venous catheter care. *Int. Crit. Care Nurs.* **21**(2), 99–109.

Townsend, S., Dellinger, R.P. Levy, M.M. *et al.* (2005) *Implementing the Surviving Sepsis Campaign.* Society of Critical Care Medicine, Des Plaines.

Trask, B.C., Rote, N.S., and Huether, S.E. (2006) Innate immunity: Inflammation. In: McCance, K.L. and Huether, S.E. (Editors) *Pathophysiology. The Biologic Basis for Disease in Adults and Children*, 5th edn. Elsevier Mosby, St. Louis.

Vila, J. and Martinez, J.A. (2007) Opportunistic infections in the intensive care unit: A microbiologic overview. In: Rello, J., Killef, M., Diaz, E., and Rodriguez, A. (eds) *Infectious Diseases in Critical Care*, 2nd edn. Springer, Berlin.

Vincent, J.L., Abraham, E., Annane, D. et al. (2002) Reducing mortality in sepsis: New directions. *Crit. Care* **6**(suppl 3), S1–18. (online) Available at: http://ccforum.com/content/6/S3/S1 (accessed 06.07.2008).

West, S.L. (2006) Physical assessment: Whose role is it anyway? Nurs. *Crit. Care* **11**(4), 161–7.

Wheatley, I. (2006) The practice of taking level 1 patient observations. *Int. Crit. Care Nurs.* **22**(2), 115–21.

World Health Organisation (2008) *Five Moments for Hand Hygiene.* (online) Available at: http://www.who.int/gpsc/tools/Five_moments/en/index.html (accessed 22.10.2008).

Chapter 9

Psycho-social assessment, care, and support

Heather Baid

Chapter contents

Physical, mental, and social well-being are all directly linked to one another, contributing to overall health. Acute care nursing involves addressing the holistic needs of the whole person and not only physical health needs. The aim of this chapter is to explore:

- psychological and social consequences of acute illness/injury
- effective communication
- assessment of the mental and social health of acute care patients
- nursing interventions for psycho-social care and support
- needs of the family/significant others in acute care
- caring for the patient with a mental illness in acute care
- transcultural nursing care.

Learning outcomes

This chapter will enable you to:

- examine the skills and techniques needed to effectively communicate with others in a hospital setting
- explain the impact of an acute illness/injury on a patient's mental and social well-being
- critically analyse a systematic approach to assessing a patient's mental health using an ABC approach (affective, behaviour, and cognition)
- critically analyse a systematic approach to assessing a patient's mental capacity and explain the relevance of the Mental Capacity Act to acute care nursing
- discuss the interplay between physical, mental, and social well-being
- critically analyse a systematic approach to assessing a patient's social health
- identify proactive measures for supporting the mental and social well-being of acute care patients
- evaluate the needs of the family/significant others in acute care and identify strategies for promoting family-centred nursing care
- explore the relevance of transcultural nursing care within acute care
- examine post-discharge planning for the social needs of acute care patients
- evaluate the impact of substance misuse with acute care patients
- differentiate between delirium, dementia, and depression.

Introduction

Health, as defined by the World Health Organization (2003), is 'a state of complete physical, mental and social well-being and not merely the absence of disease or infirmity'. This model of health is illustrated in Figure 9.1 and demonstrates how physical well-being both influences and is influenced by mental and social well-being. The relevance for acute care nurses is to recognize the impact of physical illness/injury on the patient's mental and social well-being. In addition, dysfunction across the mental or social domains will have a negative effect on physical health with the physical illness/injury then surfacing as a secondary problem from an underpinning psycho-social issue. Acute care nursing should thus take a comprehensive approach that incorporates caring for all aspects of health, not only physical well-being.

Rather than considering health or lack of health as absolute states, a continuum exists with various degrees of illness and wellness and a central neutral point where no signs or symptoms of disease appear (Travis 2004). To the left of neutral, a person is moving towards worsening states of health and to the right, improving states of wellness. At the far right of the continuum, a person can achieve high level wellness by actively promoting health through wellness-oriented actions. This continuum can be applied to all contributing factors of health across the physical, mental, and social domains.

An influential theory on a holistic view of health is Maslow's hierarchy of needs (Maslow 1943), which acknowledges that all people have a series of incremental needs which must be met to be fully satisfied. Physiological needs are the first fundamental level followed by safety needs that includes physical health and well-being. Social needs then follow involving emotionally based relationships with friends and family. Esteem and self-actualization are higher level needs brought about once the lower level needs have been achieved. The implication for acute care nurses is to view their patients as still having various physical, mental, and social needs whilst in hospital that are all essential aspects of the nature of human beings.

The core subject of this chapter is the assessment and management of the psycho-social needs of acute care patients. Prior to exploring the mental health and social health systems, the principles of communication skills will be examined because although effective communication skills

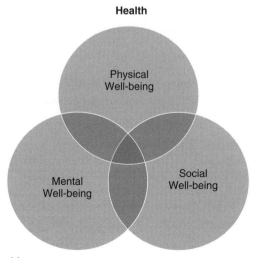

Figure 9.1 Model of health.

are important throughout all aspects of nursing practice, they are particularly important during the psycho-social assessment and interventions. The chapter will conclude by examining the specific conditions of delirium, dementia, and depression within acute care.

Communication skills

Nursing is a profession which requires a high level of interpersonal skills due to the continual communication with others. In acute care, nurses converse with a variety of people on a daily basis, including members of the healthcare team, families, carers, and of course the patients themselves. Proficient communication skills are vital for not only acquiring necessary information from the patient while taking a health history, conducting a physical assessment, or evaluating the effectiveness of nursing interventions, but are also essential for helping the patient and family to feel at ease during the hospital stay and establishing trusting relationships. The importance of communication is recognized by the Department of Health (2004) as the first core dimension of the Knowledge and Skills Framework and underpins all other aspects of health care.

Barriers to communication may prevent the nurse from fully achieving the purpose of a conversation with the patient. For instance, the patient may speak another language, technical terms are used that the patient does not understand, the patient has a sensory impairment such as poor hearing or sight, or a cognitive impairment is present from a head injury, dementia, learning disability, or mental illness. In the acute care setting, there are also a variety of factors that create an unsuitable environment for effectively communicating with a patient. There may be other people in the room which makes it difficult to discuss confidential information of a personal and sensitive nature. Standing over the patient who is lying in a hospital bed and the nurse wearing a uniform creates an authoritarian atmosphere and power difference between the nurse and the patient. Finally, the patient could be experiencing physical discomfort that is distracting from having a discussion.

Although some barriers to communication are unavoidable, there may be other measures the nurse can take to improve the environment and manner in which the conversation with the patient is being taken. Perhaps the most significant way a nurse can improve having a discussion with a patient is to prioritize time for the conversation to occur. With acute care nursing practice being incredibly fast-paced and busy, talking with patients can become lost among the multitude of nursing interventions and responsibilities. In order to prevent a task-oriented approach to nursing that does not involve communicating with patients, the nurse can ensure an adequate amount of time is allocated for speaking to patients with the nurse's full attention.

Both verbal and non-verbal techniques can be used to improve on the communication skills used by the acute care nurse:

- verbal communication skills:
  - questioning—open ended (broad), open ended (focused), close ended, leading
  - facilitation—acknowledging, willingness to share the patient's feelings
  - empathy—viewing the situation from the patient's perspective
  - clarification—ensuring the patient's story is fully understood
  - summarizing—demonstrating the nurse has been listening, highlighting key aspects of the conversation, and preventing any misconceptions by the nurse or patient

- non-verbal communication skills:
  - listening—active and passive
  - silence
  - touch

- hand gestures
- eye contact
- posture
- facial expression.

By using these types of verbal and non-verbal communication skills during a patient assessment and while implementing nursing intervention, the psycho-social care of the patient is enhanced, which in return helps to support the patient's mental and social well-being.

Mental health

There are numerous aspects of mental well-being, with each person having a unique, individual inner self. A comprehensive approach considering a holistic view of mental health includes the following types of assessment, which will be discussed in detail in this chapter:

- ABC: affective, behaviour, cognition
- mental capacity
- association between mental illness and physical illness
- spirituality.

ABC mental health assessment

The assessment of a patient's mental health status can be undertaken rapidly yet in a systematic manner by following an ABC approach: affective, behaviour, and cognition. 'Affective' refers to the patient's feelings, 'behaviour' involves the patient's appearance and actions, and 'cognition' is the patient's thinking pattern (see Table 9.1).

Table 9.1 ABC mental health assessment

A	Affective	Affect—objective interpretation of patient's feelings
		Mood—subjective information from patient about feelings
		Feelings, e.g. happiness, optimism, euphoria, sadness, anger, depression, guilt, excitement, nervousness, worry, pessimism, anxiety, disappointment, frustration, loneliness
B	Behaviour	Personal hygiene
		Eye contact during conversation
		Abnormal physical movements, e.g. pacing, repetitive actions
		Volume and manner of speech
		Appropriate actions for situation/setting
		Reduced/overactive activity
C	Cognition	Alertness
		Orientation to person, place, and time
		Attention, concentration
		Memory—short term, long term
		Speech content
		Appropriate use of language

Affective

The affective dimension of mental health focuses on the patient's feelings and emotions. An objective assessment can be made by the nurse on how the patient 'appears' to be feeling. This type of interpretation is referred to as affect and reflects the nurse's perception of the patient's emotions based on non-verbal communication. For example, a nurse could identify a flat affect based upon an observation that the patient looked depressed. However, if the patient provided a statement such as 'I feel very low', this could be documented as the patient's mood because it is subjective information in the patient's own words. Similarly, a heightened affect would reflect exaggerated feelings of euphoria. Finding out how a patient is feeling is an important aspect of an assessment because it informs the nurse of the emotional health of the patient as well as how the patient is coping with physical ill-health and hospitalization.

Behaviour and appearance

There are a variety of behavioural changes indicating there may be a problem with a patient's mental health status. Interpretation of behaviour is a subjective judgement made by the assessor, however, which should take into account past mental health history as well as the context of each individual situation. For instance, inappropriate clothing or lack of hygiene could show that a patient lacked insight into personal appearance but may not necessarily indicate a significant mental health problem. An inability to maintain eye contact or interaction during conversation could be a sign of depression or could be the cultural norm for some people. Repetitive physical movements may be a sign of a physical health problem such as a tremor or may suggest a mental health disorder such as with incessant pacing or hand washing. It is not the content of speech but the behaviour of 'how' a patient speaks that could be considered in terms of speech being clear and delivered in an audible manner. Abnormal speech behaviour would be noted with mumbling, shouting, aggression, or indeed absent speech where a patient does not respond at all.

Cognition

There is considerable overlap between a mental health assessment and a neurological assessment (see Chapter 4) while evaluating the patient's cognitive functioning because abnormal 'thinking' could indicate either a neurological illness/injury or a mental health disorder. Although differentiating between the two and diagnosing the underlying medical issue may not fall under the responsibility of the acute care nurse, a full initial nursing assessment benefits from a comprehensive overview of the cognitive functioning of the patient to establish a baseline. Ongoing assessment of cognition allows for trends to be monitored and for valuable patient information to be communicated to the medical practitioner responsible for diagnosis of the physical/mental health problem. The acute care nurse will then be contributing to multidisciplinary teamwork with the nursing assessment offering valuable aspects of patient information.

As described in Chapter 4, the Glasgow Coma Scale is a well-established tool for assessing the neurological body system with the verbal response focusing on cognition. Similar to the initial questioning for the verbal response while undertaking a Glasgow Coma Scale, assessing cognition from a mental health perspective will consider the patient's orientation to person, place, and time as well as any signs of confusion or abnormality with alertness. A further screening tool for identifying cognitive dysfunction is the Mini Mental State Examination (Folstein *et al.* 1975), which uses a series of questions to evaluate orientation, registration, attention, calculation, recall, and language.

This focused ABC mental health assessment can be used routinely on all patients in acute care and not just those patients with a history of a mental health disorder. In particular, the affective aspect of the assessment will help to determine how the patient is feeling as a result of their physical health problem and hospitalization. Examples of potential psychological consequences of physical illness/injury include:

+ altered body image
+ fear
+ anxiety
+ sadness
+ hopelessness
+ powerlessness
+ loneliness.

The clinical health problem or hospitalization may also have an emotional impact on the person by creating a feeling of loss from impaired:

+ mobility
+ independence
+ role(s)
+ responsibilities
+ occupation
+ ability to work
+ ability to travel
+ ability to partake in social activities and hobbies.

In addition to the ABC assessment, more details about a patient's mental health can come from assessing thought processes, thought content, perceptions, insight, and judgement (see Table 9.2). During the mental health assessment, it may become apparent that the patient is at risk for self-harm or suicide, which would warrant a more detailed risk assessment and immediate referral on to appropriate mental health services.

Table 9.2 Mental health assessment

	Definition	**Examples of abnormality**
Thought processes	Quantity, flow, and form of thoughts	Rapid/slow thinking Disorganized thinking pattern
Thought content	Substance of thinking	Delusions—false beliefs Obsessions Phobias Preoccupations
Perceptions	Awareness of sensations: sight, smell, hearing, touch, taste	Hallucination—false sensation without any external stimulus, e.g. seeing an image which is not truly there Pseudohallucination—experienced internally, e.g. hearing voices inside the person's head Illusion—false sensation with an external stimulus, e.g. distortion of a visual image
Insight	Understanding of health and illness	Inability to recognize that a clinical problem is present Non-compliance with treatment
Judgement	Capacity to make sound decisions	Impaired decision making which affects the person's safety or safety of others

Mental capacity assessment

Mental capacity is defined as the ability to make a fully informed, responsible decision for oneself at the time the decision needs to be taken (Office of the Public Guardian 2008a). This requires having an adequate understanding of all aspects of the decision making and an ability to cognitively retain this information. Thus, people who lack capacity are unable to make decisions or take particular actions for themselves, leaving them vulnerable and dependent on others for support of health and social care needs.

The Mental Capacity Act 2005 became fully effective in 2007 and provides a legal framework for decision making on behalf of people who lack mental capacity (Department for Constitutional Affairs 2007a). The fundamental goal of the Act is to protect people who are unable to competently make their own decisions but the Act also serves as guiding advice for those involved in caring for patients who lack capacity. In addition, the Act promotes a collaborative approach whereby people who lack mental capacity are encouraged to take part in decisions that are affecting them.

There are five statutory principles underpinning the Mental Capacity Act 2005 (Department for Constitutional Affairs 2005, p. 1–2):

1 'A person must be assumed to have capacity unless it is established that he lacks capacity.

2 A person is not to be treated as unable to make a decision unless all practicable steps to help him to do so have been taken without success.

3 A person is not to be treated as unable to make a decision merely because he makes an unwise decision.

4 An act done, or decision made, under this Act for or on behalf of a person who lacks capacity must be done, or made, in his best interests.

5 Before the act is done, or the decision is made, regard must be had to whether the purpose for which it is needed can be as effectively achieved in a way that is less restrictive of the person's rights and freedom of action'.

An assessment of mental capacity begins with the two-stage test of capacity by asking two fundamental questions (Department for Constitutional Affairs 2007a):

1 Is there an impairment of the mind or brain, or is there a disturbance affecting the way the mind or brain functions (either temporary or permanent)?

2 If yes, does the impairment or disturbance prevent the person from being able to make a decision at the time it needs to be made?

The Mental Capacity Act Code of Practice (Department for Constitutional Affairs 2007a) suggests further assessment of a person's ability to make a decision can include evaluating whether the person is able to:

1 understand the relevant information about the decision and why the decision needs to be made

2 understand the likely consequences to occur if the decision is made or not made

3 retain, use, and weigh up the information needed for the decision

4 communicate the final decision made (through speech, writing, sign language, or other means that may require support from a translator or speech and language therapist).

If a person lacks capacity for one particular decision at one moment in time, this does not mean an inability to make decisions in general or to make this same decision in the future if the loss of capacity changes over time. The loss of capacity can be partial or temporary, and a person may also have the capacity for one type of issue but not others.

Examples of reasons why a person may have impaired functioning of the mind or brain include:

♦ mental illness

♦ significant learning disability

♦ traumatic brain injury

♦ stroke

♦ dementia

♦ delirium

♦ physical or medical conditions causing altered cognition or level of consciousness

♦ substance misuse—alcohol, recreational drugs, medication overdose.

However, patients with the previously listed conditions may in fact have full mental capacity and should not be judged based on the past medical or mental health history. Each individual person should be assessed as a unique person based on the ability to demonstrate full mental capacity at the time when the decision needs to be made.

There are a variety of roles, responsibilities, and means for advance decision making recognized in the Mental Capacity Act 2005 in order for people lacking mental capacity to have full legal representation and protection of their best interest. Acute care nurses should have an awareness of these features of the Act, including the following terminology: Lasting Power of Attorney (LPA), Deputy, Court of Protection, Public Guardian, Office of the Public Guardian, Independent Mental Capacity Advocate (IMCA), Advance Decisions, and Deprivation of Liberty Safeguards. See Table 9.3 for a summary definition of each of these terms and comparisons between the different representative roles.

Lasting Power of Attorney

The LPA is a legal document registered with the Office of the Public Guardian (2008b), which allows for decisions to be made by somebody else (Attorney) on behalf of a person who lacks

Table 9.3 Summary of terminology from the Mental Capacity Act 2005

Mental capacity	The ability to make a fully informed, responsible decision for oneself at the time the decision needs to be taken
Lasting Power of Attorney	Legal document where a person appoints somebody else to make decisions on his/her behalf if mental capacity is lost
Deputy	Appointed by the Court of Protection to represent and make decisions for a person who does not have mental capacity
Court of Protection	Specialist Court with jurisdiction over the property, finances, and personal welfare of people who lack mental capacity
Office of the Public Guardian	Registers, oversees, and investigates complaints about Lasting Power of Attorneys and Court appointed Deputies
Independent Mental Capacity Advocate	Represents and protects vulnerable people who lack mental capacity and have no family/friends to support decision making
Advance decisions	Decision to refuse specific treatment under designated circumstances made in advance of losing mental capacity
Deprivation of Liberty Safeguards	Measures to ensure any deprivation of liberty of people who lack mental capacity is done in a legal manner

mental capacity (Donor). An unregistered LPA does not give the attorney the right to make a decision on behalf of a Donor and is not considered legal until it is registered with the Office of the Public Guardian. The Donor can register the LPA when they still have full mental capacity or the Attorney can apply to register the LPA at a later date. The following people contribute to the LPA:

- Donor
  - Makes the LPA to have somebody else make decisions about his/her personal welfare, property, and affairs if/when there is a loss of mental capacity.
- Attorney(s)
  - Appointed by the Donor to make decisions on his/her behalf when the Donor is lacking mental capacity.
- Named person(s)
  - Chosen by the Donor and is notified when an application is made to register the LPA.
  - Safeguard measure to protect the Donor because the named person(s) has the right to object to the registration of the LPA if there are concerns.
- Certificate provider
  - Chosen by the Donor to complete a Part B Certificate in the LPA form which confirms that the Donor understands the LPA and was not under any pressure to make it.
  - Further safeguard measure to protect the Donor.
- Witness
  - Signs the LPA form to confirm the signature and date of the Donor and Attorney(s) on the LPA form are true.
  - Final safeguard measure.

Court of Protection

The Court of Protection is a new specialist Court established by the Mental Capacity Act 2005, which has the same powers, rights, privileges, and authority as the High Court for issues related to mental capacity (Office of the Public Guardian 2008e). Specifically, the Court of Protection is able to:

- determine whether a person has mental capacity and is able to make decisions for him/herself
- make decisions about the finances or welfare on behalf of a person who lacks mental capacity
- appoint Deputies to make decisions on behalf of a person who lacks mental capacity
- decide whether an LPA is valid
- remove Deputies or Attorneys who are not fulfilling their role and responsibilities
- hear cases about objections to register an LPA.

Deputy

A Deputy will be appointed by and be accountable to the Court of Protection when decisions need to be made on behalf of somebody who lacks mental capacity. The Deputy must agree to taking on the role and responsibilities involved in representing a person who lacks mental capacity and the role is supervised and supported by the Office of the Public Guardian (2008c). There is only a need for a Deputy when essential actions for personal welfare cannot be carried out without Court of Protection approval and no other way can be found for settling a matter in the person's best interest about his/her personal welfare. The IMCA service will also be required if the Deputy's authority is limited to property/affairs, there is serious decision making about medical treatment or long-term accommodation, or there are no family members or friends to represent the person.

According to the Office of the Public Guardian (2008c), the Deputy should always:

♦ act and make decisions in the person's best interest

♦ make decisions only for those issues which are authorized by the Court order

♦ be aware of and follow the guidance provided by the Code of Practice

♦ ensure the Act's five statutory principles are adhered to

♦ maintain high standards of care while acting on the person's behalf.

Public Guardian

The Public Guardian oversees and manages the Office of the Public Guardian, which was established in 2007 as an agency of the Ministry of Justice and is responsible for registering LPAs and supervising Court of Protection appointed Deputies. The Office of the Public Guardian (2008f) also investigates complaints about an Attorney or Deputy and works closely with other organizations to ensure any allegations of abuse are looked into and acted upon.

Independent Mental Capacity Advocate

Under the Mental Capacity Act 2005, an NHS body or local authority has a legal duty to appoint an IMCA if a person lacking capacity has nobody other than paid staff to assist with serious decision making regarding serious medical treatment or changes in long-term accommodation (Department of Health 2007; Lee 2007). NHS and local authority staff also have the power, but not a duty, to appoint an IMCA when it is felt one would be beneficial during care reviews or adult protection procedures. The Office of the Public Guardian (2008d) provides guidance for safeguarding vulnerable adults with a new protocol, guidelines, and policy that help to promote best practice while preventing and managing adult protection situations.

The IMCA Service was launched in 2007 to ensure vulnerable people who lack capacity and who do not have family or friends are fully supported when significant decisions regarding their health and social care are being made (Department for Constitutional Affairs 2007a). The decision maker is a health or social care professional who is planning healthcare treatment or a change in long-term accommodation for an adult who lacks capacity. A decision maker may also be considering making a decision on behalf of the person who lacks capacity meaning if there are no family or friends available for advice and consultation as to the person's best interest, an IMCA would be necessary.

Decisions about serious medical treatment needing an IMCA include:

♦ new treatment

♦ stopping current treatment

♦ withholding treatment that could be offered

♦ or whether there is any of the following:

  • A single treatment with a fine balance between the benefits, burdens, and risks

  • A choice of treatments without one being an obvious and clear best option

  • proposed treatment with the potential for serious consequences (e.g. interventions causing severe pain/distress and reduced mobility, or those with an impact on future life choices such as the ability to conceive children).

Referral to the IMCA service will be necessary for decision making regarding a change in accommodation if a person lacking mental capacity moves into:

- hospital for a predicted stay of longer than 28 days
- residential accommodation for a predicted stay of longer than 8 weeks (including a care home, nursing home, sheltered housing, ordinary housing, housing association, or hostel).

The IMCA should be:

- independent without any connection to the person's carers or health and social care services
- fully knowledgeable with the Act
- supportive and representative of the person when there is no family or friends to assist with serious decision making
- able to voice the person's views, wishes, feelings, values, and beliefs, and make sure the person's rights are upheld throughout the decision-making process
- able to ensure the person is aware of all relevant information for the issue being decided on and help the person to explore choices, options, and services available
- able to check that principles of the Act have been followed, including best interests, and seek a second medical opinion if necessary.

Advance decisions

An advance decision allows somebody with full mental capacity to refuse specified medical treatment for a time in the future when the person may no longer be capable of consenting or refusing treatment (Department for Constitutional Affairs 2007a). The advance decision must be valid and applicable for the current circumstances and context. As they are legally binding, advance decisions must be followed by healthcare professionals as long as the maker of the advance decision is an adult (18 years or older) with full mental capacity at the time the decision is made and the advance decision clearly identifies which treatments are being refused under what circumstances.

An advance decision can only decline treatment and cannot be used to request specific treatment or ask for life to be ended. The Mental Capacity Act 2005 provides criteria for an advance decision to refuse life-sustaining treatment (Department for Constitutional Affairs 2007a). This type of advance decision must be in writing, contain the signatures of the maker and a witness, and be verified with a statement by the maker indicating which specific treatment is not wanted even if the maker's life is at risk (Office of the Public Guardian 2008g). An advance decision to refuse life-sustaining treatment can be signed on behalf of the maker if the maker is unable to sign for him/herself. The Court of Protection may step in to make a decision about refusing treatment when there is a sincere doubt or disagreement about whether an advance decision exists or is valid and applicable. However, the Court of Protection is not able to overturn or change a valid and applicable advance decision (Office of the Public Guardian 2008e).

Healthcare professionals are legally protected from liability if they:

- stop or withhold treatment when it is reasonable to believe that a valid and applicable advance decision exists
- continue with treatment when they do not know that an advance decision exists or are not satisfied that it is valid and applicable.

Deprivation of liberty safeguards

Decision making on behalf of people who lack mental capacity has the potential to take away personal freedom and choice that constitutes a deprivation of liberty. This may be in the person's best interest and necessary to protect the person's health and safety or to ensure the safety of others. However, this situation should be avoided at all costs. There are new deprivation of liberty safeguards introduced into the Mental Capacity Act 2005 by the Mental Health Act 2007, which provide a legal framework for depriving the liberty of patients in hospitals and care homes (Department for Constitutional Affairs 2007b).

The deprivation of liberty safeguard measures have come about to prevent breaches of the European Convention of Human Rights as seen with the case of H.L. versus the United Kingdom (Dute 2005). Commonly called the 'Bournewood judgment', this case revealed an autistic man admitted to hospital against his wish who lacked the mental capacity to make decisions for himself regarding healthcare treatment. Although decisions were made in his best interest, there were no legal systems in place to ensure that the process of denying personal liberty was carried out in a legitimate manner or any means to challenge the decision making. As such, the European Court of Human Rights recommended that people without mental capacity should only be deprived of liberty through a lawful process where safeguards and precautions are in place to prevent illegal detention and to allow rapid access to a court where the detention can be reviewed if necessary (Ministry of Justice 2008).

The legislation for the deprivation of liberty safeguards took effect as of April 2009 and will offer protection for people without mental capacity who need to be cared for in a restrictive way to receive the care that is in their best interest (Ministry of Justice 2008). Further guidance about the implications of these new safeguards for hospitals and care homes and the relevance for acute care is provided by the Department of Health (2008a) through consultation reports, briefing leaflets, newsletters, staff training programmes, and documentation forms.

Association between physical assessment findings and mental illness

Once a mental health assessment and mental capacity assessment have been completed, it is useful to consider whether there is a relationship between any abnormalities in physical health and a mental health disorder. There are a variety of physical assessment findings that can be caused from an underlying mental health illness rather than a primary physical health problem. Acute care nurses are not necessarily responsible for diagnosing either a physical or mental illness/injury but an understanding of how clinical signs and symptoms are associated with various mental health problems will aid the nurse in the interpretation of a holistic assessment.

The following is a list of physical signs and symptoms that could be directly caused by either a mental health disorder or from a medication prescribed for a mental health disorder:

- sleep disturbances
- dizziness
- poor memory
- impaired speech
- seizures
- facial muscle weakness
- sensory disturbances—vision, hearing, smell, touch, taste
- hyperventilation
- tachycardia
- bradycardia
- palpitations
- nausea and vomiting

+ appetite gain/loss
+ weight gain/loss
+ loss of sexual interest
+ amenorrhoea.

Relationship between physical health and mental health

There is a very strong correlation between mental health disorders and physical health problems of both an acute and a chronic nature. Patients with mental illness are more likely to experience major physical illness, develop serious physical illness earlier in life, and die of physical illness sooner compared with the general population (Disability Rights Commission 2007; Fitch *et al.* 2008). Despite the higher incidence of physical health problems among those with mental illness, people with a mental health disorder are also less likely to receive health screening, health promotion, or access physical health services (Robson & Gray 2007).

Possible reasons explaining why poor physical health is associated with mental illness are:

+ side effects of psychiatric medications
+ unhealthy lifestyle: diet, smoking, substance misuse, lack of exercise
+ poor access to health promotion services
+ poor follow-up from physical health services
+ lack of insight into physical health problems
+ lack of understanding about the mental illness from other healthcare professionals.

See Table 9.4 for a summary of relevant statistics indicating the high incidence of physical illness among patients with mental illness.

Although hospital nurses are caring for patients admitted because of a physical illness/injury, an awareness of this association between mental illness and poor physical health will help acute care nurses to appreciate the increased health risks for their patients who happen to have a mental health disorder. A holistic approach to assessing patients with a history of mental illness should then include health screening for further physical problems. The acute care nurse may not have the time, capacity, or resources to act upon secondary health problems identified with their patients but referrals can be made to other healthcare services for suitable follow up. Similarly, the acute care nurse may identify clinically significant abnormality of the mental health system and liaising with mental health services will help to ensure that the mental health needs are being met while the patient remains in an acute hospital.

Spirituality

Along with thoughts, feelings, and emotions, an additional dimension to a person's psychological being is spirituality. The term 'spirituality' is very subjective, can be interpreted in different ways, and is often interchanged with the term 'religion'. McBrien (2005) defines spirituality as a person's search for meaning and purpose in life compared with religion, which is a set of beliefs, customs, and practices of an individual or group. Spirituality is a component of a person's inner self which therefore has an impact on mental well-being and contributes to the overall health status.

The Nursing and Midwifery Council (NMC) identifies assessing and documenting the spiritual needs of a patient as one of the standards of proficiency for nursing practice (NMC 2004). Much has been written about the role of the nurse in assessing the patient's spirituality ranging from how this is an essential aspect of holistic nursing care to the difficulties nurses face due to a lack of time,

Table 9.4 Physical health and mental health

Fenton & Stover (2006)	People with depression: Twice as likely to develop type II diabetes Three times more likely to have a stroke Five times more likely to have a myocardial infarction
Rethink (2008)	People with schizophrenia and bipolar disorder: Two to four times more likely to have cardiovascular disease Two to four times more likely to have respiratory disease Five times more likely to have diabetes Eight times more likely to have hepatitis C Fifteen times more likely to have HIV
Kwok & Cheung (2007)	People with learning disabilities have increased levels of mental and physical health needs and have a high incidence of: epilepsy dementia polypharmacy
Disability Rights Commission (2006)	People with schizophrenia: Twice as likely to develop bowel cancer, which is the second most common cause of cancer death in the UK 42% more likely to develop breast cancer (women) High incidence of obesity, smoking, heart disease, diabetes, respiratory disease, and stroke
Black Mental Health UK (2008); Mental Health Foundation (2004)	Black and ethnic minorities: More likely to be diagnosed with mental health problems More likely to experience poor outcome from mental health treatment Higher inequities in access to healthcare services Higher rates of psychoses Higher rates of diabetes and hypertension

confidence, or understanding about how to intervene with the patient's spiritual needs without feeling intrusive (McSherry & Ross 2002; McSherry & Watson 2002; MacLaren 2004; Narayanasamy 2004; Ledger 2005; Swift *et al.* 2007; Timmins & Kelly 2008). The use of a spiritual assessment tool helps to provide a structured, systematic approach and will be most effective if the tool is easy to follow, not time consuming, adaptable, understandable by both the nurse and the patient, and applicable to all spiritual belief systems (McSherry & Ross 2002). Guidance on supporting both the religious and the spiritual needs of patients in the NHS is provided by the Department of Health (2003a) with a designated framework for chaplaincy-spiritual care services.

Social health

A patient's social well-being is influenced by numerous factors including family, friends, culture, ethnicity, traditions, customs, religion, occupation, education, and housing. The misuse of substances such as alcohol and recreational drugs also has implications for affecting a person's social health status. These aspects of a social health assessment and care will now be examined in detail as relevant for acute care nursing:

- family, friends, and significant others
- cultural needs

+ post-discharge social care needs
+ substance misuse.

Family, friends, and significant others

Holistic nursing practice involves caring for the patient within the context of a family unit because there is a direct relationship between individual patient health and family health, with the patient's well-being having a significant impact on the well-being of the family (International Council of Nurses 2002). Rather than assuming a patient's family to be biological relations, family is best defined by the patient who may consider friends, carers, neighbours, or other significant people as 'family'. Hanson (2001, p. 6) captures the essence of the term family by explaining family is 'two or more individuals who depend on one another for emotional, physical, and economical support'. Underpinning this definition is the concept that family is self-defined by the patient as those people who provide support and/or who the patient supports. The relevance for the acute care nurse is to incorporate an assessment of who the patient views as family (relatives and/or non-relations) into the nursing assessment.

In addition, a comprehensive family assessment is useful for the acute care nurse to be able to:

+ identify the next of kin for the patient's healthcare record
+ recognize people who may be able to provide emotional support for the patient
+ find out if the patient is the main care giver for someone who will subsequently need to have social support put into place while the patient remains in hospital
+ establish which family members the patient would like information to be passed on to about the patient's health status to protect patient confidentiality while at the same time helping to keep the family well informed
+ be aware of how the family is coping with the patient's health problem as well as any nursing interventions that may help to support the family
+ provide education and health promotion information for any aspects of patient care the family member(s) is able to be involved with either while the patient is in hospital or for after the patient is discharged
+ discover information about the patient's preferences and unique needs if the patient is not able to communicate.

 Family-centred health care promotes a partnership arrangement among the patient, family, and providers using four core principles (Institute for Family-Centered Care 2008):

1   Dignity and respect
    • Listening to and honouring the patient and family's perspectives and choices.

2   Information sharing
    • Providing timely, accurate, and unbiased information to the patient and family to keep them up to date and well informed.

3   Participation
    • Encouraging patients and families to participate in care and decision making as they choose.

4   Collaboration
    • Inviting patients and families to be representative stakeholders and collaborate with healthcare leaders during service and policy development.

By incorporating these four principles into the assessment and provision of acute services, nurses will be adhering to family-centred health care within the hospital setting. Particular situations requiring close attention to the needs of the family in acute care include immediately following the patient's admission to hospital, after significant medical events (e.g. major surgery or cardiac arrest), before discharge, and during end-of-life care.

Hospital visiting times have long been established for a variety of reasons such as preventing the spread of infection, ensuring healthcare interventions are not disrupted, and allowing patients to not become stressed or tired from having visitors. There remains much debate, however, on whether there is sufficient evidence to support restricted visiting hours with some areas in acute care taking either a 'flexible' or 'open' approach to visiting times (Ismail & Mulley 2007). The Department of Health, Social Services and Public Safety (2008) have recently provided guiding principles to help hospitals develop visiting policies. These principles aim to support patient visiting where health care is provided in a safe and timely manner and the privacy and dignity of patients are maintained.

Transcultural nursing

Today's society is a multifaceted, rich, dynamic mix of people from many different countries, cultures, and ethnic groups. As such, patients in acute care have a variety of cultural backgrounds influencing their philosophy and practices in relation to health and illness. Transcultural nursing embraces this diversity and provides culturally sensitive nursing care in ways that are meaningful for the patient (Leininger & McFarland 2002). Integrated into transcultural nursing is the concept of cultural competence, which is the ability to understand and interact with people across different cultures.

Key characteristics of cultural competence include the nurse having the following knowledge, skills, and attitude (Purnell 2005):

- insight and awareness of the nurse's own culture without allowing this to influence people from other backgrounds
- knowledge about and understanding for the patient's culture and the meaning of health and illness for this culture
- acceptance and respect for cultural differences
- not making an assumption that the patient's beliefs, values, and practices are the same as the nurse
- being open to experiencing other cultural encounters
- being flexible in the provision of nursing care that can be adapted to suit the patient's cultural needs.

See Table 9.5 for an overview of a cultural assessment suitable for acute care with some suggested questions to guide the nurse in determining information about various aspects of the patient's culture. It is important to assess each patient as an individual who may or may not follow the typical practices of the culture the patient comes from. Rather than stereotyping a patient and making assumptions, an accurate cultural assessment is best tailored to identify the beliefs, values, rituals, and practices that are important to this particular patient.

For palliative care patients, a focused cultural assessment will provide the nurse with information about the patient and family's wishes regarding end-of-life care. An understanding of the patient's health beliefs about pain, grief, and death itself will help the nurse to plan appropriate care that is tailored to the patient's requests and cultural needs. The cultural assessment for the palliative care patient will also recognize how the patient and family would like the immediate post-death period to be managed. Although there are rituals and practices about post-death care associated with different cultures (e.g. washing the patient, clothing to be worn, facing a certain direction, or prayers to be given), the patient's personal beliefs may or may not match the identified cultural background which requires nurses to remain open to each person's unique belief system about end-of-life care.

Table 9.5 Cultural assessment

	Patient questions	Other considerations
Language	What is your preferred language?	Is a translator needed to communicate with the patient at a basic level for conversation? Is a translator needed to communicate at an advanced level in order for the patient to be able to discuss healthcare information, remain fully informed, and participate in decision making? If the patient does not speak or understand English, can a translation chart be made of key words necessary for the patient to be able to communicate in acute care (e.g. pain, hungry, thirsty, short of breath, dizzy)?
Diet	Do you have any dietary requirements? Are there specific food items or drinks you take for your illness?	Do any special diets need to be ordered for the patient (e.g. kosher, halal, vegetarian, vegan, allergies)? Does the patient/family provide their own specific food items or drinks as therapy for the illness? Are there any medications or intravenous solutions to be avoided because of specific dietary requests (e.g. gelatine, eggs, dairy products)?
Religion	Is religion important to you? If so, would you like to share what religion you are affiliated with? Do you have any religious practices or restrictions that you would like discussed and shared with other healthcare professionals for your time in hospital? Would you like to be visited by the chaplain/spiritual care services?	Are there specific religious practices or restrictions that influence the healthcare being provided in acute care? Is there relevant information about the patient's religious practice/beliefs that the patient would like the healthcare team to be aware of? Do any referrals need to be made to the chaplain/spiritual care services?

Post-discharge social care needs

Depending on the severity of the healthcare problem and length of stay in hospital, a patient may require support and guidance for social care needs as part of the discharge planning. An assessment of the patient's ability to function outside of the hospital setting will reveal whether the patient is able to:

• achieve activities of daily living

• return to the previous accommodation

+ safely cohabitate in the available accommodation
+ undertake previous occupational role if the patient had been working
+ participate in social activities
+ receive psychological and emotional support from others.

In addition to assessing for physical and mental health needs, discharge planning therefore requires evaluating the need for interventions to help the patient's social needs for after the patient has been discharged from hospital. Although the acute care nurse may not be directly intervening with necessary actions identified in the social care needs assessment, referrals can be made for follow up from appropriate people such as occupational therapy, physiotherapy, social work, district nursing, intermediate care, spiritual care services, mental health services, nursing home, and voluntary organizations.

Substance misuse

The inappropriate use of substances, such as alcohol, recreational drugs, or other prescribed medications, not only causes numerous physical health problems, but also significantly impacts on a patient's mental and social well-being. As a result, reducing substance misuse to improve the overall health status of individual people and populations has been the goal of a number of international (World Health Organization 2009a, b) and national policies (Department of Health 2008b; National Treatment Agency for Substance Misuse 2008). See Table 9.6 for a summary of recent statistics regarding alcohol consumption and the effect of alcohol on health in the UK in recent years.

Current recommendations from the Department of Health (2008b) for 'sensible drinking' advises adult women to not regularly drink more than 2–3 units of alcohol/day and adult men

Table 9.6 Statistical data on effect of alcohol on health in England (National Audit Office 2008; The NHS Information Centre 2008)

Alcohol consumption	40% of men and 33% of women drink more than the daily recommended number of units at least once/week
	23% of men and 15% of women drink more than twice the daily recommended number of units at least twice/week
	31% of men drink on average more than 21 units/week and 20% of women drink on average more than 14 units/week
Alcohol related ill health and mortality	In 2007, 112,267 prescriptions for drugs used in alcohol treatment—an increase of 20% since 2003
	In 2006, there were 6,517 deaths directly linked to alcohol with 2/3 being men—an increase of 19% since 2001
	In 2006/07, there were 57,142 NHS hospital admissions with primary diagnosis related to alcohol—an increase of 52% since 1995/96
	In 2006/07, there were 207,788 NHS hospital admissions with a primary or secondary diagnosis related to alcohol—more than doubled from 93,459 in 1995/96
	Number of admissions with a primary or secondary diagnosis of alcoholic liver disease has more than tripled since 1995/96
Alcohol related costs	In 2008, estimated cost of alcohol misuse on the health service was between £2.7 billion/year
	In 2007, alcohol was 60% more affordable in the UK than in 1980
	In 2006/07, just over half of violent attacks causing wounds and minor injuries were under the influence of alcohol

3–4 units of alcohol/day. Alcohol screening is used to identify drinking that goes beyond these recommended levels with terminology about alcohol intake used as follows (Department of Health 2008b; World Health Organization 2009b):

♦ Sensible drinking

• Drinking in a manner that is not likely to cause significant risk or harm to the drinker or other people.

♦ Hazardous drinking

• Drinking above the recognized recommended drinking levels but not yet causing harm although there is a risk of physical, mental, or social harm.

♦ Harmful drinking

• Drinking above the recognized recommended drinking levels, causing harm to physical, mental, and/or social health.

♦ Dependent drinking

• Drinking above the recognized recommended drinking levels at a harmful level along with signs and symptoms of alcohol dependence.

♦ Chronic drinking

• Drinking large amounts of alcohol on a regular basis—difficult to quantify but 50 units/week for men and 35 units/week for women is the benchmark.

♦ Binge drinking

• Drinking large amounts of alcohol over short period of time, leading to drunkenness with immediate and short-term risks for harm.

See Table 9.7 for various alcohol screening tools used within healthcare practice with standardized questions that help to provide an objective, structured, and more accurate assessment of alcohol consumption compared with simply asking the patient a general question about use of alcohol.

Screening for substance misuse is undertaken in acute care to identify whether alcohol or drugs are causing the primary physical health problem (reason why the patient was admitted to hospital) or causing secondary physical health problems (clinical signs and symptoms other than those from the admitting illness/injury). Screening will also help to determine whether the patient is at risk for going through alcohol/drug withdrawal while staying in hospital and to evaluate whether alcohol or drugs are currently having a negative impact on the patient's social well-being. Furthermore, if the screening reveals a possibility of substance misuse, there is an opportunity for the acute care nurse to plan health promotion interventions and referral to specialist substance misuse services for follow-up care following discharge from hospital.

Table 9.7 Alcohol screening tools

AUDIT	The Alcohol Use Disorders Identification Test	Babor *et al.* (2001)
FAST	FAST Screening Tool	Hodgson *et al.* (2002); Health Development Agency (2002)
CAGE	Cut down, Annoy, Guilty, Eye Opener	Mayfield *et al.* (1974)
Five-Shot	Five-Shot Screening Tool	Seppa *et al.* (1998)
PAT	Paddington Alcohol Test	Smith *et al.* (1996)

Along with subjective information from the patient determined through an alcohol screening history, alcohol withdrawal syndrome may present with the following signs and symptoms occurring on average 24 h after the patient's last alcoholic drink:

- sweating
- nausea and vomiting
- headache
- tremors
- agitation
- anxiety
- sensory disturbances—visual, auditory, tactile.

Delirium tremens (DTs) typically occurs between 48 and 72 h from the time of the patient's last alcoholic drink, with symptoms of:

- confusion
- delirium
- hallucinations
- disorientation
- hypertension
- tachycardia
- tachypnoea
- tremors.

A benzodiazepine is the treatment of choice for alcohol withdrawal syndrome and DTs, and is administered according to severity of clinical presentation and response (Kelly & Saucier 2004). Ongoing assessment of the patient and review of whether withdrawal symptoms are resolving is needed to determine whether the patient can be managed in the acute care setting as planned or if referral to specialist substance misuse services is required.

Common disorders influencing psycho-social health

Cognitive impairment from delirium, dementia, or depression is frequently found with acute care patients and with an increased risk for developing in people aged 65 years or older (Pountney 2007). The clinical signs and symptoms of these three different conditions can be very similar, causing confusion for the healthcare team as to what is the underlying cause of the problem. Further difficulty in assessing and managing older patients with impaired cognition comes when there is a combination of delirium, dementia, or depression. These conditions will now be explored in terms of the nursing assessment and management in acute care to differentiate the relevance of each for acute care nursing.

Delirium

Delirium is an acute, reversible cognitive disorder that develops quickly (hours to days) and fluctuates over a period of time. Delirium is characterized by a disruption in the normal sleep–wake cycle and results in either increased or decreased psychomotor activity. The delirious patient may be hyperactive (agitated), hypoactive (quiet and withdrawn), or a combination of both types of delirium. As there is increased morbidity, mortality, length of hospital stay, and financial cost from delirium, there has been increased awareness and priority given to assessing for and managing delirium in acute care in recent years. At the time of publication, new national guidelines for delirium from the National Institute for Health and Clinical Excellence (NICE) were still being written and are expected to be available for 2010.

There are a numerous causes of delirium in acute care, making it difficult to identify the actual cause when multiple potential reasons for the patient to develop delirium coexist. In fact, any acute illness and a large number of medications will cause delirium, although common precipitants (associated causes) include:

+ medications—sedatives, analgesics, antidepressants, poly-pharmacy
+ substance misuse—alcohol, drugs, other medications
+ alcohol/drug withdrawal
+ infection—urinary tract infection, pneumonia, sepsis
+ neurological—stroke, head injury, epilepsy
+ cardiovascular—reduced cardiac output, hypotension, anaemia
+ respiratory—hypoxia
+ renal—fluid deficit, electrolyte imbalance
+ endocrine/metabolic disorders—thyroid, acid/base imbalance.

There are also a variety of risk factors for developing delirium:

+ age (elderly)
+ alcoholism
+ pre-existing cognitive impairment
+ depression
+ hypertension
+ smoking
+ sensory impairment—vision, hearing
+ immobilizations
+ sleep disturbances
+ high severity of illness
+ change in normal environment.

Patient presentation

The assessment findings that could potentially indicate delirium include:

+ altered level of consciousness
+ disorientation to person, place, or time
+ poor concentration
+ lack of attention
+ poor short-term memory
+ delusions
+ hallucinations
+ altered sleep patterns
+ lethargic or restless/agitated

- incoherent speech
- emotional or personality changes.

Clearly these signs and symptoms could be caused by many other neurological or mental health disorders. The interpretation of clinical assessment findings requires the nurse to critically analyse the current situation in relation to the fundamental definition of delirium as an acute, fluctuating episode of cognitive impairment. A baseline of cognitive functioning is crucial to compare to. Discussion with family members, carers, other nurses, and medical colleagues will also prove useful while attempting to determine whether a patient is experiencing delirium. Finally, there are screening tools developed for identifying delirium, including the Confusion Assessment Method (CAM) (Inouye *et al*. 1990), the NEECHAM Scale (Neelon *et al*. 1996), and the Nursing Delirium Screening Scale (Nu-DESC) (Gaudreau *et al*. 2005).

Nursing management

Management of delirium should always begin with consideration for the cause of the delirium to plan care that is aimed at resolving the underpinning clinical problem that has brought on the delirium (Table 9.8). Preventative measures for patients at a high risk for developing delirium (e.g. elderly patient moved from a nursing home, patient with sensory impairment, or postoperative patient receiving analgesia) can also be taken, for instance involving the family to reassure and reorientate the patient, ensuring a patient with sensory deficits has necessary aids within reach such as hearing aids or glasses, and reducing noise levels at night to promote regular sleeping patterns.

Although pharmacological management of delirium should be avoided if at all possible, when delirium is exacerbating to the point of physical harm for the patient or others, medications may be required. Discussion with the medical team and pharmacist will be beneficial both for reviewing current medications that may be causing the delirium and to decide what type of medication is best suited to relieve severe agitation.

Dementia

Dementia is characterized by a progressive, irreversible deterioration in mental function from chronic conditions such as Alzheimer's disease, vascular dementia, dementia with Lewy bodies, frontotemporal dementia, and Parkinson's disease (NICE 2006) (Table 9.9). The main distinguishing feature of dementia differentiating it from delirium is that it is a chronic syndrome as compared with a reversible, acute abnormality in cognition. A patient may not be necessarily admitted into acute care because of dementia but a high percentage of hospitalized patients have dementia as a secondary health problem that requires acute care nurses to have a comprehensive understanding of its features and management.

Patient presentation

Patients with dementia have a wide range of signs and symptoms such as:

- disorientation to person, place, and time
- confused speech
- loss of memory
- hallucinations
- delusions
- anxiety

- agitation
- aggression
- agitation
- wandering
- hoarding
- loss of sexual inhibition
- apathy
- shouting
- change in personality
- language impairment.

Table 9.8 Delirium

Potential problem	Nursing care
Altered level of consciousness	Undertake a neurological assessment (see Chapter 4) to rule out a physical neurological illness/injury Monitor Glasgow Coma Scale regularly to assess for any change or deterioration in level of consciousness Monitor vital signs and physiological functioning of other body systems to rule out other physical illnesses/injuries that may be causing delirium Report any change in level of consciousness or physiological abnormalities to medical team
Severe agitation	Assess the safety of patient and the safety of others in the current environment Provide reassurance and support to try and calm the patient Remove any stimulants that appear to be causing the agitation Orientate patient with personal, familiar objects Ensure necessary aids for communication are available to the patient if there are sensory deficits Arrange for a translator if there is a language barrier Assess for pain, nausea, or other discomfort and treat as appropriate Ambulate/sit patient out of bed if possible Review current medications for potential causes of agitation and discuss with doctor and pharmacist medical management of delirium
Physical harm to self or others	Do not use mechanical restraints if at all possible Consider interventions for agitation as listed above Discuss with doctor and pharmacist medical management of delirium
Altered sleep	Promote regular day and night routines, including light during the day and darkness at night Provide clock or watch in order for patient to remain orientated to the 24-h day
Distressed family	Provide reassurance and support for family members Provide education and information about the patient condition, including delirium Encourage family to be involved in care as appropriate to help comfort the patient and allow for family interaction
Fluid/nutritional deficit	Monitor input and output of food/fluid to ensure patient is receiving adequate hydration and nutrition Monitor for signs and symptoms of fluid deficit Encourage and help with oral intake if the patient is unable or not willing to eat and drink

Table 9.9 Dementia

Potential problem	Nursing care
Reduced ability to achieve activities of daily living	Establish baseline from patient, notes, carers, or family members about normal daily functioning of the patient and ability to achieve activities of daily living Assess patient's current ability for personal hygiene, eating/drinking independently, toileting, and mobilizing and plan nursing interventions as appropriate
Cognitive impairment	Discuss daily routine and schedule with patient and review regularly to help patient orientate to hospital routine Frequent reminders of day, time, location, and names of healthcare providers Clear sign of patient's location in hospital setting (e.g. patient's name on door and near bed) Memory cues using family photos, clock, and calendar Stimulation through activities with volunteers, television, radio, and reading (Gillis & MacDonald 2006)
Severe agitation	Assess the safety of patient and the safety of others in the current environment Provide reassurance and support to try and calm the patient Remove any stimulants that appear to be causing the agitation Orientate patient with personal, familiar objects Ensure that necessary aids for communication are available to the patient if there are sensory deficits Arrange for a translator if there is a language barrier Assess for pain, nausea, discomfort, hunger, or thirst and treat as appropriate Assess for potential causes of agitation other than dementia (e.g. infection, hypoxia, neurological illness/injury) Review current medications for potential causes of agitation and discuss with doctor and pharmacist medical management of agitation as necessary
Physical harm to self or others	Do not use mechanical restraints if at all possible Consider interventions for agitation as listed above Discuss with doctor and pharmacist medical management of harmful behaviour
Distressed family	Provide reassurance and support for family members Provide education and information about the patient condition, including delirium Encourage family to be involved in care as appropriate to help comfort the patient and allow for family interaction Provide information from NICE (2006) on dementia in the format for patients, carers, and the public Provide information about national, local, and online family support groups for family members of people with dementia

Nursing management

The nursing care of the patient with dementia in the acute care setting will focus on supporting the patient to achieve activities of daily living to the best of the patient's abilities as affected by the dementia. A patient with dementia may become agitated and distressed with a change in environment thus displaying abnormal behaviour and worsening cognitive functioning after being admitted to hospital. It is important to rule out similar signs and symptoms that overlap with delirium to ensure that the patient is not experiencing an acute episode of cognitive impairment over and above the underlying dementia (e.g. from a urinary tract infection). If a patient requires medications to control harmful behaviour, NICE (2006) recommends offering the oral route first and to avoid intravenous administration. When the oral route is not possible or not effective, an intramuscular injection of haloperidol, lorazepam, or olanzapine with preferably just one medication used (NICE 2006). For patients with dementia who are being discharged from hospital, the Department of Health (2003b) provides a checklist to help with discharge arrangements and ensure the patient's physical, mental, and social health needs are being met.

Depression

Depression is defined by NICE (2004) as a low mood or loss of interest that is typically accompanied by one or more of the following: low energy, changes in appetite, weight or sleep pattern, poor concentration, feelings of guilt or worthlessness, and suicidal ideation. In general hospital settings, patients should be screened for depression if they have a past history of depression, significant physical illness causing disability, or other mental health problems such as dementia. A two-question screening test as recommended by NICE (2004, p. 6) includes:

- 'During the last month, have you often been bothered by feeling down, depressed, or hopeless?'

and

- 'During the last month, have you often been bothered by having little interest or pleasure in doing things?'

Patient presentation

As a mood disorder, depression typically presents with features such as:

- low mood
- feelings of sadness and guilt
- loss of enjoyment
- poor memory and concentration
- tiredness and fatigue
- suicidal thoughts or plans for suicide
- delusions.

Nursing management

The entirety of managing patients with depression, both in and out of the hospital setting, is beyond the scope of this book. However, the nursing management of a patient in acute care who has a mental health disorder is to focus on identifying abnormality of the mental health system and referring on to the acute care medical team and specialist mental health services as necessary. Specialist care is particularly important if: the diagnosis of depression is uncertain, there are multiple physical problems, there is a suicide risk, the patient has not previously responded to first-line treatment or if there are psychotic symptoms such as delusions (Department of Health 2008c).

Depression is highlighted as the final condition discussed in this chapter because of the high prevalence of depression with people experiencing chronic illness and disability as well as those with dementia and the elderly (Department of Health 2008c). Although the acute care nurse may not be directly planning interventions to act upon severe states of clinical depression, many patients in acute care experience feelings of sadness and loss as a result of the illness or injury causing hospital admission. Integrated into the nursing care for all patients can be an assessment of mental and social well-being as previously described in this chapter. Empathetic communication

Clinical link 9.1 (see Appendix for answers)

A 70-year-old female patient has been admitted to a medical ward from A&E, where she was brought in by ambulance after a neighbour had found her confused and wandering in the street. The admitting diagnosis was a suspected urinary tract infection based on the initial urinalysis result completed in A&E, although the full microbiology report is still pending from the urine culture and sensitivity.

The A&E nurse was able to pass on some social history details about the patient that were obtained from the neighbour who came into the A&E earlier in the day. The neighbour has since gone home but the handover report from the A&E nurse offered the following information:

♦ has lived alone since husband died 4 years ago

♦ has three adult children (two daughters who live abroad and one son who lives locally)

♦ independent with activities of daily living, although neighbour reports the outside of patient's house has not been attended to over the past 6 months (grass is very overgrown and the patient no longer keeps a garden although she did for many years)

♦ normally not confused but neighbour states he had an 'unusual' conversation with the patient a few months ago when she locked herself out of the house and appeared to have forgotten where she was

♦ remains active with her church activities and belongs to a weekly bridge group.

You undertake an assessment of the patient which reveals the following:

♦ temperature 37.2°C, BP 140/80 mmHg, pulse 110 beats/min, respirations 20 breaths/min, oxygen saturations 97% on room air

♦ agitated, restless, and unable to maintain eye contact

♦ oriented to person but disoriented to place and time

♦ mumbling to herself and unable to answer questions appropriately or follow commands

♦ pupils equal, round, and reactive to light

♦ mucous membranes pink but dry with coated tongue

♦ moving all limbs spontaneously with equal strength and movement

♦ skin pink, warm, and dry with capillary refill <2 s

♦ breath sounds clear throughout all lung fields

♦ respirations regular and easy without use of accessory muscles

♦ pedal pulses palpable with bilateral oedema present up to ankles

♦ abdomen round but soft with active bowel sounds

♦ skin intact with no apparent wounds or rashes

♦ wears glasses and a hearing aid to left ear.

Identify aspects from the health history and assessment findings which indicate that this patient may be experiencing delirium, depression, and/or dementia. What investigations and treatments does this patient appear to need? How would you support the psychosocial needs of the patient?

skills and interventions to help patients feel emotionally supported will also help patients experiencing low states of mood.

End of chapter test

The learning you gained from this chapter can be assessed by working through an evaluation of your knowledge and skill in undertaking a psychosocial assessment as well as suitable interventions for acting on the psychosocial assessment findings.

Knowledge assessment

Evaluate your understanding of these aspects of psychosocial assessment and care:

♦ Provide a definition for 'health', including the components that contribute to a person's health status.

♦ Rationalize why effective communication skills are necessary for acute care nursing practice.

♦ Identify verbal and non-verbal communication skills that can be used while interacting with patients, family members, or others.

♦ Explain the process of an ABC mental health assessment.

♦ Recognize common abnormalities in affect, behaviour, or cognition.

♦ Define mental capacity.

♦ Identify four key abilities a person with full mental capacity should be able to demonstrate.

♦ List the five statutory principles underpinning the Mental Health Act 2005.

♦ Describe the two-stage test of capacity.

♦ Differentiate between Lasting Power of Attorney, Deputy, Court of Protection, Public Guardian, Office of the Public Guardian, IMCA, Advance Decisions, and Deprivation of Liberty Safeguards.

♦ Explain the relevance for assessing the mental capacity of patients within acute care.

♦ Identify physical signs and symptoms that could be secondary to a mental health disorder or a side effect from a medication prescribed for a mental health disorder.

♦ Evaluate why patients with mental illness are at risk for poor physical health.

♦ Differentiate between spirituality and religion, and explain why assessing and documenting the spiritual needs of a patient is an acute care nursing responsibility.

♦ Recognize four core principles of family-centred nursing care.

♦ Explain the concept of transcultural nursing, including key characteristics of a nurse with cultural competence.

♦ Evaluate the assessment of post-discharge social care needs of a patient.

♦ Rationalize why screening for substance misuse is necessary in acute care.

♦ Describe different alcohol screening tools, recognizing their advantages and disadvantages.

♦ Compare and contrast alcohol withdrawl syndrome from DTs, including clinical signs and symptoms for both.

♦ Provide a definition for delirium, dementia, and depression and how they are all managed in acute care.

Skills assessment

Under the guidance of your practice mentor/supervisor, undertake these actions to evaluate your ability to undertake a psychosocial assessment and plan appropriate actions.

- ◆ Complete a health history of a patient utilizing a variety of verbal and non-verbal communication skills.
- ◆ Assess a patient's mental health status, including:
  - ABC assessment
  - mental capacity assessment
  - physical assessment interpreting whether there is any association between physical abnormalities and a mental health disorder
  - spirituality assessment.
- ◆ Assess a patient's social health status, including:
  - family, friends, and significant others
  - cultural needs
  - post-discharge social care needs
  - substance misuse.
- ◆ Identify abnormalities found during the psychosocial assessment, interpret these findings within the context of the patient situation, and plan interventions as necessary.
- ◆ Document the psychosocial assessment and nursing care plan with associated actions.
- ◆ Evaluate all actions with nursing care plan updated as needed.
- ◆ Explain the local practice where you work with visiting times and any situations when flexibility is used to allow visitors outside of set visiting hours.
- ◆ Find relevant hospital policies related to the psychosocial system, including:
  - visiting times
  - substance misuse
  - spiritual care services
  - end-of-life care.
- ◆ Explain how to refer to the following services:
  - social work
  - chaplaincy/spiritual care
  - mental health team
  - occupational therapy
  - district nursing
  - GP practices
  - voluntary organizations.

References

Babor, T.F., Higgins-Biddle, J.C., Saunders, J.B., and Monterio, M.G. (2001) *AUDIT: The Alcohol Use Disorders Identification Test.* (online). Available at: http://whqlibdoc.who.int/hq/2001/WHO_MSD_MSB_01.6 a.pdf (accessed 03 Aug 2009).

Black Mental Health UK. (2008) Alan Johnson to tackle widening health gap. *Black Mental Health UK.* (Online). Available at: http://www.blackmentalhealth.org.uk/index.php?option=com_content&task=view&id=343&Itemid=117 (accessed 03 Aug 2009).

Department for Constitutional Affairs (2005) *Mental Capacity Act 2005.* (Online). Available at: http://www.opsi.gov.uk/acts/acts2005/pdf/ukpga_20050009_en.pdf (accessed 03 Aug 2009).

Department for Constitutional Affairs (2007a) *Mental Capacity Act 2005: Code of Practice.* The Stationary Office, London.

Department for Constitutional Affairs (2007b) *Mental Health Act 2007.* (Online). Available at: http://www.opsi.gov.uk/acts/acts2007/ukpga_20070012_en_1 (accessed 03 Aug 2009).

Department of Health (2003a) *NHS Chaplaincy Meeting the Religious and Spiritual Needs of Patients.* (Online). Available at: http://www.dh.gov.uk/en/Publicationsandstatistics/Publications/PublicationsPolicyAndGuidance/DH_4073108 (accessed 03 Aug 2009).

Department of Health (2003b) Discharge from Hospital: Getting it right for people with dementia. A supplementary checklist to help with planning the discharge from acute general hospital settings of people with dementia. (Online). Available at: http://www.dh.gov.uk/en/Publicationsandstatistics/Publications/PublicationsPolicyAndGuidance/DH_4007881 (accessed 03 Aug 2009).

Department of Health (2004) *The NHS Knowledge and Skills Framework* (NHS KSF) and the Development Review Process. (Online). Available at: http://www.dh.gov.uk/en/Publicationsandstatistics/Publications/PublicationsPolicyAndGuidance/DH_4090843 (accessed 03 Aug 2009).

Department of Health (2007) *Independent Mental Capacity Advocate (IMCA) Service.* (Online). Available at: http://www.dh.gov.uk/en/SocialCare/Deliveringadultsocialcare/MentalCapacity/IMCA/index.htm (accessed 03 Aug 2009).

Department of Health (2008a) *The Mental Capacity Act 2005 Deprivation of Liberty Safeguards.* (Online). Available at: http://www.dh.gov.uk/en/SocialCare/Deliveringadultsocialcare/MentalCapacity/MentalCapacityActDeprivationofLibertySafeguards/index.htm (accessed 03 Aug 2009).

Department of Health (2008b) *Safe. Sensible. Social. The Government's Alcohol Strategy.* (Online). Available at: http://www.dh.gov.uk/en/Publichealth/Healthimprovement/Alcoholmisuse/DH_085386 (accessed 03 Aug 2009).

Department of Health (2008c) *Depression.* (Online). Available at: http://www.dh.gov.uk/en/Publicationsandstatistics/Publications/PublicationsPolicyAndGuidance/Browsable/DH_4901990 (accessed 03 Aug 2009).

Department of Health, Social Services and Public Safety (2008) *Guiding Principles for the Production of Hospital Visiting Policies.* (Online). Available at: http://www.dhsspsni.gov.uk/visiting_policies_-_june_2008.pdf (accessed 03 Aug 2009).

Disability Rights Commission (2006) *Equal Treatment: Closing the Gap. Formal Investigation into Physical Health Inequalities Experienced by People with Learning Disabilities or Mental Health Problems.* Disability Rights Commission, London.

Disability Rights Commission. (2007) Equal Treatment: Closing the Gap—One Year On. (Online). Available at: http://www.learningdisabilitiesuk.org.uk/docs/DRCrpt.pdf (accessed 03 Aug 2009).

Dute, J. (2005) ECHR 2005/1 Case of H. L. v. United Kingdom, 5 October 2004, no. 45508/99 (Fourth Section). *Eur. J. Health Law.* **12**, 77–90.

Fenton, W.S. and Stover, E.S. (2006) Mood disorders: Cardiovascular and diabetes comorbidity. *Curr. Opin. Psychiatr.* **19**(4), 421–427.

Fitch, C., R. Daw, N. Balmer, K. Gray, and M. Skipper. (2008) *Fair Deal for Mental Health.* Royal College of Psychiatrists, London.

Folstein, M.F., Folstein, S.E., and McHugh, P.R. (1975) 'Mini-mental state.' A practical method for grading the cognitive state of patients for the clinician. *J. Psychiatr. Res.* **12**(3), 189–98.

Gaudreau, J.D., Gagnon, P., Harel, F. *et al.* (2005) Fast, systematic, and continuous delirium assessment in hospitalized patients: The nursing delirium screening scale. *J. Pain Symp. Manag.* **29**, 368–75.

Gillis, A.J. and MacDonald, B. (2006) Unmasking delirium. *Canad. Nurse* **102**(9), 19–24.

Hanson, S.M. (2001) Family health care nursing: An introduction. In: Hanson, S.M. (ed.), *Family Health Care Nursing: Theory*, Practice, and Research, 2nd edn, pp. 3–35. F.A. Davis, Philadelphia.

Health Development Agency (2002) *Manual for the Fast Alcohol Screening Tool (FAST)*. Health Development Agency, London. (Online). Available at: http://www.nice.org.uk/niceMedia/documents/manual_fastalcohol.pdf (accessed 03 Aug 2009).

Hodgson, R.J., Alwyn, T., John, B. *et al.* (2002) The FAST Screening Test. *Alcohol Alcoholism.* **37**, 61–66.

Inouye SK, van Dyck CH, Alessi CA *et al.* (1990) Clarifying confusion: The confusion assessment method. A new method for detection of delirium. *Ann. Int. Med.* **113**, 941–8.

International Council of Nurses (2002) *Nurses Always There For You: Caring For Families. Information and Action Tool Kit*. International Council of Nurses, Geneva.

Institute for Family-Centered Care (2008) *What is Patient and Family Centered Health Care?* (Online). Available at: http://www.familycenteredcare.org/faq.html (accessed 03 Aug 2009).

Ismail, S. and Mulley, G. (2007) Visiting times. *BMJ.* **335**, 1316–7.

Kelly, A. and Saucier, J. (2004) Is your patient suffering from alcohol withdrawl?. *RN.* **67**(2), 27–31.

Kwok, H. and Cheung, P.W.H. (2007) Co-morbidity of psychiatric disorder and medical illness in people with intellectual disabilities. *Curr. Opin. Psychiatr.* **20**(5), 443–449.

Ledger, S.D. (2005) The duty of nurses to meet patients' spiritual and/or religious needs. *Br. J. Nurs.* **14**(4), 220–225.

Lee, S. (2007) *Making Decisions: The Independent Mental Capacity Advocate (IMCA) Service*. (Online). Available at: http://www.dca.gov.uk/legal-policy/mental-capacity/mibooklets/booklet06.pdf (accessed 03 Aug 2009).

Leininger, M. and McFarland, M.R. (2002) *Transcultural Nursing: Concepts, Theories, Research and Practice*, 3rd edn. McGraw-Hill, New York.

MacLaren, J. (2004) A kaleidoscope of understandings: Spiritual nursing in a multi-faith society. *J. Adv. Nurs.* **45**(5), 457–64.

Maslow, A.H. (1943) A theory of human motivation. *Psychol. Rev.* **50**, 370–96.

Mayfield, D., McLeod, G., and Hall, P. (1974) The CAGE questionnaire: Validation of a new alcoholism instrument. *Am. J. Psychiatr.* **131**, 1121–3.

McBrien, B. (2005) A concept analysis of spirituality. *Br. J. Nurs.* **15**(1), 42–45.

McSherry,W. and Ross, L. (2002) Dilemmas in spiritual assessment: Considerations for nursing practice. *J. Adv. Nurs.* **38**(5), 479–88.

McSherry, W. and Watson, R. (2002) Spirituality in nursing care: Evidence of a gap between theory and practice. *J. Clin. Nurs.* **11**, 843–4.

Mental Health Foundation (2004) Black and minority ethnic communities and mental health. *Mental Health Foundation.* (Online). Available at: http://www.mentalhealth.org.uk/information/mental-health-a-z/black-minority-ethnic-communities/ (accessed 03 Aug 2009).

Ministry of Justice (2008) *Deprivation of Liberty Safeguards: Code of Practice to Supplement the Main Mental Capacity Act 2005 Code of Practice*. (Online). Available at: http://www.dh.gov.uk/en/Publicationsandstatistics/Publications/PublicationsPolicyAndGuidance/DH_085476 (accessed 03 Aug 2009).

Narayanasamy, A. (2004) Spiritual coping mechanisms in chronically ill patients. *Br. J. Nurs.* **11**(22), 1461–70.

National Audit Office (2008) *Reducing Alcohol Harm: Health Services in England for Alcohol Misuse*. (Online). Available at: http://www.nao.org.uk/publications/0708/reducing_alcohol_harm.aspx (accessed 03 Aug 2009).

National Treatment Agency for Substance Misuse (2008) *Good Practice in Harm Reduction*. (Online). Available at: http://www.nta.nhs.uk/publications/documents/nta_good_practice_in_harm_reduction_1108.pdf (accessed 03 Aug 2009).

NICE (2004) *Depression: Management of Depression in Primary and Secondary Care*. National Institute for Health and Clinical Excellence, London, (Online). Available at: http://www.nice.org.uk/CG023 (accessed 03 Aug 2009).

NICE (2006) *Dementia: Supporting People with Dementia and Their Carers in Health and Social Care*. National Institute for Health and Clinical Excellence, London. (Online). Available at: http://www.nice.org.uk/Guidance/CG42 (accessed 03 Aug 2009).

Neelon, V., Champagne, M., Carlson, J., and Funk, S. (1996) The NEECHAM confusion scale: Construction, validation, and clinical testing. *Nurs. Res.* **45**(6), 324–330.

Nursing and Midwifery Council (2004) *Standards of Proficiency for Pre-registration Nursing Education*. Nursing and Midwifery Council, London.

Office of the Public Guardian (2008a) *What Mental Capacity Is*. (Online). Available at: http://www.publicguardian.gov.uk/mca/what.htm (accessed 03 Aug 2009).

Office of the Public Guardian (2008b) *Lasting Power of Attorney*. (Online). Available at: http://www.publicguardian.gov.uk/arrangements/lpa.htm (accessed 03 Aug 2009).

Office of the Public Guardian (2008c) *Court Appointed Deputy—the Role and Duties*. (Online). Available at: http://www.publicguardian.gov.uk/decisions/deputy-roles-responsibilities.htm (accessed 03 Aug 2009).

Office of the Public Guardian (2008d) *Vulnerable Adults to Get Better Protection*. (Online). Available at: http://www.publicguardian.gov.uk/about/843.htm (accessed 03 Aug 2009).

Office of the Public Guardian (2008e) *Court of Protection*. (Online). Available at: http://www.publicguardian.gov.uk/about/court-of-protection.htm (accessed 03 Aug 2009).

Office of the Public Guardian (2008f) *The Public Guardian*. (Online). Available at: http://www.publicguardian.gov.uk/about/public-guardian.htm (accessed 03 Aug 2009).

Office of the Public Guardian (2008g) *Making Decisions: A Guide for People Who Work in Health and Social Care*. (Online). Available at: http://www.publicguardian.gov.uk/docs/making-decisions-opg603-1207.pdf (accessed 03 Aug 2009).

Pountney, D. (2007). Dementia, delirium, or depression?. *Nurs. Older People*. **19**(5), 12–14.

Purnell, L. (2005). The Purnell Model for cultural competence. *J. Multicultural Nurs. Health*. **11**(2), 7–15.

Rethink (2008). *What's the Physical Health Problem?* (Online). Available at: http://www.rethink.org/how_we_can_help/campaigning_for_change/opening_doors/physical_health/whats_the_physical.html (accessed 03 Aug 2009).

Robson, D. and Gray, R. (2007) Serious mental illness and physical health problems: A discussion paper. *Int. J. Nurs. Stud.* **44**, 457–66.

Seppa, K., Lepisto, J., and Sillanaukee, P. (1998) Five-shot questionnaire on heavy drinking. *Alcohol. Clin. Exp. Res.* **22**, 1788–91.

Smith, S. G. T., Touquet, R., Wright, S., and Das Gupta, N. (1996) Detection of alcohol misusing patients in accident and emergency departments: The Paddington alcohol test (PAT). *J. Acci. Emerg. Med.* **13**(5), 308–12.

Swift, C., Calcutawalla, S., and Elliot, R. (2007) Nursing attitudes towards recording of religious and spiritual data. *Br. J. Nurs.* **16**(20), 1279–82.

The NHS Information Centre (2008) *Statistics on Alcohol: England, 2008*. (Online). Available at: http://www.ic.nhs.uk/webfiles/publications/alcoholeng2008/Statistics%20on%20Alcohol-%20England%202008%20final%20format%20v7.pdf (accessed 03 Aug 2009).

Timmins, F. and Kelly, J. (2008). Spiritual assessment in intensive and cardiac care nursing. *Nurs. Crit. Care* **13**(3), 124–131.

Travis, J.W. (2004). Refining the Illness-wellness Continuum: (Online). Available at: http://www.thewellspring.com/flex/introduction-to-wellness/2443/refining-the-illness-wellness-continuum.cfm (accessed 03 Aug 2009).

World Health Organization (2003) *WHO Definition of Health*. (Online). Available at: http://www.who.int/about/definition/en/print.html (accessed 03 Aug 2009).

World Health Organization (2009a) *Substance Abuse.* (Online). Available at: http://www.who.int/topics/substance_abuse/en/ (accessed 03 Aug 2009).

World Health Organization (2009b) *Alcohol.* (Online). Available at: http://www.who.int/topics/alcohol_drinking/en/ (accessed 03 Aug 2009).

Bibliography

British Medical Association (2007) *Withholding and Withdrawing Life-prolonging Medical Treatment: Guidance for Decision Making.* 3rd edn. Blackwell Publishing, London.

Department for Constitutional Affairs (2005) *The Mental Capacity Act 2005.* (Online). Available at: http://www.opsi.gov.uk/acts/acts2005/pdf/ukpga_20050009_en.pdf (accessed 03 Aug 2009).

Department of Health (2005) *Independent Mental Capacity Advocates.* (Online). Available at: http://www.dh.gov.uk/en/SocialCare/Deliveringadultsocialcare/MentalCapacity/IMCA/index.htm (accessed 03 Aug 2009).

Ellis, R.B., Gates, B., and Kenworthy, N. (2003) *Interpersonal Communication in Nursing: Theory and Practice.* 2nd edn. Elsevier, London.

Falconer, C. (2007) *Foreword to the Mental Capacity Act Code of Practice.* (Online). Available at: http://www.dca.gov.uk/legal-policy/mental-capacity/mca-cp.pdf (accessed 03 Aug 2009).

Lynch, T. (2008) The Mental Capacity Act 1: Advance decisions. *Nurs. Times.* **104**, 42, 28–9.

Lynch, T. (2008) The Mental Capacity Act 2: patient advocacy and ethics. *Nurs. Times.* **104**, 43, 26–7.

McSherry, W. (2006) *Making Sense of Spirituality in Nursing and Health Care Practice: An Interactive Approach.* 2nd edn. Jessica Kingsley Publishers, London.

Sims, J., Kristian, M.R., and Iphofen, R. (2007). Profile of secondary care attendees with identified alcohol misuse problems. *Drugs Alcohol Today.* **7**(1), 16–24.

Sully, P. and Dallas, J. (2002). *Essential Communication Skills for Nursing Practice.* Elsevier Mosby, Edinburgh.

White, G. (2006) *Talking About Spirituality in Health Care Practice: A Resource for the Multi-professional Health Care Team.* Jessica Kingsley Publishers, London.

Wright, L.M. and Leahey, M. (2005) *Nurses and Families: A Guide to Gamily Assessment and Intervention.* 4th edn. F.A. Davis, Philadelphia.

Chapter 10

Blood investigations in acute care

Gary Creed

Chapter contents

Acutely ill patient management frequently involves the sampling and analysis of blood and urine tests. Investigations may be used diagnostically to either confirm or eliminate likelihood of disease or used therapeutically to guide treatment. It is estimated that the data received by clinicians from medical laboratories constitute 70–80% of the information they rely on to make major medical diagnoses (Blann 2008). It is essential therefore to have a broad understanding of routine laboratory investigations. This chapter will examine:

♦ urea and electrolytes, including sodium, potassium, urea, and creatinine

♦ estimated glomerular filtration rate (eGFR)

♦ liver function tests

♦ cardiac function tests (cardiac markers)

♦ glucose

♦ amylase

♦ magnesium

♦ calcium

♦ full blood count to include white blood cells, red blood cells, haemoglobin, and platelets

♦ marker of infection and inflammation: C-reactive protein (CRP)

♦ coagulation assessment.

Learning outcomes

This chapter will enable you to:

♦ understand most frequently requested blood tests

♦ examine the underpinning physiology that causes changes in blood results

♦ develop knowledge related to normal blood values

♦ identify where blood results are abnormal

♦ examine conditions that may cause derangements in blood results

♦ discuss patient management.

Introduction

This chapter aims to provide help and guidance in understanding the majority of the normal blood tests requested by clinicians to aid the assessment of a patient's clinical diagnosis and treatment.

REFERENCE LABORATORY RANGES | 307

The most frequently requested routine blood tests in the acute care setting conveniently fall into one of three groups:

♦ haematology

♦ chemical pathology

♦ haemostasis (coagulation).

It is impossible to fully understand laboratory tests without a sure grounding in physiology. Within this chapter there will be clear explanation of the associated physiology required to understand each test and its associated problems.

Reference laboratory ranges

The interpretation of any clinical laboratory test involves comparing the patient's results with the test's 'reference range'. The first step in determining a normal range is to define the population to which the range will apply. A large number of individuals who are thought representative of the 'normal' population will be tested for a particular laboratory test. Careful consideration is required as to whether sex, age, and ethnical subpopulations affect this derivation. The reference range is then derived mathematically. In this way, ranges quoted by labs will represent the values found in 95% of individuals in the chosen 'normal' group.

Examination of test results from different populations highlights that 'normal' for one group is not necessarily normal for another. Increasingly results will be provided with a normal range suitable for the demography of the particular patient, i.e. a male normal range for blood from a man. Indeed, ethnical issues may also need to be reflected in the normal range, for example creatinine and estimated GFR derivation are dependent on age, sex, and ethnicity.

It is important to consider that results from blood investigations may impact on patient treatment. The result must always be considered within the clinical context and take into consideration the patient's past medical history, current medication, and the results of any other investigations (Higgins 2007).

Please note that there may be slight variations in the reference ranges cited in this text and reference ranges within individual local areas. It is vital that practitioners view patients' blood results in relation to their hospitals' central laboratory reference ranges rather than those included in this book.

Assessment of fluid balance and renal function

Creatinine, urea, and electrolytes

♦ Normal/reference range

♦ Sodium: 135–145 mmol/L

♦ Potassium: 3.4–5.1 mmol/L

♦ Urea: 1.7–8.3 mmol/L

♦ Creatinine: female 45–105 umol/L, male 59–122 umol/L

♦ eGFR: >90 mL/min

Creatinine, urea, and electrolytes are the most commonly requested biochemical tests in clinical practice and may be used to screen for an electrolyte or pH imbalance and to monitor the effect of treatment on a known imbalance. Electrolytes are minerals that are found in body tissues and blood in the form of dissolved salts. As electrically charged particles, electrolytes help move nutrients into and wastes out of the body's cells, maintain water balance, and stabilize the body's acid/base. Electrolytes are usually measured as part of a renal profile that measures the main electrolytes in the body, sodium (Na$^+$), potassium (K$^+$), together with creatinine and urea. Most of the body's sodium is found in the extracellular fluid (ECF), where it helps to regulate water homeostasis. Potassium is found mainly in the intracellular fluid. Importantly, 98% of the potassium found within the body is located in skeletal muscle. A small but vital amount of potassium is found in the plasma. Monitoring potassium is important as small changes in the K$^+$ level can affect the heart's rhythm and ability to contract. Chloride travels in and out of the cells to help maintain electrical neutrality, and its level usually mirrors that of sodium. The main job of bicarbonate, which is excreted and reabsorbed by the kidneys, is to help maintain a stable pH level and, secondarily, to help maintain electrical neutrality.

Since electrolytes are often abnormal in a variety of acute and chronic illnesses, they are the most frequently requested profile in hospitalized patients.

Sodium

Sodium is present in all body fluids and its homeostasis is maintained within a very small concentration range by:

♦ producing hormones that can increase or decrease sodium losses in urine, including natriuretic peptides and aldosterone

♦ producing antidiuretic hormone that prevents water loss

♦ controlling thirst (even a 1% increase in blood sodium will make patients extremely thirsty)

♦ administration of appropriate intravenous fluids.

Abnormal blood sodium is usually due to abnormalities with one or more of the above. When the level of sodium in the blood changes, the water content in the body compartments also change (see Chapter 7).

Blood sodium is usually monitored in acute illness and may be abnormal in many diseases; clinicians may request this test if the patient has symptoms involving the brain, lungs, liver, heart, kidney, thyroid, or adrenal glands.

Urine sodium levels are typically tested in patients who have abnormal blood sodium levels, to help determine whether an imbalance is due to taking in too much sodium or losing too much sodium. It may be used to see if a patient with high blood pressure is consuming too much salt. It is often used in patients with abnormal kidney function to help the clinician determine the cause of kidney disease, which can help guide treatment (Kumar & Berl 1998).

Hyponatraemia

Decreased blood sodium concentration is called hyponatraemia and is usually due to sodium loss (diarrhoea, vomiting, excessive sweating, diuretic administration, kidney disease, or Addison's disease). In some cases, it is due to excess fluids in the body (excessive fluid/water intake/administration, heart failure, cirrhosis, and kidney diseases that cause protein loss) and malnutrition. In a number of diseases (particularly those involving the brain and the lungs, many kinds of cancer, and with some drugs) the body secretes increased levels of anti-diuretic hormone, causing the patient to retain fluid. (Peng 2004). Hyponatraemia is rarely due to decreased sodium intake.

Drugs such as diuretics, sulphonylureas (diabetic drugs), angiotensin-converting enzyme (ACE) inhibitors, heparin, non steroidal anti inflammatory drugs, tricyclic antidepressants, and vasopressin, among others, can decrease sodium levels (Adrogue & Madias 2000).

If sodium levels fall rapidly, the patient may feel weak and tired and in severe cases, experience confusion or lose consciousness. When sodium falls slowly, however, symptoms may be mild or absent highlighting the significance of checking sodium levels even if convincing symptoms are absent (Lee et al. 2000).

Hypernatraemia

Increased blood sodium concentration is referred to as hypernatraemia and is almost always due to excessive loss of water without adequate water intake. Symptoms include dry mucous membranes, thirst, agitation, restlessness, acting irrationally, and coma or convulsions if levels rise extremely high. In rare cases, hypernatraemia may be due to increased salt intake without enough water, Cushing's syndrome, or too little anti-diuretic hormone (diabetes insipidus).

Recent trauma, surgery, or shock may increase sodium levels because blood flow to the kidneys is decreased. Drugs such as lithium and anabolic steroids may increase sodium levels; this is uncommon with most other drugs.

Potassium

Potassium is present in all body fluids, but the highest concentration of potassium is in the intracellular fluid, with only a very small amount in the serum or plasma component of the blood. Abnormal concentration can alter the function of the nerves and muscles, for example in extreme cases patients may experience heart rhythm disturbances or the heart muscle may even lose its ability to contract.

Blood potassium levels are routinely measured in those who take diuretics or heart medications, and in the investigation of high blood pressure and kidney disease. It is also used to monitor patients on kidney dialysis or diuretic therapy, and patients receiving intravenous infusions.

Hyperkalaemia

A raised blood potassium level is called hyperkalaemia. This may indicate:

- kidney disease
- Addison's disease
- injury to tissue
- infection
- diabetes
- excessive intravenous potassium intake (in patients on an intravenous infusion).

Certain drugs can also cause hyperkalaemia in a small percentage of patients. These include non-steroidal anti-inflammatory drugs (such as ibuprofen); beta-blockers, ACE inhibitors and potassium-sparing diuretics (Evans 2005; Schafer & Wolford 2005).

The way that blood is taken and handled may cause the potassium level in the sample to be falsely high. If the patient clenches and relaxes their fist a lot while blood is being collected, this can make potassium rise. If blood comes out of the veins too fast or too slow, the blood cells can burst (haemolyse) and release potassium into the blood, giving a falsely raised potassium result. Some tubes that are used to collect blood into contain potassium salts as a preservative. If blood is collected into one of these by mistake potassium will be falsely high. Potassium can also be elevated if the specimen takes a long while to travel from the GP surgery or hospital ward to the central laboratory (Gennari 1998; Rastergar & Soleimani 2001).

Hypokalaemia

A low blood level of potassium is called hypokalaemia. This may occur in a number of conditions, including:

- vomiting
- diarrhoea

+ deficient potassium intake (this is rare)

+ inappropriate intravenous fluid administration.

Low potassium is commonly due to diuretics, which will require potassium level to be checked regularly. If the patient has diabetes, potassium concentration may fall after insulin dose, particularly if blood glucose levels have been poorly managed. Serum potassium levels may also be depleted during the administration of intravenous salbutamol (Caraway & Olsson 2008).

A patient's acid–base status will produce marked variations in potassium concentration. Acidosis will promote the movement of potassium from the intracellular fluid to the ECF, leading to an increase in serum potassium concentration and possible hyperkalaemia. Alkalotic patients however show a movement of potassium from the ECF into the intracellular fluid, leading to a decrease in serum potassium concentration and possible hypokalaemia.

Urea

When protein is broken down by normal metabolism ammonia is produced, which is neurotoxic and hepato-toxic. In order for safe excretion ammonia is converted by the liver into urea, which can safely be removed in urine. If liver function is compromised urea levels will be affected. Healthy kidneys eliminate more than 90% of the urea the body produces, so blood levels indicate the effectiveness of renal function. Urea and creatinine levels are used to evaluate kidney function and to monitor patients with kidney failure or those receiving dialysis.

Urea is often requested with creatinine:

+ if kidney problems are suspected

+ to monitor treatment of kidney disease

+ to monitor kidney function while on certain drugs.

High urea levels suggest impaired kidney function, which may be due to acute or chronic kidney disease. However, there are many things besides kidney disease that can affect urea levels, such as decreased blood flow to the kidneys if clinical shock is present.

Low urea levels are not common and are not usually a cause for concern. They can be seen in severe liver disease or malnutrition. Urea levels increase with age and also with the amount of protein in the diet. High-protein diets may cause abnormally high urea levels. Very low-protein diets can cause abnormally low urea. Drugs that impair kidney function may increase urea levels.

Urea levels increase with age, and are also slightly higher in men. Urea levels are normally slightly lower in pregnancy, especially in the last few months when the foetus is using large amounts of protein for growth (Zuccaro 1998; Waikar & Bonventre 2006).

Creatinine

Creatinine is produced in muscles when a compound called creatine spontaneously breaks down. Creatine is used to produce the energy needed to contract muscles and it is produced at a relatively constant rate. Almost all creatinine is excreted by the kidneys, so blood levels are a good measure of renal function, with increased sensitivity to urea.

A combination of blood and urine creatinine levels may be used to calculate a 'creatinine clearance'. This measures how effectively the kidneys are filtering small molecules like creatinine from the bloodstream (see Chapter 5). Increased creatinine levels in the blood suggest diseases that affect kidney function. These can include:

+ glomerulonephritis

+ pyelonephritis

- acute tubular necrosis
- urinary tract obstruction
- reduced blood flow to the kidney due to shock.

Creatinine can also increase as a result of muscle injury. Low levels of creatinine are not common and are not usually a cause for concern. As creatinine levels are related to the amount of muscle the person has, low levels may be a consequence of decreased muscle mass (such as in the elderly), but may also be occasionally found in advanced liver disease.

Since creatinine levels are in proportion to muscle mass, women tend to have lower levels. In general, creatinine levels will stay the same if the patient maintains a normal diet. However, eating large amounts of meat may cause short-lived increases in blood creatinine levels. Taking creatinine supplements may also increase creatinine. General moderate exercise will not affect creatinine levels. Creatinine levels relate to both muscle mass and to kidney function. As an individual's age increases, muscle mass tends to decrease but the kidneys tend to function less effectively. The net result is not much change in creatinine levels in the blood as patients get older (Hilton 2006; Schrier 2006, 2008).

Estimated glomerular filtration rate (calculated creatinine clearance)

For a more definitive assessment of kidney function, or to monitor changes in kidney function measurement of creatinine clearance is preferred. Creatinine clearance can be calculated using age, weight, gender, and serum creatinine; in some formulae, race is also used in the calculation.

Measured creatinine clearance, which gives an assessment of glomerular filtration rate (GFR), is calculated from serum and urine creatinine levels. This requires a blood sample and normally a 24-h collection of urine. Creatinine clearance gives an assessment of GFR, which in turn is a measure of kidney function.

Calculated creatinine clearance is an estimate of creatinine clearance based on the serum creatinine value only and used when it is either not practical or possible to collect 24-h urine. Creatinine clearance is a more accurate way to detect changes in kidney status than measurement of serum urea and creatinine, which are easier to do but cannot pick up early damage to the kidneys. If kidney damage is detected early, it may be possible to prevent further damage. The calculation of eGFR that has been adopted in the UK uses a formula that uses the concentration of creatinine in blood, the age and sex of the patient, and their ethnic original.

Since April 2006 eGFR, 'estimated GFR' or calculated creatinine clearance has been routinely offered by the majority of UK laboratories. It has been introduced to improve the detection of early kidney damage so that measures can be taken to stop or at least slow the progression to more severe kidney damage. eGFR is suitable for most patients who are 18 or more years old, not pregnant or malnourished, and do not have acute kidney damage. GPs and UK laboratories are now using eGFR to look for the presence of kidney damage in various 'at risk groups', including people with diabetes, blood vessel disease, heart problems, high blood pressure, obstructions to urine flow, and in patients taking some commonly prescribed drugs, including diuretics and a variety of drugs used to treat high blood pressure.

A normal result means that kidney disease is less likely, while a low value suggests that some kidney damage has occurred. Creatinine clearance results are usually evaluated in the same way. Sometimes, in very early kidney damage (especially when the kidneys are damaged by diabetes), measured or estimated clearance may actually be high, indicating that the kidneys are working harder than normal. Creatinine clearance can increase during pregnancy.

Clinical link 10.1 (see Appendix for answers)

Fred Smith is a 76-year-old man admitted to the medical assessment unit following prolonged history of vomiting. His observations are:

BP: 120/60

HR: 102

CVP 2

RR: 21

A blood test is requested and the results show:

NA: 147

K: 4.0

Urea: 9.8

Creatinine: 122

Discuss these results alongside this patient's presenting symptoms. What treatment is most appropriate?

Direct measurement of the GFR is complicated and requires experienced personnel. The most commonly used method for determining the GFR is the creatinine clearance method mentioned above (Smith & Shilpak 2006; Beauuvieux & Barthie 2007; McDonough 2007).

Assessment of liver function

Normal/reference range

♦ Alanine transaminase (ALT): <55 IU/L

♦ Aspartate transaminase (AST): <35 IU/L

♦ Alkaline phosphatase (ALP): 31–129 IU/L

♦ Gamma glutamyl transferase (GGT): <72 IU/L

♦ Albumin: 35–52 g/L

♦ Total protein: 64–86 g/L

♦ Bilirubin: <17umol/L

Liver function tests

Liver function tests are used to detect liver damage or disease. Combinations of up to five tests are measured at the same time on a blood sample (Gopal & Rosen 2000; Skelly & James 2001; Smellie & Ryder 2006).

Alanine aminotransferase

Alanine aminotransferase (ALT) is an enzyme found mostly in the liver; smaller amounts are also found in the kidneys, heart, and muscles. Under normal conditions, ALT levels in the blood are low. When the liver is damaged, ALT is released into the bloodstream, usually before more obvious symptoms of liver damage occur, such as jaundice. It is an especially useful test in patients with hepatitis.

The ALT test detects liver injury. ALT values are usually assessed along with the values found for other enzymes, such as alkaline phosphatase (ALP) and aspartate aminotransferase (AST), to help determine which form of liver disease is present.

ALT is used to evaluate a patient who has symptoms of a liver disorder. ALT can also be used to assess for:

◆ hepatitis

◆ alcohol abuse

◆ familial liver disease

◆ drug abuse or prescription drugs with known hepatic toxicity.

In people with mild symptoms, such as tiredness or loss of energy, ALT may be tested to make sure that they do not have chronic (long-term) liver disease. ALT is often used to evaluate the treatment of patients who have liver disease.

Very high levels of ALT (more than 10 times the highest normal level) are usually due to acute hepatitis, often due to a virus infection. In acute hepatitis, ALT levels usually stay high for about 1–2 months, but can take as long as 3–6 months to return to normal. ALT levels are usually not as high in chronic hepatitis.

Intra muscular injections and strenuous exercise may increase ALT levels. Certain drugs may raise ALT levels by causing liver damage in a very small percentage of patients taking the drug. This is true of both prescription drugs and some 'natural' health products (West & Brousil 2006; Sanai *et al.* 2008).

Alkaline phosphatase

Alkaline phosphatase (ALP) is found in high levels in bone and liver. Smaller amounts of ALP are found in the placenta of pregnant women and in the intestines. Each of these body parts makes different forms of ALP (isoenzymes). If a patient has high levels of ALP, and clinical indicators are inconclusive, ALP isoenzyme tests might be requested to try to determine the cause.

When a patient has evidence of liver disease, very high ALP levels can indicate that the bile ducts are partially or totally blocked or inflamed. Often, ALP is high in patients with cancer that has spread to the liver or the bones. If patients with bone or liver cancer respond to treatment, ALP levels decrease. If other liver function tests such as bilirubin, gamma-glutamyl transferase (GGT), or alanine aminotransferase (ALT) are also raised, this usually indicates that the ALP is coming from the liver.

However, if calcium and phosphate measurements are abnormal, this suggests that the ALP might be coming from bone. ALP can also be raised in bone diseases such as Paget's disease (where bones become enlarged and deformed) or in certain bone cancers.

Pregnancy can increase ALP levels. Children have higher ALP levels because their bones are growing, and ALP is often very high during the 'growth spurt', which occurs at different ages in males and females.

Eating a meal can increase the ALP level slightly for a few hours in some people. Ideally, the test should be done after fasting overnight. Some drugs may increase ALP levels, especially some of the drugs used to treat psychiatric problems, but significant increases are rare (Boyd & Delost 1998; Corathers 2006).

Aspartate aminotransferase

Aspartate aminotransferase (AST) is an enzyme found mostly in the heart and liver, and to a lesser extent in other muscles. When heart, liver, or muscle cells are injured, they release AST into the blood. Even though AST is found in heart and other muscles, another enzyme, creatine kinase (CK), is present in much higher amounts and is usually used to detect heart or muscle injury.

Very high levels of AST (more than 10 times the highest normal level) are usually due to a rapidly developing liver disease (acute hepatitis), which is often due to a viral infection. In acute hepatitis, AST levels usually stay elevated for about 1–2 months, but can take as long as 3–6 months to return to normal. In chronic hepatitis AST levels are usually not as high, often less than four times the highest normal level. In chronic hepatitis, AST often varies between normal and slightly increased, so doctors might request the test regularly to determine the pattern of change. When liver damage is due to alcohol, AST often increases much more than ALT (this is a pattern seen with few other liver diseases). AST can be increased from break up of red blood cells (haemolysis), and is increased after myocardial infarctions and with muscle injury.

Pregnancy may decrease AST levels. An intramuscular injection or even strenuous exercise may increase AST levels. In rare instances, some drugs can damage the liver or muscle, increasing AST levels. This is true of both prescription drugs and some 'natural' health products (Limdi & Hyde 2003).

Total bilirubin

Bilirubin is an orange-yellow pigment found in bile. It is formed when haemoglobin, breaks down. Small amounts of bilirubin are present in blood from damaged or old red cells that have died. When bilirubin levels are high, jaundice occurs, and further testing is needed to determine the cause. Too much bilirubin may mean that too many red cells are being destroyed or that the liver is incapable of removing bilirubin from the blood.

Bilirubin is measured to diagnose and/or monitor liver diseases. Levels can be used to monitor the progression of jaundice and to determine if it is the result of red blood cell breakdown or liver disease. This can be done by measuring two different chemical forms of bilirubin: direct (or con-jugated) and indirect (or unconjugated). If the direct bilirubin is elevated there may be some kind of blockage of the liver or bile duct, perhaps due to gallstones, hepatitis, trauma, a drug reaction, or long-term alcohol abuse. If the indirect bilirubin is increased, haemolysis (undesirable break-down of red blood cells) may be the cause. Increases in bilirubin may be due to metabolic prob-lems, obstruction of the bile duct, physical or chemical damage to the liver (cirrhosis), or an inherited abnormality.

Albumin

Albumin is used to screen for liver or kidney disease or to evaluate nutritional status, especially in hospitalized patients. Albumin is frequently requested if there are obvious symptoms of liver or kidney disease, if the patient has suffered recent, rapid weight change, or prior to planned surgery.

Albumin is the most abundant protein in the blood plasma. It keeps fluid from leaking out of blood vessels, nourishes tissues, and carries hormones, vitamins, drugs, and ions throughout the body. Albumin is made in the liver and is sensitive to liver damage. The level of albumin in the blood drops with hepatic damage, nephrotic syndrome, when a patient is malnourished, if there is severe inflammation, or clinical shock. Albumin increases when a person is dehydrated. Low albumin levels may also suggest conditions in which the body does not properly absorb and digest protein, such as Crohn's disease. Patients with prolonged diarrhoea can develop abnormal albumin levels.

High albumin levels usually reflect dehydration. Certain drugs increase albumin in blood, including anabolic steroids, androgens, growth hormones, and insulin. If the patient is receiving large amounts of intravenous fluids, the results of this test may be inaccurate because of the effects of haemodilution (McCluskey et al. 1996; Vincent 2003).

Gamma-glutamyl transferase

Gamma-glutamyl transferase (GGT) is an enzyme found mainly in the liver and is normally present in low levels in the blood. When the liver is injured or the flow of bile is obstructed, the GGT level rises. It is therefore a useful marker for detecting bile duct problems.

Clinicians may also use the test to help find out the reason for a raised level of ALP. Both ALP and GGT are elevated in disease of the bile ducts and in some liver diseases, but only ALP will be elevated in bone disease. If the GGT level is normal in a person with a high ALP, the cause is most likely to be bone disease. GGT can also be used to screen for alcohol abuse (it will be elevated in about 75% of long-term drinkers).

GGT is increased in most diseases that cause damage to the liver or bile ducts, but is usually not helpful in distinguishing between different causes of liver damage.

In patients with a history of alcohol abuse who are undergoing treatment, GGT may be used to check that the person is following the treatment programme properly. Elevated levels may be due to liver disease, but they may also be due to congestive heart failure, and use of many prescription and non-prescription drugs including non-steroidal anti-inflammatory drugs, lipid-lowering drugs, antibiotics, histamine blockers (such as ranitidine), antifungal agents, anticonvulsants, antidepressants, and hormones such as testosterone. Oral contraceptives can decrease GGT levels.

Even small amounts of alcohol within 24 h of test being performed may cause a temporary increase in the GGT. Smoking can also increase GGT. Levels of GGT increase with age in women, but not in men, and are predominantly higher in men.

Cardiac markers

Normal values

- Troponin T: negative ng/mL
- Troponin I: 0.01–0.03 ng/mL
- Total CK: <160 IU/L female, <250 IU/L male
- CK-MB: <4.0%
- Myoglobin: 25–58 ng/mL female, 28–72 ng/mL male

Troponins

Troponins are a family of proteins found in skeletal and heart muscle fibres. The three different types of troponin are troponin C (TnC), troponin T (TnT), and troponin I (TnI). Together, these three proteins regulate muscular contraction. Two of the proteins, TnI and TnT, occur in a form that is found only in the heart. These cardiac-specific troponins, called cTnI and cTnT, are normally undetectable in the blood. When there is damage to heart muscle cells, cardiac troponins I and T are released into the circulation. The more damage there is, the greater the concentration of cardiac troponins I and T in the blood.

When a patient has a myocardial infarction, levels of troponin can become elevated in the blood within 3 or 4 h after injury and may remain elevated for 10–14 days. Troponin measurements are performed when a patient presents with chest pain to help determine whether a myocardial infarction or other damage to their heart muscle has occurred. Either a troponin I or a troponin T test will be measured.

Troponins are occasionally requested with other cardiac biomarkers, such as CK-MB or myoglobin. However, troponins are the preferred tests for a suspected infarct because they are more specific for heart injury than tests that may become positive in skeletal muscle injury and remain elevated for a longer period of time.

Chest pain can be due to heart-related issues, indigestion, strain on chest muscles, or other causes. In a myocardial infarction, heart muscle cells die and release their contents, which include troponin, myoglobin, and CK. In acute coronary syndrome (ACS), the heart cells may also release troponin. Studies have shown that people who have ACS and an abnormal troponin, but normal CK, CK-MB, and myoglobin, have a higher risk of having a myocardial infarction or other serious heart problem in the next few months. Many clinicians now check troponin in patients with ACS to identify those who may benefit from such treatments as angioplasty or cardiac bypass surgery.

In patients with ACS, a troponin test may be requested if the patient's symptoms; get worse, occur when the patient is at rest, and/or the patient is no longer at ease with treatment. These are all signs that ACS is developing, which increases the risk of infarct or other serious heart problems in the future (Hamm *et al.* 1997).

Troponin values can remain high for 1–2 weeks after a myocardial infarction. The test is not generally affected by damage to other muscles, so intramuscular injections, accidents, strenuous exercise, and drugs that can damage muscle do not affect troponin levels.

Increased troponin concentrations should not be used by themselves to diagnose or rule out a myocardial infarction. A physical examination, clinical history, and electrocardiogram (ECG) are also important. Some patients who have a myocardial infarct will have normal troponin concentrations, and some people with increased troponin concentrations have no apparent heart injury. Troponin levels may also be elevated with acute or chronic conditions such as myocarditis, congestive heart failure, severe infections, kidney disease, and certain chronic inflammatory conditions of muscles and skin (Adams & Bodor 1993; DeFillipi & Tocchi 2000; Beishuizen & Hartemink 2005; Babuin & Jaffe 2005; Bagwe *et al.* 2007).

Creatine kinase

CK is an enzyme found in the heart, brain, and skeletal muscle. CK occurs in three major forms, called isoenzymes:

- CK-MB (found mostly in heart muscle)
- CK-BB (found mostly in brain)
- CK-MM (found in heart and skeletal muscle).

CK in the blood comes mainly from skeletal muscles. The CK in brain almost never gets into the bloodstream without obvious clinical signs and symptoms. CK levels rise when skeletal or cardiac muscle cells are injured. In the first 4–6 h after a myocardial infarction, CK in blood begins to rise. It reaches its highest level after about 18–24 h, and returns to normal in about 2–3 days. CK can also indicate whether skeletal muscle damage has occurred.

Patients who have greater muscle mass have higher CK levels (e.g. a young fit male will have more muscle mass and hence a higher CK level than an elderly female), and Afro-Caribbeans may have higher CK levels than other ethnic groups. Raised CK levels can also be seen in those with hypothyroidism. Very heavy exercise can increase CK. Other forms of muscle damage, such as from a fall, a car accident, surgery, or after an injection, can also increase CK. Alcohol slightly increases CK.

CK-MB

CK-MB is found mostly in heart muscle. It rises when there is any damage to heart muscle cells. CK-MB levels, along with total CK, are tested in patients who have chest pain to diagnose myocardial infarct. A high total CK could indicate damage to either the heart or other muscles, but because CK-MB is specific to the heart, a high CK-MB suggests that the damage was to heart muscle.

CK-MB above the reference range suggests possible myocardial infarction. A high CK with a low CK-MB suggests significant skeletal muscles were damaged.

Patients with renal failure can have high CK-MB levels without having had infarction. Rarely, long-term muscle disease, low thyroid hormone levels, and alcohol abuse can increase CK-MB, producing changes similar to those seen in a myocardial infarct (Hines *et al.* 1993).

Myoglobin

Myoglobin is a protein found in heart and skeletal muscle. While haemoglobin brings oxygen to most of the body, myoglobin traps oxygen in muscle to allow muscle cells to work properly. When heart or skeletal muscle is damaged, myoglobin is released into the blood. Myoglobin is a small protein, and it leaks out of cells soon after injury. Myoglobin levels start to rise within 1–3 h of a myocardial infarction or other muscle injury, reach their highest values by about 8–12 h, and generally fall back to normal by about 1 day after the injury occurred.

Myoglobin tests may be used in patients with chest pain who are suspected of having had an infarct, particularly if the ECG does not give definitive results. When myoglobin rises, there has been very recent injury to the heart or skeletal muscle tissue. If myoglobin does not increase at that point, an infarct is very unlikely, unless the patient has had chest pain for more than 24 h. As myoglobin is also found in other muscles, high levels usually require troponin or CK-MB determination to indicate whether the damage was to myocardial or skeletal muscle. High levels can occur in accidents, seizures, surgery, or muscular disease.

Increased myoglobin levels can occur after intramuscular injections or strenuous exercise. As the kidneys remove myoglobin from the blood, myoglobin levels may be high in patients with renal failure. Rarely, heavy alcohol abuse and certain drugs can cause muscle injury and increase myoglobin (Hofmann *et al.* 2007).

Additional laboratory tests in acute illness

Normal ranges

Glucose: 3.3–5.5 mmol/L

Magnesium: 0.65–1.05 mmol/L

Calcium: 2.15–2.60 mmol/L

Phosphate: 0.8–1.45 mmol/L

Amylase: <110 IU/L

Lactate: 0.4–1.2 mmol/L

CRP: <5 mg/L

Glucose

Glucose is a six-carbon sugar that acts as the main source of energy for the body. Most of the body's cells require glucose for energy production; the brain and nervous system cells rely on glucose for energy, and can only function when glucose levels in the blood remain within a certain range.

The body's use of glucose depends on the availability of insulin, a hormone produced by the pancreas. Insulin acts to control the transport of glucose into the body's cells to be used for energy. Insulin also directs the liver to store excess glucose as glycogen for short-term energy storage and promotes the synthesis of fats, which form the basis of a longer-term store of energy.

Normally blood glucose levels rise slightly after a meal, and insulin is released to lower them, with the amount of insulin released dependent on the size and content of the meal. If blood glucose levels drop too low, such as might occur between meals or after a strenuous exercise, glucagon (another hormone from the pancreas) is produced to facilitate release of glucose stores from the liver, raising the blood glucose levels. If the glucagon/insulin system is working properly the amount of glucose in the blood remains fairly stable.

Hyperglycaemia and hypoglycaemia, caused by a variety of conditions, are both debilitating to normal body homeostasis. Severe, sudden high or low blood glucose levels can be life threatening, causing organ failure, brain damage, coma, and, in extreme cases, death. Long-term high blood glucose levels can cause progressive damage to body organs such as the kidneys, eyes, blood vessels, heart, and nerves. Untreated hyperglycaemia that arises during pregnancy (gestational diabetes) can cause mothers to give birth to large babies who may have low glucose levels. Long-term hypoglycaemia can lead to brain and nerve damage.

Patients with diabetes monitor their own blood glucose levels, often several times a day, to determine how far above or below normal their glucose is and to determine what oral medications or insulin injections they may need. In those with suspected hypoglycaemia, glucose levels are used to help confirm a diagnosis. With known diabetics, clinicians will use glucose levels in conjunction with other tests such as haemoglobin A1C (HbA1 C) to monitor glucose control over a period of time.

Blood glucose concentration may be determined as part of a routine examination, especially in those people at high risk of developing diabetes, i.e. those with a family history of diabetes, those who are overweight, and those who are more than 45 years old. It may also be used to help diagnose diabetes when someone has symptoms of hyperglycaemia such as:

♦ increased thirst

♦ increased urination

♦ tiredness

♦ blurred vision

♦ slow-healing infections.

Glucose may also be tested when a person has symptoms of hypoglycaemia, such as:

♦ sweating

♦ hunger

♦ trembling

♦ anxiety

♦ confusion.

Glucose testing is also done in emergency settings to determine if low or high glucose is contributing to symptoms such as fainting and unconsciousness.

Fasting blood glucose concentration (collected after an 8–10 h fast) is used to screen for and diagnose diabetes. The following information summarizes the meaning of the fasting blood glucose results:

♦ from 3.6–6.0 mmol/L: normal fasting glucose

♦ from 6.1–6.9 mmol/L: impaired fasting glucose

♦ 7.0 mmol/L and above: probable diabetes.

Some of the other diseases and conditions that can result in elevated glucose levels include:

- acromegaly
- acute stress
- long-term kidney disease
- Cushing's syndrome
- drugs, including corticosteroids, tricyclic antidepressants, diuretics, and adrenaline
- excessive food intake
- hyperthyroidism
- pancreatic cancer
- pancreatitis.

Low glucose levels are also seen with:

- adrenal disease (Addison's disease)
- alcohol consumption
- drugs, for example anabolic steroids
- extensive liver disease
- hypopituitarism
- hypothyroidism
- insulin overdose
- insulinomas
- starvation.

Hypoglycaemia is characterized by a drop in blood glucose to a level where first it causes nervous system symptoms (sweating, palpitations, hunger, trembling, and anxiety). It then begins to affect the brain (causing confusion, hallucinations, blurred vision, and sometimes even coma and death). An actual diagnosis of hypoglycaemia requires satisfying the following three criteria:

- documented low glucose levels (<2.5 mmol/L)
- symptoms of hypoglycaemia
- reversal of the symptoms when blood glucose levels are returned to normal.

Patients with fasting hypoglycaemia may require intravenous glucose or administration of intramuscular glucagon. Glucose will only show up in the urine if it is at sufficiently high levels in the blood (usually above 10 mmol/L). This exceeds the renal threshold for glucose and the excess is excreted into the urine. Renal impairment may also lead to excretion of glucose in the urine. Urine glucose may sometimes be used as a rough indicator of high glucose levels, and if it is detected further blood glucose tests should then be carried out (Van den Berghe *et al.* 2001; Dandona & Mohanty 2005; Braunschweig & Jensen 2006).

Magnesium

Magnesium is an electrolyte that is found in every cell. It is vital to energy production, muscle contraction, nerve function, and maintenance of strong bones. About half of the body's magnesium is combined with calcium and phosphorus to form bone. Normally, only 1% of the total magnesium found in the body is present in blood. The body maintains magnesium levels in its blood, cells, and bone by regulating how much it absorbs from the intestines and by how much it excretes or conserves in the kidneys.

Since a low magnesium level can, over time, cause persistently low calcium and potassium levels, it may be checked to help diagnose problems with calcium, potassium, phosphorus, and/or parathyroid hormone (PTH) (involved with calcium regulation).

Magnesium levels may be measured frequently to monitor the response to oral or intravenous magnesium supplements and may be used, along with calcium and phosphorus testing, to monitor calcium supplementation.

Magnesium testing may be requested as a follow-up to persistently low levels of calcium and potassium. It may also be requested if symptoms of an abnormally low magnesium level, such as muscle weakness, twitching, cramping, confusion, cardiac arrhythmias, and seizures, are present. Low levels of magnesium (hypomagnesaemia) in the bloodstream may mean that the patients are:

+ not getting enough magnesium in diet/nutrition
+ not absorbing enough magnesium
+ excreting too much magnesium.

Deficiencies may be due to:

+ low dietary intake
+ gastrointestinal disorders
+ uncontrolled diabetes
+ hypoparathyroidism
+ long-term diuretic use
+ prolonged diarrhoea
+ surgery
+ severe burns
+ toxaemia of pregnancy.

Increased levels of magnesium are rarely due to dietary/nutritional sources and are usually the result of an excretion problem or excessive supplementation. Increased levels are seen in:

+ kidney failure
+ hyperparathyroidism
+ hypothyroidism
+ dehydration
+ diabetic acidosis on first presentation
+ Addison's disease
+ use of magnesium-containing antacids or laxatives.

Magnesium blood levels may be low normally in the second and third months of pregnancy (Tong 2005).

Calcium

Calcium is one of the most important electrolytes in the body. About 99% of it is found in the bones, and most of the rest circulates in the blood. Roughly, half of the calcium is referred to as 'free' (or 'ionized'), and is active within the body; the remaining half, referred to as 'bound' calcium, is attached to protein and other compounds, and is inactive. Most commonly, the total amount of calcium in the bloodstream is determined, which reflects both the active and the inactive forms of calcium. If measurement of the ionized form of calcium is needed, special sample handling is required, although this can be determined using most modern blood gas analysers. Urine calcium tells how much calcium is being excreted by the kidneys.

Blood calcium is tested to help diagnosis, and to monitor conditions relating to the bones, heart, nerves, and kidneys. Clinicians may achieve a better understanding of the patient's condition by comparing calcium and phosphate result at the same time. For example, when PTH from the parathyroid gland is released, calcium levels rise and phosphate falls. However, in kidney disease, high phosphate levels and low calcium levels are often seen. Depending on the levels, these two tests can help clinician decide whether a parathyroid disorder is present.

Directly measuring 'free' calcium can be valuable in certain situations where the total calcium level is likely to be misleading, for example during major surgery (particularly after a blood transfusion), in critically ill patients, and when protein levels are abnormal. Large fluctuations in free calcium can cause the heart to slow down or to beat too rapidly, can cause muscles to go into spasm, cause confusion, or even coma.

Calcium can be used as a diagnostic test if patient present with symptoms that suggest:

+ kidney stones
+ bone disease
+ neurological disorders.

Clinicians may request a calcium test if:

+ kidney disease is present
+ clinical symptoms of hypercalcaemia, such as tiredness, weakness, loss of appetite, nausea, vomiting, constipation, abdominal pain, urinary frequency, and increased thirst are present
+ clinical symptoms of hypocalcaemia, such as cramps in the abdomen, muscle cramps, or tingling fingers are present; or
+ established diseases that can be associated with abnormal blood calcium are present.

A high calcium level is called hypercalcaemia. This is usually caused by:

+ hyperparathyroidism: this condition is usually caused by a benign tumour on the parathyroid gland. This form of hypercalcaemia is usually mild and can be present for many years before being noticed.
+ cancer: cancer can cause hypercalcaemia when it spreads to the bones, which releases calcium into the blood, or when cancer causes a hormone similar to PTH to increase calcium levels.

Other causes of hypercalcaemia include:

+ hyperthyroidism
+ sarcoidosis
+ tuberculosis
+ fractures
+ excess vitamin D intake
+ kidney transplant
+ diuretics
+ high-protein levels.

Taking thiazide diuretic drugs (drugs that encourage urination) is the most common drug-induced reason for a high calcium level (Baker & Worthley 2002).

Hypocalcaemia can be caused by many conditions:

- low-protein levels
- hypoparathyroidism
- decreased dietary intake of calcium
- decreased levels of vitamin D
- magnesium deficiency
- too much phosphate
- acute inflammation of the pancreas
- chronic kidney disease
- calcium ions becoming bound to protein (alkalosis)
- bone disease
- malnutrition
- alcoholism.

Phosphate

In the body, phosphorus is combined with oxygen to form a variety of phosphates (PO_4). Phosphates are vital for energy production, muscle and nerve function, and bone growth. They also play an important role as a buffer, helping to maintain the body's acid–base balance. About 70–80% of the phosphates are combined with calcium to help form bones and teeth, about 10% are found in muscle, and about 1% is in nerve tissue. The rest are found within cells throughout the body, where they are mainly used to store energy; about 1% of total body phosphate is found within plasma. Most phosphate in the body comes from dietary sources. The body maintains phosphate levels in the blood by regulating how much it absorbs from the intestines and how much it excretes or conserves in the kidneys.

Blood phosphate concentration can be helpful in people who are malnourished or who are being treated for ketoacidosis. Phosphate concentration is used to help diagnose and evaluate the severity of conditions and diseases that affect the digestive system and interfere with the absorption of phosphate, calcium, and magnesium. Testing also can help to diagnose disorders that affect the kidneys and interfere with mineral excretion and conservation. Phosphate levels are carefully monitored in people with kidney failure.

Although abnormal phosphate levels usually cause no symptoms (with the exception of very low levels), phosphate testing often is performed as a follow-up to an abnormal calcium level and/or related symptoms, such as fatigue, muscle weakness, cramps, or bone problems.

Dietary deficiencies in phosphate are rare but may be seen with alcoholism and malnutrition. Low levels of phosphate (hypophosphataemia) may also be due to or associated with:

- hypercalcaemia (high levels of calcium), especially when due to high levels of PTH
- overuse of diuretics
- severe burns
- diabetic ketoacidosis after treatment
- hypothyroidism
- hypokalaemia

♦ chronic antacid use

♦ rickets and osteomalacia.

Higher than normal levels of phosphate (hyperphosphataemia) may be due to or associated with:

♦ kidney failure

♦ hypoparathyroidism

♦ hypocalcaemia

♦ diabetic ketoacidosis on first presentation

♦ phosphate supplementation.

Very low levels of phosphate are rare but require swift medical attention. Test results may be affected by the use of enemas and laxatives containing sodium phosphate, excess vitamin D supplements, and by intravenous glucose administration (McClatchey 2001; Baker & Worthley 2002).

Amylase

Amylase is an enzyme made mainly by the pancreas. It is released from the pancreas into the digestive tract to help digest starch. It is usually present in the blood in small quantities. When cells in the pancreas are injured or if the pancreatic duct is blocked (by a gallstone or rarely by a tumour), increased amounts of amylase find their way into the bloodstream.

Amylase levels in blood are used to diagnose acute pancreatitis (inflammation of the pancreas) and other pancreatic diseases. The swift rise of amylase at the beginning of a pancreatitis attack, and its fall after about 2 days, helps to pinpoint this diagnosis. Amylase is sometimes, although rarely used in the diagnosis and follow-up of cancer of the pancreas, gallbladder disease, and mumps. Amylase may be requested by the clinician when possible symptoms of a pancreatic disorder, such as severe abdominal pain, fever, loss of appetite, or nausea, are present.

In acute pancreatitis, amylase levels are usually very high, often 5–10 times normal. Increased amylase levels may also indicate cancer of the pancreas, gallbladder disease, a perforated ulcer, obstruction of the intestinal tract, mumps, or ectopic pregnancy. Chronic (long-term) pancreatitis is often associated with alcoholism. It may also be caused by trauma to the pancreas or associated with genetic abnormalities such as cystic fibrosis. Amylase levels may be moderately elevated with chronic pancreatitis or may be decreased when the cells that produce amylase in the pancreas become damaged or destroyed.

Some drugs that may cause amylase to rise include aspirin, diuretics, and oral contraceptives, steroids such as corticosteroids, indometacin, and opiates (Pezzilli *et al.* 2005).

Lactate

Measurement of blood lactate is commonly performed in the critical and acute care setting. Increased lactate production during resuscitated stress states such as sepsis, trauma, or burns occurs as the result of enhanced anaerobic glycolysis. The degree of hyperlactataemia directly correlates with the severity of the stress response to critical illness.

The major cellular sources of lactate are monocytes (macrophages) and neutrophils: these phagocytes demonstrate enhanced glycolysis during stress. The major organ sites of lactate production in shock include the muscle and the gut, whereas during stress, lung, gut, and wounds are the major sources of lactate.

In acutely ill patients, both shock and stress lactate may be produced concurrently. In addition, conditions in which lactate clearance is impaired, for example acute or chronic hepatic dysfunction, will result in a greater degree of hyperlactataemia for a given lactate production.

Blood lactate levels have been shown to adequately reflect the presence and persistence of tissue hypoxia in acutely and critically ill patients. In acutely unwell patients, increased blood lactate levels and the persistence of hyperlactataemia have been associated with significant morbidity and mortality. Hyperlactatataemia is not necessarily coincident with metabolic acidosis; however, the combination carries the worst prognosis, with an in-hospital mortality rate varying between 50 and 80%.

The most common causes of hyperlactataemia are:

♦ shock

♦ sepsis

♦ malignancy

♦ burns

♦ trauma.

Less common aetiologies include:

♦ antiretrovirals

♦ parenteral beta agonists

♦ hypoglycaemia.

Lactate may be artificially raised if there is a delay in sample analysis in patients with high leukocyte counts. Blood lactate concentration is useful as a prognostic index in patients with circulatory shock and failure of lactate clearance has been shown to be a reliable predictor of the development of multiple system organ failure and death after trauma or in sepsis (see Chapter 8).

Lactate analysis has proved useful in the triage of trauma patients since the degree of lactate elevation correlates with the severity of injury. Elevated lactate levels in patients with chest pain have been found to identify critical cardiac illness. In patients with acute myocardial infarction elevated lactate are found to predict development of shock.

Blood lactate determination is also a key component of the Surviving Sepsis Campaign care bundle, where blood lactate greater than 2 mmol/L indicates likely evidence of sepsis and greater than 4 mmols/L indicates lactic acidosis. It is important in the recognition of severe sepsis and serial measurements may demonstrate response or lack of response to resuscitation. (Kirshenbaum *et al.* 1998; Bakker 1999; Mizcock 2002; Carter 2007).

Markers of infection and inflammation

C-reactive protein

CRP is an acute phase protein made by the liver and released into the blood within a few hours after the start of an infection or inflammation. Increased levels are observed after a myocardial infarction, in sepsis, and after a surgical procedure. It is often the first evidence of inflammation or an infection in the body. Its rise in the blood often precedes pain, fever, or other clinical indicators. The level of CRP can jump a thousand-fold in response to inflammation and can be valuable in monitoring disease activity.

CRP is useful in assessing patients with:

♦ sepsis

♦ inflammatory bowel disease

+ some forms of arthritis

+ autoimmune diseases

+ pelvic inflammatory disease

+ and in assessing patients post operatively.

While CRP is not specific enough to diagnose a particular disease, it does serve as a general marker for infection and inflammation. A high CRP level suggests the presence of acute infection or inflammation—most infections and inflammations result in CRP levels above 10 mg/L (Pepys 2001).

CRP levels can be elevated in the later stages of pregnancy, with use of birth control pills, or in women taking hormone replacement therapy. Higher levels of CRP have also been observed in the obese. Another test to monitor inflammation is called the erythrocyte sedimentation rate (ESR). Both CRP and ESR are elevated in the presence of inflammation; however, CRP appears and disappears sooner than changes in the ESR. CRP levels may therefore fall to normal if patient is treated effectively, whereas ESR may remain abnormal for a prolonged timeframe.

Haematological assessment of the acutely unwell

Full blood count

Full blood count (FBC) is used as a broad screening test to check for anaemia irrespective of cause, infection, possible clotting disorders, and many other diseases. It is actually a panel of tests that examines different functional aspects of blood.

Many patients will have baseline FBC tests to help determine their general health status. If they are healthy and they have cell populations that are within normal limits, then they may not require another FBC until their health status changes or until their clinical condition deteriorates. FBC normally includes:

+ white blood cell (WBC) count

+ red blood cell (RBC) count

+ haemoglobin (Hb)

+ haematocrit (HCT).

Clinical link 10.2 (see Appendix for answers)

Mrs Smith is a 45-year-old lady admitted with pneumonia. Her observations are:

BP: 110/50

HR: 120

RR 22

Temperature: 38.6°C

A blood test is requested and the results are:

Lactate 4.5

CRP: 10

WCC 20

Discuss these results in the light of her presenting condition.

White blood cells (leukocytes)

Normal range

WBC: $4.0–11.0 \times 10^9$/L

Neutrophils: $1.5–8.0 \times 10^9$/L

Lymphocytes: $1.2–3.5 \times 10^9$/L

Monocytes: $0.2–1.0 \times 10^9$/L

Eosinophils: $0–0.4 \times 10^9$/L

Basophils: $0–0.2 \times 10^9$/L

The WBC count indicates the number of WBCs in a sample of blood. This count may indicate the presence of illness. WBCs are made in the bone marrow and protect the body against infection and aid in the immune response. If an infection develops, WBCs attack and destroy the bacteria causing the infection.

Conditions or drugs that weaken the immune system, such as HIV infection or chemotherapy, cause a decrease in WBCs. The WBC count is used to suggest the presence of an infection, an allergy, or leukaemia. It is also used to help monitor the body's response to various treatments and to monitor bone marrow function.

An elevated number of WBCs are called leukocytosis. This can result from bacterial infections, inflammation, leukaemia, trauma, or stress. A WBC count of $11.0–17.0 \times 10^9$/L cells would be considered mild-to-moderate leukocytosis. A decreased WBC count is called leukopenia. It can result from many different situations, such as chemotherapy, radiation therapy, or diseases of the immune system. A count of $3.0–5.0 \times 10^9$/L cells would be considered mild leukopenia. In some acutely ill septic patients an overwhelming infection can lead to a significantly low WBC count (see sepsis diagnosis criteria Chapter 8), which significantly increases patient morbidity and mortality.

The WBC count tends to be lower in the morning and higher in the late afternoon. WBC counts are age related. On average, normal newborns and infants have higher WBC counts than adults. It is not uncommon for the elderly to fail to develop leukocytosis as a response to infection. Treatment depends on the cause. Infections usually cause increased WBC counts and may be treated with antibiotics. Some diseases cause decreased counts and may be treated simply with bed rest. Leukaemias require chemotherapy and other treatments (Higgins 2007; Blann 2008).

Differential WBC

There are five types of WBCs, each with different functions: neutrophils, lymphocytes, monocytes, eosinophils, and basophils. The differential reveals if these cells are present in normal proportion to one another, if one cell type is increased or decreased, or if immature or abnormal cells are present. This information is helpful in diagnosing specific types of illnesses that affect the immune system. WBC differential assesses the ability of the body to respond to and fight infection. It also detects the severity of allergic reactions, parasitic and other types of infection, and drug reactions. It can also identify some types of leukaemia or lymphoma. WBC differential indicates the quantity of each type of WBC that is present.

- *Neutrophils* can increase in response to bacterial infection, inflammatory disease, steroid medication, or more rarely leukaemia. Decreased neutrophil levels may be the result of severe infection or other conditions, such as responses to various medications or chemotherapy.
- *Eosinophils* can increase in response to allergic disorders, inflammation of the skin, and parasitic infections. They can also occur in response to some infections or to various bone marrow malignancies.

+ *Basophils* can increase in cases of leukaemia, long-standing inflammation, the presence of a hypersensitivity reaction to food, or radiation therapy.

+ *Lymphocytes* can increase in cases of bacterial or viral infection, leukaemia, lymphoma, or radiation therapy. Decreased lymphocyte levels are common in later life but can also indicate steroid mediation, stress, lupus, and HIV infection.

+ *Monocyte* levels can increase in certain leukaemias, in response to infection and inflammatory disorders. Decreased monocyte levels can indicate bone marrow injury or failure and some forms of leukaemia.

Eating, physical activity, and stress may alter WBC differential values. Long-term exposure to toxic chemicals (e.g. some solvents, petroleum products, and insecticides) can increase the risk of an abnormal differential (Higgins 2007; Blann 2008).

Red blood cell parameters

Normal range

Red blood cell count (RBC): $4.5–6.5 \times 10^{12}$/L female, $3.8–5.8 \times 10^{12}$/L male

Haemoglobin: 11.5–16.5 g/dL female, 13.5–18.0 g/dL male

Haematocrit: 0.37–0.47 (37–47 %) female, 0.4–0.54 (40–54 %) male

Red blood cells

Red blood cells originate in the bone marrow and carry oxygen from the lungs to the cells and transport carbon dioxide from the cells to the lungs. Women tend to have lower RBC counts and levels tend to decrease with age. When the value decreases by more than 10% of the expected normal value, the patient is said to be anaemic. RBC count is used to evaluate any type of decrease in red blood cells (anaemia) or increase in red blood cells (polycythaemia).

A high RBC count may indicate congenital heart disease, dehydration, obstructive lung disease, or bone marrow over-production. An increase in red blood cell count is often seen in chronic obstructive pulmonary disease (COPD). A low RBC count may indicate anaemia, bleeding, kidney disease, bone marrow failure (for instance from radiation or a tumour), malnutrition, or other causes. A low count may also indicate nutritional deficiencies of iron, folate, vitamin B12, and vitamin B6.

Normal decreases in red blood cells are seen during pregnancy as a result of normal body fluid increases that dilute them. Living at high altitudes causes an increase in RBC counts. Tiredness, dizziness, and altered mental state may indicate a low RBC count. Fainting, pallor (loss of normal skin colour), and shortness of breath also can indicate low RBCs (Lyons 2008).

Haemoglobin

The amount of haemoglobin in the bloodstream is a good indication of the blood's ability to carry oxygen throughout your body. Haemoglobin carries oxygen to cells from the lungs. If haemoglobin levels are low, this is termed *anaemia*, a condition in which the body is not getting enough oxygen, causing fatigue and weakness.

Haemoglobin measurement as part of a full blood count test is used to:

+ detect and measure the severity of anaemia or polycythaemia

+ monitor the response to treatment

+ help make decisions about blood transfusion

+ monitor patients with ongoing bleeding problems.

Normal values in an adult are influenced by the age, sex, and ethnic origin in the person. Above-normal haemoglobin levels may be the result of:

♦ dehydration

♦ excess production of RBCs in the bone marrow

♦ severe lung disease.

Below-normal haemoglobin levels may be the result of:

♦ iron deficiency

♦ inherited haemoglobin defects

♦ bone marrow failure

♦ bleeding

♦ vitamin and mineral deficiencies

♦ kidney disease

♦ chronic illness

♦ bone marrow cancer.

Haemoglobin decreases slightly during normal pregnancy. Haemoglobin levels peak around 8 a.m. and are lowest around 8 p.m. each day. Heavy smokers have higher haemoglobin levels than non-smokers.

Treatment depends on the cause. Some types of anaemia are treated with iron, folic acid, or vitamin B12 or B6 supplements. If the decrease is significant the clinician will consider blood transfusion (generally if Hb falls below 8 g/dL). Women of childbearing age may have temporary decreases during menstrual periods and pregnancy (Eckhart 2001).

Haematocrit (haematocrit/packed cell volume)

Blood is a mixture of cells and plasma. The packed cell volume (PCV)/HCT is a measurement of the proportion of blood that is made up of cells. The value is expressed as a percentage or fraction of cells in blood. For example, a PCV of 40% means that there are 40 mL of cells in 100 mL of blood.

The PCV/HCT is raised when the number of red blood cells increases or when the blood volume is reduced, as in dehydration. The PCV falls to less than normal, indicating anaemia, when your body decreases its production of RBCs or increases its destruction of RBCs (Kenning 2003). The PCV may decrease following fluid resuscitation or if excessive intravenous fluid replacement occurs.

This test is used to evaluate:

♦ anaemia

♦ polycythaemia

♦ dehydration

♦ need for blood transfusion

♦ the effectiveness of transfusion.

The PCV/HCT is repeated at regular intervals for many conditions, including:

♦ diagnosis and treatment of anaemia

♦ recovery from dehydration

♦ monitoring of ongoing bleeding.

A decreased PCV indicates anaemia, such as that caused by iron deficiency. Further testing may be necessary to determine the exact cause of the anaemia. Other conditions that can result in a low PCV include vitamin or mineral deficiencies, recent bleeding, cirrhosis of the liver, and malignancies.

The most common cause of increased PCV is dehydration, and with adequate fluid intake, the PCV returns to normal. However, it may reflect a condition called *polycythaemia vera*—that is, when a person has more than the normal number of RBCs due to a problem with the bone marrow. More commonly polycythaemia is a compensation for inadequate lung function (the bone marrow manufactures more RBCs to carry enough oxygen throughout your body).

Platelet parameters

Normal range

Platelet count: $150\text{--}450 \times 10^9/\text{L}$

Platelet count

Platelets are tiny fragments of cells made in the bone marrow that circulate in the blood. As they are very sticky, they are the first components to be activated when there has been an injury to a blood vessel and begin the formation of a 'blood clot'. Abnormal platelet counts or abnormally shaped platelets are associated with bleeding disorders and other bone marrow diseases, such as leukaemia.

In an adult, a normal count is about 150,000–450,000 platelets per microlitre of blood. Patients who have a bone marrow disease, such as leukaemia or other cancer in the bone marrow, often experience excessive bleeding, which is generally due to a significantly decreased number of platelets (thrombocytopenia). Low numbers of platelets may occur in some patients with long-term bleeding problems, thus reducing the supply of platelets. Individuals with autoimmune disorders, e.g. lupus, can cause the destruction of platelets. Patients undergoing chemotherapy may also have a decreased platelet count.

More commonly (up to 1% of the population), easy bruising or bleeding may be due to an inherited disease called von Willebrand's disease. Von Willebrand's disease is due an abnormality, either quantitative or qualitative, of von Willebrand factor, which functions as the carrier protein for factor VIII. In addition, von Willebrand factor is required for normal platelet adhesion. Von Willebrand factor functions on both primary and secondary haemostasis.

Many cases go undiagnosed due to the mild nature of the disease; however, the more severe form can be devastating. If platelet levels fall below 20,000 per microlitre, spontaneous bleeding may occur and is considered a risk.

A pronounced and/or significant reduction in platelet count may be due to heparin-induced thrombocytopaenia (HIT) without or with thrombosis in patients on thromboprophylaxis and all nurses giving heparin on the wards should be aware of this condition. HIT is defined as a decrease in platelet count during or shortly following exposure to heparin. It is associated with significant morbidity and mortality if unrecognized.

Increased platelet counts (thrombocytosis) may be seen in individuals who show no significant medical problems or in myeloproliferative disorders. Some may have a tendency to bleed due to the lack of stickiness of the platelets, yet in others, the platelets retain their stickiness but, because they are increased in number, tend to stick to each other, forming a clump that can get stuck within a blood vessel and cause damage.

Living in high altitudes may cause increased platelet levels, as can strenuous exercise. Decreased levels may be seen in women before menstruation. Drugs that may cause increased platelet levels include oestrogen and oral contraceptives.

Clinical link 10.3 (see Appendix for answers)

Mr Hill is a 56-year-old man who has returned to the ward post surgery. He has a wound drain in situ (drainage increasing) and his observations are:

BP: 120/86

HR: 105

RR: 23

Temperature: 36°C

He is complaining of pain and blood is leaking from his wound site. A FBC is requested and the results are:

RBC: 3.9

Hb: 10

HCT: 33

Discuss these results in relation to his presenting condition.

The use of steroids may stimulate an increase in platelet production. Bruising for no apparent reason, bleeding from the nose, mouth, or rectum also without obvious injury, or the inability to stop a small wound from bleeding within a reasonable period of time, a large numbers of pinpoint dots of blood (petechiae) or larger flat collections of blood (purpura) under the skin, may all indicate a platelet deficiency.

Elevated platelet levels can lead to blood clots. The greater danger is bleeding that will not stop or continues for an abnormally long time, due to a low platelet count.

Assessment of coagulation in acute illness

Normal range

Prothrombin time (PT): 12.6–15.6 s

International normalized ratio (INR): 0.89–1.10

Activated partial thromboplastin time (APTT): 29.5–34.5 s

aPTT ratio: 0.95–1.11

Fibrinogen: 2.10–2.90 g/dL

D-dimer: <300 µg/L

Prothrombin time/INR

Most laboratories report PT results that have been adjusted to the INR. The INR test is most often used to check how well anticoagulant tablets such as warfarin are working. Warfarin prevents the formation of clots by directly acting on vitamin K, which is important in the synthesis of four essential clotting factors. If these factors are not produced clots are not formed. This is particularly important in patients with heart conditions such as atrial fibrillation or artificial valves, or in patients with a history of recurrent blood clots. The drug's effectiveness can be determined by how much it prolongs the PT (measured in seconds), or increases the INR (a standardized ratio of the patient's PT versus a normal sample).

If the patient is prescribed an anticoagulant drug, the INR will be regularly determined to ensure that the dosage is correct and that the INR is appropriately increased. In addition, PT or INR may be used on a patient who is not taking anticoagulant drugs—to check for a bleeding disorder, liver disease or vitamin K deficiency, or to ensure clotting ability before surgery.

♦ Patients on anticoagulant drugs usually have a target INR of 2.0–3.0 (i.e. a PT two to three times as long as in a normal patient, using standardized conditions).

♦ For some patients who have a high risk of clot formation, the INR needs to be higher: about 3.0–4.0.

Antibiotics, aspirin, and cimetidine can increase PT. Barbiturates, oral contraceptives, and hormone-replacement therapy, and vitamin K—either in a multivitamin or liquid nutrition supplement—can decrease PT. The use of diuretics and antihistamines and the onset of illness or allergies can alter results. Blood collection technique and the difficulty in obtaining the blood sample can also affect test results (Marques & Fritsma 2006).

Activated partial thromboplastin time

The activated partial thromboplastin time (aPTT or PTT) is a measure of the functionality of the intrinsic and common pathways of the coagulation cascade. The body uses the coagulation cascade to produce blood clots to seal off injuries to blood vessels and tissues, to prevent further blood loss, and to give the damaged areas time to heal.

The cascade consists of a group of coagulation factors. These proteins are activated sequentially along either the extrinsic (tissue related) or intrinsic (blood vessel related) pathways. The branches of the pathway then come together into the common pathway, and complete their task with the formation of a stable blood clot. When a person starts bleeding, these three pathways have to work together.

Each component of the coagulation cascade must be functioning properly and be presenting in sufficient quantity for normal blood clot formation. If there is an inherited or acquired deficiency in one or more of the factors, or if the factors are functioning abnormally, then stable clot formation will be inhibited and excessive bleeding and/or clotting may occur.

The aPTT test is used when a patient has unexplained bleeding or clotting. Along with the PT test (which evaluates the extrinsic and common pathways of the coagulation cascade), the aPTT is often used as a starting place when investigating the cause of a bleeding or thrombotic (blood clot) episode. It is often used with recurrent miscarriages. The aPTT and PT tests are also used as pre-surgical screens for bleeding tendencies. The aPTT is also used to monitor heparin anticoagulant therapy. However, it cannot monitor therapy with newer low molecular weight heparin (LMWH). LMWH effect is usually predictable from the dose and only occasionally needs to be measured, using an anti-Xa test.

The aPTT may be requested, along with PT/INR, when a patient presents with unexplained bleeding or bruising, or a thromboembolism (blood clot). It may be useful to look for complications of some diseases, such as disseminated intravascular coagulation (DIC). DIC can occur in severe infections or some cases of cancer, causing both bleeding and clotting as coagulation factors are activated and used up at a rapid rate. The aPTT may also increase in liver disease, as the liver is the source of most coagulation factors. When the patient has had a thrombotic episode or recurrent miscarriages, an aPTT may be ordered.

The aPTT may be used as part of a pre-surgical evaluation for bleeding tendencies, especially if the surgery carries an increased risk of blood loss and/or if the patient has a clinical history of bleeding—such as nosebleeds and bruising that may indicate the presence of an inherited or acquired factor deficiency or of an acquired inhibitor. When a patient is on intravenous or injection heparin therapy, the aPTT is ordered at regular intervals to monitor the degree of anticoagulation. When a person is switched from heparin therapy to longer-term warfarin therapy, the two are overlapped and both the aPTT and the PT are monitored until the patient has stabilized.

Normal aPTTs may reflect normal clotting function but moderate single factor deficiencies may still exist. They will not be reflected in the aPTT until they have decreased to 30–40% of normal.

A decreased aPTT may result when coagulation factor VIII is elevated. This may occur during an acute phase reaction and is the blood's reaction to acute tissue inflammation or trauma. This is usually a temporary change. When the condition causing the acute phase reaction is resolved the aPTT will return to normal.

Prolonged aPTT tests may be due to:

+ pre-analytical problems, which may include:

  • insufficient sample—there must be enough blood collected and the anticoagulant to blood ratio must be 9:1

  • patients with high or low HCT levels may have an altered aPTT

  • heparin contamination

  • clotted blood samples

+ inherited or acquired factor deficiencies: some factor deficiencies cause bleeding; others prolong the aPTT in vitro but do not cause bleeding and have little clinical significance

+ warfarin and heparin anticoagulation therapy.

Platelet counts should always be monitored during heparin therapy to detect HIT promptly (McGhee 2003; Marques & Fritsma 2006).

D-dimer

D-dimer is performed when symptoms of a disease or condition that causes acute and/or chronic inappropriate blood clot formation, such as deep vein thrombosis (DVT), pulmonary embolism (PE), or disseminated intravascular coagulation (DIC), are present and to monitor the progress and treatment of DIC and other thrombotic conditions.

When a vein or artery is injured and begins to leak blood, a sequence of clotting steps and factors (called the coagulation cascade) is activated by the body to limit bleeding and create a blood clot to plug the hole. During this process, threads of a protein called fibrin are produced. These threads are cross-linked (glued together by a protein called thrombin) to form a fibrin net that catches platelets and helps hold the forming blood clot together at the site of the injury. Once the area has had time to heal, the body uses a protein called plasmin to break the clot (thrombus) into small pieces so that it can be removed. The fragments of the disintegrating clot are called fibrin degradation products (FDPs). One of the FDPs produced is D-dimer, which consists of variously sized pieces of cross-linked fibrin. D-dimer is normally undetectable in the blood and is produced only after a clot has formed and is in the process of being broken down.

D-dimer tests are requested, along with imaging scans, to help exclude, diagnose, and monitor diseases and conditions that cause hypercoagulability, a tendency to clot inappropriately. One of the most common of these conditions is DVT, which involves clot formation in the deep veins of the body, most frequently in the legs. These clots may grow very large and block blood flow in the legs, causing swelling, pain, and tissue damage. It is possible for a piece of the clot to break off and travel to other parts of the body, where the clot can lodge in the lung vasculature (PE).

Most clots travel in the body's veins, but clotting can also sometimes occur in the oxygen-carrying arteries. The combination of these two parts of thrombosis is sometimes referred to as venous thromboembolism (VTE). If a blood clot blocks the flow of blood to a vital organ, such as a kidney, the brain, or the heart, it may cause irreversible damage (infarction) and can lead to organ failure. D-dimer levels are generally requested to make sure that they are not elevated.

Measurements of D-dimer may also be requested, to help diagnose DIC (DIC). DIC is a complex acute condition that can arise from a variety of situations, including: some surgical procedures, burns, infections, cancer, liver disease, poisonous snake bites, and postpartum (after the delivery of a baby). With DIC, clotting factors are activated and then used up throughout the body. This creates numerous minute or larger blood clots and at the same time leaves the patient vulnerable to excessive bleeding. Steps are taken to support the patient, while the underlying problem is addressed and the underlying condition resolved. D-dimer levels may be used to monitor the effectiveness of DIC treatment.

D-dimer may be requested when a patient has symptoms of DVT, such as leg pain, tenderness, oedema, discolouration, or symptoms of PE, such as breathlessness, cough, and lung-related chest pain. D-dimer is especially useful when the clinician suspects that something other than DVT or PE is causing the symptoms. It is a quick, non-invasive way for the clinician to help exclude abnormal or excess clotting.

A positive D-dimer indicates the presence of an abnormally high level of cross-linked FDP in your body. It tells the clinician that there has been significant clot (thrombus) formation and breakdown in the body, but it does not identify the location or cause. An elevated D-dimer may be due to a VTE or DIC but it may also be due to a recent surgery, or trauma, infection, liver or kidney disease, pregnancy and diseases of pregnancy such as eclampsia, heart disease, and some cancers.

A normal D-dimer test means that it is most unlikely that an acute blood clot or disease causing abnormal clot formation and breakdown is present. Most clinicians agree that a negative D-dimer is most valid and useful when the test is done on patients who are considered to be low risk. The test is used to help exclude a clot as the cause of symptoms.

Anticoagulant therapy can cause a false-negative D-dimer. D-dimer concentrations may rise in the elderly, and false positives may be seen with high levels of rheumatoid factor (a protein seen in patients with rheumatoid arthritis). Substances such as lipaemia (a large amount of fats in the blood) and raised bilirubin can also cause false positives as can haemolysis (rupturing of RBCs) caused by improper collection and handling (Volschan & Mesquita. 2005; Dewar *et al.* 2008). D-dimer levels may be normal if the clot has been in situ for more than 10 days and is stable, therefore a detailed history and when symptoms were first apparent is vital.

A final point

This chapter has highlighted the vast array of blood and urine tests that may be of use in the diagnosis, treatment, and management of acute illness. It has identified and discussed the most frequently requested tests and the implications of the results.

It is vital, however, that the results must always be considered within the clinical context and take into consideration the patient's past medical history, current medication, and the results of any other of investigations (Higgins 2007). Local policies should always be referred to gain blood specimens (the taking of blood specimens is beyond the scope of this chapter and local policy should be adhered to). Results should always be discussed with medical team and laboratory staff before any changes to patient's treatment are instigated.

End of chapter test

It is important that you understand both the theory related to blood tests and the implications that this may have for your patient. In order to test your knowledge and apply this knowledge to clinical practice you should undertake the following assessment with an appropriately trained member of staff in clinical practice. If you are unable to answer any questions it may be helpful to revisit the section in this chapter.

Knowledge assessment

Work with your mentor/supervisor in practice and ask them to test your knowledge in relation to the following. Incorrect answers/lack of knowledge will require further revision/re-reading of this chapter.

+ Describe a 'normal reference range' and its significance in clinical practice.
+ Discuss when urea, creatinine, and electrolytes may be requested.
+ Identify potential problems that may cause changes to urea, creatinine, and electrolytes.
+ Discuss the significance of GFR and why it may be required in practice.
+ Identify groups of patients who may have abnormal liver function tests.
+ Analyse which cardiac markers are most useful and discuss why.
+ Identify clinical signs of hypo and hyperglycaemia.
+ Discuss clinical conditions that may cause hypo/hyperglycaemia.
+ Discuss the significance of lactate measurement.
+ Describe which markers of infection/inflammation are useful in clinical practice.
+ Analyse factors that may cause changes to full blood count.
+ Provide rationale for examining Hb alongside HCT results.
+ Identify which tests should be used to assess coagulation in acute illness.
+ Discuss the relevance of D-dimmers in diagnosing PE and DVT.
+ Identify which other factors must be taken into account when interpreting blood results.
+ Discuss when urgent blood sampling may be required.
+ Understand health and safety issues related to blood sampling.

Skills assessment

Work with your mentor/supervisor in practice and ask them to assess your ability to care for patients requiring blood tests using the following criteria where appropriate. Note: You may not be able to demonstrate all these skills. Ask your mentor/supervisor to give you feedback on areas that you did well and areas that may require improving.

+ Identifies when blood sampling is required.
+ Identifies correct blood test/tests for the patient.
+ Discusses need for blood test with medical staff.
+ Takes blood in accordance with local policy demonstrating an understanding of:
  • infection control measures
  • health and safety issues
  • Department of Health guidelines
  • patient consent
  • documentation/labelling policies
  • correct use of blood bottles
  • correct blood sampling technique
  • psychological issues associated with blood sampling
  • liaison with medical, portering, and laboratory staff.

♦ Demonstrates understanding of local policy and applies to practice.

♦ Communicates with laboratory staff and porters re collection and analysis of blood specimen.

♦ Follows local procedure if urgent blood test and results required.

♦ Demonstrates ability to access blood results (following local policy) in a timely manner.

♦ Documents results according to local policy.

♦ Interprets results alongside clinical data.

♦ Identifies abnormal blood results that require urgent attention and follows correct procedure to escalate concern.

♦ Reports changes to medical staff.

♦ Liaises with medical staff about changes to patient treatment.

♦ Changes medical treatment as directed by medical staff.

♦ Ensures clear documentation trail in patients nursing and medical notes.

♦ Explains results to patient in terms that they are able to understand.

(Adapted from University of Brighton skills template, Author Gary Creed)

References

Adrogue, H.J. and Madias, N.E. (2000) Hypernatremia. *N. Engl. J. Med.* **342**, 1493–9.

Adams, J.E. and Bodor, G.S. (1993) Cardiac troponin I marker with high specificity for cardiac injury. *Circulation.* **88**, 101–6.

Babuin, L. and Jaffe, S. (2005) Troponin; the biomarker of choice for the detection of cardiac injury. *Can. Med. Assoc. J.* **173**, 1191–202.

Bagwe, S., Sachdeva, R., and Mehta, J.L. (2007) High risk ACS patient and cardiac biomarkers in the emergency department, where do we stand? *Eur. Heart J.* **28**, 1043–4.

Baker, S.B. and Worthley, L.I.G. (2002) The essentials of calcium, magnesium and phophate metabolism. *Crit. Care Resuscitation.* **4**, 301–6.

Bakker, J. (1999) Blood lactate levels. *Curr. Opin. Crit. Care.* **5**, 234.

Beauuvieux, M.C. and Barthie, N. (2007) New predictive equations improve monitoring of kidney function in patients with diabetes. *Diabet. Care.* **30**, 1988–94.

Beishuizen, A. and Hartemink, K.J. (2005) Circulating cardiovascular markers and mediators in acute illness. *Clin. Chim. Acta.* **354**, 21–34.

Blann, A. (2008) *Routine Blood Results Explained.* 2nd edn. M&K Publishing, Keswick.

Braunschweig, C. and Jensen, G.L. (2006) Hyperglycaemia, nutrition support and acute illness. *J. Parenteral Enteral Nutr.* **30**, 175–6.

Boyd, J.L. and Delost, M.E. (1998) Calcium, phosphorus and ALP values in elderly subjects. *Clin. Lab. Sci.* **11**, 223–7.

Caraway, T.C. and Olsson, J.M. (2008) Hypokalemia. *Paediatr. Rev.* **29**, 50–1.

Carter, C. (2007) Implementing the severe sepsis care bundle outside the ICU by outreach. *Nurs. Crit. Care.* **12**, 225–30.

Corathers, S.D. (2006) Focus on diagnosis; the alkaline phosphatase level. *Paediatr. Rev.* **27**, 383–4.

Dandona, P. and Mohanty, P. (2005) Insulin infusion in acute illness. *J. Clin. Invest.* **115**, 2069–72.

DeFillipi, C.R. and Tocchi, M. (2000) Cardiac troponin T in chest pain unit patients with ischaemic ECG changes: Angiographic correlates and long term clinical outcomes. *J. Am. Coll. Cardiol.* **35**, 1827–34.

Dewar, C., Selby, C., and Jamieson, K. (2008) Emergency department nurse-based outpatient diagnosis of DVT using an evidence based protocol. *Emerg. Med. J.* **25**, 411–6.

Eckhart, K.U. (2001) Anaemia in critical illness. *Wien Klin Wochenschr.* **113**, 84–9.

Evans, K.J. (2005) Hyperkalemia a review. *J. Int. Care Med.* **20**, 272–90.

Gennari, F.J. (1998) Hypokalemia. *N. Engl. J. Med.* **339**, 451–8.

Gopal, D.V. and Rosen, H.R. (2000) Abnormal findings in liver function tests; interpreting results to narrow the diagnosis and establish a prognosis. *Postgraduate Med.* **101**, 7s–11s.

Hamm, C.W., Goldman, B.U., and Heeschen, C. (1997) Emergency room triage of patients with acute chest pain by means of rapid testing for troponin T and troponin I. *N. Engl. J. Med.* **337**, 1648–9.

Higgins, C. (2007) *Understanding Laboratory Investigations for Nurses and Health Professionals.* 2nd edn. Blackwell Publishing, Oxford.

Hilton, R. (2006) Acute renal failure. *Br. Med. J.* **333**, 786–90.

Hines, J.E., Kehely, A.M., and Thomson, J.N. (1993) Creatine kinase in acute illness. *Lancet.* **342**, 1120–1.

Hofmann, D., Buettner, M., and Rissner, F. (2007) Prognostic value of serum myoglobin in patients after cardiac surgery. *J. Anaesth.* **21**, 304–10.

Kenning, G.I. (2003) Anaemia in the ICU, tolerance or therapy? Poster Presentation Euroanaesthesia.

Kirshenbaum, L.A., Astiz, M.E., and Rackow, E.C. (1998) Interpretation of blood lactate in patients with sepsis. *Lancet.* **352**, 921–2.

Kumar, S. and Berl, T. (1998) Sodium. *Lancet.* **352**, 220–8.

Lee, C.T., Guo, H.R., and Chen, J.B. (2000) Hyponatraemia in the emergency department. *Am. J. Emerg. Med.* **18**, 264–8.

Limdi, J.K. and Hyde, G.M. (2003) Evaluation of abnormal liver function. *Postgraduate Med. J.* **79**, 307–12.

Lyons, W.S. (2008) Blood banks under siege. *Chest.* **134**, 214–5.

Marques, B. and Fritsma, G.A. (2006) *Quick Guide to Coagulation Testing.* American Association of Clinical Chemistry Press, Washington, DC.

McClatchey, D. (2001) *Clinical Laboratory Medicine*, 2nd edn. Lippincott, Williams and Wilkins, Philadelphia.

McCluskey, A., Thomas, A.N., and Bowles, B.J. (1996) The prognostic value of serial measurements of albumin concentration in patients admitted to an intensive care unit. *Anaesthesia.* **51**, 724–7.

McDonough, D.P. (2007) New Jersey's experience: Mandatory estimated GFR reporting. *Clin. J. Am. Soc. Nephrol.* **2**, 1355–9.

McGhee, M.F. (2003) *Guide to Laboratory Investigations.* 3rd edn. Radcliffe Publishing, Abingdon.

Mizcock, B.A. (2002) Point of care testing of blood lactate. *J. Lab. Med.* **26**, 77–81.

Peng, K. (2004) Management of hyponatremia. *Am. Fam. Phys.* **69**, 2387–94.

Pepys, M.B. (2001) The renaissance of C reactive protein. *BMJ.* **322**, 4–6.

Pezzilli, R., Billi, P., Miglioli, M., and Gullo, L. (2005) Serum amylase and lipase concentrations and lipase/amylase ratio in assessment of etiology of acute pancreatitis. *Digest. Dis. Sci.* **38**, 1265–9.

Rastergar, A. and Soleimani, M. (2001) Hypokalaemia and hyperkalaemia. *Postgraduate Med. J.* **77**, 759–64.

Sanai, F.M., Benmousa, A., and Hussani-Al, H. (2008) Is serum ALT level a reliable marker of histological disease in chronic hepatitis C infection? *Liver Int.* **28**, 1011–8.

Schafer, T.J. and Wolford, R.W. (2005) Disorders of potassium emergency. *Med. Clin. North Am.* **23**, 723–47.

Schrier, R.W. (2006) Role of diminished renal function in cardiovascular mortality; marker or pathogenic factor? *J. Am. Coll. Cardiol.* **47**, 1–8.

Schrier, R.W. (2008) Blood urea nitrogen and serum creatinine. *Circulation.* **1**, 2–5.

Skelly, M.M. and James, P.D. (2001) Findings on liver biopsy to investigate abnormal liver function tests in the absence of diagnostic serology. *J. Hepatol.* **35**, 195–9.

Smellie, W.S. and Ryder, S.D. (2006) Biochemical liver function tests. *BMJ.* **333**, 481–3.

Smith, G.L. and Shilpak, M.G. (2006) Serum urea, creatinine and estimators of renal function mortality in older patients with cardiovascular disease. *Arch. Int. Med.* **166**, 1134–42.

Tong, G.M. (2005) Magnesium deficiency in critical illness. *J. Int. Care Med.* **1**, 3–17.

Van den Berghe, G., Wouters, P., and Weekers, F. (2001) Intensive insulin therapy in critically ill patients. *N. Engl. J. Med.* **345**, 1359–67.

Vincent, J.L. (2003) Hypoalbuminaemia in acute illness. *Ann. Surg.* **237**, 319–34.

Volschan, A. and Mesquita, E.T. (2005) D-dimer for myocardial infarction diagnosis in patients with ACS admitted to a chest pain unit. *Crit. Care.* **9**, 15.

Waikar, S.S. and Bonventre, J.V. (2006) Can we rely on blood urea as a biomarker to determine when to initiate dialysis. *Clin. J. Am. Soc. Nephrol.* **1**, 993–4.

West, J. and Brousil, J. (2006) Elevated ALT in patients with diabetes mellitus. *Quart. J. Med.* **99**, 871–6.

Zuccaro, G. (1998) Management of the adult patient with acute lower gastrointestinal bleeding. *Am. J. Gastroenterol.* **93**, 1202–6.

Chapter 11

Assessment tools and track-and-trigger systems

Fiona Creed, Jackie Dawson, and Kaye Looker

Chapter contents

The need to quickly assess and treat acutely ill patients is beyond dispute. Reports such as the Department of Health's Comprehensive Critical Care (2000) highlighted the need for an early warning or track-and-trigger system to ensure timely and appropriate assessment and early escalation of the patient who is deteriorating. The development of these tools has rapidly spread throughout the UK, but has been idiosyncratic therefore there is a current drive for a national early warning score. Understanding of the development, use, and effectiveness of these tools is essential when caring for acutely ill adults.

This chapter will examine:

+ the need for appropriate patient assessment
+ the types of assessment tool available
+ assessment using the ALERT® framework
+ assessment using track-and-trigger scoring systems
+ parameters measured in track-and-trigger scoring systems
+ the evidence for using a track-and-trigger tool
+ the limitations of these assessment tools
+ evaluation of track-and-trigger tools
+ future developments
+ the development of a national modified early warning score.

Learning outcomes

This chapter will enable you to:

+ understand the need for assessment tools
+ look at the main types of tool available
+ understand changes that may occur in variables
+ become aware of the nurses role in track-and-trigger systems
+ analyse the need for early and appropriate escalation
+ know the limitations of these tools
+ consider future developments.

Introduction of a systematic assessment tool

The need to adequately assess the patient who is deteriorating is stressed throughout the literature. Several significant assessment tools have been developed to assist in the identification, assessment, and escalation of the acutely ill adult. One of the most important developments is the introduction of a systematic assessment framework (Smith 2003). The ALERT® framework was introduced by Dr Gary Smith at Portsmouth and provided health professionals with a straightforward framework for rapid assessment of the patient who is deteriorating. On the basis of the ABC assessment that has been used in resuscitation training and practice for many years it was welcomed as a tool for all ward based staff in recognizing, and more importantly in rescuing, the critically ill ward patient.

This framework encourages practitioners to use a stepwise approach to the assessment of the acutely ill adult. It uses an alphabetical system to ensure that patients are quickly and systematically assessed. The system allows systematic review of the acutely ill adult by following a simplistic tool focusing on assessment of:

+ airway
+ breathing
+ circulation
+ disability
+ exposure/everything else/escalation.

The tool encourages practitioners to focus on potentially life-threatening problems first using a 'look, listen, and feel approach', gradually assessing more complex problems if the patient is sufficiently stable enough (Jevon 2007). The following steps are incorporated into the assessment:

Step 1: Airway Look, listen, and feel for signs of airway obstruction. This could include complete obstruction of airway (silent) or partial obstruction of airway. Partial obstruction may result in gurgling, snoring, stridor, or wheeze. Any obstruction of the airway requires urgent attention. Use of airway adjuncts may be appropriate and emergency action should be taken if any airway obstruction is present.

Step 2: Breathing Look, listen, and feel to assess breathing. Alongside counting respirations the patient should be observed for signs of respiratory distress or respiratory suppression. This will involve noting chest movement, respiratory pattern and depth, chest auscultation, palpation, and percussion. Saturations and position of trachea should also be evaluated. Full respiratory assessment is detailed in Chapter 2.

Step 3: Circulation Look, listen, and feel to assess the circulation. The patient should have the strength and rate of the pulse assessed. In addition, the practitioner should assess colour and temperature of the skin, capillary refill time, blood pressure, and ECG. It is also useful to assess for signs of reduced cardiac output (deteriorating levels of consciousness, poor urine output) and examine patient for signs of haemorrhage (Jevon 2007). It is important that fluid balance is assessed here as this is often the cause of clinical deterioration. Full cardiovascular assessment is detailed in Chapter 3; fluid assessment is detailed in Chapter 7.

Step 4: Disability Neurological assessment should be conducted using the AVPU scale. More detailed assessment using the Glasgow Coma Scale may be appropriate. Full neurological assessment is detailed in Chapter 4.

Step 5: Exposure/everything else/escalation The patient should be exposed ensuring dignity is maintained and potential for heat loss reduced. This will facilitate a thorough examination of the deteriorating patient (Smith 2003). The examination should focus upon the suspected cause of deterioration, for example examine calves of legs for swelling if pulmonary embolism suspected, wound drains, abdominal girth if bleeding is suspected, or skin for presence of urticaria if anaphylaxis suspected (Jevon 2007). Alongside exposure the practitioner should consider 'everything else' that may be contributing to the patient's deterioration. This could include:

♦ taking a full history

♦ reviewing notes/observation charts

♦ identifying trends from the observation charts

♦ administering medication, where appropriate

♦ review of laboratory results/12-lead ECG recordings

♦ reviewing anything that may impact on the patient's condition.

Appropriate use of the ALERT® framework should ensure that the level of the patient is quickly assessed and action plan relating to future management determined. It is also vital that all findings are accurately documented in the patient's records (see Chapter 16) and that the patient's deterioration is quickly escalated to an appropriate level (see section on escalation of the patient later in this chapter).

Alongside the need for an immediate assessment tool when the patient is deteriorating there was also a drive to develop assessment tools that could quickly identify those patients who had either deteriorated or were at risk of subsequent deterioration. This initiative encouraged outreach services to begin to develop tools that could identify sick or potentially sick patients and led to the development of track-and-trigger scoring systems.

The introduction of track-and-trigger systems

Track-and-trigger systems are primarily a monitoring tool that alerts the user to any abnormality in physiological parameters by firstly tracking the parameters as they are recorded and then triggering a warning if they are outside of the expected range. Track-and-trigger systems were initially developed in response to studies that clearly showed cardiac arrest victims had abnormal physiological signs before the event (Wood & Smith 1999). The premise behind track-and-trigger systems is that they are usually drawn from routine observations and require little additional workload for ward staff (Gao *et al.* 2007). Track-and-trigger systems may be referred to locally as patient at risk scores (PARS), early warning scores (EWS), or modified early warning scores (MEWS). However, to avoid confusion the term track-and-trigger system will be used throughout this chapter.

Track-and-trigger tools were widely developed and implemented in response to the Comprehensive Critical Care Report (Department of Health 2000) alongside the development of critical care outreach services (see Chapter 12). This document highlighted the need for the support of patients by outreach services and was one of the first reports to highlight the need for outreach services to develop warning systems for patients whose condition was deteriorating.

Subsequent guidelines from NICE (2007) have recommended that all acute care trusts should implement track-and-trigger scoring systems for all patients in acute hospital wards. These guidelines explicitly identify the need for:

♦ the use of track-and-trigger scores on all patients

♦ the need for track-and-trigger systems to be linked to an appropriate escalation policy

♦ a graded response strategy to be developed alongside track-and-trigger systems.

The introduction of track-and-trigger systems has varied widely throughout the UK and little evidence exists to identify which scoring system is the best (see evaluation of track-and-trigger systems later in the chapter). There is a drive towards a national early warning scoring system to be implemented (see future developments of track-and-trigger systems later in this chapter). NICE (2007) have identified the use of a number of track-and-trigger tools and have identified that the tools currently in use are dependent on measurement of:

♦ single parameters:
  • These are used to trigger a response if one of the physiological variables changes sufficiently to 'trigger' a response. This approach is used commonly by medical emergency teams (MET, see Chapter 12)

♦ multiple parameters:
  • These are used to trigger a response if there are more than one abnormal physiological variable. Multiple parameter tools will 'trigger' a response if there is a change in a combination of identified parameters, for example if three out of six measured variables have changed. This approach is commonly used in patient at risk teams (PART, see Chapter 12).

♦ aggregate parameters:
  • In this system measured variables are given a weighted response meaning that changes to some observations are deemed more indicative of deterioration than others, for example respiration score more highly than other observational changes. Again as in multiple parameters it is dependent on multiple changes being identified as abnormal. This approach is commonly used in EWS or MEWS.

♦ combination approaches
  • In this system an aggregate score is used but any single parameter may trigger a response in its own right if scoring at the highest level.

NICE (2007) have reinforced the need to measure multiple parameters in track-and-trigger systems, using an aggregate approach that allows a graded response. They have identified the need to include the following parameters:

♦ heart rate

♦ respiratory rate

♦ systolic blood pressure

♦ levels of consciousness

♦ oxygen saturations

♦ temperature.

They have highlighted that each of these parameters may change in response to acute illness and by tracking small changes in the early stages of acute illness we may be able to identify those patients at risk of further deterioration and implement intervention at an earlier stage.

Most track-and-trigger systems allocate numerical values to each physiological parameter, including respiratory rate, pulse, blood pressure, temperature, conscious level, and sometimes oxygen saturations and urine output. The numerical score will increase as the parameter falls outside of the normal range and the further the parameter is from normal the higher the score. A normal value for any given parameter will normally score a zero. The total of all the abnormal values is added together (aggregate score) and if this value is greater than that recommended for that patient then the patient is said to have 'triggered' on the track-and-trigger system. An example of a track-and-trigger tool is given in Table 11.1.

The significance of variables measured on track-and-trigger tools

The changes that can be anticipated in the early stages of acute illness will be briefly identified but you are reminded that more in depth rationale for changes can be found in the earlier systems-based chapters and you may wish to refresh your knowledge of each systems assessment.

Table 11.1 Adult patient observation chart

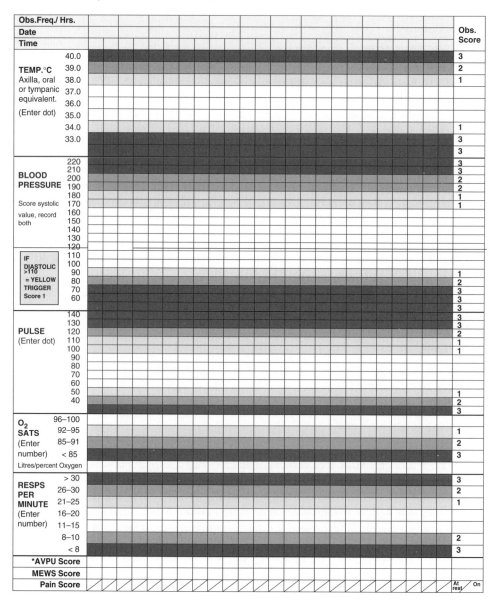

Changes in respiratory rate

One of the most significant variables assessed in all track-and-trigger tools is that of respiration recording. Respiratory rate should be recorded on all patients in an acute hospital area and respirations should be counted for a full minute when the patient has rested. Normal respirations should range between 10 and 17 breaths per minute and any deviation from this may indicate that the patient's condition is deteriorating (Docherty & Coote 2006a). Respiratory rates higher or lower than expected values will trigger a score, the score will increase as the respiratory rate deviates away from normal values.

Alongside simple rate counting the practitioner should note changes in respiratory rate, increased workload of breathing, use of accessory muscles, lung expansion, and colour of the patient (however, for simplicity these factors are not included on the track-and-trigger score). Practitioners should also be alert to patients who report feelings of dyspnoea or simply state that they can't breathe (Smith 2003).

A number of studies have drawn tight correlation between respiratory deterioration and subsequent patient deterioration. This is because respiratory changes are the most sensitive indicator of any deterioration and most patients will exhibit respiratory changes up to 24 h before life-threatening events (Cretikos et al. 2008).

The need for accurate in-depth respiratory assessment is discussed in Chapter 2. However, simple respiration counting can highlight the body's need to both increase oxygen uptake and delivery or remove carbon dioxide. The respiratory system also has an important role in the regulation of acid–base balance and respiration may increase in the presence of a metabolic acidosis in an attempt to remove volatile acid to neutralize pH or the prevention of an accumulation of carbon dioxide (see Chapter 2 for in-depth explanation). It is also influenced by the central nervous system and respiratory suppression may highlight factors such as accidental drug overdose (such as opiates) or CNS damage that require early intervention.

The respiratory system provides an important physiological indicator that something is deteriorating in a patient. The respiratory system has the ability to highlight metabolic and respiratory disturbances and is therefore a key predictor of adverse events (Cretikos et al. 2008).

Alarmingly, however, there is strong evidence that this is the most frequently omitted observation (National Patient Safety Agency 2007; Cretikos et al. 2008). Suggestions for the reasons behind this abound. It should be noted that on a ward environment the respiratory rate has to be counted manually by nursing staff. This may be the reason that this parameter was frequently not recorded on an observation chart as it involves discreetly observing the patients chest for at least 30 s. Anecdotally, student practitioners report finding respiratory monitoring a difficult process and feel uncomfortable in directly observing this important observation.

Subbe et al. (2003) made the observation that changes in blood pressure and pulse are comparatively small and the significance of these changes could be easily missed. It was noted that relative changes in respiratory rate are of much greater magnitude and therefore more likely to be better at discriminating between stable patients and those at risk.

Cretikos et al. (2008) identify the need for all practitioners to be made aware of the need to adequately assess respiratory rate and to understand its significance as a marker of serious illness. They argue that measurement of the rate of respiration does not require complex technology and is not time-consuming. Cretikos et al. (2008) highlight the need for an increased educational emphasis on the significance of respiratory recording stressing the usefulness of this marker and they suggest that all staff should:

♦ record respirations on all patients at least once a day, more if the patient is deteriorating, and that all sets of observations should include respiratory rate recording

♦ understand that pulse oximetry is not a replacement for respiration recording

♦ ensure that patients whose respiratory rate is greater than 24 breaths per minute should be closely monitored and regularly reviewed

♦ ensure that patients whose respiratory rate is greater than 27 breaths per minute at rest should receive immediate medical review

♦ that if patients have a respiratory rate of greater than 24 breaths per minute and other signs of physiological instability (e.g. hypotension, reduced levels of consciousness, tachycardia) they should also be reviewed immediately.

An example of how changes in respiratory rate can aid detection of acute illness is given in Box 11.1.

Changes in heart rate

The pulse is another important vital sign as this may again show early signs of deterioration. The pulse should be counted for a full minute, ideally using the radial pulse as this is most easily accessible on all patients. If your patient's condition has deteriorated this pulse may be difficult to palpate and use of a central pulse may be required, e.g. the femoral or carotid pulse. The pulse should be recorded when the patient has rested. Acute illness may elicit changes to the pulse therefore the nurse should note the heart rate, strength of the pulse, and regularity of the pulse. Pulse estimations must never be taken from the pulse oximeter as this may record the pulse unreliably and will not highlight any irregularities (see Chapter 3 for further details on cardiovascular assessment).

Acutely ill patients may become tachycardic (heart rate greater than 100) or bradycardic (heart rate slower than 60). Variations from the normal anticipated heart rate will automatically trigger a score; the score will increase as the pulse deviates away from normal values.

Tachycardia normally occurs in response to a compensatory mechanism and may indicate hypovolaemia, infection, arrhythmias, cardiac damage, or it may be related to electrolyte imbalance.

Box 11.1

Patient A was admitted to an acute surgical ward for elective hemicolectomy for confirmed bowel cancer. She had an uneventful operation with only minimal blood loss and remained stable throughout. Patient A continued to make a satisfactory recovery until day 5 postoperatively, when her respiratory rate increased and the patient complained of feeling unwell. As per the track-and-trigger chart the observations were recorded more frequently and the patient was reviewed and examined by the medical staff.

Blood and blood cultures were taken and intravenous fluids were recommenced, although no definitive diagnosis was made. Patient A's observations continued to deteriorate, her respiratory rate increased, and her blood pressure decreased. At this point the nursing staff contacted critical care outreach. A full assessment was made, including arterial blood gas and ECG, the senior surgical team were contacted and X-rays taken. The investigations indicated a perforation and the patient was taken back to theatre, where she was found to have faecal peritonitis. The patient was transferred to critical care postoperatively and eventually made a full recovery from her surgery. The track-and-trigger chart highlighted the early signs of deterioration, allowing the staff to act on the MEWS, which resulted in the patient receiving assessment and optimum treatment in a timely manner.

Tachycardia is generally a sign of sympathetic activation in acute illness and caused by the release of catecholamines (adrenaline and noradrenaline) in an attempt to provide an increased cardiac output during episodes of acute illness (Cooper & Cramp 2003). It may be accompanied by hypotension (a late physiological indicator of shock) and by pallor, clamminess, and sweating (stimulated by release of catecholamines). Tachycardia is a later sign than changes in respiration and changes may be subtle at first (Subbe *et al.* 2003). Goldhill *et al.* (1999) reviewed observation charts following patient's admission to the intensive treatment unit (ITU) and noted that whilst respiratory rate changes had occurred, often 24 h before admission to ITU, heart rate changes did not follow the same pattern.

Bradycardia may be caused by certain drugs, cardiac damage, and diseased cardiac conduction pathways or raised intracranial pressure (Docherty & Coote 2006b). Severe bradycardia will have a direct effect on blood pressure and this may drop dramatically. Tachycardia and bradycardia must be quickly reported. Patients with tachycardia/bradycardia may benefit from continuous ECG measurement and this should be instigated immediately if you are concerned about the patient's heart rate or rhythm. It may be beneficial, if the patient is sufficiently stable, to record a 12-lead ECG whilst waiting for review from the medical staff.

Heart rate changes will have a physiological impact on blood pressure and it is essential that the nurse compares changes in heart rate alongside changes in blood pressure.

Changes in blood pressure

Blood pressure changes may occur in acutely ill patients and it is vital that blood pressure is recorded accurately in acute settings. It is now common practice to use electronic blood pressure recorders to speed up clinical assessment, but some areas still use manual sphygmomanometers. Where these are used it is important that the correct technique is adopted and that staff are competent in their use. Normal blood pressure ranges from a systolic of 100–139 mmHg and a diastolic pressure of 60–90 mmHg (British Hypertension Society 2007).

Although hypertension is clearly an issue in clinical practice, because of the potential long-term detrimental effect, it is not usually considered on track-and-trigger systems and will only trigger a response if excessively high.

Track-and-trigger scoring systems generally try to identify hypotension and will trigger a score if the blood pressure is lower than expected values—the score will increase as the blood pressure deviates away from normal values. Score values are only attributed to systolic blood pressure and will generally begin to trigger a score if the systolic pressure falls below 100 mmHg. As blood pressure begins to fall organ perfusion decreases and clinical signs of poor perfusion such as decreased urine output may be present (Docherty & Coote 2006b). Mean arterial pressure is a more reliable indicator of organ perfusion and perfusion will reduce if MAP drops below 60 mmHg.

In acutely ill patients hypotension normally occurs as a result of shock, usually alongside tachycardia. It is important to recognize that hypotension occurs as a very late sign of shock. In the initial and compensatory stages of shock the sympathetic nervous system will trigger the release of catecholamines (adrenaline and noradrenaline) that will initially stabilize blood pressure. Blood pressure will further be stabilized by release of hormones that encourage the retention of fluid and further vasoconstriction. Examination of the stages of shock (see Table 11.2) identify that hypotension occurs only in the progressive stage of shock, by which time the patient is acutely unwell and needs urgent attention.

Blood pressure changes should be promptly notified and urgent medical attention sought if the patient is presenting with other signs that may indicate the progression of shock (see Table 11.2). It should be noted that electronic measuring devices for blood pressure may be unreliable if the patient is hypotensive and manual recordings may be preferable.

Table 11.2 Stages of shock

Stage of shock	Symptoms
Initial stage	Very little noticeable change, Increase in respiratory rate
Compensatory stage	Slight increase or unchanged blood pressure, Increasing diastolic pressure, Tachycardia, Increased respirations, Cool peripheries
Progressive stage	Hypotension, Tachycardia, Increased respirations, Pallor, Sweating, Decreased levels of consciousness
Refractory stage	Organ dysfunction, Death if untreated.

Changes in levels of consciousness

Consciousness is a dynamic state and monitoring of conscious levels may provide indicators that the patient's condition is deteriorating. Levels of consciousness may be affected by acute illness either in response to reduced oxygen or blood flow to the central nervous system or accumulations of carbon dioxide and other substances (such as drugs) that are detrimental to the central nervous system.

Assessment of conscious levels needs to be fast in acute illness and most track-and-trigger systems use the AVPU system to determine consciousness. Patients' conscious levels are based on speedy assessment of whether they are:

A **a**lert

V awake to **v**erbal stimulus

P awake to **p**ain

U **u**nconscious

A full neurological assessment (see Chapter 4) is usually only deemed necessary if the patient's levels of consciousness have rapidly deteriorated or there is evidence that loss of consciousness is linked to a neurological problem.

Most track-and-trigger scoring systems will attribute a score if consciousness is affected or if the patient is showing signs of new confusion/agitation. It is usually useful to record a blood glucose level if consciousness is impaired (as this is the most frequent cause of reduced levels of consciousness in the ward patient).

Practitioners should be aware of the need to maintain the patient's airway if levels of consciousness are reduced, the insertion of an oropharyngeal or nasopharyngeal airway may be required until consciousness returns, and careful positioning of the patient should prevent aspiration if consciousness is severely affected. Urgent medical attention should be sought if the patient is only responsive to pain or is unconscious.

Changes in oxygen saturation

Oxygen saturation changes are a recent addition to some track-and-trigger scoring systems. Normal oxygen saturation is generally held to be above 97% on room air (Jevon 2007). Variations from the normal anticipated saturation will automatically trigger a score that will increase as saturation drops below normal values.

The NICE (2007) guidelines emphasized the need to record oxygen saturation changes as a core initiator on all track-and-trigger systems. However, the recent addition of this important parameter is not simplistic as it is a difficult parameter to provide a score for. The usefulness of oxygen saturations as a value is dependent on the amount of oxygen the patient is receiving. If a patients saturations are 90% on room air this is potentially less of a concern than identical saturations on a patient receiving high-flow oxygen via a non-rebreath mask (approx. 85%). There has therefore been considerable discussion on whether absolute saturation values (e.g. 90%) should be attributed a score value or whether an attempt should be made to compare saturation values to the amount of oxygen the patient is receiving. Inclusion of complex parameters (i.e. scoring saturations in relation to inspired oxygen saturation) may make the track-and-trigger scoring system more complex and, perhaps, more prone to error if additional calculation is required.

Alongside the complexities of comparing oxygen requirement and oxygen saturation Cretikos *et al.* (2008) identify the potential drawbacks of saturation as a reliable measure of acute illness and highlight poor understanding about the potential limitations of saturation in clinical practice. Cretikos *et al.* (2008) identify confusion over the meaning of oxygen saturation, suggesting that nurses appear to view saturation results as an indicator of adequate ventilation (it is not!). A number of factors have been shown to affect the reliability of oxygen saturation results in acute illness, these include:

+ poor peripheral perfusion (often associated with acute illness)
+ low cardiac output states (often associated with acute illness)
+ anaemia
+ presence of carboxyhaemoglobin
+ hypothermia
+ cardiac arrhythmias
+ dark skin pigmentation
+ false or painted nails
+ incorrect probe/incorrect probe position.

Alongside incorrect readings practitioners should be aware that saturation recordings do not reflect carbon dioxide levels and patients with relatively normal saturations may have high carbon dioxide levels (hypercarbia) present.

NICE (2007) also identify the need to recognize the potential limitations of oxygen saturation monitoring but highlight that studies have shown saturation in some incidences to have a correlation to deterioration and admission to ITU (Cuthbertson *et al.* 2007).

Practitioners should ensure that the saturation probe is moved at regular intervals (as poor blood flow due to compression may reduce reliability), ensure that the probe is positioned correctly away from bright light, and ensure that the correct probe is used. Practitioners should check for capillary refill and peripheral shutdown and consider the effects of this on the reliability of the saturation result. In addition, practitioners should be aware of other situations where saturation may be an unreliable measurement of oxygenation.

Changes in temperature

Temperature is an important variable in acute illness and all track-and-trigger systems will provide a score for temperature. Variations from the normal anticipated temperature will automatically trigger a score that will increase as temperature deviates from normal values. Monitoring of temperature highlights if the patient is hypothermic or pyrexial. Most track-and-trigger scoring systems will only trigger a score if the patient's temperature is below 35 or above 38.5°C.

Hypothermia will achieve a score if the temperature falls below 35°C. Potential causes of hypothermia should be evaluated and include:

+ environmental factors
+ exposure

♦ large fluid replacement

♦ post surgery

♦ extra corporeal blood circulation (e.g. dialysis).

The practitioner should monitor for side effects of hypothermia (cardiac arrhythmias, blood coagulopathies, hypotension, etc.) and attempt to slowly increase core body temperature.

The monitoring of pyrexia is especially significant in the acutely ill patient and temperature above 38.5° C should begin the process of evaluation for infection. Whilst it is recognized that there may be other causes for pyrexia, it is important to exclude infection as the root cause. It is well recognized that sepsis is poorly identified in acutely ill patients and appropriate escalation of septic patients is vital. Full details about the diagnosis and management of sepsis in acute care are discussed in Chapter 8. However, the need for appropriate treatment is stressed by the surviving sepsis campaign (http://www.survivingsepsis.org) and includes the following recommendations:

♦ timely diagnosis

♦ administration of broad spectrum antibiotics within 1 h of diagnosis

♦ measurement of serum lactate

♦ evaluation of blood cultures

♦ early fluid resuscitation

♦ early goal-directed therapy.

Pyrexia alongside tachycardia, increased respiratory rate, and alterations to blood pressure and peripheral temperature requires speedy intervention. The changes to blood pressure and peripheral temperature will be dependent on the stage of the sepsis. Simplistically these are:

♦ early stages of sepsis: normal or slightly high blood pressure with an increasing pulse pressure, patient feels peripherally and centrally warm

♦ late stages of sepsis: low blood pressure, patient feels peripherally cool despite high central temperature.

Other significant variables

Alongside the core variables suggested by NICE some track-and-trigger systems include the evaluation of other variables. The use of these variables will differ considerably between trusts and scores may be attributed to variations in urine output or levels of pain. Additional blood test results may be used to help inform the medical team but are not usually ascribed a value on track-and-trigger systems.

Changes to fluid balance

The use of changes to fluid balance, specifically urine output, is deemed important in some trusts. Track-and-trigger systems may attribute a score to a reducing urine output (excessive urine output as seen in some conditions such as diabetes inspidus is not scored). The kidneys are susceptible to acute illness and reduction in urine output may highlight that either:

♦ the body is attempting to conserve fluid to increase cardiac output and blood pressure

♦ the kidneys are not adequately perfused (usually if the mean arterial pressure is below 60 mmHg).

NICE (2007) do not recommend that urine output is included in the core variables of a track-and-trigger system as its sensitivity is reliant on accurate measurement of urinary output. This is only possible if the patient has a urinary catheter in situ. Many patients, in the early stages of deterioration are not catheterized and periodic measurement of urine output may be unreliable.

Practitioners should be aware that knowledge of patient's fluid balance is fundamental to the assessment of acutely ill patients. It is therefore essential that a fluid balance chart is recorded for all acutely ill patients and that fluid balance (i.e. input minus output) should be recorded frequently throughout the shift to determine the patients current fluid status (see Chapter 7 on fluid management).

Changes in pain levels

Pain assessment is of importance in acute care. Assessment of pain has been included in some scoring systems but again is not recommended as a core variable by NICE (2007).

It is important to monitor pain levels in acutely ill patients for a number of reasons:

+ Practitioners have a professional and ethical duty to ensure that adequate analgesia is provided to all patients.

+ The presence of pain may adversely affect some of the core variables. Heart rate and respiratory rate may be increased in the presence of pain and it is useful to exclude pain as the cause for any changes documented.

+ Analgesia may directly affect the core variables, in particular opiate-based analgesia may cause hypotension, bradycardia, or tachycardia and may cause respiratory depression. Side effects of analgesia require careful monitoring in the acute patient.

+ Increases in pain levels may be signs of the patient's condition worsening, for example patients post abdominal surgery may develop increased levels of pain if they are haemorrhaging.

Pain assessment is clearly relevant in assessment of the acutely ill adult but it may not receive a numerical value if it is not part of the track-and-trigger system.

Changes in blood analysis

Blood results may enable the medical staff to make a differential diagnosis. There are a large number of blood results that may be requested when caring for an acutely ill adult (see Chapter 10 on blood investigations). However, the complexity and range of blood results available prohibit their use on a track-and-trigger scoring system. Commonly requested blood tests in acute situations include:

+ suspected bleeding: full blood count, clotting studies

+ suspected infection: full blood count (white cell count and neutrophils), C-reactive protein, blood lactate

+ suspected respiratory problems: full blood count, arterial blood gas analysis

+ fluid overload: full blood count (haematocrit), urea, and electrolytes

+ suspected pulmonary embolism: full blood count, clotting studies, D-dimers.

This list is not extensive and other blood tests and investigations may be requested by the medical team. It is useful to locate recent blood results for the patient wherever possible as the medical team may require these to make a differential diagnosis.

Developing plans for monitoring patients

Alongside the development of the track-and-trigger systems, NICE (2007) also highlighted the importance of developing plans for monitoring patients. NICE (2007) identified the need to ensure that all patients in acute wards were monitored using a track-and-trigger scoring system at least once every 12 h. However, the frequency of observations should increase appropriately if the patient's condition deteriorates.

The frequency of observations may vary between trusts and between individual patients, but recommendations from the National Patient Safety Agency (2007) identify the need for trusts to have clear guidelines in place in relation to monitoring plans for patients whose condition is deteriorating. These guidelines should detail the frequency of observations to be recorded and the type of observations required. Monitoring plans should avoid ambiguous terms such as 'monitor the patient more often' and use objective measurable terms that will facilitate later audits, for example if MEWS = 2 increase observations to 30 min. Monitoring plans should be linked to an escalation of concern protocol.

Escalation of concern

One of the main necessities in clinical practice is for any track-and-trigger system to be linked to a reliable escalation policy. The purpose of the track-and-trigger system is to identify those patients who are giving cause for concern and using that information to effectively escalate that concern to an appropriate person. Timely and appropriate escalation of concern will enable timely and effective treatment to the patient who is deteriorating.

The speed of the escalation process will be dependent on the correct assessment using a track-and-trigger score. Again hospitals have each developed their own individual escalation policy and there is evidence of a variety of approaches being used in clinical practice. It is, however, essential that each practitioner within the NHS is aware of the trust's individual escalation process. Some guidance in relation to escalation of concern has been provided by NICE (2007). The guidelines highlight the need to develop localized strategies that will be effective for each individual trust; however, they suggest that escalation of concern should be graded and linked to three areas of concern:

♦ Low score/concern

Patients scoring low scores should have the frequency of their observations increased as a matter of course. The concern about the patient should be escalated to the nurse in charge.

♦ Medium score/concern

Where patients score medium scores areas of concern should be escalated to the primary medical team wherever possible. This may be difficult out of hours, but the team responsible for covering that patient should be informed. At the same time the areas of concern should be escalated to those professionals within the trust with critical/acute care core competencies. This will clearly vary between trusts, and may involve escalation of concern to outreach services, hospital at night team, site managers, etc.

♦ High score/concern

Where the patient's score is high there should be immediate escalation of concern to an appropriate team. Again this will be trust dependent but may include MET, outreach calls, anaesthetists, and cardiac arrest teams. The urgency of this escalation should be articulated clearly and the need for an immediate response stressed.

An example of an escalation policy is included in Box 11.2.

The need for a robust escalation policy to be in place in every trust has been stressed by the NPSA report on responding to deteriorating patients (2007). This report highlights the need for each trust to establish a deterioration recognition group. This group should be multidisciplinary in nature and should link with clinical policy makers, risk assessment groups, clinical staff,

Box 11.2 Escalation process used at a local trust

Action in the event of a patient trigger

Any patients whose observations trigger *must always* be reported to the registered nurse who is responsible for the patient. A MEWS score *must* be completed for all patients who trigger. The registered nurse will then use clinical judgement to decide on the necessary course of action. For help in patient assessment, refer to the outreach folder.

The registered nurse should use the following as a guide.

If the MEWS score is 4 or more

1 Call the patient's parent team.

2 Inform the outreach team (see below).

3 Check the patient's observations (including MEWS) every 15 min—*The patient may be deteriorating*!

If the MEWS score is 1, 2, or 3.

The patient's observations (including MEWS) must be rechecked regularly to identify any deterioration.

For MEWS scores of:

1 recheck every hour

2 recheck every 30 min

3 recheck every 15 min

The registered nurse should use clinical judgement to decide how long these enhanced observations should continue.

Clinical judgement should take into account:

♦ any trends in the observations that may identify deterioration or improvement.

♦ the patient's previous history or baseline observations.

♦ any current treatment plans (including DNAR status).

managers, and educators to ensure that appropriate escalation procedures are in place and evaluated.

The NPSA have also identified (but does not endorse) a number of various educational initiatives that may improve escalation of acutely ill patients. These include:

♦ the ALERT® programme—a 1-day multiprofessional course run at most trusts

♦ acute illness management—a 1-day course aimed at standardizing approaches to assessment and management of acute illness

♦ the ill medical patients' acute care and treatment course aimed at SHOs in medicine to improve knowledge and management of sick medical patients.

The NPSA are also in the process of developing the 'foresight' training initiative aimed at using scenarios to help identify factors that may impair safe practice.

Box 11.3

Patient B was admitted with increasing sudden shortness of breath. Patient B had recently been on a long-haul journey to America, sitting in the economy section of the aircraft. There was no relevant past medical history, although patient B was overweight and had previously been a smoker. Patient B's initial observations showed a MEWS score of 9, thus making her at high risk of critical illness. This extremely high MEWS score indicated that immediate escalation to staff with critical care skills was essential.

The trust's escalation policy was followed and the critical care outreach and medical teams were contacted. On initial assessment it was clear that the patient was acutely unwell, the anaesthetic consultant was contacted and the patient was admitted to the intensive treatment unit. Patient B had suffered a massive pulmonary embolus and was mechanically ventilated but made a full recovery. The early recognition and the importance of the nursing staff appreciating that the patient required specialist care ensured assessment and intervention were commenced in a timely manner.

The need for a robust escalation system to improve communication between nursing staff and medical staff regarding patients at risk is emphasized. There is little doubt that if used and acted on it can aid the timely recognition and aid of patients. An example of how rapid assessment using track-and-trigger and appropriate escalation can save lives is included in Box 11.3.

The chain of response, a new initiative to improve assessment, treatment, and escalation

In an attempt to tighten the escalation process and make clear each staff member's role in caring for acutely ill patients the Department of Health (2008) have launched a competency framework. Within this framework there is an explicit requirement for each trust to establish a chain of response to acutely ill patients. Included within the chain of response is the need to define roles and role boundaries of all staff, in an attempt to streamline assessment, treatment, communication, and escalation of the sick patient.

The Department of Health envisages a team response to the acutely ill adult, whereby all members in that team have explicitly stated roles and competencies (although there is an acknowledgement that some ward roles may cross the boundaries within the 'chain of response'). In identifying a team approach the Department of Health have identified several roles including:

♦ non-clinical supporter

♦ recorder

♦ primary responder

♦ secondary responder

♦ tertiary responder.

These roles have been explored in depth earlier (see Chapter 1). However, the development of these roles and the 'chain of response' aims to ensure that the 'team' caring for acutely ill patients possess overall competencies to facilitate effective care. These competencies include the team's ability to:

♦ accurately record and document observations using a track-and-trigger scoring system

♦ recognize when values are abnormal and then interpret potential causes for the deviation from abnormality

Box 11.4

Mr C is a 56-year-old man admitted following a total hip replacement. He is a smoker and has been coughing frequently postoperatively.

Recorder: The healthcare assistant records his observations and informs you that his respiratory rate has increased to 34, his heart rate is 110, and his saturations 90% on 40% oxygen.

Recognizer: The band 5 staff nurse reviews the patient, notes the change in his respiration, performs a more in-depth respiratory assessment, and repositions the patient and informs outreach, requesting an immediate review. Observations increase to once every 30 min,

The primary responder: The outreach nurse reviews the patient, recognizes that the patient has acute respiratory problems and increases the oxygen concentration to 60%, ensures continuous monitoring and liaises with the registrar regarding the need for arterial blood gases and the instigation of non-invasive ventilation.

The secondary responder: The patient is reviewed by the medical team. Arterial blood gases show type 1 respiratory failure and the outreach nurse sets up continuous positive airway pressure (CPAP) ventilation. Monitoring of the patient is increased to every 15 min and 1:1 nursing instigated during the initial establishment of CPAP.

The patient remains on CPAP but fails to improve and his condition continues to deteriorate. Repeat blood gas show the development of type 2 respiratory failure. Advice is sought from the ITU team.

The tertiary response: The patient is reviewed by the ITU registrar, who notes the continued deterioration of this patient's respiratory function and organizes his immediate transfer to ITU for invasive ventilation and support.

- assess the patient and provide timely and appropriate intervention at a level that corresponds with the severity of the patient's condition
- provide intervention at three varying levels: a primary response, a secondary response, and a tertiary response
- recognize when a higher level of intervention is required
- communicate the urgency of the situation to ensure that the patient receives optimum care.

The implementation of this 'chain of response' is at developmental stages, but the net effect is illustrated in a clinical vignette (see Box 11.4).

The implementation of this new initiative is in an early stage and no audit of the effectiveness of this to improve assessment, treatment, and escalation is currently available.

Issues arising in clinical practice related to track-and-trigger tools

Whilst there appears to be a continuing need for the development of track-and-trigger systems, there is also evidence that there are other factors to consider and several clinical issues relating to the implementation of track-and-trigger systems still need to be considered.

Issue 1: Variation from normal value

An important aspect of the track-and-trigger tool is that it is based on variations of pre-defined 'normal observations' and it is important to recognize that 'normal' values will vary with age and co-morbidity. Any variable that may cause alterations to physiological measurements has the potential to cause the tool to artificially trigger when that patient may be stable.

The work of Duckitt *et al.* (2007) shows that adult patients under 55 years will have an average respiratory rate of 18, whereas patients who are older may have a respiratory rate in excess of 20 as their norm. This may mean that older patients would trigger an outreach call but still have relatively normal physiological measurements in relation to their age. It is questionable whether trigger scores should be increased in older patients to prevent unnecessary triggering of outreach calls. There is, however, no available data to substantiate this.

A recent study by Smith *et al.* (2008) examined whether it was useful to include age as a parameter on a track-and-trigger scoring system. Smith *et al.* (2008) identified that an increase in age had a direct correlation in increasing mortality rates, for example older patients had an greater risk of mortality with an increased MEWS than younger patients with a similar MEWS score. This study did not attempt to see how age could be used to change trigger parameters, but reviewed the effect of age on hospital survival. Unsurprisingly, this study drew direct correlations between age and hospital mortality following acute illness and drew the conclusion that inclusion of age could be advantageous on track-and-trigger systems, but only really in enabling them to predict mortality. The study highlighted the potential ethical issues this could raise. Inclusion of age on a track-and-trigger system would require careful implementation and evaluation.

Whilst age is clearly an important indicator of morbidity, it should be remembered that it is not the only factor that may alter normal values. The patient's current condition and medication will also have an effect on the 'normal' observations. These factors should be taken into account rather than purely relying on the numerical values allocated. For example, a cardiology patient who is on antihypertensive medication will have a low blood pressure that would 'trigger' a response. However, if the patient is warm and well perfused and passing adequate urine the trained nurse needs to make an assessment of the patient, decide whether to call the team, or document why the trigger has not been acted upon at that time.

Issue 2: Failure to identify the deteriorating patient

It is important to reflect that an early warning tool should be used as an aid to guide the medical and nursing staff. There will occasionally be patients who are clearly unwell but still do not trigger on the EWS. This is reflected in work by Gardner Thorpe *et al.* (2006), who state that patients within their small study were admitted into ITU without triggering on the early warning tool. They suggested that staff need to use professional judgement alongside the tool to ensure appropriate assessment of all patients.

Review of the MET tools highlights the use of intuitive practice as a trigger threshold. Alongside scoring individual variables the MET team can be called if the practitioner is concerned about the patient. A study by Cioffi (2000) identified that many nurses used subjective measurements such as the 'patient not looking right' and used intuitive or sixth sense to replace other more objective measurements. This view echoes work by Benner (1984), who discusses that the 'expert' nurse may use intuition to guide practice. It is clearly difficult to ascribe a numerical value for patients who appear unwell. Some trusts also include this variable on their escalation protocol. Care should be taken, if this approach is used, that the practitioner is still able to articulate the cause for concern. Medical staff may need other evidence of deterioration if a prompt review is required.

Issue 3: The need for more education

In today's climate it is widely acknowledged that the ward patients are a sicker group of people than would have been the case a few decades ago. The use of day surgery and specialized clinics has had the effect of increasing the acuity of the ward patient and it is very rare that a hospital in-patient is given time to convalesce after major surgery. The training and establishment of staff has not always reflected this increased acuity.

Cuthbertson & Smith (2007) suggest that track-and-trigger systems are not necessarily better at detecting the deteriorating patient than high-quality clinical assessment and judgement by appropriately skilled and experienced personnel. The NPSA (2007) audit identified that experience was important when carrying out observations, suggesting that experienced nurses were more able to make appropriate judgements when caring for an acutely ill patient. McArthur-Rouse (2001) highlights the potential reductionalist assessment that track-and-trigger tools may facilitate. She suggests that nurses should not be encouraged to rely on simplistic tools but develop the knowledge and skills to conduct a thorough whole-patient assessment and be able to articulate this to medical staff.

Whilst this is clearly a gold standard for all experienced registered practitioners, it should be remembered that these experienced nurses may not be instrumental in recording ward observations. The NPSA (2007) noted that a large proportion of observations were delegated to junior staff, student nurses, and healthcare assistants. They suggested that these staff may not have the experience or competence to accurately interpret the changes in observations or may not be aware of the serious nature of the changes. In particular, they noted lack of physiological knowledge that would enable the interpretation of observations. They suggested that an over-reliance on junior staff to complete observations may lead to acutely ill patients being undetected.

Issue 4: Which system to use?

Some outreach teams argue that the use of colour coding on EWS facilitates easier identification of the patient who is deteriorating. Oakey & Slade (2006) discuss the use of a colour-coded chart that emphasizes abnormal physiological measurements, therefore allowing easier identification of the deteriorating patient. They highlight that an observation chart with coloured bandings to represent the varying degree of physiological derangement is easy to use and has an immediate visual impact.

Other trusts have used the analogy of a traffic light system to aid understanding and application of a track-and-trigger system (Ryan *et al.* 2004). These systems employ a 'traffic light' system with red being severely abnormal observations, orange being moderately abnormal and green being just slightly out of range. It is argued that these tools allow early identification of the patient who is deteriorating and facilitate identification and communication of level 1 and 2 patients.

Some track-and-trigger scoring systems rely upon the numerical calculation of the MEWS and do not colour code their systems. Each deviation away from a normal value is attributed a score (as observations are in colour-coded systems) and the practitioner has to calculate the MEWS without the addition of colour bands as a visual prompt.

Much discussion surrounds the use of these systems. Those in favour of colour-coded systems point to their visual prompting and reduction in complex calculations. Oakley & Slade (2006) highlight the difficulties in the implementation of their MEWS chart when the scoring system for the calculation was based on the reverse of the chart. They highlighted that lack of colour often caused confusion over when an observation generated an at risk score. In addition, Smith & Oakey (2006) highlighted that numeracy could also be problematic in some staff and their study highlighted that correct calculations of MEWS score often decreased as the wards got busier. They also suggested that nurses' numeracy abilities were sometimes suboptimal, and reflected general numeracy trends throughout the UK. Their study identified that the nurses took more time in calculating complex MEWS scores as the patient's condition deteriorated and calculations became more complex.

Other areas have moved away from paper scoring and use hand-held computer systems to generate the MEWS score in an attempt to reduce human error in mathematical calculation. Experimental work on using a hand-held computer illustrated that the MEWS score was more reliably calculated when data were input into a hand-held device rather than when mental calculation of the MEWS was relied on (Mohammed *et al.* 2009). There is, however, no consensus over the best type of tool and work is ongoing in developing more accurate and user-friendly tools. Practitioners should, in the meantime, acknowledge the potential limitations of each of these types of tools.

Issue 5: Important measurements not considered in track-and-trigger tools

In an attempt to maintain simplicity of these tools, a number of observations that are valuable in the assessment of acutely ill patients have been omitted as they:

+ may be difficult to provide a numerical value for
+ may be affected by other conditions for example peripheral vascular disease or
+ make recordings and calculations too complex.

Most notably assessment of diastolic pressure is not used (all systems are reliant upon systolic pressure) and patients' peripheral temperature and capillary refill time are not taken into account.

Omission of diastolic pressure in these systems is unfortunate as it prevents very early indicators of shock to be noted. In highlighting the significance of blood pressure as a variable in track-and-trigger systems, it was highlighted that changes to systolic pressure occur when compensatory mechanisms have failed (see Table 11.2). Diastolic pressure is a useful measurement in identifying patients who are in the compensatory stages of hypovolaemic shock. In these patients diastolic pressure will initially rise alongside a falling pulse pressure. This may provide an earlier indicator of shock and the significance of diastolic pressure should be appreciated by ward staff. To an extent, failure to include it as part of a track-and-trigger score may further detract from understanding of this important variable as an indicator of early hypovolaemia.

Most systems also do not use peripheral temperature or capillary refill as indicators of deterioration. In acute illness physiological changes occur in an attempt to maintain homeostasis. Table 11.2 also highlights that cool peripheral temperature, caused by the release of catecholamines, will cause vasodilatation in hypovolaemic patients during the compensatory stages of shock as a result of sympathetic activation (Cooper & Cramp 2003). Attempts have been made to use skin temperature as a non-invasive marker of haemodynamic status (Schey *et al.* 2009). This small-scale study identified that assessment of cool peripheries could be used to make assumptions about haemodynamic status. However, practitioners should be cautious in patients with a history of peripheral vascular disease. This important physiological sign is often overlooked in clinical practice but does provide important early indicators of the presence of hypovolaemia in some patients.

Whilst it is inappropriate to recommend the inclusion of these as they generally make assessment more complex for inexperienced staff, it is important that the necessity for speedy assessment does not ignore the significance of a more holistic assessment of the acutely ill adult (McArthur-Rouse 2001) and the acknowledgement that these can enhance patient assessment as they provide valuable early indicators of deterioration.

Issue 6: Failure to record observations

A major problem area surrounding the use of track-and-trigger systems is the failure to appropriately record observations. In their 2007 report, the NPSA identified a number of problem areas, including:

+ low priority given to the recording of observations, leading to them being viewed as a menial task that needs to be completed

- complacency over the recording of observations as staff may not always expect well patients to deteriorate
- frequency of observations may not be reviewed even in cases of deterioration and sometimes observations are excessively recorded on stable patients who do not require frequent monitoring
- failure to fully complete MEWS charts or total up scores, leading to inaccurate records; regrettably the NPSA still found problems associated with the recording of respiration despite greater emphasis on this important observation.

Where observations were recorded appropriately staff reported problems with the sensitivity of the trigger, meaning that many patients were inappropriately escalated. This led to staff reporting feelings of 'trigger fatigue', which reduced the staff's responsiveness to the MEWS score as an indicator of deterioration.

The need to record observations and ensure that they are a priority is emphasized by the NPSA (2007) and Patient Safety First (2008). Both of these bodies highlight the need for:

- accurate recording of observations for all patients
- training for all staff about the need for assessment and interpretation of results
- local protocols for the assessment of physiological measurements
- assessment of key observational skills to be judged against core competencies (Department of Health 2008)
- staff to recognize the importance of recording and interpreting clinical observations.

The need to adequately audit the recording of observations as part of an ongoing monitoring process is stressed by the NPSA and the Patient Safety First campaign.

Evaluation of track-and-trigger tools

Whilst there is anecdotal evidence that track-and-trigger systems appear valuable in practice, it is important to ensure that these new tools are evaluated appropriately. Several studies have been undertaken in an attempt to evaluate the use of track-and-trigger systems and various aspects have been evaluated. Studies have examined:

- the use of single/multivariable track-and-trigger systems
- the reliability of track-and-trigger assessment tools
- the sensitivity of track-and-trigger tools.

Single parameter versus multiple/aggregate parameters

The use of a single parameter certainly simplifies the process of track and trigger and may offer some benefits. Studies on the MET calling criteria, that is the deterioration of one physiological variable, have highlighted that the simplicity of this system allows more rapid identification of the patient who is deteriorating. This system is reliant on the immediate reporting of a change in any observation that is sufficient enough to trigger a response. Whilst this approach certainly appears to increase the number of medical emergency calls (MERIT 2005) it must be emphasized that using a single parameter has a number of limitations. In its systematic review of the evidence of single parameter scoring systems NICE (2007) identifies that whilst use of a single parameter system offers more reproducible results, it has a number of significant limitations. It limits the progress of a patient to be tracked, as effective tracking is reliant on examining a number of factors. It also highlighted that when used in the clinical situation single parameters may trigger unnecessary calls to outreach teams and potentially miss patients who are acutely unwell. Because of these limitations single parameter systems are not used widely in the UK and most systems include other parameters in any track-and-trigger systems as multimodal systems are thought to capture more patients by using an aggregate score.

Multiparameter tools are considered by many to be superior to assessing a single change in the patient's condition and allow for more accurate tracking of the patient's condition (NICE 2007). These tools examine a number of changes in the patient's physiological status and examination of the literature suggests that the reliability of the tool to identify the patient who is deteriorating increases with the number of affected variables, that is the more abnormal results the quicker the patient may be identified. These tools are, however, prone to human error and miscalculation as they are inherently more complex than single parameter tools. They may also not identify patients who only have changes in one parameter. The reliability of these tools appears to increase with severity of illness (sick patients will be recognized more quickly than those with only moderate deterioration).

The use of aggregate scores to trigger a response has also been examined. Aggregate scores, for example MEWS, have been widely adopted throughout the UK. The advantage of the aggregate systems was that they allowed a graded response to the patient. Ideally, there needs to be some form of algorithm or calling cascade for the ward nurses to follow once a patient has triggered and this should take the form of a 'graded' response, that is

♦ if MEWS ≥ 4 call the parent team and/or critical care outreach within 15 min

♦ if MEWS = 2–3 repeat the observations within 15 min and inform the nurse in charge

♦ if MEWS = 1, inform a trained nurse and repeat observations within an hour.

However, the complexity and potential for human error were highlighted as areas of weakness of an aggregate tool (NICE 2007).

Reliability of track-and-trigger scoring

The ability for differing nurses to obtain the same or similar results when using track-and-trigger tools has also been examined. In a small-scale study by Subbe *et al.* (2006) the use of three differing types of track-and-trigger systems were examined in an attempt to identify which system was the most reliable offering reproducible results. In the examination of single and multiple parameter tools Subbe *et al.* (2006) highlighted that the more simplistic the tool the greater the reliability. The researchers found that a single parameter tool provided more consistent results than tools that used multiple parameters. Interestingly, reliability of the tool decreased as the tools became more complex and allowed the inclusion of several parameters. The MEWs score was the most complex assessment tool assessed and there appeared to be a marked difference in scores attributed by different assessors. The study did identify, however, that irrespective of scores attributed each system showed better agreement on triggers for escalation than aggregate scores.

Sensitivity of track-and-trigger systems

Gao *et al.* (2007) undertook one of the first systematic reviews of track-and-trigger systems and highlighted that whilst they were a useful tool in practice there were limitations. One of the main limitations of the tools was the level of sensitivity. Sensitivity is a measurement of how accurate the tool is in identifying at risk or acutely ill patients. The majority of tools tested had poor sensitivity, this meant that they were unable to always identify those patients who were acutely ill or who had the potential to deteriorate. Gao *et al.* (2007) suggested that this was because many of the tools had not been robustly tested and suggested that further research and development of tools was required. They suggested that most tools were only useful if used as an adjunct to clinical judgement.

Wide-scale evaluation of track-and-trigger systems

More recently, the Intensive Care National Audit Research Committee (ICNARC) have commissioned a study evaluating track-and-trigger assessment tools (Rowan *et al.* 2009). This is the first national wide scale audit and some useful data have been produced by this evaluation. The audit identified that almost all acute trusts now had some form of track-and-trigger scoring system and that this was usually, but not always, linked to an escalation policy or response algorithm.

Disappointingly, most of track-and-trigger tools had not been robustly tested and there was little supportive evidence that they were valid or reliable. Examination of the tools highlighted that there was not one tool that had been robustly tested to level 1 research criteria. The study showed that the majority of the tools had low sensitivity. They highlighted that this sensitivity may have been affected by the rapid deterioration of some, but not all, patients and may reflect the standard of physiological measurement in some cases. Examination of the trigger suggested that this may in cases be set too high and that if the trigger were lowered more patients might be identified, thereby increasing the sensitivity of the tool. It should be remembered, however, that decreasing the trigger may cause unnecessary calls to outreach.

From a staff perspective the audit suggested that staff found the track-and-trigger tools useful and welcomed them as an adjunct to patient assessment. The usefulness of this, however, has to be countered with the potential for staff to 'over-rely' on track-and-trigger tools as a replacement for sound clinical judgement. The study found that poor documentation in relation to track-and-trigger tools was still evident in some areas. Some staff attempted to link this to the use of health-care assistance in recording observations, but the study highlighted that healthcare assistants usually adhered to the track-and-trigger tool and response algorithm more closely than registered nurses in some areas.

The study was unable to collect data in relation to response times and this would have been useful in determining whether escalation processes and track-and-trigger scoring systems had an effect on the response time to a patient who is deteriorating.

The study concluded that because of the low sensitivity of the track-and-trigger tools examined it was not possible to rely on these tools to identify all acutely ill patients. It suggested that reducing the trigger for a response may be of benefit but identified that this would have resource and cost implications. It suggested that it was unlikely that a tool would be developed that was sensitive enough to identify all of the acutely ill patients in ward areas. However, in areas where the tool has been developed well it plays an important role in improving the pathway of an acutely ill patient.

The future of track-and-trigger tools

Rowan *et al.* (2009) made a number of recommendations for future practice. They identified the need to continue with the development of track-and-trigger scoring systems, despite the low sensitivity and lack of robust evaluation of some tools, pointing out that there was insufficient evidence to suggest that they should be discontinued.

They recommended that track-and-trigger tools should continue to be developed and audited despite these inherent flaws for a number of reasons, including:

♦ the tools reinforce the need for accurate assessment of the patient
♦ the tool helps educate staff about the likely changes in physiological measurements in acutely ill patients

♦ the tool, when used with a response algorithm, reinforces the need for a non-negotiable response from senior staff.

They highlighted, however, that the tools should be seen as an aid to, not a replacement for, sound clinical judgement. They suggested that the tools worked best if combined with:

♦ sound education of all staff completing the tool

♦ recognition that complete and regular recording of observations is required to enhance the reliability of the tool

♦ a rapid and appropriate response from experienced staff.

They again identified a need for further evaluation and audit of tools and suggested that where tools were failing trusts should review them and implement a tool that may work in that area instead.

These suggestions for improvement echo the recommendations from the National Outreach Forum (2007) that identified the need to audit track-and-trigger tools. They recommended that the audit should include evaluation of documentation, response times to triggers, and the number of critical care admissions triggered. It becomes clear that further evaluation will play an important part in the continuation of track-and-trigger systems. These systems remain in their infancy and more robust testing is clearly required.

The development of a national track-and-trigger tool

The evaluations of track-and-trigger assessment tools have to date concentrated on the audit of a number of isolated locally developed tools that have been individually developed by each trust.

More recently, however, there has been a continued drive towards the development of a national tool that could be implemented and evaluated nationally. This tool is currently being developed for use in the UK but is yet to be widely implemented.

References

Benner, P. (1984) *From Novice to Expert, Excellence and Power in Clinical Nursing.* Addison Wesley, California.

Cioffi, J. (2000) Recognition of patients who require emergency assistance: a descriptive study. *Heart Lung.* **29**, 262–8.

Cooper, N. and Cramp, P. (2003) *Essential Guide to Acute Care.* BMJ Books, London.

Cretikos, M., Bellamo, R., Hillman, K. *et al.* (2008). Respiratory rate as an indicator of acute illness. *Med. J. Australia.* **188**(11), 657–9.

Cuthbertson, B., Boroujerdi, M., McKie, L. *et al.* (2007) Can physiological parameters and early warning scoring systems allow early recognition of the deteriorating surgical patient? *Crit. Care Med.* **35**, 402–9.

Cuthbertson, B. and Smith, G. (2007) Editorial II. A warning on early warning scores. *Br. J. Anaesth.* **98**(6), 704–6.

Department of Health (2000) Comprehensive Critical Care, a Review of Adult Critical Care Services. HMSO, London.

Department of Health (2008) *Competencies for Recognising and Responding to Acutely Ill Adults in Hospital.* Draft guidelines for consultation DOH, HMSO, London.

Docherty, B. and Coote, S. (2006a) Respiratory assessment as part of a track and trigger. *Nurs. Times* **102**(44), 28–31.

Docherty, B. and Coote, S. (2006b) Monitoring the pulse as part of a track and trigger. *Nurs. Times* **102**(43), 28–31.

Duckitt, R.W., Buxton, R., Walker, J. and Cheek, H. (2007) Worthing physiological scoring system: Derivation and validation of a physiological warning score for medical admissions. *Br. J. Anaesth.* **98**(6), 769–74.

Garner-Thorpe, J., Love, N., Wrightson, J. *et al.* (2006) The value of Modified Early Warning Scores in patients: A Prospective Observational Study. *Ann. Roy. Coll. Surg. England.* **88**(6), 571–5.

Gao, H., McDonnel, A., Harrison, D.D. *et al.* (2007) Ststematic review and evaluation of physiological track and trigger warning systems for identifying patients at risk on the ward. *Int. Care Med.* **33**, 667–79.

Goldhill, D., Worthington, L., Mulcahy, A. *et al.* (1999) The patient at risk team: Identifying and managing seriously ill ward patients. *Anaesthia.* **54**(0), 853–60.

Jevon, P. (2007) *Treating the Critically Ill Patient.* Blackwell Publishing, Oxford.

McArthur-Rouse, F. (2001) Critical care outreach services and early warning scoring systems: A review if the literature. *J Adv. Nurs.* **36**(5), 696–704.

MERIT Study Investigators (2005) Introduction of the medical emergency team(met): a cluster-randomised controlled trial. *Lancet.* **365**, 2091–7.

Mohammed, M., Hayton, R., Clements, G. *et al.* (2009) Improving accuracy and efficiency of early warning scores in acute care. *Br. J. Nurs.* **18**(1), 18–24.

National Outreach Forum (2007) *Critical Care Outreach Services-Indicators of Service Achievement and Good Practice.* National Outreach Forum, London.

National Patient Safety Agency (2007) *Safer Care for the Acutely Ill Patient: Learning from Serious Incidents.* National Patient Safety Agency, London.

NICE (2007) *Acutely Ill Patients in Hospital: Recognition of and Response to Acute Illness of Adults in Hospital.* HMSO, London.

Oakey, R. and Slade, V. (2006) Physiological observation track and trigger system. *Nurs. Standard.* **20**(27), 48–54.

Patient Safety First (2008) *The 'How to guide' for Reducing Harm from Deterioration.* Patient safety first campaign, London.

Rowan., K., Adam, S., Ball,C. *et al.* (2009) *Evaluation of Outreach Services in Critical Care.* Intensive Care National Audit and Research Committee, London.

Ryan, H., Cadman, C. and Hann, L. (2004) Setting standards for assessment of ward patients at risk of deterioration. *Br. J. Nurs.* **13**(20), 1186–90.

Schey, B., Williams, D. and Bucknall, T. (2009) Skin temperature as a non invasive marker of haemodynamic and perfusion status in adult critical care surgical patients: an observational study. *Int. Crit. Care Nurs.* **25**, 31–7.

Smith, G. (2003) *ALERT: Acute Life Threatening Events, Treatment and Recognition.* 2nd edn. University of Portsmouth, Portsmouth.

Smith,G., Prytherch, D., Schmidt, P. and Featherstone, P. (2008) Review and performance of aggregate weighted "track and trigger" systems. *J Resuscitation.* **77**, 170–9.

Smith, A. and Oakey, R. (2006) Incidence and significance of errors in a patient track and trigger system during an outbreak of Legionnaires disease: retrospective case note analysis. *Anesthesia.* **61**(3), 222–8.

Subbe, C.P., Slater, A., Menon, D. and Gemmell, L. (2006) Validation of physiological scoring systems in the accident and emergency dept. *Emer. Med.* **23**, 841–5.

Subbe, C., Gao, H., and Harrison, D. (2003) Reproducibility of physiological track and trigger warning systems for identifying patients at risk on the ward. *Int. Care Med.* **33**, 619–24.

Wood, J. and Smith, A. (1999) Active management should prevent cardiopulmonary arrest. *BMJ.* **7175**(318), 51–2.

Chapter 12

The role of outreach

Fiona Creed, with contributions from Ruth Creasy, Corinne Elliott, Sylvia Hedges, and Joanna Thorpe

Chapter contents

The development of critical care outreach teams was recommended in the Department of Health (2000) report *Comprehensive Critical Care: A Review of Adult Critical Care Services*. Since this publication, many NHS trusts have instigated a variety of outreach services to meet the report's requirements. Development of these services has been idiosyncratic and there are a wide range of services throughout the UK. These services are continuing to develop and are viewed by many as an essential part of providing care for acutely ill patients. The NICE (2007) guidelines highlight the need to develop outreach services in all acute trusts, with services offering 24 h cover 7 days a week. This chapter will enable you to understand how outreach services may assist in management of the acutely ill patient and will explore:

+ the development and evolution of critical care outreach services
+ other developments that support acute care delivery
+ the remit of the outreach service
+ the education role of outreach teams
+ outreach service role in developing critical care follow-up services
+ auditing and evaluating outreach services
+ potential limitations of outreach services
+ future development of outreach services.

Learning outcomes

This chapter will enable you to:

+ review the rationale for setting up outreach services
+ understand the role of the outreach service
+ recognize the need for collaboration with outreach services
+ analyse how outreach may help ward staff manage acutely ill patients
+ reflect on the need to evaluate outreach services.

The introduction and evolution of outreach

Patients whose condition deteriorates are among the sickest in a hospital and require highly skilled multidisciplinary teams (Department of Health 2005). Critical care outreach services are a relatively new development within the critical care service, which aim to ensure that the needs of all critically ill patients are met, irrespective of their location.

Outreach was developed in response to concerns about the care of critically ill patients on the ward. Several studies have identified that patients admitted to the intensive care unit (ICU) from the wards had received suboptimal care and in some cases the admissions were preventable (McQuillan *et al.* 1998; McGloin *et al.* 1999). Patients who suffered an in-hospital cardiac arrest frequently had abnormal physiological values in the preceding hours (Wood & Smith 1999).

McQuillan *et al.* (1998) studied the prevalence, nature, causes, and consequences of suboptimal care before ICU admission. In this study, only 20% of cases were well managed before ICU with the majority receiving suboptimal care. ICU admission was thought to be late in 69% of cases and potentially avoidable in 41%. The main causes of suboptimal care were identified as failure of organization, lack of knowledge, failure to appreciate clinical urgency, lack of supervision, and failure to seek advice. Suboptimal care before ICU admission was also shown to increase mortality.

In April 1999, the Department of Health commissioned a review of adult critical care services and set up an expert working party to develop a framework for the modernization of critical care services. The Audit Commission's report, *Critical to Success*, emphasized the idea of the patient at risk and recommended better training of medical and nursing staff, early warning scoring systems, and introduced the idea of critical care outreach teams.

Critical care outreach services were introduced throughout the UK in the later half of 2000 and early 2001 following the publication of the Department of Health's report *Comprehensive Critical Care: A Review of Adult Critical Care Services*. This document outlined a 5-year modernization programme and set out a new approach to critical care that was based on patients' needs rather than their location in the hospital. It also recommended that critical care services should be provided not only for patients who are already critically ill, but also for patients who are at risk of critical illness.

The role of outreach services/differing types of services

The primary role of outreach services is to ensure that all patients at risk of deterioration or patients who are deteriorating have timely treatment in the most suitable area of the hospital. Critical care networks and NHS trusts have been encouraged to develop their own locally customized service (NICE 2007). This has meant that different hospitals have developed differing approaches to this such as medical emergency teams (METs), patient at risk teams (PARTs), and hospital at night teams rather than developing a unified approach. Review of the literature highlights that there have been several differing systems established to help identify the deteriorating patient. All have the common aim of early recognition and treatment of the patient who is deteriorating and provide a systems approach to improving care. The three most commonly cited examples are hospitalists (largely USA based), MET (largely Australia based), and outreach in the UK (incorporating PARTs).

Hospitalists

Hospitalist services are not used in the UK but are seen in the USA. It refers to a system where medical staff are employed specifically to specialize in acute medicine and treat patients who either deteriorate or are at risk of deterioration. It is unlikely that this system is compatible with current UK healthcare delivery systems as it is reliant on the costly employment of additional medical staff to supplement the generalist teams. In addition, the healthcare delivery service in the UK is very different to services in North America, restricting the transferability of such a service to the UK.

The medical emergency team

The concept of the MET originated in Australia. The MET generally consists of nursing and medical staff and is a predominantly medically focused and run service. The MET is made up of highly trained medical/nursing professionals who offer a quick response to the patient who is deteriorating. The team respond rapidly to patient deterioration with the aim of improving further deterioration or even death (Valentine & Skirton 2006).

The team-based approach relies heavily on the use of abnormal physiological parameters to trigger concern to the ward staff. MET calling criteria include:

- airway problems
- respiratory changes
- cardiovascular changes
- neurological changes.

Interestingly, the MET calling criteria also include a category that the staff are concerned about a patient. A study by Cioffi (2000) identified that many nurses used subjective measurements of 'patient not looking right' and intuitive or sixth sense to replace other more objective measurements.

There is not a wealth of data supporting the success of MET, but evaluations have highlighted that staff feel more empowered to make decisions and take proactive action. Statistically, however, the establishment of these teams has had little impact on cardiac arrest numbers, unplanned admissions to ITU, and unexpected deaths (Valentine & Skirton 2006).

Patient at risk teams

These teams are very similar to the METs from Australia and are used in a number of hospitals throughout the UK. The PART aims to improve the care to the deteriorating ward patient by providing advice and support to the ward medical and nursing staff, and by facilitating early intensive care unit admission if this is deemed necessary. The PART may also prevent unnecessary admissions, which will release the valuable critical care beds for the patients with the greater need.

The aim of the PART is to respond to patients admitted to wards who fulfilled certain criteria. These criteria include either changes to certain physiological criteria or subjective opinions that patients are causing concern. There will undoubtedly be patients who do not trigger on early warning charts that are clearly unwell. This is reflected in the work by Gardner Thorpe et al. (2006), who stated that patients within their study group were admitted to the critical care unit without actually triggering on the observation track-and-trigger chart, augmenting the view that a 'feeling' of a senior nurse or a doctor should be the default rather than simply relying on scoring systems alone (Subbe et al. 2006).

Critical care outreach teams

These teams are used predominantly in the UK and have built on the foundation of the Australian-based MET. There are very many similarities between these teams and outreach services. Whilst the MET's main objective is rapid assessment and treatment of the patient using an external group of specialists, the aim of outreach is to identify and manage patients at risk using collaborative and educational methods (Bright et al. 2004). The main aims of outreach services are to empower ward staff to care for acutely ill patients by offering regular support and education.

The quick expansion and development of critical care outreach teams has meant that outreach services vary throughout the UK and may include several differing healthcare professionals.

They are predominantly nurse-led services that are usually linked to the critical care areas and run with support from the critical care medical staff. In some trusts specialist nurse consultant roles have been established. Nurse consultant outreach nurses have been instrumental in the establishment, implementation, and eventual audit of outreach services throughout their trust.

Until the intensive care society created guidance for the establishment of outreach services in 2002 there was little standardization between services and variations in parity of service and team membership occurred. The Intensive Care Society (2002) defines outreach services as a multidisciplinary approach to the identification of patients at risk of critical illness or deterioration (and those recovering from acute illness). It should ideally be collaboration between critical care departments and other departments within the hospital to ensure continuity and appropriateness of care regardless of location. The service should be developed as a partnership aimed at prevention by education and action.

The Intensive Care Society (2002) stress that outreach services should not be used as a replacement for inadequate service provision, including:

- lack of ITU beds
- inadequate ward resources
- poor skill mixes on wards
- lack of experienced staff/supervision for staff.

A recent survey has identified that most NHS trusts (73%) now have a form of outreach (Rowan et al. 2007). However, the provision and services offered by the teams varies dramatically, with some teams offering 24 h cover 7 days a week and others with a much more restrictive service. Where outreach teams do exist they employ, on average, two whole-time equivalents, necessitating predominantly daytime outreach services only (Welch 2003). In areas where outreach has been well funded services are able to provide continuous 24-h cover (however, this has occurred in only a limited number of trusts).

The National Outreach Forum (2007) have identified a lack of a unified approach to outreach services in the UK, but they have agreed that the general principles of an outreach service involve timely detection of the patient who is deteriorating and appropriate intervention. They have highlighted that the objectives of any type of outreach service should be:

- to improve the quality of acute patient care, patient experience, and to reduce adverse clinical events
- to enhance clinical staff confidence and competence to care for acutely ill patients through education, training, and skills development
- to improve organizational aspects of acute care delivery to ensure a trust-wide approach to the delivery of acute care.

In addition to highlighting the objectives of an outreach service the National Outreach Forum (2007) have also been instrumental in developing a pathway framework for care of the acutely ill adult that may be implemented by outreach services (this complements the NICE guidelines 2007) and have identified possible variables that may be used for auditing outreach services (see section on audit later in this chapter).

The pathway of care for the acutely ill adult has been separated into three distinct phases:

- recognition and management of the acutely ill adult on ward areas
- clinical involvement in care following discharge from critical care or after a period of acute illness
- support and outpatient services post discharge home from hospital

In addition to this NICE (2007) identify that the over-riding aims of all of these types of outreach services are to:

♦ avert admissions to critical care

♦ facilitate timely admissions to critical care areas and discharges back to the ward

♦ share critical care skills and experience via educational pathways

♦ promote continuity of care

♦ ensure there is evaluation and audit of outreach services.

Outreach teams have taken a variety of approaches in an attempt to meet the aims highlighted by the Department of Health (2000) and NICE (2007). Review of the literature highlights that all outreach teams appear to use these five main aims to develop their services.

Aim 1: Aversion of admission to ITU/supporting ward staff

The shortages of critical care beds (Department of Health 2000) and the evolving concept of critical care without walls means that acutely ill patients should receive the treatment they require wherever they are and that treatment should focus on need rather than geographical location. The initial vision was that the outreach team would be able to avert any admissions to ITU and ensure that patients whose condition had deteriorated could be nursed in a ward area with support from the outreach services.

Evaluation of outreach referrals highlights that ward staff commonly seek support with four main groups of patients (Cutler 2006):

♦ those with respiratory problems

♦ those with hypotension

♦ those with altered renal function

♦ those with deteriorated levels of consciousness.

Alongside these common problems audit by outreach has also identified that support is often required in similar areas. Coad & Haines (1999) identified that ward nurses often needed support with:

♦ haemodynamic assessment

♦ cardiovascular drug therapy

♦ medical equipment

♦ fluid and electrolyte replacement/management

♦ management and care of tracheostomies

♦ high-flow oxygen

♦ non-invasive ventilation and continuous positive airway pressure (CPAP)

♦ understanding arterial blood gases.

A study by Chellel *et al.* (2006) identified that the outreach team were deemed to have a number of important roles in supporting ward staff in the recognition and management of acutely ill patients. This research identified a number of themes surrounding the roles undertaken by outreach. The themes included:

♦ Action

Outreach teams were perceived by ward staff as being able to focus on 'getting things done' and ensuring that appropriate care was delivered and treatment decisions were quickly made.

An important role of outreach was to ensure that there were immediate physical interventions in care and appropriate treatment decisions made. Often the role of the outreach nurse also focused upon delivery of basic 'hands on care', for example mouth care and bed linen changes, as well as the more advanced roles of blood gas sampling and coordination of other services. The significance of provision and setting up of appropriate equipment was also an important outreach intervention and outreach were often involved in familiarizing staff with equipment and ensuring equipment that was not commonly used in some ward areas, for example non-invasive ventilation, was set up correctly. Participants in the study also highlighted that the outreach team were often more able to expedite clinical decision making by ensuring that clinical discussions occurred at an appropriate level.

- ♦ Focusing on the patient
  The outreach team were perceived to be able to focus on one patient and their problems, whilst the ward nurse still had a number of other patients in her care. Concentration on one patient led to the ability to make a much more detailed and accurate assessment of the patient's condition and need for intervention, enabling the outreach nurse to ensure appropriate patient management. Outreach staff were perceived by the ward to have more time to intervene than ward staff did and greater flexibility in their working arrangements. This ability to focus enabled the outreach staff to ensure appropriate and timely intervention.

- ♦ Orchestration
  Outreach teams were perceived to be able to quickly access other members of the multidisciplinary team and ensure effective coordination either face to face or by phone. There was a perception that outreach had more influence in the multidisciplinary team than more junior ward staff. A key factor in this orchestration appeared to revolve around communication and use of appropriate language to articulate the severity of the patient's condition. The ward staff perceived that outreach had more authority and respect, and were able to quickly gain a response from the medical staff.

- ♦ Clinical expertise
  Outreach teams were perceived as experts in the field of nursing the critically ill. Ward staff acknowledged that most members of the outreach team were highly skilled critical care nurses who were keen to share their skills to improve patient care. They were often viewed as experts in their field and staff who could be relied on, a helpful resource when assessing, caring, and treating deterioration.

Chellel *et al.* (2006) acknowledged that aversion of admissions to ITU also included supporting ward staff and clinicians to make appropriate decisions about care. Not all patients referred to the outreach team are suitable for admission to ITU and outreach teams have a role in facilitating discussion regarding palliation rather than instigation of aggressive treatment therapies. In some instances ceiling treatments may be set whereby care is delivered to a point, for example CPAP would be commenced but would not be extended to full invasive ventilation. Outreach was often involved in encouraging teams to consider the resuscitation status of acutely ill adults, again in an attempt to prevent unnecessary admissions to ITU and to ensure that patients received palliative care rather than unnecessary invasive treatment.

A similar study by Valentine & Skirton (2006) also identified that the ward staff generally found outreach services to be supportive to ward staff. In response to a questionnaire the majority of the participants felt that outreach services main role is to support ward staff by acting as a resource, providing help and advice. Ward staff often viewed outreach services as a bridge between themselves and the critical care staff. It was highlighted that ward staff felt outreach opinion carried more weight and enabled ward nurses concerns about patients to be heard. The majority of respondents appeared to value outreach's teams supporting them when caring for acutely ill and deteriorating patients. An example of how outreach has been able to assist ward staff in a clinical situation is highlighted in Box 12.1.

Box 12.1 Clinical example of outreach intervention

Patient scenario discussing the role of outreach in assessing an acutely ill patient.

Outreach was called to review a 69-year-old man who had been very recently diagnosed with acute myeloid leukaemia. The staff nurse was concerned because the patient had low oxygen saturations and a distended abdomen. Initial advice was given over the phone about placing the patient on a reservoir bag with 15 L oxygen per minute.

On arrival on the ward the outreach nurse immediately went to the patient to carry out an initial assessment, using the ALERT system. It is essential that the patient's airway, breathing, and circulation are assessed to ensure that the safety of the patient and prevent further deterioration.

The outreach nurse recognized that the patient was clearly unwell. The observations made by the outreach nurse found the following:

Airway: The patient had a clear airway and was able to talk in short sentences.

Breathing: Respiratory rate was 28, chest movement equal. Auscultation found equal air entry although bases were quiet bilaterally, probably due to abdominal distension splinting the diaphragm. Oxygen saturations were unable to be obtained with pulse oximetry due to poor peripheral perfusion. The patient was receiving oxygen 15 L per min via a non-re-breath mask as advised by outreach.

Circulation: Weak peripheral pulses with a pulse rate of 146. The patient was pale, cold, and clammy and had prolonged capillary refill time. Blood pressure was 117/70. No fluid chart was available to assess fluid balance or urine output. The patient denied any chest pain. Disability. Patient was alert but distressed and anxious.

Expose and examine: Patient had a hard, tense, distended abdomen but was not complaining of any pain due to recent analgesia. No other findings of note. At the time of outreach assessment the patient had a MEWS of 5; this had not been previously recorded and may have alerted nursing staff earlier to the deterioration in the patient's condition.

The medical doctors on call had arrived by this time and outreach advised continuing high-flow oxygen and giving a fluid challenge of 500 mL gelofusin while further tests were carried out, including ABG, full set of blood tests and an ECG. Outreach also advised an urgent surgical review regarding the patient's tense abdomen.

An arterial blood gas was obtained and the results were:

PH 7.41.

PCO_2 2.74.

PO_2 26.46.

HCO_3 15.6.

BE −11.6.

Lactate 12.64.

The outreach nurse immediately recognized a severe metabolic acidosis with respiratory compensation. However, a junior doctor, who was concerned that the patient was hyperventilating and blowing off too much carbon dioxide, missed the metabolic acidosis completely! Following the ABG result the outreach nurse informed the medical registrar and called the anaesthetic registrar to review the patient without delay. Outreach had appreciated the clinical

---

Box 12.1 Clinical example of outreach Intervantion *(continued)*

urgency and the need for prompt treatment requiring critical care input. A raised lactate is associated with increased mortality and a base deficit of more than −4 mmol/L is associated with an in hospital mortality of 70% if not corrected within 24 h. The outreach nurse was able to give a clear report to the anaesthetic register, who came to review the patient within a few minutes (Cooper & Cramp 2003).

During this time the outreach nurse continually reassessed the patient, including response to each fluid challenge given.

Further blood results were obtained which showed that the patient had a pancytopenia with an HB 5.6, WCC 4.5, and platelets of 16. Outreach assisted the ward nurses and medical doctors in ordering the necessary blood products, including packed red cells, platelets, and fresh frozen plasma.

Both the anaesthetic and surgical registrars agreed that the patient needed an emergency laparotomy as he had an acute abdomen of unknown aetiology. However, as the patient was too unstable to go straight to theatre and would also require correction of his blood clotting before surgery, he needed to be transferred to the ICU for optimization before surgery.

The outreach nurse liased with the ITU to facilitate a timely admission and together with the anaesthetist was able to transfer the patient safely and quickly to ITU, where he was ventilated and given further fluid resuscitation and blood products.

At laparotomy the patient was found to have 6 L of frank blood and clots within his peritoneal cavity, no clear bleeding point was found so the cause was though to be due to coagulopathy. He returned to the ITU where he gradually improved and was discharged back to the ward 7 days later.

He continued to be visited by outreach nurses during follow-up visits, thus providing continuity of care until he was assessed as being a level 0 patient requiring basic ward care only.

The National Outreach Forum (2007) highlighted that the use of outreach teams on the wards could bring about a number of potential benefits, including:

◆ reduction in inappropriate admission to critical care

◆ reduction in admissions to critical care caused by omissions in care delivery or failure to appropriately assess an acutely ill patient

◆ reduction in the number of readmissions to critical care areas caused by inappropriate care or omissions in care.

They also highlighted the need to assess patients for admission to ITU and facilitate a timely admission to critical care for those level 2/3 patients who could not be cared for in the general ward area.

Aim 2: Facilitate timely ITU admissions

The National Outreach Forum (2007) identifies the need for the deteriorating patient, in need of ITU support, to be transferred to an appropriate area as quickly as possible. They highlight that this should be achieved in an appropriate time frame that is consistent with the needs of that particular patient, for example the sicker the patient/risk of deterioration the quicker the patient needs to be transferred. Wherever possible it has been suggested that transfer should occur within an hour of the patient's condition been acknowledged as requiring ITU admission. Admission should not be delayed where there are sufficient resources for the ITU to receive that patient.

However, in some cases this is not always possible as there may be insufficient beds/staff in ITU or the acceptance of the deteriorating patient may be conditional on another patient being discharged. On some occasions the ITU may have a considerable delay in providing appropriate resources/admission and this may necessitate transfer of the patient to another area within the hospital or transfer to another hospital that has an available ITU bed.

Outreach has a role in these circumstances in assisting with patient care and providing appropriate supervision for nurses who are caring for these patients in an inappropriate environment. Outreach services also have a role in assisting with the safe and timely transfer of the level 2/3 patient to a critical care area (see Chapter 14).

The National Outreach Forum (2007) identifies the need for treatment options to be discussed with the patient and their family/carers if this is possible. Some ITU admissions may be averted if appropriate evaluation of the suitability of ITU is discussed before admission. Outreach services clearly have a role in facilitating these discussions and helping to identify which patients are not suitable for ITU admission and subsequent applications of do not resuscitate orders (McArthur-Rouse 2001).

Aim 2a: Facilitating transfers back to the ward

The need for appropriate care and support following transfer from ITU has clearly been identified as a role of the outreach team (NICE 2007). This group of patients are particularly vulnerable (the physical and psychological needs of this group of patients and their families are discussed extensively in Chapter 15). Again the role in facilitating transfers is varied and may include:

+ planning of transfer
+ communication in relation to transfer
+ visiting ward areas post transfer from ITU.

Some outreach teams have been instrumental in improving transfer planning and developing transfer communication and care plans to facilitate a seamless transfer back to the ward area. The NICE (2007) guidelines stress the importance of effective documentation and appropriate written plans of care following discharge from ITU. Work in developing written plans of care and appropriate transfer planning is still in the early stages and there is no evidence within the literature evaluating the success of such initiatives.

Other teams are involved in visiting ITU patients post transfer. In reviewing the nurse-led service in her trust Carr (2002) highlights the benefits of providing nurse-led services to patients post transfer from ITU. She identifies the importance of visiting patients post ITU to follow-up their progress on the ward. She also highlights the importance of discussing ongoing management problems and providing education for staff in relation to specific problem areas such as tracheostomy management.

Carr (2002) suggests that ward visits can help promote continuity of care, improve communication channels, and enhance the experience of transition for patients and their families. She suggests that these visits may enable earlier recognition of patients at risk of deterioration post discharge and may enable earlier discharge back to the ward if appropriate support is available. Further evaluation and audit of this important role, however, is required.

Aim 3: Developing educational support for ward nurses

The comprehensive critical care document (2000) highlighted that all staff caring for the acutely ill patient should be provided with sufficient education and skills to enable them to provide effective care. The document identified that a significant part of the outreach team's role would be to address the educational needs of the multidisciplinary team in caring for the sick patient, through the development of training programmes and information sharing in clinical and academic settings.

The perceived problem

It is argued that current nurse education does not always equip staff with the knowledge and skills required to care for the acutely ill patient in hospital, particularly if the patient is nursed outside of a designated critical care area and the staff do not have frequent contact with acutely ill patients (Welch 2003). The National Outreach Forum (2007) identifies the need for appropriate education for all hospital staff. It is suggested that all acute care staff should be able to recognize basic signs of deterioration and understand the need for timely intervention and treatment (Welch 2003). More recently there has been lobbying for acute care competencies and the Department of Health competencies have been developed to guide the development of generic competencies that all ward staff caring for acutely ill patients should possess. Outreach clearly has a role in:

- providing education to ward staff
- enabling the implementation of the new Department of Health competencies
- development of competence assessment strategies for ward staff.

In identifying the acute care pathways, the National Outreach Forum (2007) identified the need for all three phases of the acute pathway (recognition of deterioration, discharge to the wards, follow-up following discharge) to be grounded in education. It was noted that each of these distinct phases had an educational role for the outreach nurse or involved the outreach team liaising with other educationalists.

Evaluation of the outreach team's educational role highlights the differing types of education outreach teams may be involved in. These include:

- informal/ad hoc clinical education
- formal education systems
- liaising with higher education institutes to develop accredited educational programmes.

Informal and ad hoc clinical education

Recognition of the need for education at ward level is central to the role of the outreach team. However, supporting learning in clinical practice is a multifactorial complex issue and involves developing close working relationships with ward areas to assess their learning needs and offer educational support where it is needed.

An initial remit of the outreach teams was to develop early warning systems, which specify observation levels, assist with recognition of the deteriorating patient, and clearly identify a process to call for help from outreach or medical teams (see Chapter 11). Outreach has had an important role in developing early warning scores and facilitating the introduction of these systems (McArthur-Rouse 2001).

In addition to the development of early warning scores the remit of outreach was also to develop teaching at the bedside for ward staff. Because of the complexities associated with bedside teaching whilst caring for a patient who is deteriorating, a number of educational approaches may need to be adopted by the teams.

In an acute emergency situation, where there is an absence of skilled medical staff, the outreach practitioner would be likely to take a lead in the situation and the learners develop their knowledge through observation and reflection after the event.

However, in the less critical situation the outreach practitioner may adopt a more facilitative role that supports the ward nurse in developing systematic patient assessment skills. The outreach practitioner may provide guidance about the use of assessment processes as the A, B, C, D, E approach advocated by Smith (2003).

Education away from the bedside, but remaining within the clinical area, is another important role. Assessment of clinical skills and demonstrations of equipment such as central venous pressure monitoring, tracheostomy equipment, and non-invasive ventilators are essential to provide a safe patient environment. Subject areas taught are usually driven by the needs of the ward area, for instance approaching a ward with a rigid plan to teach fluid management when the real need, at that time, is the care of the patient with a tracheostomy would be inappropriate and damaging to team relationships.

Alongside supporting trained nurses in clinical practice outreach has also been instrumental in the development of competencies for healthcare assistants (HCAs). It is often the HCAs who are left to complete patient observations, it is therefore important that outreach play a role in producing a competency frameworks that ensure safe practice of the HCAs in undertaking and understanding their role in the assessment of the sick patient.

Formal education sessions

The provision of formal study days is an important aspect of the educational role. The development of in-house training days such as Acute Life-threatening Events, Recognition and Treatment (ALERT®), tracheostomy study days, and identification of the sick patient study days are led by the outreach team and encourage lecturers from different areas of the multidisciplinary team to work together.

In most trusts the courses provided are open to all members of the multidisciplinary team and attended by such individuals as HCAs, medical and nursing students, nurses, junior doctors, physiotherapist, and speech and language team members.

Encouraging access to other courses

In addition to planning formal and informal education sessions outreach also has a substantial role in the development of accredited programmes and in encouraging practitioners to attend these programmes to facilitate further development of knowledge and skills.

Several universities have established acute care modules for ward nurses such as identifying the critically ill patient and caring for the acutely ill adult modules. Increasingly post registration acute care pathways are being developed to enable bespoke educational packages to be developed for the ward nurse. These provide a more formal programme inclusive of classroom-based teaching and competency-based assessments within the ward environment.

The initial Department of Health's framework (2000) identified that all ward nurses should attend a high dependency programme. This has been interpreted by many trusts as the attendance at 1- or 2-day study programmes. The review of comprehensive critical care (Department of Health 2005) re-examined provision of education and indicated that attendance at trust days was sufficient. However, there is still widespread agreement surrounding the importance and value of longer, more formalized courses (Welch 2003). These courses, however, require staff to be released from practice, often for 10–15 days over the period of the modules. This clearly has financial implications to ward areas releasing staff to attend these valuable courses (see Chapter 17 for further details of educational programmes).

Continuing the educational role of the outreach team

It is important to have trust support in the development of future educational initiatives. The success of these outreach educational programmes to improve the care of the critically ill patient within the ward environment is reliant on continuous acknowledgement of the need for educational input to improve services. Success of initiatives will be hindered without support from shareholders and government. Courses can be provided, but staff need to be released to attend. Trust policies need to recognize a specified level of post-registration skills that need to be accomplished and provide resources to enable national drives such as the development of core acute care competencies (Department of Health 2009).

Aim 4: Continuity of care, team communication, and escalation of concern

The importance of continuity of care and effective communication cannot be over emphasized in the care of the critically ill patient. Patients who are acutely ill need care to be delivered in a timely manner; if they are already showing signs of deterioration they need doctors and nurses to communicate their concerns quickly.

Evaluation of the literature highlights that poor communication issues may be instrumental in the failure to appropriately escalate concerns to the correct level in a timely manner (National Confidential Enquiry into Patient Outcome and Death 2005; National Patient Safety Agency 2007). In a recent study the National Patient Safety Agency (2007) identified communication issues as the biggest problem in failure to escalate concern about a sick patient. The study identified a number of reasons for poor communication, highlighting several reoccurring themes. Some communication breakdown appeared to be evident during handover and staff may not adequately inform each other of the patient's current condition. Communication problems were also seen to occur more frequently in outlying patients, where confusion often existed as to which team member should be notified of deterioration in the patient's condition. Communication between nurses and medical staff appeared to be particularly problematic and it was suggested that nurses may not communicate clearly enough or may not be able to convey the urgency of the situation over the telephone.

The medical staff questioned by the National Patient Safety Agency (2007) appeared to have similar problems and found it difficult to assess the urgency of the situation over the telephone, especially if they did not know the patient or if they were provided with insufficient detail about the patient's condition.

Problems also appeared to occur in written communication, further compounding the problem. Written communication and plans of care for acutely ill patients were often incomplete or absent from written notes (National Patient Safety Agency 2007). Doctors also appeared to make the assumption that if instructions were written in the medical notes that the nurses would have time to read them; nurses were sometimes unaware of written instructions. The study highlighted that the combination of these communication issues often caused delays in care for acutely ill patients.

The study highlighted the need for all staff who care for sick patients to be able to communicate information succinctly and assertively to gain an appropriate and timely response. It appeared that often staff may not know who to contact and this appeared to delay escalation of concern.

Studies have highlighted the significant role that the outreach team play in effective communication (Chellel et al. 2006). Outreach staff were identified, by ward staff, to have effective communication that allowed the relevant information to be passed on to the appropriate person. One factor of effective communication appeared to be the use of appropriate language that enables timely recognition of the significance and severity of the patient's condition. The ITU background of the outreach team may enable them to be more familiar and fluent in medical terminology, enabling expression of concern in an authoritative manner (Chellel et al. 2006). An additional factor was the persistence in communicating with the medical teams. Outreach nurses cited examples of continually referring through the medical hierarchy until the patient was appropriately reviewed. It was argued that junior ward nurses may lack the confidence to contact more senior medical staff.

Table 12.1 SBAR communication tool

SBAR communication tool
Situation
Identify yourself and ward area
State patients name and rationale for calling
State concern
Background
Provide background information, including patient's history, reason for admission, a brief summary of treatment to date (e.g. medications, blood results, diagnostic test results)
Assessment
Provide assessment information, including most recent observations, MEWS or PARS, GCS, fluid balance, mental state any suspicions about diagnosis may also be provided
Recommendation
Explain what you require the doctor/outreach team to do and clarify your expectations, e.g. I would like the patient reviewed within 30 min.
Document who you have spoken to and their response.

The need to ensure that concerns are escalated to the appropriate person in a timely manner is vital to the management of acute illness. Indeed, the new Department of Health competencies stress the need for effective communication in their development of the 'chain of response' to acute deterioration. A recent innovation by some outreach teams is the use of structured communication tools to facilitate effective escalation of concern. The NHS have been instrumental in developing the SBAR (Situation, background, assessment, recommendation) tool to facilitate communication between healthcare professionals. It is a tool developed initially by the military and aviation authorities, and adapted for use within the NHS for many situations, including the escalation of concern (NHS Institute for Innovation and Improvement 2008). The SBAR tool has been used by some outreach departments to facilitate communication using SBAR principles see Table 12.1.

Implementation of the SBAR tool by outreach teams is in its early stages and there is no robust evidence to support its introduction, but the principles of the tool certainly seem to address known communication deficits.

Alongside escalation of concern, outreach nurses have a tertiary role in ensuring effective communication between teams. It is important that the outreach team appreciate the importance of ensuring that all members of the multidisciplinary team are involved in the care of the patient. It is important to remember that the patient's medical team have a responsibility for instigating and delivering care and should be kept informed of any changes in the patients condition. The outreach team have an important role in the coordination of treatment plans for the critically ill patient in the ward setting as they work closely with the critical care team and alongside the parent team.

Outreach also plays an important role in communication with wards and patients post discharge from ITU. Many teams have been instrumental in developing handover sheets to facilitate communication between ITU and the ward once the patient is discharged. They also act as a communication link between the ITU and the ward when the patient initially returns to the ward.

Aim 5: Outreach team's role in follow-up clinics

Studies suggest that a significant number of patients face many physical and psychological problems following discharge from ITU (Rattray & Crocker 2007). These issues are discussed extensively in Chapter 15.

Traditionally, ITU patients would have been discharged home from hospital for subsequent referral to GP and outpatient services, but often these staff may not have sufficient awareness of the potential problems the patient faces and may not be able to provide appropriate support. More recently, however, medical staff and nurses have seen the importance of viewing an admission to ITU as a continuum, and there is a belief that specialists in intensive care (such as the outreach nurse) have a role to play in subsequent care. Many critical care services offer follow-up clinics following discharge to enable support and planning of subsequent treatment, providing an opportunity to assess and facilitate longer-term recovery from critical illness (Rattray & Crocker 2007).

The National Outreach Forum (2007) echoes this view and highlights the need for ongoing care following discharge home from hospital. They maintain that outreach services should incorporate:

♦ physical assessment and referral to specialist rehabilitation teams if necessary
♦ psychological/cognitive assessment and appropriate psychiatric/psychological support if necessary
♦ assessment of any residual effects of critical illness, such as neuropathies.

The report also highlights the benefits of being able to provide auditable statistics from outreach clinics that extended beyond mortality/morbidity rates, therefore facilitating the collection of useful data about the long-term consequences of critical illness. The quality of life post ITU is often difficult to measure and many of the clinics that are well established also use 'quality of life' data collection tools to enhance the audit/data collection. These tools allow for collection of data about the patient's experiences and how the individual perceives their quality of life has been affected. Quality of life post ITU is to an extent a subjective issue and there are several tools available for attempting to assess this in follow-up clinics.

There are a number of approaches used in the establishment of follow-up services. They may be led by doctors (intensivists), nurses (usually outreach but occasionally ITU nurses), or involve multidisciplinary team involvement. In many cases these clinics are nurse led as the financial implications are an important consideration in a modern health economy and nurse-led clinics are cheaper to implement than those involving all members of the multidisciplinary team (Sharland 2002). They are often held once or twice a month and criteria will be identified for inviting patients (usually those who have spent more than 4 days in ITU). Patients and their families may attend on a one-off basis or may be invited over a period of time such as 2 months, 6 months, and 12 months post discharge home. Sharland (2002) highlights that 2 months post discharge appears to be a particularly difficult time for the patient. She identifies that the main aims of the follow up are to:

♦ enable patients and families to understand their period of critical illness
♦ provide information re rehabilitation
♦ provide advice and support for patients and their families
♦ identify any ongoing problems/ issues
♦ promote a quality service
♦ provide feedback to the ITU staff about the patient's progress.

Patients often require clarification about details of their ITU stay and enjoy having their questions answered. In some cases it is beneficial for the patient to revisit ITU to enable them to put their frightening memories into perspective (Sharland 2002).

Waldmann's (2002) study examined the benefits of critical care follow-up services to the patients and found that 99% of his respondents found them a useful experience. They found having their questions answered by somebody who understood their experience and discussion of their own personal problems following discharge from ITU to be extremely useful. Other patients felt that they benefited from counselling services offered by the follow-up clinic and referral to other specialists. Interestingly, the patients also felt that they were helping ITU staff by providing feedback. Indeed, Sharland (2002) identifies that a number of changes have been made to nursing practice following follow-up clinic reviews, including:

+ ensuring clocks and boards are visible to patients

+ development of an after intensive care booklet for patients and their families

+ change in ITU discharges processes to facilitate the transition to the ward

+ follow-up teams to visit patient on ward following discharge from ITU

+ development of ITU discharge letters for patient's GP

+ changes in ITU staff attitudes and care delivery patterns as a result of greater awareness of patient's needs, such as encouraging normal day–night cycle, more frequent mouth care.

Some follow-up clinics have evolved to offer bereavement follow-up services for patient's relatives. The clinics have found that relatives often require information and support about the events that led to the death of their family member. Provision and support to these families is viewed as crucial to their grieving process as it enables the families to fully understand and obtain a more realistic impression about the events leading to the loss of their loved one (Hall Smith *et al.* 1997).

The current provision of follow-up clinics is inconsistent in the UK. Approximately only 30% of hospitals offer follow-up services following a period of critical illness. The National Outreach Forum (2007) highlight the need for follow-up service standards to be set to ensure that all patients who have been critically ill can access a clinic if it is required.

Audit and evaluation of services

The potential benefits to the ward of outreach services may imply that the service should be extended so that the goals established by National Confidential Enquiry into Patient Outcome and Death (2005) and NICE (2007) of 24-h continuous outreach cover may be achieved. However, the widespread implementation of such a service has huge financial implications to the NHS in the UK.

The need to audit the effectiveness of critical care outreach services has been stressed in the literature (Valentine & Skirton 2006). Audit will provide valuable data about the effectiveness of the outreach service and may begin to answer the question of whether outreach services warrant the huge financial resources that are involved in supplying the recommended 24-h, 7-day-a-week cover that is stipulated in most reports (National Confidential Enquiry into Patient Outcome and Death 2005; NICE 2007).

The nature and wide variation of the trust-led outreach services make audit a difficult concept as it is unclear how auditing should progress. There are suggestions that audit could involve the following criteria:

+ data about critical care outreach interventions

+ ITU admission rates

+ readmission to ITU

+ morbidity and mortality statistics.

It is difficult, however, to quantify all of the purposes of outreach as it is impossible to effectively measure how many clinical deteriorations have been averted (Valentine & Skirton 2006).

Several authors have attempted to audit/evaluate individual outreach services and a number of studies are available in the literature. It is important to stress that this type of audit process is in its infancy and most audits make recommendations for further audit to take place.

An initial evaluation of METs in Australia (on which the outreach service in the UK is based) identified very little effect on survival statistics. The MERIT (2005) study identified whether the introduction of a MET affected/influenced patient outcome. It was the first wide-scale study evaluating the impact of METs on patient outcome and the teams were frequently called to visit acutely ill patients in the ward areas. It concluded that the MET system had a significant impact on demand and received a large number of emergency referrals. Disappointingly, it did not influence the number of cardiac arrest calls, unplanned ITU admissions, or unexpected deaths on the wards.

Similar studies have been conducted examining the effect of outreach services in the UK. Many of these studies have been small and concentrated on the evaluation of localized services.

Ball *et al.* (2003) audited their outreach teams by evaluating the following criteria:

- the effect of outreach teams on survival to discharge home
- readmission to critical care.

The study examined these indicators in relation to previous hospital statistics (using retrospective analysis) in relation to survival to discharge home and readmission to ITU. The study highlighted no significant difference in the range of patients admitted to ITU during the audit period. However, it demonstrated that there was a significant increase in survival to discharge home rates and a significant decrease in readmission to ITU rates. It concluded that critical care teams appeared to have an impact on survival to discharge home rates and readmission to ITU rates.

A second audit by Valentine & Skirton (2006) provided quantitative (numerical data) and qualitative (opinions and value statements) data about the use of outreach teams as it attempted to audit:

- usage of outreach services
- perceptions of staff about outreach services
- acceptability of outreach services
- potential for improvement to outreach services.

From a statistical perspective the audit identified that the service was utilized by the ward staff and that a significant number of referrals were made to the outreach team during the audit process. It highlighted that the highest number of referrals to outreach were from critical care areas (A&E, medical assessment unit, and theatres) and surgical wards.

From a qualitative perspective the audit highlighted that the ward staff appeared to favour the introduction of an outreach service with most rating the service as useful or very useful. Most staff felt that the outreach service was useful in providing help and advice, and the majority of respondents felt that outreach was a useful resource to enhance clinical care. Respondents particularly valued the implementation of educational aspects of outreach such as introduction of the Acute Life Threatening Events, Recognition and Treatment programmes (ALERT®) and the introduction of track-and-trigger scoring systems. The participants felt that increasing the hours that the outreach service was available would be beneficial but it was recognized that this had serious resource implications and would be dependent on further audit results. The study concluded that outreach services appeared to be perceived as beneficial but more study/audit/evaluation of services was required. It identified a need to evaluate the impact of outreach services on patient outcome and the acceptability of the service to the patient and their experience of care.

The need to audit outreach services is stressed by the National Outreach Forum (2007). In their stakeholders' forum report they included parameters that they felt would enhance the audit process. They suggested that standards for outreach services should be developed and audited against specific criteria. The criteria included:

♦ evaluation of the patient referral pathway

♦ evaluation of documentation and whether documentation of acute illness episodes was complete

♦ local mortality rates linked to track-and-trigger scores

♦ response times to referrals

♦ appropriateness to interventions

♦ critical care admission statistics

♦ patient/carer and staff evaluations of the service.

The first substantial review/audit of critical care services was conducted by the Intensive Care National Audit Research Committee (ICNARC) in 2007 (Rowan *et al.* 2009). It audited the impact of critical care outreach services throughout the UK and was the first large-scale research project examining outreach provision in the UK.

The audit highlighted the overwhelming variations in the provision of outreach services, identifying considerable differences in the composition and availability of outreach teams and the types of roles undertaken by the teams. It identified that the recommendations for continuous 24-h outreach provision was not met and several areas failed to meet minimum staffing requirements. In reviewing previous studies exploring the impact of outreach Rowan *et al.* (2009) identified that most studies were uncontrolled and used poor research methodology.

One of the positive aspects of outreach was that the presence of an outreach team was associated with a significant decrease in resuscitation rates, out of hours admissions to ITU, and the acuity of patients when admitted to ITU (based on ICNARC physiology scoring parameters). These findings were consistent with small-scale research conducted in the UK (Ball *et al.* 2003; Valentine & Skirton 2006). However, the MERIT study (2005) that examined the impact of MET in Australia did not reflect this finding and reported no statistically significant change in resuscitation rates following introduction of METs.

However, the study identified that other anticipated outcomes relating to the introduction of critical care outreach services had not been achieved and the study reflected a very mixed picture of the use of outreach services, with no identified characteristics for an optimal outreach service.

The study attempted to provide an estimate of the economic cost of outreach services per patient. It restricted its calculations to the cost of an outreach visit post discharge from ITU and estimated that the average cost per patient visit was £115. They again highlighted that there was no published economic evaluations of outreach services, yet trusts appeared to be keen to provide a service despite this.

Most of the outreach teams offered some sort of educational service to ward staff, although the educational role varied considerably between teams. Several of the respondents identified education as a problematic area. The study identified agreement with the need to develop critical care skills for ward nurses but identified large problems in the retention of such skills. It highlighted that the expertise of the critical care outreach team was founded in daily exposure and many years of practical experience in caring for acutely ill adults. It questioned whether it was feasible or achievable to expect ward nurses to attain acute care skills when they were not always exposed to them on a frequent basis. It highlighted the need to modify educational objectives and attempt to focus on improving knowledge about acute illness and its presentation rather than on acquiring critical care skills.

The study praised the entrepreneurial nature of many of the founders of outreach services (predominantly nurse leaders) and stressed that all respondents were committed to the future development of the service and had invested extensive time, effort, and resources in the development of their individual services.

The study concluded that audit of outreach was complex because of the variable nature of service provision throughout the UK. It highlighted that there appeared to be:

+ improved recognition of acute illness, initial management, and escalation of patients
+ a significant impact upon morale, ward staff clinical skills, and confidence

The study was unable, however, to either prove or disprove the relative benefits of outreach services and stressed the need for further evaluation, especially in relation to the financial implications of outreach services. It concluded that ultimately management of the acutely ill patient should be the responsibility of appropriately trained professionals who possess in-depth knowledge and skills.

The development of critical care networks

It is important to recognize that although the implementation of outreach services has occurred individually in each trust, the development and audit of outreach services has been overseen by groups of trusts combined together to form critical care networks. The concept of a critical care network arose from the Department of Health comprehensive critical care report (Department of Health 2000) that not only identified the need to develop outreach services but identified the need for these services to be developed alongside the critical care network.

The critical care networks have the objective of trying to provide and commission work together to meet the needs of all critically ill patients in one particular geographical location. The initial aims of each network were to:

+ assess critical care needs in that geographical location
+ encourage development of general and specialist services
+ standardize practice through the network through locally agreed standards and protocols
+ commission appropriate resources throughout the network
+ undertake comparative audit throughout the network (Department of Health 2000).

The role of critical care networks in trying to standardize service provision in their geographical locations and evaluate services is an important and ongoing role.

Potential limitations of outreach services

Alongside benefits of the outreach services a number of studies/authors have commented on the potential detrimental effect to the wards of the implementation of outreach services.

In her review of the literature McArthur-Rouse (2001) identified concerns that the presence of critical care outreach services has the potential to 'de-skill' ward nurses as they may become increasingly reliant on external sources to assess and manage acutely ill patients. This has potential to increase the need for more dedicated level 2 (high-dependency beds) as ward nurses may become increasingly reluctant to manage sick patients in general ward areas. McArthur-Rouse (2001) also reflects the view that the fragmentation of acute care delivery may be introduced by involving yet another specialist team into the patient's care. Widespread use of outreach services may fragment care further as the patient's care is devolved between ward nurses and doctors and specialist outreach teams.

A similar view is echoed by Chellel *et al.* (2006), who expressed concern that the impetus to handover sick patients to outreach, in order to reduce the already heavy workload of ward staff, may lead to potential misuse of an outreach service and potential de-skilling of the ward nurse. Chellel *et al.* (2006) highlighted the need to develop ward staff's leadership qualities, alongside the need for cultural change and a greater emphasis on education for both pre-registration and post-registration practitioners.

Chellel *et al.* (2006) suggested that outreach teams had become a necessary development because of the complexities of ward staffing deficiencies. She argued that managers were treating the symptoms of suboptimal ward care but did not tackle the issues that caused suboptimal care initially. This stance is echoed by Rafferty *et al.* (2006), who highlighted the detrimental impact low ward staffing levels had on patient outcome. This study identified that in patients in wards where the patient-to-nurse ratio was high there was a mortality rate increase of 26% in comparison to wards with a lower patient to staff ratio. It could be argued that outreach is only part of the answer to suboptimal ward care. Other managerial issues surrounding appropriate ward staffing levels need to be addressed.

Some medical staff maintain that the approach taken by the UK to encourage management of the patient alongside the outreach team on a general ward area may not be appropriate. Hillman (2004) suggests, in reviewing the METs in Australia, that acute care is a speciality in its own right and it is unreasonable and impractical to expect ward nurses and doctors to acquire and maintain the level of skills required. He suggests that ward staff are encouraged to promptly recognize and refer patients to a specialist team. This point is reiterated by ICNARC (Rowan *et al.* 2009), who also identify the difficulties in ward staff learning and retaining critical care skills when they only have occasional exposure to acute and critical care situations.

A significant problem in relation to the further development of outreach services is that of funding. The funding of outreach services as Welch (2003) identifies is problematic and may be worsened by changes to funding of critical care areas. Funding of outreach throughout the UK is variable and the emphasis placed on development of services varies extensively from trust to trust (even where trusts are in the same critical care network). Funding is a clear issue that needs resolution if outreach services are to continue.

The future of outreach services

Despite some of the potential limitations and lack of robust evidence, the majority of reports appear to favour the continued evolution and development of critical care outreach services. Rowan *et al.*'s (2009) extensive audit highlights that despite the lack of robust validation there is no evidence suggesting that outreach should be discontinued and they suggest the need for continued development of outreach services.

Some of the flaws of the current system lie in the policy that called for introduction of an outreach concept with little guidance as to how this could be most effectively developed (Rowan *et al.* 2009). The researchers suggest that continuation of outreach services is vital in all acute trusts and that development should be matched to local need. The audit highlighted the need for all areas to use robust track-and-trigger systems (see Chapter 11), utilize a response algorithm and ensure that ward staff are competent in the assessment and management of acutely ill patients and their families.

The lack of a consistent outreach model is problematic and has inhibited the reviewers to make a recommendation about a specific service model for outreach services. Rowan *et al.* (2009) have suggested that the development of trust-specific outreach models may continue in the near future as changes are dependent on appropriate funding of a single model and there is no robust evidence demonstrating any single model of outreach to be preferable.

It is clear that any future development of outreach services will clearly have funding issues. Rowan *et al.* (2009) point to the newly implemented resource allocation strategy for critical illness. This strategy will audit critical care usage and make resource allocation dependent on critical care use. Critical care usage statistics will be generated only if the patient is in a designated critical care area. This may lead to reduction in resources for outreach as sick patients kept on a general ward will not generate statistical critical care data and may threaten the income of critical care, reducing the incentive to nurse critical care patients on general wards. The impact of this income-generation scheme on outreach services will clearly require careful evaluation.

It is evident, however, that NICE (2007) continue to reinforce the requirement for the development of outreach services with the provision to be extended to 24-h service, 7 days a week in all acute care trusts. It is likely that the outreach team will play a large role in the development and assessment of the newly developed acute care competencies (Department of Health 2009). It appears unlikely that with the current drivers to develop outreach that the service will not be appropriately funded. However, the need to provide effective and robust evaluation of these services to secure funding is echoed throughout the literature (Ball *et al.* 2003; Welch 2003; Bright *et al.* 2006; Valentine & Skirton 2006).

End of chapter test

This test should be completed after you have read Chapters 11 and 12 as information from both of these chapters is required to ensure a coordinated approach to the patient who is deteriorating. It is important that you understand both the theory related to the role of outreach, use of patient assessment tools, and effective escalation of the patient. In order to test your knowledge and apply this knowledge to clinical practice you should undertake the following assessment with an appropriately trained member of staff in clinical practice. If you are unable to answer any questions it may be helpful to revisit the section in Chapter 11 or 12.

Knowledge assessment

Work with your mentor/supervisor in practice and ask them to test your knowledge in relation to the following. Incorrect answers/lack of knowledge will require further revision/re-reading of Chapter 11 or 12.

- Examine rationale for provision of outreach services.
- Identify model of outreach used within own hospital area.
- Describe main objectives of outreach services.
- Analyse need for support from outreach services.
- Discuss why track-and-trigger systems were introduced.
- Identify trust's track-and-trigger system.
- Analyse which changes in track-and-trigger parameters may cause concern, providing rationale for answer.
- Explain why aggregate scoring systems are seen as the most appropriate tool and explores why these are recommended by NICE.
- Analyse advantages and disadvantages of using track-and-trigger systems to enhance patient assessment.
- Discuss limitations of trust's track-and-trigger tool.
- Discuss situations in which outreach intervention would be appropriate.

- Discuss situations that should trigger emergency call to medical/outreach staff.
- Analyse the trust's escalation policy and discuss how appropriate escalation of concern may be facilitated.
- Discuss potential problems with communication of concern about a patient.
- Describe use of SBAR tool to improve escalation of concern.
- Discuss outreach's role in follow-up of ITU patients.
- Analyse evidence base for continuation of outreach services.
- Identify benefits of outreach services for the ward nurse.
- Analyse the need for a documented monitoring plan.
- Analyse the need for whole-team review of patient.
- Discuss their own accountability in relation to caring for the acutely ill adult.
- Understand their own role in the 'chain of response'.

Skills assessment

Work with your mentor/supervisor in practice and ask them to assess your ability to work alongside the outreach services to enhance care of the patient whose condition is deteriorating using the following criteria where appropriate. Note: You may not be able to demonstrate all these skills. Ask your mentor/supervisor to give you feedback on areas that you did well and areas that may require improving.

- Explains need for assessment to the patient and gains patient's consent.
- Communicates effectively with patient throughout assessment, offering reassurance as necessary.
- Assesses patient using hospital's track-and-trigger system and own nursing knowledge of deteriorating patients.
- Is able to use ABCDE approach to assessment alongside track-and-trigger and other assessment tools.
- Analyses assessment details and provides rationale for concern about patient.
- Utilizes track-and-trigger system to assess the need for patient escalation
- Follows local policy in relation to escalation of acutely ill patient.
- Collates other information that may be useful to obtain (blood results, fluid balance, pain score, GCS, etc.).
- Communicates areas of concern using SBAR principles to appropriate practitioner and documents concerns in nursing notes.
- Articulates need for fast intervention and provides time frame for review to medical staff/outreach services.
- Emphasizes the need for a written action plan if patient is deteriorating.
- Communicates effectively when staff arrive to review patient, identifying specific areas of concern.
- Works well as a team member in enabling a coordinated response to the patient who is deteriorating.
- Communicates with other members of the ward team.

- Participates in the whole-team review of the patient and changes care as directed by medical team/outreach.
- Ensures any changes in care are delivered in a timely manner.
- Ensures appropriate additional monitoring as requested by outreach/medical staff.
- Recognizes the need to reassess the patient following intervention.
- Reassesses patient and informs team of continuing areas of concern about the patient.
- Is able to participate in effective decision making and ongoing planning of care.
- Is able to recognize own sphere of competence and identify when assistance is required from senior practitioners.
- Is able to lead other members of staff where appropriate.
- Is able to assist in decision making regarding appropriateness of treatment.
- Informs patient's next of kin about any patient deterioration.
- Maintains patient assessment until patient either stabilizes or is transferred to another area.
- Documents all changes to care and interventions in patient's notes.

References

Ball, C., Kirby, M., and Williams, S. (2003) Effect of the critical care outreach team on patient survival to discharge from hospital and readmission to critical care: Non randomised population based study. *BMJ* **327**, 1014–7.

Bright, D., Walker, W., and Bion, J. (2004) Clinical review: Outreach—a strategy for improving the care of the acutely ill hospitalized patient. *Crit. Care.* **8**, 33–40.

Carr, K. (2002) In: Griffiths, R.D. and Jones, C. (2002) *Intensive Care After Care.* Butterworth Heinemann, Oxford.

Chellel, A., Higgs, D., and Scholes, J. (2006) An evaluation of the contribution of critical care outreach to the clinical management of the critically ill ward patient in two NHS trusts. *Nurs. Crit. Care.* **11**(1), 42–51.

Cioffi, J. (2000) Recognition of patients who require emergency assistance: A descriptive study. *Heart Lung.* **29**, 262–268.

Coad, S. and Haines, S. (1999) Supporting staff caring for critically ill patients in acute care areas. *Nurs. Crit. Care.* **4**, 245–8.

Cooper, N. and Cramp, P. (2003) *Essential Guide to Acute Care.* BMJ Books, London.

Cutler, L. (2006) IN: Cutler, L. and Robson, W. (2006). *Critical Care Outreach.* Wiley, Chichester.

Department of Health (2000) *Comprehensive Critical Care, a Review of Adult Critical Care Services.* The Stationary Office, London.

Department of Health (2005) *Quality Critical Care – Beyond Comprehensive Critical Care.* The Stationary Office, London.

Department of Health (2009) *Competencies for Recognising and Responding to Acutely Ill Adults in Hospital.* Draft guidelines for consultation. The Stationary Office, London.

Gardner Thorpe, J., Love, N., Wrightson, J. *et al.* (2006) The value of modified early warning scores in patients: A prospective observational study. *Ann. Roy. Coll. Surg. England.* **88**(6), 571–5.

Hall Smith, J., Ball, C., and Coakley, J. (1997) Follow up services and the development of a clinical nurse specialist. *Int. Care Int. Crit. Care Nurs.* **13**, 243–8.

Hillman, K. (2004) Expanding critical care monitoring beyond the intensive care unit. *Crit. Care.* **8**(1), 9–10.

Intensive Care Society (2002) *The Intensive Care Standards for the Introduction of Outreach Services.* Intensive Care Society, London.

McArthur-Rouse, F. (2001) Critical care outreach services and early warning scoring systems: a review if the literature. *J. Adv. Nurs.* **36**(5), 696–704.

McGloin, H., Adam, S.K., and Singer, M. (1999) Unexpected deaths and referrals to Intensive Care of patient on general wards: are some potentially avoidable? *J. Roy. Coll. Phys.* **33**, 255–9.

McQuillan, P., Pilkington, S., and Allan, A. (1998) Confidential enquiry into quality of care before admission to intensive care. *BMJ.* **316**, 1853–8.

MERIT Study Investigators (2005) Introduction of the medical emergency team(met): a cluster-randomised controlled trial. *Lancet.* **365**, 2091–7.

National Confidential Enquiry into Patient Outcome and Death (2005) *An Acute Problem?*: National Confidential Enquiry into Patient Outcome and Death, London.

National Health Service Innovations and Improvements (2008) *No Delays Achiever, Service Improvement Tools (SBAR).* NHS, London.

National Outreach Forum (2007) *Critical Care Outreach Services-Indicators of Service Achievement and Good Practice.* National Outreach Forum, London.

National Patient Safety Agency (2007) *Safer Care for the Acutely Ill Patient: Learning From Serious Incidents.* National Patient Safety Agency, London.

NICE (2007) *Acutely Ill Patients In-Hospital: Recognition of and Response to Acute Illness of Adults In-Hospital.* The Stationary Office, London.

Rafferty, A.M., Clarke, S.P., Coles,J. *et al.* (2007) Outcomes of variations in-hospital staffing in English hospitals: cross sectional analysis of survey data and discharge records. *Int. J Nurs. Stud.* **44**(12), 175–82.

Rattray, J. and Crocker, C. (2007) The intensive care follow up clinic: Current provision and future direction. *Nurs. Crit. Care.* **12**(1), 1–3.

Rowan, K., Adam, S., Ball, C. et al. (2009) *Evaluation of Outreach Services in Critical Care.* Intensive Care National Audit and Research Committee, London.

Sharland, C. (2002) In: Griffiths, R.D. and Jones, C. (2002) *Intensive Care After Care.* Butterworth Heinemann, Oxford.

Smith, G. (2003) *ALERT: Acute Life Threatening Events, Treatment and Recognition.* 2nd edn. University of Portsmouth, Portsmouth.

Subbe, C.P., Slater, A., Menon, D., and Gemmell, L. (2006) Validation of physiological scoring systems in the accident and emergency dept. *Emerg. Med.* **23**, 841–5.

Valentine, J. and Skirton, S. (2006) Critical care outreach: A meaningful evaluation *Nurs. Crit. Care.* **11**(6), 288–96.

Waldmann, C. (2002) In: Griffiths, R.D. and Jones, C. (2002) *Int. Care After Care.* Butterworth Heinemann, Oxford.

Welch, J. (2003) Critical care outreach—The story so far. *Int. Crit. Care Nurs.* **20**, 1–5.

Wood, J. & Smith, A. (1999) Active management should prevent cardiopulmonary arrest. *BMJ.* **7175**(318), 51–2.

Chapter 13

Acute emergency situations

Lorna East

Chapter contents

Maximizing survival from cardiac arrest in hospital requires a coordinated and rapid response, skilled practitioners performing resuscitation procedures correctly, and utilizing evidence-based guidelines. This chapter will therefore examine:

+ causes and prevention of acute emergency situations
+ initial assessment of the patient in acute emergency situations
+ management of the patient in cardiac arrest
+ management of the patient with anaphylaxis
+ management of the patient in peri-arrest arrhythmias
+ post-resuscitation care
+ decisions relating to cardiopulmonary resuscitation(CPR)/ethics and resuscitation
+ family presence during resuscitation.

Learning outcomes

This chapter will enable you to:

+ be able to define cardiac arrest and CPR
+ explore a structured approach to assessing an acutely sick patient
+ identify early recognition and cardiac arrest prevention in acute care patients
+ identify causes of cardiac arrest
+ identify all the known cardiac arrest rhythms and differentiate the management for shockable versus non-shockable arrests
+ consider the assessment, diagnosis, and management of the patient in cardiac arrest
+ understand the importance of chest compressions and early defibrillation
+ be familiar with management of peri-arrest arrhythmias, including pacing and synchronized cardioversion
+ evaluate the nursing management of a patient with anaphylaxis.

An essential part of nursing in an acute care area is to be fully prepared to deal promptly and effectively with any acute emergency situation. More acutely ill patients are being cared for within ward environments, which places an ever-increasing need for staff to be competent and confident in the care and management of those at risk of cardiac arrest. Approximately 80% of cardiac arrests are predictable, with patients displaying adverse clinical signs in the few hours preceding the event. Strategies to prevent cardiac arrest are therefore paramount. The assessment of simple vital signs helps to predict cardiorespiratory arrest (Resuscitation Council (UK) 2006a,b). Recognition of adverse signs from the deteriorating patient, calling for early expert assistance and intervention of key therapies such as airway management, oxygen, and fluid resuscitation, must therefore aim to prevent cardiac arrest occurring in the first instance. It is clear that the current and future focus on resuscitation must be to ensure that all healthcare professionals are able to recognize the deteriorating patient and to be able to activate the early warning or track-and-trigger response systems in place, within our acute hospitals. (Further information can be obtained from Chapter 11 on track-and-trigger systems.)

> It is crucially important that acute care skills are taken to the patient in a timely manner so that survival from cardiac arrests within our hospitals can significantly improve.

Recognition and prevention of cardiac arrest

Nurses today are practising more advanced assessment skills than ever before. It is vital, however, that the basics are not forgotten (Cox *et al.* 2006). Evidence suggests that patients who become acutely unwell in hospital may still receive suboptimal care (McQuillan *et al.* 1998; NICE 2007). They also identified that communication and documentation are often poor, experience might be lacking, and provision of critical care expertise, including admission to critical care areas, could be delayed.

A third of patients who have a false cardiac arrest call will die subsequently (Cashman 2002). The National Confidential Enquiry into Patient Outcome and Death (National Confidential Enquiry into Patient Outcome and Death 2005) found that with patients who died, staff demonstrated the inability to seek advice and even appreciate any sense of clinical urgency. Evidence-based practice emphasizes the necessity for effective communication and collaboration between nursing and medical teams (Cutler 2002). The introduction of medical emergency teams (METs) has been associated with improvement in the rate of documentation of vital signs (Chen *et al.* 2009).

Early recognition therefore prevents:

- cardiac arrests and deaths
- inappropriate resuscitation attempts
- admissions to ITU (Resuscitation Council (UK) 2006a,b)

Over the last few years, early recognition and cardiac arrest prevention has been a heavily weighted component of hospital resuscitation training programmes (ALERT™ 2003, Advanced Life Support 2006, Intermediate Life Support 2006). Greater emphasis is now placed on earlier recognition of the deteriorating patient (National Confidential Enquiry into Patient Outcome and Death 2005; National Patient Safety Agency (National Patient Safety Agency 2007; NICE 2007). Using a framework ensures the identification of the life-threatening needs and care to be prioritized in a structured airway, breathing, circulation, disability, and exposure (ABCDE) approach (Smith 2000; Resuscitation Council (UK) 2005). The aim of initial treatment is to keep the patient alive and achieve some clinical improvement to buy time for further treatment (Resuscitation Council (UK) 2006b). Many hospitals have already put effective strategies in place so that patients at risk of critical illness and cardiorespiratory arrest can be identified (see Chapter 11).

ABCDE approach

In general, the clinical signs of critical illness are similar whatever the underlying process is before they reflect failing respirations, cardiovascular, and neurological systems, that is ABCDE problems (Resuscitation Council (UK) 2006a,b).

This rapid assessment is performed in a structured order so that life-threatening symptoms can be dealt with along the way. If at any stage through the assessment life-threatening signs are evident, the emergency team, depending on your local trust policy, must be called; recognize when you need extra help and call for help early (Resuscitation Council (UK) 2006a,b).

Situations that are likely to result in serious harm should be dealt with first. For instance, a blocked airway should be prioritized before breathing or circulation difficulties and these areas must be assessed and supported in order of priority. Guidelines on the ABCDE approach are now embedded in current resuscitation documentation (Resuscitation Council (UK) 2006a,b) adapted originally from the ALERT™ course (Smith 2003):

- Airway
- Breathing
- Circulation
- Disability
- Exposure.

Airway

It is vital to look, listen, and feel in the assessment of the airway (Box 13.1). Gurgling noises may indicate fluid or vomit in the airway, which will need removing with a wide bore suction catheter (yankeur) and working suction. It is important not to push the suction too far down into the airway as it may cause more harm. It may cause trauma and/or laryngospasm and you may potentially be faced with an obstructed airway. Remember just to suction what you can see. Any concerns with the airway at all and the call must be put out. Stridor is a high-pitched noise, which occurs on inspiration indicating a partially obstructed airway. This can be caused by inflammation or swelling of the upper airway or by the presence of a foreign body by irritation of the vocal cords. This can also occur sometimes when patients are waking up from an anaesthetic or heavy sedation.

Simple measures will almost always open an obstructed airway using airways manoeuvres (see Figure 13.1).

Breathing

Evidence of respiratory distress or inadequate ventilation can also be determined using a simple 'look, listen, feel' approach (Smith 2003).

Box 13.1 Airway assessment in the acutely ill patient

- Is the airway patent? Is the patient talking or mumbling?
- Are there any added noises/sounds?
- Is suction required?
- What is the patient's colour?
- Are airway opening manoeuvres required? Consider c-spine.
- Apply O_2 high flow.
- Check oropharyngeal/nasopharyngeal airways.

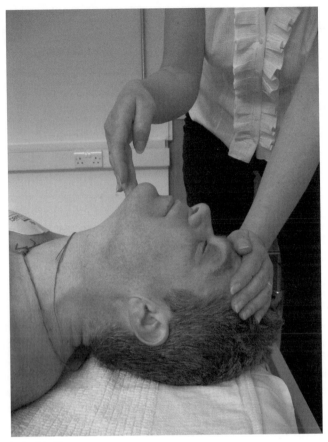

Figure 13.1 Head tilt/chin lift.

Along with the assessments identified in Box 13.2 it is essential that the patient is ventilating adequately. If the patient's ventilations are inadequate, then the heart rate will increase, the skin colour will deteriorate, become grey/pale, and even cyanosed. This is a peri-arrest sign. The patient may also become anxious, restless, or even drowsy if ventilation is inadequate because oxygen to the brain is significantly reduced.

Again, simple measures can be applied, for example sitting your patient upright if possible to optimize oxygenation and ventilation. All acutely ill patients should receive oxygen and it is important to treat all underlying causes of respiratory problems. The emergency team must be called immediately if acute life-threatening conditions occur, such as acute asthma and/ or pulmonary oedema. (See Chapter 2 for a detailed discussion of respiratory assessment and care.)

Circulation

It is important to assess the patient's circulatory status using the same look, listen, and feel approach (Box 13.3). In almost all medical and surgical emergencies, hypovolaemia should be considered the primary cause of shock until proven otherwise (Smith 2003; Resuscitation Council (UK) 2006a,b). If the patient has a normal blood pressure it does not exclude shock, severe blood loss, or critical illness. (For further information see Chapters 3 and 7.)

Box 13.2 Breathing assessment in the acutely ill patient

- Rate.
- Effort.
- Depth.
- Bilateral chest movement and equal air entry.
- Breath sounds/added sounds.
- O_2 saturations (Note: This does not detect raised CO_2)/ABGs.
- Colour.
- Sweating/clammy.
- Use of accessory muscles.
- Position of patient.

Disability (neurological)

A rapid assessment of the patient's neurological function should follow a quick reassessment of ABC. See Box 13.4 for neurological assessment. (Read Chapter 4 on neurological assessment and care.)

Exposure

Finally, 'a top to toe' look at the patient should be conducted, to check that no other cause of their acute episode has been missed (see Box 13.5).

The aim of treating the acutely ill patient is the early anticipation and detection of abnormal physiology at a stage before organ failure is established and to initiate simple preventative therapies and interventions (Smith 2003).

Box 13.3 Circulation assessment in the acutely ill patient

- Reassess airway and breathing.
- Pulses: peripheral/central? Rate? Rhythm? Volume?
- Peripheral circulation: Cool? Clammy? Warm/hot?
- Capillary refill time.
- Blood pressure.
- Any blood/fluid loss? Wounds? Drains? Dressings? Arterial lines? Haemorrhage control.
- CVP.
- Urine output.
- 12-lead ECG interpretation.
- Need intravenous access? Take bloods.
- Fluid challenge.

Box 13.4 Disability (neurological) assessment in the acutely ill patient

- ♦ Reassess ABC. Is it still hypoxic or hypotensive?
- ♦ AVPU (Alert, responds to Voice, responds to Pain, Unresponsive).
- ♦ Blood sugar.
- ♦ Pupil(s) reaction.
- ♦ Posture.
- ♦ Anxious? Restless? Aggressive? Fidgety?
- ♦ Airway secure? Left lateral position (if C spine ok).
- ♦ Look at drug chart/blood results.

Cardiac arrest: causes, rhythms, and the 'chain of survival'

Cardiac arrest can be defined as the cessation of circulation along with absent signs of life such as normal respirations or movement. The patient will have loss of consciousness, and become unresponsive and lifeless. Respiratory effort will be absent or gasping, along with an absent pulse in a major artery (carotid or femoral).

Sudden cardiac arrest is responsible for more than 60% of adult deaths from coronary heart disease. Other causes can be viewed in Box 13.6. In 2006, a report of cardiac arrest epidemiology showed in-hospital mortality rates were 67% out of 19,819 adult patients (Nadkarni *et al.* 2006). A study in the UK of 24,132 patients admitted to critical care units after cardiac arrest produced a similar figure of 71% mortality (Nolan *et al.* 2007).

Although evidence-based resuscitation knowledge, practice, and technology has advanced over the past 40 years, these numbers remain extremely poor. Those who survive to discharge tend to come from arrests with a primary ventricular fibrillation (VF) or pulseless ventricular tachycardia (VT). The annual incidence of a VF/VT arrest is 17 per 100,000 patients and survival to hospital discharge is 21.2% (Resuscitation Council (UK) 2005). Treatment for these arrest rhythms is prompt defibrillation. Defibrillation is the only treatment for sustained ventricular arrhythmias.

Survival to discharge for ALL cardiac arrest rhythms is only 10.7% (Nolan *et al.* 2005). Box 13.7 identifies all four cardiac arrest rhythms.

Box 13.5 Exposure in the acutely ill patient

- ♦ Rashes? Wounds? Lines?
- ♦ Top to toe look.
- ♦ Signs of deep vein thrombosis?
- ♦ Central temperature.
- ♦ Maintain dignity.
- ♦ Reassess ABCDE.

Clinical link 13.1 (see Appendix for answers)

Part A

A 43-year-old patient has been admitted to hospital with anaemia, cause unknown. She returns to the ward after having an endoscopy procedure. She is supine in the bed. Your initial assessment reveals respirations 10/min, heart rate 115 and regular, blood pressure 130/80, central temperature 36.3 C and O_2 saturations 86%. She is pale and clammy. She is responding to voice.

♦ What would your immediate actions be and why?

♦ What other assessments would you consider?

Part B

After your initial intervention and treatment her condition appeared to improve. However, on your return with more help to change her position and to recheck further observations, you notice she is cyanosed around her lips and a noise is coming from her airway.

♦ What are your priorities for this patient?

♦ What interventions/actions will you take?

♦ Can you list all the signs of complete and partial airway obstruction?

Box 13.6 Causes of cardiorespiratory arrest in acute care

♦ Airway obstruction.

♦ Hypoxia.

♦ Anaphylaxis.

♦ Pulmonary embolism.

♦ Hypovolaemia (sepsis and/or haemorrhage).

♦ Acute coronary syndrome.

♦ Metabolic and electrolyte disturbances.

♦ Cardiac arrhythmias.

♦ Drugs (i.e. anti-arrhythmics; opiates).

♦ Neurological insult (i.e. CVA; head injury).

♦ Tension pneumothorax.

Box 13.7 The four cardiac arrest rhythms

These two rhythms together are known as the *shockable* cardiac arrest rhythms:

♦ ventricular fibrillation

♦ ventricular tachycardia (pulseless).

These two rhythms are known as the *non-shockable* cardiac arrest rhythms:

♦ pulseless electrical activity (PEA)

♦ asystole (including p-wave asystole)

Chain of survival

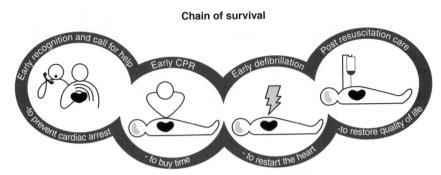

Figure 13.2 Chain of survival (European Resuscitation Council 2005).

The 'chain of survival' (Cummins *et al.* 1991) concept still remains true to current recommendations, with emphasis on swift implementation of good quality chest compressions and early defibrillation (Figure 13.2). Effectiveness of defibrillation falls rapidly with even small delays to treatment. The chain is only as strong as its weakest link. To optimize the chances of a successful outcome, each link in the chain needs to be strong.

Cardiopulmonary resuscitation

CPR is an emergency procedure required for someone in cardiac arrest. It combines techniques of providing external chest compressions creating artificial blood circulation and delivering artificial respirations to create lung inflation and oxygen delivery. A combination of these more modern techniques have been used over the past 50 years, but have been fine tuned according to current evidence-based medicine. CPR may have been known in theory, if not in practice, for hundreds or even thousands of years. The first ever written account of a resuscitation attempt was in fact that of Elijah the prophet, who warmed a dead boy's body and placed his mouth over the boy's mouth.

CPR is unlikely to restart the heart but is a holding measure delaying cell death. Irreversible tissue death occurs within 4–5 min if resuscitation attempts are not commenced. Good quality CPR will extend this very brief window in order for advanced life support (ALS) techniques to be implemented. The brain and the heart will be oxygenated, albeit to only approximately 30% of normal cardiac output. The aim therefore is for a successful resuscitation attempt to occur without permanent brain damage.

Why resuscitation guidelines?

Although the birth of a modern approach to CPR was described in the 1950s/1960s, the Resuscitation Council (UK) was not formed until 1981. It recognized that the greatest challenge was to spread the word of CPR and to promote, educate, and encourage the healthcare workers and more recently lay people in the skills of resuscitation. The Resuscitation Council (UK) is continually reviewing the literature to provide evidence-based national standards and guidelines for resuscitation. International reviews of resuscitation science occur every 5 years, usually resulting in new European and UK guidelines. More importantly in recent years resuscitation guidelines around the world are now broadly similar (Paradis *et al.* 2007).

It is important to remember that guidelines do not define the only way that resuscitation should be achieved but represent a widely accepted view of how resuscitation can be undertaken both safely and effectively (Nolan *et al.* 2005). The current guidelines published in 2005

(Resuscitation Council (UK) 2005) were introduced to simplify the teaching process and to encourage retention of skills. Main changes included an increase of chest compressions during CPR. This is based on studies that show circulating blood increases during chest compressions and even minimal delays of 10–20 s can reduce the chances of successful defibrillation (Nolan *et al.* 2006). Future guidelines aim to be introduced after 2010 and you are advised to check them for any radical changes.

Resuscitation equipment

In every emergency situation a speedy response is crucial. It is vital that all essential equipment is ready, accessible, works, and is in date. A designated trolley must be set up and should only be used in an emergency and checked on a daily basis. It must be restocked and checked again after use. Your hospital's own resuscitation department should advise a checklist; it is important that an agreed system is in place and monitored. The defibrillator must also be checked according to the manufacturer's guidelines. Any faults must be reported to your maintenance team. To avoid the machine's battery failing it is important to ensure that the machine is always plugged into the mains, ready for use. Most manufacturers recommend that ECG and defibrillator electrodes should not be opened until required for use.

Despite acute care bed areas being facilitated with individual suction and bedside piped oxygen facility, an emergency mobile suction unit, and spare oxygen cylinder (which must be over half full) must be readily available as a backup. In theory, any patient, relative, or member of staff could collapse outside of a bed space area. The equipment must be checked daily as well as the bedside units at the start of a shift. The suction units must be tested that they are working (will create suction up to 300 mmHg) and that enough tubing is available so it can reach with ample room. A wide bore suction catheter should also be attached ready for use (after the suction has been tested). There must also be a non-rebreathe oxygen mask and reservoir device available (see Figure 13.3) and ideally a single patient use bag–valve–mask (BVM) unit with its own oxygen tubing, ready at each bed space (only necessary in the high dependency unit areas). All bed spaces must be kept tidy and free from clutter, so that the resuscitation team can easily and swiftly access the patient safely from all sides of the bed if required.

In-hospital resuscitation

The public expect that clinical staff can undertake CPR (Resuscitation Council (UK) 2006a). All healthcare professionals should be able to recognize cardiorespiratory arrest, call for help, and start CPR (see Box 13.8).

Staff should do what they have been trained to do, using skills in which they are trained and competent (Nolan *et al.* 2005; Department of Health 2008 a). (See Chapter 1 regarding Department of Health competencies.)

Safety

Your personal safety and that of the resuscitation team members is the first priority during any resuscitation attempt (Resuscitation Council (UK) 2006a,b). It is really important that protective equipment is used with gloves and aprons as standard. A sharps box must be readily available on the emergency trolley and staff must be fastidious in their use and disposal.

Call for help early

It is vital to shout 'Help!' whilst approaching the patient having assessed it is safe to do so. Your colleagues are therefore alerted to assist you and more importantly your experienced senior nurses

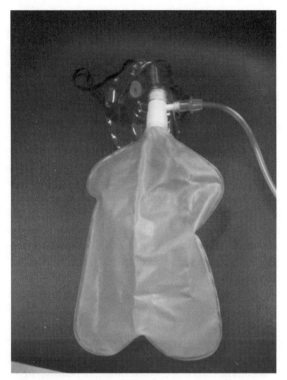

Figure 13.3 Non rebreathe mask with reservoir device.

will also be there to help. The single rescuer must always ensure that help is coming (Resuscitation Council (UK) 2006a,b) and therefore emergency buzzers should also be deployed.

Responsive patient

Check the patient's responsiveness with a gentle shake and ask loudly, 'Are you alright?' (Resuscitation Council (UK) 2006a,b). If there is a response, assess the patient using the ABCDE approach (Resuscitation Council (UK) 2006a,b) and call either the MET or outreach team depending what policy is in place in your trust. (See Chapter 11 on track-and-trigger systems). Ensure that the patient has high-flow oxygen, sit them upright if tolerated, insert a cannula, and

---

Box 13.8 Sequence of events in hospital cardiac arrest

In hospital, all healthcare professionals should:

♦ immediately recognize cardiorespiratory arrest

♦ ensure that emergency team has been despatched using standard number (e.g. 2222)

♦ commence CPR immediately; using airway adjuncts once arrived: pocket mask or two person technique BVM

♦ defibrillate, if indicated, and attempt this within 3 min.

Resuscitation Council (UK) (2006a,b)

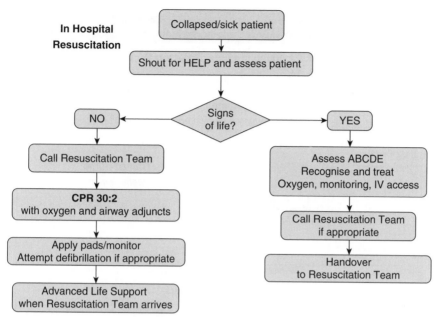

In Hospital Resuscitation

Collapsed/sick patient

↓

Shout for HELP and assess patient

↓

Signs of life?

NO → → YES

NO path:

Call Resuscitation Team

↓

CPR 30:2
with oxygen and airway adjuncts

↓

Apply pads/monitor
Attempt defibrillation if appropriate

↓

Advanced Life Support
when Resuscitation Team arrives

YES path:

Assess ABCDE
Recognise and treat
Oxygen, monitoring, IV access

↓

Call Resuscitation Team
if appropriate

↓

Handover
to Resuscitation Team

Figure 13.4 In-hospital algorithm (Resuscitation Council (UK) 2006) (with kind permission from the Resuscitation Council (UK)).

start blood pressure, ECG, and O_2 saturation monitoring. Be prepared to handover to the team when they arrive. Always ensure that medical notes are available and observation and fluid charts visible (see Figure 13.4).

Unresponsive patient

If the patient does not respond, the nurse must perform a quick and timely ABC assessment to confirm cardiac arrest. Ideally, the patient should be flat on their back. As recommended by the Resuscitation Council (UK) (2006a,b), keeping the airway open with either head tilt chin lift (see Figure 13.1) or jaw thrust (in c spine injury patients), ensures that it is clear from any obstruction. The rescuer needs to determine if the patient is breathing normally or has any other signs of life (i.e. coughing, moving) for no longer than 10 s. Gasping or very slow or noisy breathing is abnormal and not adequate. It is essential to look for normal rise and fall of the chest wall, listen for breath sounds, and feel for air on your cheek. As acute care nurses it would be expected that you should assess the circulation at the same time, therefore check for normal breathing, signs of life, and a carotid pulse check simultaneously.

The cardiac arrest call of 2222 (UK, but ensure that you are familiar with your trust number) has to be made immediately and practical resuscitative measures commenced. Box 13.9 demonstrates the key personnel involved in a cardiac arrest procedure and their position and roles.

Fortunately within acute care areas staff members are usually within closer working distances and many actions can be performed at the same time. One nurse can make the call, one can bring the resuscitation trolley with the defibrillator, and one can start immediate chest compressions. Qualified nursing staff must be able to carry out a wide range of resuscitation procedures, including the use of a defibrillator (Department of Health 2002, 2008a). Whilst the defibrillator is being brought to the resuscitation attempt, chest compressions must be ongoing. Only if there were adequate personnel with the correct equipment would the compressions be halted, to allow

Box 13.9 Cardiac arrest team members, roles, and positions

F1, foundation year 1 doctor; F2, foundation year 2 doctor; IV, intravenous; ODP, operating department practitioner; BLS, basic life support.

Anaesthetist ± ODP
Airway protection & ventilation/oxygenation

F1/2 Doctor
IV access & drugs

Trained nurse
Defibrillation

Patient

X2 BLS providers

Good quality chest compressions

Porter
(back up defibrillator)

Senior nurse
*documentation &
audit form (may
be required for
family presence)*

Team Leader
On-call medical doctor/ALS provider

pocket mask or BVM ventilation to occur. Without effective head tilt chin lift and a good effective tight seal, ventilations will not be successful and the patient's chest will not rise and fall (see Figure 13.5). If this is the case, chest compressions *must not* stop in order for any more ventilatory attempts until the next group of uninterrupted 30 compressions. The only time immediate interruption should occur is when the rescuer is ready to assess the heart rhythm to determine whether it is shockable or non-shockable or if there are signs of life from the patient. If the patient is in VF or pulseless VT then immediate safe defibrillation must occur. For non-VF/non-VT arrest rhythms, compressions and ventilations at 30:2 must resume.

Remember if there is *no* evidence of normal breathing, coughing, and/or any movement, then there are *no* signs of life: this is a *cardiac arrest*. If there are any doubts you *must* ensure that help and equipment, including a defibrillator and pocket mask, is coming and commence immediate CPR, starting with 30 chest compressions then two ventilations.

If there is any doubt the nurse must commence CPR, as delays in chest compressions will affect a positive outcome. It must be noted that starting CPR on a very sick patient with a low cardiac output is unlikely to be harmful and may even be beneficial (Resuscitation Council (UK) 2006b).

It is important to remember that if you have taken your patient to the MRI or CT scanning areas or are transferring your patient to another area within the hospital, you may have to call the resuscitation team yourself. This must be done *prior* to commencing resuscitation measures if you are

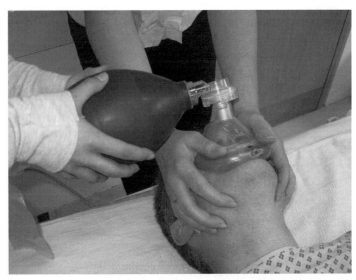

Figure 13.5 Bag–valve–mask ventilation showing two person technique.

the single responder. It is also the nurse who is responsible when chaperoning patients to these areas, therefore take adequate equipment in the event of their patient's condition deteriorating (see Chapter 14 on safe transfer of the acutely ill). These patients should, on any transfer, have a defibrillator/monitor, suction equipment, and a pocket mask, with a full oxygen cylinder, in the event of a cardiac arrest occurring outside the acute care area. Within some NHS trusts the portering staff may be trained in chest compression only CPR, in which case they could commence this immediately whilst the single rescuer (the acute care nurse) makes the call. Fortunately within NHS trusts basic life support skills are mandatory for all healthcare professionals. This arguably makes it a little less stressful for the nurse, if anything sudden should occur outside of their acute care area.

Chest compressions

These have been called external cardiac massage or cardiac massage in the past but this can be extremely misleading, as a great amount of effort is required to perform them correctly and to be as effective as possible for the patient. Chest compressions need to be at the correct rate, depth, and position, with the patient lying on their back face up, ideally on a solid surface. They must be performed using a vertical force directing in the middle of the patient's sternum. The old method of measuring with two fingers is simply wasting time. Two hands should be on the centre of the chest (sternum) with straight arms, elbows locked, and shoulders directly over the patient. If the patient is on the floor, the nurse must ensure that their knees are as close to the patient as possible. This will allow optimum position (see Figure 13.6). Remember to lower any hospital beds or trolleys as low as possible to optimize good quality compressions. It is also important to deflate low air loss mattresses using the CPR handle or button. The sternum must be compressed hard and fast. The depth should be 4–5 cm (2 inches) and the rate 100 a minute (almost 2 every second!). The rate refers to the speed at which the compressions are given and not the total number delivered each minute (Handley *et al.* 2005). Ideally, try not to allow your fingers to press on the chest wall over the ribs. The heels of your hands are much stronger. With the wrists bent and fingers up, it allows better force to be applied (see Figure 3.7). After each compression the pressure must be released, but without taking away the hand position. Compression and release should take the same time and this should avoid any jerky compressions. *Use 30 compressions to 2 ventilations.*

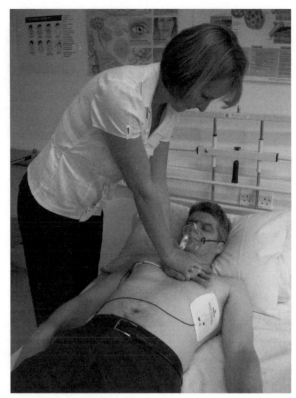

Figure 13.6 Body/hand position for chest compressions.

The only times the ratio of compressions changes are:

♦ When first commencing CPR and waiting for the resuscitation trolley to arrive, continuous compressions should prevail unless there are signs of life.

♦ When the patient is already intubated and has a secure airway, compressions should be continuous. The patient will be ventilated independently of the compressions, so it becomes asynchronous.

♦ For basic life support purposes *if you are not in the hospital setting*: if you are not able or are unwilling to give rescue breaths, give chest compressions only (Handley *et al.* 2005).

Chest compressions provide critical but small blood flow to the brain and heart. They also increase the likelihood that a defibrillatory shock will terminate VF (Nolan *et al.* 2005). This is achieved by increasing intrathoracic pressure within the chest cavity and also by directly pushing down on the heart itself. Paradis *et al.* (1989) were only able to show that mean arterial pressure seldom exceeded 40 mmHg. However, almost a third of cardiac output is still being created with good quality chest compressions. Minimizing chest compression interruptions cannot be over emphasized. To reduce fatigue, it is important to change the individual undertaking compressions every 2 min (Resuscitation Council (UK) 2006a,b).

Advanced life support

The current guidelines published in 2005 (Resuscitation Council (UK) 2005) were introduced to simplify the teaching process and to encourage retention of skills. The main changes of more chest compressions during CPR are based on studies showing circulating blood increases during

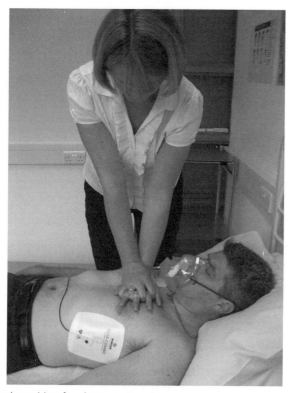

Figure 13.7 Hand/body position for chest compressions.

chest compressions. Even delays of 10–20 s can reduce the chances of successful defibrillation (Nolan *et al.* 2006) (Figure 13.8).

Evidence suggests that patients who have sudden cardiac arrests comprise 1.5–3.0/1,000 admissions (Resuscitation Council (UK) 2005) are in shockable cardiac arrest rhythms (VF/VT) and tend to be nursed in areas such as A&Es, critical care units, and cardiac high dependency areas. Patients in intensive care and general ward areas tend to have non-shockable arrest rhythms (asystole and PEA) and survival to discharge in these groups is extremely poor. In about two-thirds of in-hospital cardiac arrests, the first monitored rhythm is asystole or PEA (Nolan *et al.* 2006).

Management of shockable arrest rhythms

Ventricular fibrillation

- A chaotic bizarre disorganized waveform. No recognizable QRS complex.
- The ventricles are fibrillating like a plate of jelly. There is absence of any ventricular contraction, hence immediate loss of output and sudden cardiac arrest occurs.
- VF may present in a 'fine' or 'coarse' form as highlighted in Figures 13.9 and 13.10.

Ventricular tachycardia (pulseless VT)

- Fast, broad regular complexes.
- Treat as ventricular fibrillation until proven otherwise.

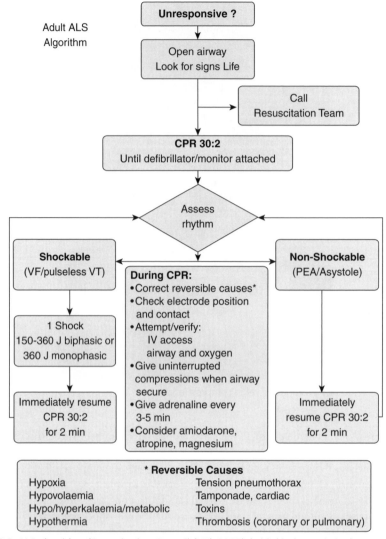

Figure 13.8 ALS algorithm (Resuscitation Council (UK) 2005) (with kind permission).

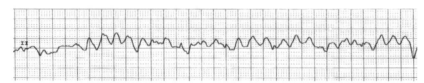

Figure 13.9 Fine ventricular fibrillation.

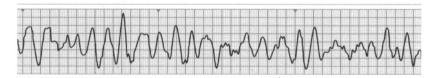

Figure 13.10 Coarse ventricular fibrillation.

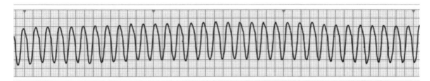

Figure 13.11 Ventricular tachycardia.

♦ Most patients cannot tolerate this rhythm for very long, if at all. The ventricles are contracting so fast that venous return is impeded and the patient will be in cardiac arrest.
♦ VT will often deteriorate into VF if not managed effectively.
♦ VT with a pulse is a peri-arrest situation, which will be discussed later.

As soon as the defibrillator arrives, the rhythm needs to be assessed once the paddles or adhesive hands-free pads have been applied. If VF (Figures 13.9 and 13.10) or VT (Figure 13.11) has been confirmed then charge immediately and give *one shock*. For biphasic machines this will be 150–360 J depending on each hospital policy (and according to manufacturer's recommendations) or 360 J for older monophasic defibrillators. Immediately after the shock is delivered chest compressions must resume and a pulse check is not recommended at this stage. Evidence suggests that it is very rare for a pulse to be present *immediately*, even if a perfusing rhythm has been restored (Rea *et al.* 2005). A delay in trying to palpate a pulse will only compromise the patient if it has not been restored (Figure 13.12).

After 2 min of CPR, it is prudent to quickly glance at the monitor to do a rhythm check. If it is still VF/VT then a second shock must be given (150–360 J) and then 2 more uninterrupted minutes of CPR *unless* there are obvious signs of life. After 2 more minutes pause for a third rhythm check and if it is still VF/VT, give 1 mg adrenaline followed by the third shock at 150–360 J (biphasic) (or 360 J monophasic). If VF/VT continues after the next 2 min of CPR give 300 mg amiodarone just before the fourth shock. Continue in the drug–shock–CPR-rhythm sequence with adrenaline returning just before the fifth shock. It is given therefore in every other loop regardless of the arrest rhythm until return of spontaneous circulation (ROSC) is achieved. Check the monitor only if there are obvious signs of life from the patient, for example movement, coughing, groaning, and normal breathing. If a recognized and organized rhythm is evident then an ABC assessment must be made, but for no longer than 10 s. If normal breathing and pulse is absent and without signs of life, recommence chest compressions and follow the non-shockable arm of the algorithm (asystole/PEA). If a pulse is present and there are signs of life, reassess ABCDE optimizing patient care, post arrest (see Table 13.1).

Defibrillation

Defibrillation is the application of a direct current (DC) electric shock through paddles or large sticky electrode pads to the heart via the chest wall (see Figure 13.13). It is a quick shock with extremely high energy aiming to terminate life-threatening tachy-arrhythmias. The energy, which is measured in joules, creates mass depolarization of the myocardium. It halters the chaotic arrhythmia by prolonging refractoriness therefore fibrillation wave fronts. This allows the

```
DRUG-SINGLE SHOCK-CPR-RHYTHM CHECK
            SEQUENCE
```

Figure 13.12 'Drug-single shock—CPR-rhythm check' sequence (European Resuscitation Council 2005; Resuscitation Council (UK) 2006).

Table 13.1 Post-resuscitation care: patient assessment and treatment after return of spontaneous circulation

Problem area	Assessment	Nursing care/intervention
Airway and breathing Aim: a patent airway, good oxygenation and ventilation	Look, listen, and feel Rate and effort of breathing Added sounds/noises Equal chest movement Pulse oximetry/ABGs Colour Chest X-ray: overall picture also for lines, fractures, and tubes Mental state Sweating/clammy	Head tilt/chin lift Oro/nasopharyngeal airway Suction as required using a wide bore suction catheter High-flow O_2 via non-rebreathe. Aim sats 90% BVM ventilation (two-person technique) if respirations 6 Prepare equipment for intubation and escalation of care/ITU Nasogastric tube if intubated Document observations and MEWS scores
Circulation Aim: maintain adequate cardiac output/organ perfusion and arrhythmia control	Monitor heart rate and rhythm Central/peripheral pulses and temperature/capillary refill time Observe colour Blood pressure Adequate intravenous access Assess recent blood results CVP/arterial lines and monitor Assess drains/wounds Urine output	Attach to heart monitor Cannulate into two large veins and send bloods Aim blood pressure systolic 100 mmHg Evaluate 12 lead recording/contact cardiology physicians/?PCI Urinary catheter insertion and hourly measurements Take blood cultures if pyrexial Administer fluids as prescribed Replace electrolytes as prescribed Documentation and care bundles Blood group and save/note location of O negative blood if required
Disability: Aim: maintain brain perfusion and optimise neurological recovery	AVPU/GCS Pupils Posture/limb movements Blood sugar	Blood sugar control and monitoring (aim normoglycaemic); may require sliding scale Regular neurological observations If GCS 8 prepare equipment to secure airway Seizure control/sedation as prescribed if required Ensure communication is maintained to patient with reduced conscious level
Exposure: Aim: to ensure any other underlying causes are excluded	Temperature Skin Lesions/wounds/holes/rashes Any bleeding areas/points Assess for DVT	Full observation of patient top to toe maintaining dignity at all times Control any bleeding points Send any infective looking sources for microscopy, culture, and sensitivity from wound swabs, lesions, pus from any source. Administer analgesia as prescribed and monitor effect Maintain privacy and dignity

ABGs, arterial blood gases; BVM, bag valve mask; ITU, intensive therapy unit; MEWS, modified early warning score; CVP, central venous pressure; PCI, percutaneous coronary intervention; AVPU, Alert, responds to Voice, responds to Pain, Unresponsive; GCS, Glasgow Coma Score; DVT, deep vein thrombosis.

natural pacemaker, the sino-atrial node, to take over the normal electrical function of the heart and therefore maintain mechanical stability.

In 1947, the first human was defibrillated successfully directly on the heart itself, which is called internal defibrillation. Dr Paul Zoll in 1956 was the first to be successful in closed chest defibrillation. Initially, the defibrillators were used with alternating current (AC) and changing to DC

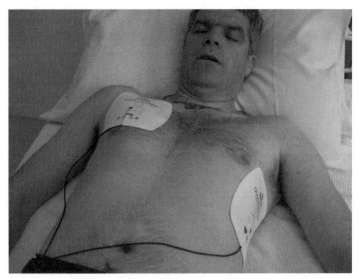

Figure 13.13 Hands-free pad position for defibrillation.

shocks meant that they could be battery operated, portable, and also proved to have fewer side effects. 1980 witnessed the first implanted internal defibrillator in Baltimore, USA. Over the past 10 years further information has become available from the defibrillators themselves, in predicting the success of defibrillation using ECG analysis. Evidence suggests that higher VF amplitude and frequency correlates to success, along with minimizing interruption of chest compressions and the number of shocks delivered.

Early defibrillation has been demonstrated to be the key factor in the treatment of cardiac arrest (Kloeck *et al.* 1997; Resuscitation Council (UK) 2006a,b). There are several types of defibrillators and all healthcare professionals should be trained in the safe use of their particular model.

Manual defibrillators

It is beneficial to have manual-type defibrillators in acute care areas as they can also be used as a transfer monitor, have added facilities for synchronized cardioversion, and provide external pacing, which may be required in the peri-arrest management (see peri-arrest). The user has to interpret the rhythm and makes the decision to defibrillate. The joules must also be set by the user, the charge button deployed, and, in turn, the shock button when it is safe to do so.

Automated external defibrillators

Automated external defibrillators (AEDs) analyse the rhythm and decide if a shock is required. If it is they will charge up the machine and then indicate to the user when the shock is ready to be delivered. The user then pushes the shock button when it is safe to do so. AEDs are used in the community setting. With a widespread increase in public access defibrillation programmes, many more lives will undoubtedly be saved (Box 13.10 and Figure 13.13).

Implantable cardiac defibrillators

Implantable cardiac defibrillators (ICD) look very similar to pacemakers. They are implanted in a subcutaneous pocket and will detect a life-threatening arrhythmia and either attempt to over-drive pace or deliver a shock. This can be very distressing and painful for patients if shocks are

> ## Box 13.10 Hands-free pad position for defibrillation
>
> ◆ Top pad/adhesive electrode below the right clavicle to the right of the sternum, thus avoiding large bone mass.
> ◆ Lower electrode/apical pad because it lies closer to the apex of the heart. It should be placed just below the left nipple, avoiding breast tissue in mid-axillary line (in line to V6).

discharged unnecessarily, which can sometimes happen. The healthcare team can care for and touch the patient in a normal manner as they are at no risk of feeling or getting a shock themselves. For the patient's well being and comfort the critical care unit or cardiac departments within your trust should have large magnets available, which when placed over the ICD will deactivate it. This should only be performed in an emergency situation and it is essential that the trust's electropysiologist or cardiac consultant review the patient as soon as possible.

There are also a number of important safety issues with which you should be familiar in relation to defibrillation—these are identified in Table 13.2.

Table 13.2 Defibrillation safety

Defibrillation preparation and safety	Intervention
Team and self	The person using the defibrillator must take responsibility for ensuring the area is safe. Visual checks all around the bedspace must be performed in addition to warning all to 'stand clear' before the machine is charged
	Ensure that neither you nor anyone else are not touching the patient or bed and beware of any stray clothing such as, ties, coats, or dangling stethoscopes
Oxygen	Remove any O_2 mask and place at least 1 m away
	Leave connected to closed circuit unless ventilator unable to achieve adequate tidal volumes due to chest compressions
Hands-free pads/hand-held paddles	Use of large adhesive electrodes (hands free) rather than held paddles may reduce risk of sparks
	Only charge defibrillator when paddles/pads are on the patient's chest
Chest hair	Can reduce chance of successful defibrillation as impedance can be reduced with a lot of chest hair
	The patient will need to be shaved very rapidly using razor from trolley, this should be performed only where the pads/paddles need to be placed
	Remember to minimize interruptions on chest compressions therefore the second rescuer will need to quickly shave the chest areas
Drug patches	Remove any transdermal drug patches as they may create unnecessary impedance to defibrillation
	They may also cause burns to the patient
Fluids	Ensure no-one is left holding attached bags of fluids, as there is an indirect risk to that person
	Be aware of wet surroundings; make sure patient's chest is dry and ensure team are not all standing in puddles of fluid

Biphasic technology

Technology has improved and modern biphasic defibrillators have been shown to be superior to older models. They are based on the technology from ICDs. The polarity of the electrical current is reversed part way through defibrillation. A longer refractory period is created that will block any stubborn fibrillating wave fronts. Machines are getting smaller, more sophisticated, and easier to use, and the future is very exciting. As a consequence, nurses today are much happier to be trained in this skill and every acute care nurse has the duty and responsibility to ensure that they are (Department of Health 2002). Resuscitation skills are practical ones and are best retained by regular sessions on CPR, as it is essential that hands-on practice with manikins forms an essential part of life-support training (Hamilton 2005).

Precordial thump

This is a sharp blow from a tightly clenched fist with immediate release, on the middle of the sternum. Only those who have been trained in this technique should perform this (Resuscitation Council (UK) 2006a,b). It should be performed when cardiac arrest is witnessed *and* monitored in a shockable rhythm (VF/pulseless VT). If the defibrillator is situated next to the patient then the defibrillator must be used and the precordial thump is no longer recommended. Immediately after the precordial thump, if there are no obvious signs of life or you are unsure then chest compressions must be commenced and await the defibrillator.

Consider reversible causes

After ensuring good quality chest compressions between shocks and checking that electrodes are positioned and adhered correctly, a search for other reversible causes should commence. These are known as the 4Hs and 4Ts and are identified in Table 13.3 (Resuscitation Guidelines (UK) 2006). Consider changing electrodes or defibrillator if VF/VT persists after Hs and Ts have been corrected.

Airway and ventilation

Once the anaesthetist has arrived the airway can be secured and intubation still remains the gold standard. Intubation should not take longer than 30 s. If so, a return to BVM ventilation, with or without an oropharyngeal/nasal airway, will be required. It is important for the team leader, when working through the Hs and Ts, to confirm high-flow oxygen is still attached, turned on, and that the patient's chest is rising and falling with each ventilation breath. Some hospitals do not always have anaesthetists available and alternative policies have to be put in place. Some nurses and operation department practitioners within hospitals are assessed competent in the insertion of a laryngeal mask airway, which is an acceptable alternative in these circumstances. Once the airway is secure, ventilations will be 10/min and asynchronous to compressions at 100/min.

Management of non-shockable arrest rhythms

Pulseless electrical activity

+ Cardiac electrical activity on the monitor *without* any palpable pulse/signs of life.
+ Patients can have very weak mechanical function but will be too weak to produce signs of life/pulse.
+ Often caused by reversible causes (Figures 13.14 and 13.15).

Table 13.3 Potentially reversible causes during cardiac arrest (4Hs and 4Ts)

H or T	Causes	Intervention
Hypoxia	Airway obstruction Respiratory failure Sepsis	Clear, open, suction High O_2 attached BVM, ETT gold standard Check bilateral air entry/chest movement
Hypovolamia	Haemorrhage Trauma Sepsis Gastrointestinal bleed Ruptured aortic aneurysm	2 large bore cannulas Aggressive IV fluids Blood, O negative supplies Urgent surgical referral
Hypothermia (<35°C, severe<30°C)	Exposure—collapse outside Immersion in water Ingestion of drugs/alcohol	Remove wet clothes and dry ↑ABC assessment time IV fluids at 40°C/warmed air through ventilator/hugger/Bypass if available/dialysis DC shock may not work<30°
Hyper/hypokalaemia and metabolic disorders	Renal disease Calcium channel blocker overdose Documented electrolyte imbalance	Look at current results ABG to see electrolytes Replace quickly electrolytes if low Ca chloride 10 mL 10% IV for hyperkalaemia and OD channel blockers
Tamponade	Penetrating chest trauma Myocardial infarction Cardiac surgery	Needle pericardiocentesis—long cardiac needle (and large syringe) at base of sternum towards left shoulder at 45% angle pulling back whilst inserting Ideally, under echocardiogram if on unit at time of arrest In cardiothoracic centres prepare for urgent chest opening procedure
Tension pneumothorax	History of chest trauma Asthma CVP line insertion Missed pneumothorax plus positive pressure ventilation	Absent breath sounds and chest wall rise and fall Tracheal shift—often late sign Large bore cannula mid-clavicular line second intercostal space→chest drain
Toxic/therapeutic disorders	Drug overdose A good history Industrial exposure	Protection of team National poisons unit/toxbase Rapid administration of known antidotes
Thrombo-embolic	Pulmonary embolism (surgery/pregnancy/DVT/long haul travel)	Immediate thrombolysis IV for known or high suspicion pulmonary embolism: full ALS up to 1 h

BVM, bag valve mask; ETT, endo-tracheal tube; ABC, airway, breathing, circulation; DC, direct current; OD, overdose; DVT, deep vein thrombosis; ALS, advanced life support.

Asystole

♦ The heart has absent electrical or mechanical activity.

♦ Wandering baseline (Figure 13.16). (Exact straight line could indicate the pads/leads have fallen off the patient therefore check this.)

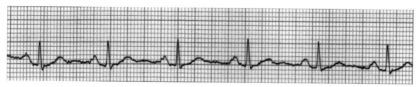

Figure 13.14 Pulseless electrical activity 1 (PEA).

Asystole with p-waves (ventricular standstill)

♦ Sino-atrial node firing and atrial contraction only (p-waves) therefore no cardiac output.

♦ Attempt pacing once sticky pads applied (Figure 13.17).

The use of chest compressions, intubation and ventilation, reversible causes, intravenous access, and adrenaline are common to both shockable and non-shockable arrest rhythms. In PEA or asystole as soon as chest compressions are underway administer 1 mg adrenaline. Ensure that the leads are attached in asystole to confirm the rhythm. In slow PEA/asystole also give atropine 3 mg. If only p-waves are visible, attempt to externally pace (see peri-arrest management).

If the cardiac arrest rhythm changes to a VF/VT shockable rhythm, change sides on the algorithm and prepare to shock the patient.

Fine VF or asystole?

If it is unclear whether the patient is in asystole or fine VF, compressions must recommence. Defibrillation at this point is no longer recommended by the Resuscitation Guidelines 2006. In fact by compressing the chest uninterrupted, the fibrillating heart should become much more responsive to defibrillation.

It is important to remember even if the patient is already being monitored, confirmation of cardiac arrest must be a clinical observation. Always treat the patient and not the monitor.

Drugs used in advanced life support

In past years a great deal of emphasis was given to the administration of drugs in resuscitation. Currently, there is much debate over the use of so many drugs and whether the evidence supports long-term survival from cardiac arrest. Drugs now play their part much further down the ALS algorithm so other crucial components are emphasized first. Provision of drug therapy must not delay defibrillation and continuous chest compressions, but it is important to secure intravenous or other access as soon as possible, if this has not already been done.

Routes

Intravenous access (IV) remains the best route for delivery of drugs during ALS. The peripheral route is easier and safer to insert than central access in an emergency and has far fewer complications.

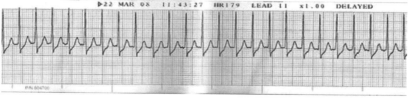

Figure 13.15 Pulseless electrical activity 2 (PEA).

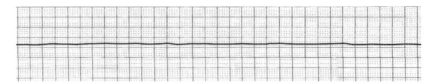

Figure 13.16 Asystole.

The *intraosseous* (*IO*) route has been advocated in paediatric guidelines and is now the second-choice route in adult guidelines. Many ambulance staff are currently undergoing training in insertion of IO needles as well as there being an increased number of medical practitioners. As this is a relatively new addition to the guidelines, many acute care staff will not yet be familiar with its use. Further information can be obtained through hospital resuscitation departments and advance life support courses. After each drug, it is important to give a 10 mL bolus of 0.9% saline or 5% dextrose after amiodarone.

The *endotracheal* (*ET*) route is the last option for some drugs during resuscitation. It is unclear as to how much of the drug is actually absorbed this way. It provides unpredictable plasma concentrations of the drug (Nolan *et al.* 2005).

Below is a list of drugs and their actions recommended by the current European Resuscitation Council (2005) and UK Resuscitation Guidelines (2006).

Adrenaline

Indication during cardiac arrest

+ First drug to be given during cardiac arrest.
+ Given to increase cerebral and coronary perfusion.

Dose

+ 1 mg IV/IO.
  (If needed ET tube dose is 3 mg diluted to 10 mL water.)
+ Half-life 3 min.

Frequency

+ Note: If VF/VT persists after two shocks then give adrenaline. Then give adrenaline every 3–5 min (every other loop).
+ For asystole/PEA give with chest compressions and every 3–5 min thereafter.

Desired effects

+ Stimulates alpha 1 and alpha 2 receptors to produce vasoconstriction.
+ Increases systemic vascular resistance during CPR, producing an increase in coronary and cerebral perfusion.

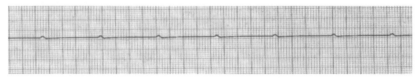

Figure 13.17 Asystole with p-waves (ventricular standstill).

Undesired effects

♦ Post arrest: increase in heart rate and force of contraction, therefore increasing the work of the heart.

♦ Subsequently increasing myocardial oxygen demand and consumption: may increase ischaemia and or infarct size.

♦ Pro-arrhythmogenic due to an increase in myocardial excitability.

Amiodarone

Indication during cardiac arrest

♦ Shock/refractory/resistant VF/pulseless VT.

Dose

♦ 300 mg IV preloaded syringe or diluted in 20 mL 5% dextrose.

Frequency

♦ One 300 mg dose recommended for use.

Desired effects

♦ Increases the entire action potential duration, therefore reducing the rate of repolarization.

♦ Reduces the excitability of all cardiac tissues by increasing the refractory period.

♦ Reduces the automaticity of the sino-atrial and atrio-ventricular nodes.

♦ Facilitation of electrical or DC cardioversion.

Undesired effects

♦ Prolongation of the Q-T interval and may therefore induce polymorphic VT, called torsades des points.

♦ Pro-arrhythmic.

♦ Extravasation may cause necrotic tissue damage, therefore ideally given via a central line. If this is not possible a large bore cannula in a large peripheral vein should be used, such as the ante cubital fossa region.

♦ Post arrest: bradycardia and hypotension.

Magnesium

Indications during cardiac arrest

♦ Hypokalaemia/hypomagnesaemia.

♦ Shock resistant/refractory VF/VT.

♦ Torsades des pointes.

♦ Digoxin toxicity.

Dose

♦ 8 mmols (2 g) as bolus in cardiac arrest over 1–2 min.

Frequency

♦ May be repeated during resuscitation attempt.

Desired effects

- Improves contraction of a stunned myocardium.
- Neurochemical transmission properties.

Undesired effects

- Post arrest: acute overdosage may cause bradycardias due to inhibition of the sino-atrial node.
- Post arrest: magnesium and calcium work against each other at the cell membrane of vascular smooth muscle, therefore an excess of magnesium or if it has been given too rapidly may cause vasodilation therefore hypotension.

Atropine

Indication during cardiac arrest

- Asystole.
- Slow PEA with rate <60 beats per minute.

Dose

- 3 mg IV once only.

Frequency

- Given as one single dose. Half-life 3 h.

Desired effects

- Blocks vagus nerve completely at the sino-atrial node (SA) and the atrio-ventricular node (AV).
- Subsequent increase in automaticity of the heart.
- Facilitating atrio-ventricular node conduction.

Undesired effects

- Post arrest: increase in heart rate.
- Subsequently increasing myocardial oxygen demand and consumption: may increase ischaemia and/or infarct size.

Calcium

Indication during cardiac arrest

- Hyperkalaemia.
- Hypocalcaemia.
- Overdose of calcium channel blockers.

Dose

- 10 mL of 10% calcium chloride IV.

Frequency

- Usually one single dose but may need to be repeated.

Desired effects

+ Protects the heart from the toxic effects of potassium in hyperkalaemia.
+ An increase of serum calcium. Will need serum levels checking post arrest.

Undesired effects

+ Does not lower serum potassium in hyperkalaemia. Dextrose and insulin pre and post arrest most effective.
+ Extravasation may cause soft tissue damage.
+ Post arrest: bradycardia and arrythmias.

Sodium bicarbonate

Indication during cardiac arrest

+ Hyperkalaemia.
+ Tricyclic overdose.
+ Consider in severe metabolic acidosis.

Dose

+ 50 mmol (50 mL of 8.4% sodium bicarbonate) IV bolus.

Frequency

+ Titrated to acid/base values (venous or arterial blood).

Desired effects

+ Acts as the buffer in a severe acidotic state. Only consider use if pH is <7.1 or base excess $\leq$10 mmols/L.
+ Some evidence to show benefit in cardiac arrest due to tricyclic anti-depressants.
+ An increased sodium load pushes potassium back into the cells.

Undesired effects

+ It causes production of carbon dioxide (CO_2), which diffuses into the cells causing a rebound intracellular acidosis.
+ Negative inotropic effect on the myocardium.
+ Produces a shift to the left on the oxygen (O_2) dissociation curve, which inhibits further oxygen delivery to the tissues (see Chapter 2).

Post-resuscitation management

ROSC is the first step in the continuum of resuscitation (Resuscitation Council (UK) 2006b). Some patients who survive cardiac arrest are resuscitated easily and quickly. They rapidly regain consciousness and resume breathing. Treatment then concentrates on preventing a recurrence. These patients may well stay on the high dependency unit for close monitoring and continuing care. However, some patients who have ROSC will remain unconscious and may or may not be able to breathe satisfactorily for themselves. They may also have poor cardiac output and will therefore be hypotensive. Treatment for these patients is aimed at restoring cardiovascular and respiratory function so that cerebral and systemic tissue perfusion is maintained. As soon as ROSC occurs, post-resuscitation care will begin and it is the final link in the chain of survival. Table 13.1

identifies patient assessment and nursing care/treatment after ROSC. This care must be altered and adapted to meet the patient's own individual needs to provide the best possible chance of leaving hospital. Most patients will be moved to an area for ongoing care and support, whether it is the intensive care unit, the cardiac catheter laboratory, or the coronary care unit.

The International Liaison Committee on Resuscitation (ILCOR) has recently published a consensus statement on a new proposed term called post-cardiac arrest syndrome (Nolan *et al.* 2008). It explains the syndrome 'incorporates a unique and complex combination of pathophysiological processes' and identified four key components:

♦ post-cardiac arrest brain injury

♦ post-cardiac arrest myocardial dysfunction

♦ systemic ischaemia/reperfusion response

♦ persistent precipitating pathology (Nolan *et al.* 2008).

ILCOR strongly believes that each component is potentially treatable but further research is needed. For further information and more in-depth reading please refer to the consensus scientific statement (Nolan *et al.* 2008).

Therapeutic hypothermia

This is an area that has already the evidence to show proven benefit. Mild hypothermia is thought to suppress chemical reactions associated with reperfusion injury (Hypothermia After Cardiac Arrest Study Group 2002). The Resuscitation Council (UK) Guidelines (2006) therefore recommend unconscious adult patients with ROSC post-VF arrest should be cooled to 32-34°C starting as soon as possible for at least 12–24 h. As acute care nurses, you will care for patients who have been discharged from intensive care and have received therapeutic hypothermia.

Percutaneous coronary intervention

Patients who show signs of acute myocardial infarction on a post-cardiac arrest 12-lead ECG will require an immediate review by the on-call cardiologist. Patients who have sustained a VT/VF arrest during or after their acute myocardial infarction are extremely at high risk and may require immediate transfer to the cardiac catheter laboratory for percutaneous coronary intervention (PCI) to ensure the best possible outcome for the patient. The term percutaneous coronary intervention (sometimes called PTCA, angioplasty, or stenting) describes a range of procedures that treat narrowing or blockages in coronary arteries, supplying blood to the heart. Thrombolysis therapy may be considered as an alternative in hospitals unable to offer PCI. Chest compression is no longer an absolute contraindication to thrombolysis therapy (see Chapter 3).

Peri-arrest arrhythmias

These rhythms are life threatening to patients if left untreated. Peri-arrest rhythms can either be narrow complex arrhythmias, originating from the atrium, or broad complex arrhythmias, which usually (but not always) originates from the ventricles.

This section will pay close attention to the recognition and treatment of an unstable patient with a bradyarrhythmia and/or tachyarrhythmia (see Chapter 3 for a general overview of rhythms and stable arrhythmia management).

> If the patient is unstable the acute care nurse must focus on initiating early treatment and calling for the appropriate help, instead of becoming too engrossed in interpreting the exact rhythm.

Peri-arrest arrhythmias are life-threatening emergency situations, therefore it is crucial that the patient is assessed first. The acute care nurse must be aware of the presence of any *adverse*

Box 13.11 Adverse signs in peri-arrest

In the peri-arrest situation many treatment principles are common to all the tachycardias (Nolan *et al.* 2005):

♦ call for help

♦ high-flow oxygen

♦ IV access

♦ blood pressure, oxygen saturations, respirations, and pulse

♦ 12-lead ECG

♦ correct any electrolyte imbalances.

signs, which will indicate the need for immediate treatment (Box 13.11) Patients who are not acutely ill can often be seen by a member of the cardiology team for advice on appropriate treatment.

Peri-arrest: bradycardia

This is defined as a heart rate of below 60 beats a minute. For many patients this can be entirely normal and is not dangerous. Athletes especially have very low resting heart rates and can often be around 40 beats a minute. Patients who are prescribed β-blockers also have lower heart rates. Severe or extreme bradycardia of below 40 beats a minute is rarely physiological and usually needs urgent treatment (Resuscitation Council (UK) 2006b).

As the heart rate falls cardiac output is increased by an increase in stroke volume (see Chapter 3), but when this compensation fails cardiac output and blood pressure fall. Coronary filling is also reduced, which will reduce blood supply to the myocardium. The patient may show signs of pallor, be sweaty or clammy, and have altered level of consciousness.

Bradyarrythmias include extreme sinus bradycardia (Figure 13.18) and first, second, and third degree atrioventricular block (Figure 13.19).

The causes of bradyarrythmias include:

♦ myocardial infarction (especially inferior wall)

♦ hypothyroidism

♦ raised intracranial pressure

♦ hypothermia

♦ electrolyte imbalances, that is hyponatraemia

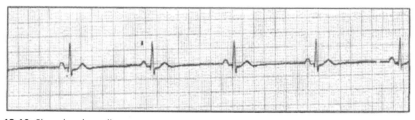

Figure 13.18 Sinus bradycardia.

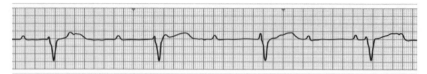

Figure 13.19 3rd Degree AV block.

♦ drug effects, particularly β-blockers and digoxin
♦ severe hypoxia
♦ severe hypovolaemia.

If the patient is at risk of asystole and/or there are any adverse signs proceed to:

♦ calling 2222 medical emergency
♦ atropine 500 μg IV increments according to response (max 3 mg)
♦ adrenaline infusion (2–10 μg/min) if required
♦ pacing

Pacing

There are four types of pacing: permanent pacing, temporary transvenous pacing, emergency external or transcutaneous pacing, and emergency percussion pacing (fist pacing). Inserting a permanent system and even a temporary transvenous wire is *invasive* and takes time, requiring skilled personnel and specialist radiological equipment. In an acute situation therefore, a quick life-saving interim measure that is *non-invasive* is required that can be started within a minute by trained nursing staff within the acute setting.

Trancutaneous pacing Non-invasive pacing is achieved easily and is an immediate treatment for bradyarrhythmia, which is a potential risk to the patient who is not responding to drug therapy (Resuscitation Council (UK) 2006b).

Large adhesive electrodes should be placed in the same place as for defibrillation or alternatively in an anterior posterior (A/P) position. A 10–200 milliamp pulse several milliseconds long can be delivered by turning on the pacing facility on the defibrillator. The aim is to achieve cardiac capture, as long as the myocardium still has some evidence of spontaneous electrical activity, by increasing the amount of milliamps until electrical capture is seen on the monitor. Most modern defibrillators placed in an acute area will have a pacing facility capable of demand pacing, whereby the patients' intrinsic QRS complexes are sensed and pacing stimuli will be delivered only if needed. To make it much easier and quicker, modern hands-free defibrillation electrodes (sticky pads) are multifunctional and are capable of monitoring the ECG, defibrillation/cardioversion, and pacing as required.

Due to the stimulation to the nerve endings and skeletal muscle it can be very uncomfortable and can cause distress and pain to conscious patients. The patient's upper body can also jerk along with each stimulus, therefore it is very important to explain what will happen in order to pre-warn the patient. Strong analgesia, for example morphine, should be prescribed by the doctor to ensure comfort.

An appropriate demand rate should be set, which is usually around 60–80 a minute. In some situations a much lower rate should be set, especially if the patient has third degree AV block with wide QRS, extreme bradycardia or at risk of ventricular standstill (p-wave asystole), for example patients in Mobitz type 2 second degree AV block (refer to Chapter 3).

External transcutaneous pacing must only be used in an acute medical emergency to gain time before more definitive treatment can be organized.

Once electrical capture has been achieved it is vital to immediately check a central pulse to ensure that mechanical capture has also occurred. This will confirm that the stimulus has created a myocardial contraction. As soon as this is confirmed expert help will arrange for urgent insertion of a temporary transvenous pacing wire. The acute care nurse must be vigilant, organized, and prepare for safe transfer to the cardiac catheter laboratory (see Chapter 14 on transfer of the acutely ill patient).

Remember it is quite safe to touch the patient during external pacing as less than 1 J is delivered through extremely well insulated electrodes/pads.

Percussion pacing This is also an emergency type of pacing. It is not as reliable as electrical pacing. It can be used if there is a delay in activating or preparing the defibrillator ready for external transcutaneous pacing.

Deliver firm repeated blows over the precordium to the side of the lower left sternal edge at about 10 cm above the chest. They should be gentle enough so that the conscious patient tolerates them. If capture does not occur, attempt to move the blows around to change the point of contact and also make them more gentle (Resuscitation Council (UK) 2006b).

Peri-arrest: tachycardia

This is defined as a heart rate of above 100 beats a minute. Sinus tachycardia, however, is not an arrhythmia. Whether the patient is stable or unstable affects the treatment options during peri-arrest arrhythmias. If the patient is *stable* they should be given drug therapy to chemically cardiovert the arrhythmia (see Chapter 3). If the patient is *unstable* and compromised (see Box 13.12; Resuscitation Council (UK) 2005) then electricity is used to cardiovert the arrhythmia (urgent synchronized cardioversion).

Tachyarrhythmias include narrow complex tachycardias, atrial flutter (Figure 13.20), atrial fibrillation (Figure 13.21), and supraventricular tachycardia (Figure 13.22). These tachycardias are usually less life threatening than broad complex tachycardias.

Causes of narrow complex tachycardia include:

- electrolyte abnormalities
- alcohol/caffeine
- myocardial infarction
- antiarrhythmic drugs

Box 13.12 Adverse signs in peri-arrest

- Systolic blood pressure < 90mmHg.
- Heart failure.
- Chest pain.
- Heart rate <40 or ≥150.
- Drowsiness/confusion.

Resuscitation Council (UK) (2005)

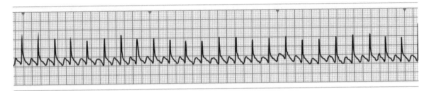

Figure 13.20 Atrial flutter.

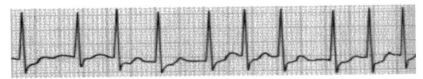

Figure 13.21 Atrial fibrillation.

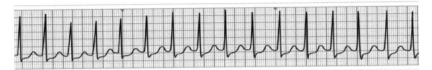

Figure 13.22 Supraventricular tachycardia.

- Wolff Parkinson White syndrome
- thyrotoxicosis
- coronary heart disease
- heart failure.

  VT is a broad complex tachycardia, the causes of which include (Figure 13.23):

- myocardial infarction
- cardiomyopathy
- long QT syndrome
- Brugada syndrome
- antiarrythmic drugs
- heart failure
- Ron T phenomenon
- electrolyte imbalances
- tricyclic antidepressant overdose.

  If the patient with broad complex tachycardia has any adverse signs proceed to:

- calling 2222 medical emergency
- support ABCs
- giving O_2, cannulating, and correcting electrolytes
- if possible perform 12 lead ECG
- synchronized DC shock three attempts (range of 80–360 J depending on trust policy and type of defibrillator used)

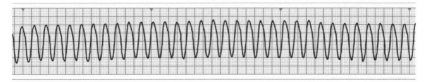

Figure 13.23 Broad complex tachycardia (ventricular tachycardia).

♦ amiodarone 300 mg IV over 10–20 min
♦ repeat DC synchronized shock.

Synchronized cardioversion for unstable tachyarrhythmias

The patient needs to be prepared for urgent synchronized cardioversion whilst the nurse waits for medical support. Full explanation and reassurance to the patient is essential. The anaesthetist will need to heavily sedate or even anaesthetize before cardioversion because it is an extremely painful procedure. In readiness for synchronized shock, the large adhesive electrodes (defib pads) will be placed on the patient's chest (see Figure 13.13). Energy levels may differ according to trust policy but usually start at less than for VF/VT cardiac arrest. Once the energy is selected on the defibrillator the synchronized button needs to be turned on. The shock delivered needs to be synchronized onto the patient's own R-wave, to avoid the DC shock affecting the unstable part of the cardiac cycle. If this occurred the patient's rhythm could deteriorate into pulseless VT or VF. All safety aspects apply as for defibrillation during cardiac arrest. The person responsible for defibrillating must ensure that all the safety checks are performed and must only deliver the shock when they are sure the rhythm is being synchronized and it is safe to do so. Once the synchronized shock is delivered the patient's central pulse must be checked in case the patient's condition has deteriorated. A cardiac monitor along with non-invasive saturation, respirations, and blood pressure monitoring must be recorded throughout and also post procedure. A repeat 12-lead ECG should be recorded to rule out myocardial infarction or other cardiac causes for the arrhythmia after the procedure. Electrolytes will also need to be checked, as shocks can cause loss of available potassium and/or magnesium within the circulation to the myocardium. The patient may need to be transferred to the coronary care unit for escalation of care.

Anaphylaxis

Anaphylaxis is an acute, severe, and life-threatening allergic reaction. The term comes from the Greek words *ana* meaning 'against' and *phylaxis* meaning 'protection'. It is undoubtedly an acute emergency and unfortunately its occurrence appears to be on the increase. Twenty deaths in the UK every year are due to anaphylaxis, but this number is probably an underestimation as many will probably be unrecognized (Resuscitation Council (UK) 2008). The American College of Allergy, Asthma and Immunology Epidemiology of Anaphylaxis Working Group (2006) established the occurrence to be 30–950 cases per 100,000 persons per year.

Common triggers

♦ Insect stings/bites: wasps, bees, and others.
♦ Foods: nuts, fish and seafood, strawberries, milk, chickpeas, bananas.
♦ Drugs: antibiotics, non-steroidal anti-inflammatory drugs, muscle relaxants, contrast medium, colloids, angiotensin-converting enzyme inhibitors.

+ Blood transfusions.

+ Others: hair dye, latex.

Anaphylaxis is triggered by something (the antigen) that sensitizes the immunoglobulin anti-bodies (IgE mediated). In many cases no cause can be identified and these are generally idiopathic and non-IgE mediated.

An allergic response triggers a quick release of many immunological mediators from mast cells. Mast cells can be found in connective tissue and are required as part of the body's normal inflammatory process within the immune system. Large quantities of released histamines, prostaglandins, and leukotrienes cause blood vessels to dilate and capillaries to leak out plasma into tissues.

Life-threatening signs and symptoms of anaphylaxis

+ Gross oedema, especially around the face (angioedema) and upper airway, causing airway obstruction.

+ Severe bronchoconstriction/bronchospasm and lung oedema (non-cardiac), causing extreme breathing difficulties, hypoxaemia, and respiratory failure.

+ Profound vasodilatation, causing severe hypotension, circulatory collapse, unconsciousness, and cardiac arrest.

+ Looks and feels unwell.

Other symptoms may include:

+ wheezing

+ urticaria (hives/rash)

+ itching

+ anxiety, 'impending doom'

+ abdominal cramps and diarrhoea

+ flushed appearance or pallour

+ runny eyes.

These other symptoms alone do *not* indicate an anaphylactic reaction but may occur alongside the life-threatening symptoms.

The Resuscitation Council (UK) updated the guidelines on anaphylaxis in 2008. Criteria for anaphylaxis (Resuscitation Council (UK) 2008) include:

+ the sudden onset and rapid progression of symptoms.

+ life-threatening airway and/or breathing and/or circulation problems.

+ skin and/or mucosal changes such as flushing, urticaria, and angioedema.

Symptoms can occur immediately, after a few minutes (usually within 5–35 min). or can be delayed up to hours after exposure. Some cases have been reported anything up to 72 h after the triggering event. Biphasive episodes may also occur whereby symptoms improve, only to worsen again, each time in a more severe fashion until they are severe enough to threaten life. Death caused by intravenous medications occurs most commonly within 5 min, but rarely over 6 h from contact with the trigger (Resuscitation Council (UK) 2008). There is also a strong link of severity of reaction and risk of death associated with patients with asthma (Pumphrey & Gowland 2007).

Nurses working within acute care must have an excellent understanding of this acute emergency situation to recognize the signs early and instigate appropriate prompt treatment.

Without appropriate care their patient may die within minutes. However, with the knowledge and prompt action according to the Resuscitation Council (UK) (2008) guidelines (Figure 13.24), patients will often make a quick and complete recovery.

Using the ABCDE approach (Resuscitation Council (UK) 2006a,b) in an acute emergency is important as anaphylaxis can be very difficult to diagnose. In any critical illness the clinical signs will always be similar, therefore adopting a structured approach will ensure life-threatening symptoms will be recognized, and treated quickly and appropriately.

As nurses, we have the responsibility to ensure that the patient has a full investigation by their medical team after the reaction has occurred, so that they are followed up as soon as possible by an allergy specialist. To help confirm diagnosis blood samples should be obtained. Mast cells degranulate in anaphylaxis, which increases levels of blood tryptase levels. Peak time is 1–2 h after start of symptoms and is back to normal at 6–8 h (Schwartz 2006), therefore it is important to take samples at the correct times. A 24-h sample or at follow up should be analysed to show baseline levels of tryptase.

Treatment

Please refer to Figure 13.24 (with kind permission from the Resuscitation Council (UK)).

It is vitally important to firstly remove the suspected trigger. As IV injections usually cause a rapid reaction, if suspicions are raised then the IV drug must be stopped immediately. With suspected food-induced anaphylaxis, attempts to make the patient vomit are not recommended by the Resuscitation Council (UK) (2008). During your ABCDE assessment it is important to remember that you are treating life-threatening problems as you find each one. Calling for support from your nurse colleagues early is essential and if the three criteria are met then a medical emergency call (or cardiac arrest call if your hospital does not have a separate MET) must be deployed.

Intramuscular (IM) adrenaline 0.5 mg (1/2 mL 1:1,000 adrenaline) should be given immediately (refer to algorithm for child doses) and can be repeated after 5 min if there is no improvement (1:10,000 IV adrenaline can be given by an intensivist/anaesthetist because they will be experienced in using IV adrenaline). The IM route is safer, easier to administer, and does not require IV access. There are no randomized-controlled trials, but there is good anecdotal evidence to support the use of adrenaline as a vasoconstrictor (on alpha agonist receptors), thereby restoring cardiac output, and as a bronchodilator (from β-2 adrenergic receptors) to dilate the bronchial airways. Adrenaline also helps by suppressing mediator release.

Ensure that the patient has high-flow oxygen via a non-rebreathe mask with reservoir. Ensure that the resuscitation trolley is nearby, with airway protecting and intubation equipment ready for the anaesthetist to use if required. Provide all monitoring available, including pulse oximetry, ECG, and blood pressure. If possible and if you are trained in cannulation skills, attempt to secure a cannula in a large vein and prepare for IV crystalloid fluid challenge.

Other medications

Antihistamines and steroids are only for second-line treatment and can be given after the acute emergency and initial resuscitation. There is no evidence to support their usage in the initial stages and they should not be given before adrenaline, oxygen, or fluids.

Cardiac arrest following anaphylaxis

If the patient has sustained a cardiac arrest, start immediate CPR and instigate in-hospital resuscitation, as already discussed earlier in this chapter. ALS remains unchanged and adrenaline doses

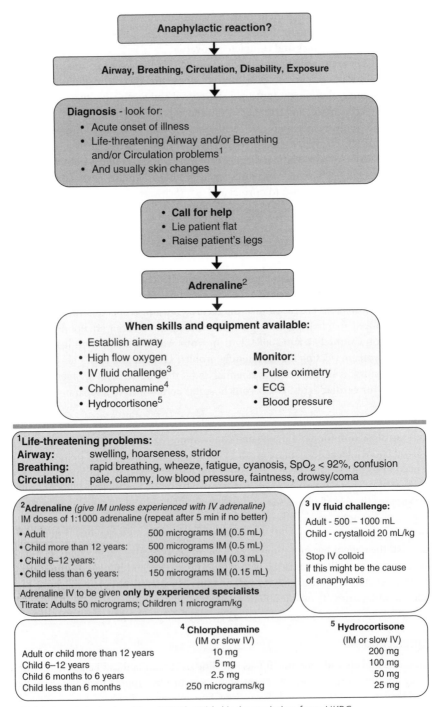

Figure 13.24 Anaphylaxis algorithm (2008). With kind permission from UKRC.

Clinical link 13.2 (see Appendix for answers)

A 23-year-old patient has been admitted with cellulitis of the left ankle after a horsefly bite he sustained playing golf last week. It has become infected. He has been admitted directly to your unit via the GP. At 14.20 the call bell goes off in the bathroom. You open the door to find the patient sitting on a chair holding his head up. He appears to be panicking, and his face and lips look swollen.

Part A

♦ What course of action and nursing care would you take?

♦ What interventions from the doctors would you anticipate?

Part B

On initial contact it may be difficult to differentiate between 'panic attack' and 'anaphylaxis'.

♦ Can you identify these differences?

and routes are stated in the ALS guidelines (2006) (see Figure 13.8). The IM route is not recommended once the patient has sustained a cardiac arrest from anaphylaxis.

Resuscitation ethics

The majority of resuscitation attempts are unsuccessful, but many lives are saved and patients go on to enjoy many more years with their friends and families. Resuscitation science continues to strive towards improving the numbers of those saved. It is clear that many resuscitation attempts that have taken place have only caused more suffering and prolonged the natural dying process (Resuscitation Council (UK) 2006b). Chest compressions and other resuscitation procedures are invasive, brutal, and, if futile, do not allow dying with dignity and peace. The consequence of inappropriate CPR is also distressing for the families and friends of the patient and for the staff too. The healthcare team, particularly the nurses, often feel frustrated and demoralized in these situations.

The evidence suggests that the views of the public are completely opposite to reality and are optimistic in the outcomes of survival from cardiac arrest (Diem *et al.* 1996). The media today appear to portray many more successful resuscitation attempts, which conveys a very unrealistic picture.

Resuscitation is a sensitive and emotive subject that needs time for discussion. Making resuscitation decisions can be distressing for patients and families. They are necessary to make it clear that in some situations, a resuscitation attempt in the event of cardiac arrest, is not appropriate. All too often it is discussed too late or not at all. Evidence suggests when cardiac arrest or death is likely, staff rarely make decisions about the patient's resuscitation status (Kause *et al.* 2004).

The Mental Capacity Act (Department of Health 2005) and the End of Life Care Strategy (Department of Health 2008b) both emphasize the importance of patient choice in medical decision making. However, this becomes very difficult when patients want to make decisions that may not be in their best interests. A joint statement from the British Medical Association, Royal College of Nursing, and the Resuscitation Council (UK) (http://www.resus.org.uk) on decisions relating to CPR state that if a person has a cardiac or respiratory arrest and is unlikely to survive, then CPR should not be attempted. However, they also state that if a patient is adamant, even when it is suggested it is likely to be futile then the patient's choice should be followed. However, at the time of the arrest, the decision should be reviewed. Final decisions will always lie with the senior doctor in charge of the patient's care and according to local trust policies on resuscitation decisions. All NHS trusts should have a resuscitation policy that respects the patient's rights, that staff understand, and is accessible to those who need to use it. Comprehensive audit and monitoring arrangements need to be in place. Do not attempt resuscitation (DNAR) is part of this policy and all staff should be aware of their local trust's policy (Department of Health 2000). The above situation should be avoided with the use of appropriate discussions and information about CPR. Patients should not, in the first instance, be offered treatment that is inappropriate or given choices that have little chance of success. DNAR must therefore be considered when the patient does not wish to have CPR and if the patient will not survive cardiac arrests even if CPR is attempted.

Acute care nurses can be directly involved in improving decision making within CPR issues. They can provide important information and encourage communication and discussions between doctors, patients, and their relatives. This will also improve communication within the team and aim to ensure decisions are made in a timely manner. Nurses can also encourage patients to speak out, encouraging them to make their own decisions. Patients have a right to be involved in their own destinies (Smith 2003). An important consideration for nurses and all multiprofessional staff are the new laws on mental capacity. Since 2005 patients' next of kin may hold power of attorney for health (see Chapter 9). Staff may see more of patients' advanced decisions through advanced directives (living wills). Some patients may have particular decisions on resuscitation and CPR. These documents should be carefully put together and signed by the appropriate people before they are legally binding. They also need to be very specific and relevant to the patient's situation. As nurses we must seek expert help when we are faced with any documents that arise from patients or their loved ones. All trusts have legal departments in place to assist with local policies. In the event of cardiac arrest when the wishes of the patient are unknown and a valid decision regarding their resuscitation has not been made, then resuscitation attempts are instigated (see Chapter 16).

Family presence

This is a very sensitive topic that has had much debate, particularly over the past 15 years, and arguably remains controversial in practice today. Many healthcare professionals hold the view that relatives should be excluded from observing resuscitation attempts because it is too stressful to observe aggressive and invasive procedures that are often futile. If they are excluded, however, this could be more stressful for the family. Family presence is now much more widely accepted and appears to be a growing trend. This may be due to more publications from professional bodies that are supporting the concept of family presence during CPR (Royal College of Nursing 2002; European Resuscitation Council Guidelines for Resuscitation 2005; Resuscitation Council (UK) 2007). Furthermore, there has been much more of a public interest in family presence during CPR expressed in the media (Blundell et al. 2004).

The nursing staff's aims should be to assist relatives to make their own decisions, support those who need to be present to help with their grieving process, whilst ensuring proper preparation and training are given to overcome resistance or hesitancy from the staff involved (Resuscitation Council (UK) 2007). There are several benefits to family presence during CPR. It is hugely important for families to see that everything was done that could be done and also that they were present during their loved one's final moments. This can be extremely comforting and also supportive to the patient in their time of need (Baskett et al. 2005).

In order to assist this process it is really important that the family is given the opportunity to choose whether or not they want to attend. Many families will automatically leave and are not aware that there is a choice. To support family members therefore, a staff member not included in the clinical resuscitation attempt should be assigned to initiate interventions to assist the family and to provide emotional and psychosocial support. It is important that this person remains with the family members throughout the process (Twibell *et al.* 2008). The Royal College of Nursing (2002) and the European Resuscitation Council (2005) both recommend the nurse is the best professional to chaperone the family. It is extremely important that the nurse is senior enough to have experience of cardiac arrests and also feels confident enough to be able to explain what procedures are occurring and why they are occurring. Preparing the family therefore is the key to a successful supportive process. It is important to stress what they are likely to see and to emphasize they are free to leave at any time. Particular instructions must be given to the family that they do not interfere with any resuscitation procedures. Nurses need to clearly explain the dangers associated with this (Baskett *et al.* 2005).

Overall the evidence sways towards family presence but in a facilitated fashion. Further research, however, would be welcomed on how family presence impacts on the patients, family members, and healthcare professionals involved.

Conclusion

Reversibility of cardiac arrest has only in recent times been made a practical reality. If patients in peri and/or cardiac arrest are to receive quality care and treatment to have a chance to survive, it is essential that management and treatment are based on sound evidence supported by clear concise guidelines. These guidelines need to be available to all involved in patient care and this, along with further staff education, training and audit of practice, will help to ensure patients receive the optimum care they deserve.

Early recognition and treatment of critically ill patients will prevent some cardiac arrests (Resuscitation Council (UK) 2006a,b). The most important factor in the survival from a cardiac arrest is the presence of a trained rescuer who is equipped to intervene (Paradis *et al.* 2007). As identified, the most effective tools of the trained rescuer are CPR and defibrillation.

The nurse working in the acute care arena will undoubtedly gain knowledge, experience, and an increased level of skill and confidence by reflecting on each acute emergency situation they face. The opportunity to regularly undertake practical updates and practice scenarios in the classroom is also essential for the retention of these skills. This will reduce stress, improve performance, and enhance their understanding. To this end acute care nurses will become a crucial component of any resuscitation team.

Patients with acute emergencies present the nurse with a wide range of problems and challenges that test knowledge, abilities, and skills. The systems of patient assessment can be easily applied to any clinical area. Using this prior knowledge, experience, and reflection in assessment and treatment will undoubtedly assist the acute care nurse with the next acutely sick patient presented. Above all it is vital to have the understanding that an emergency situation actually exists. Hopefully this chapter has given you this understanding and an increased confidence to ensure that happens.

References

American College of Allergy, Asthma and Immunology (2006) Epidemiology of anaphylaxis. *Ann Allergy Asthma Immunol.* **97**(5), 596–602.

Baskett, P.J., Steen, P.A., Bossaert, L. for European Resuscitation Council (2005) European resuscitation guidelines for resuscitation 2005 Section 8. The ethics of resuscitation and end-of-life decisions. *Resuscitation.* **67**(suppl 1), S171–180.

Blundell, A., Rich, S., Watson, A., and Dale, L. (2004) Attitudes of doctors and nurses to relatives witnessing resuscitation. *J. Roy. Coll. Phys.* **34**(2), 134–6.

Cashman, J.N. (2002) In-hospital cardiac arrest: What happens to the false arrests? *Resuscitation.* **53**, 271–6.

Chen, J., Hillman, K., Bellomom, R. *et al.* (2009) The impact of introducing medical emergency team system on the documentations of vital signs. *Resuscitation.* **80**(1), 35–43.

Cox, H., James, J., and Hunt, J. (2006) The experiences of trained nurses caring for critically ill patients within a general ward setting. *Int. Crit. Care Nurs.* **18**, 280–91.

Cummins, R.O., Ornato, J.P., Thies, W.K., and Pepe, P.E. (1991) Improving the survival from sudden cardiac arrest: The 'chain of survival' concept. *Circulation.* **83**, 1832–47.

Cutler, L. (2002) From ward based critical care to educational curriculum: a focused ethnographic case study. *Int. Crit. Care Nurs.* **18**, 280–91.

Department of Health (2000) *Health Service Circular: Resuscitation Policy.* Department of Health, London.

Department of Health (2002) *Implementing the NHS Plan—Ten Key Roles for Nurses.* The Stationary Office, London.

Department of Health (2005) *Mental Capacity Act.* The Stationary Office, London.

Department of Health (2008a) *Competencies for Recognising and Responding to Acutely Ill Patients in Hospital.* The Stationary Office, London.

Department of Health (2008b) *End of Life Care Strategy.* The Stationery Office, London.

Diem, S.J., Lantos, J.D., and Tulsky, J.A. (1996) Cardiopulmonary resuscitation on television: Miracles and misinformation. *N. Engl. J. Med.* **334**, 1578–2.

European Resuscitation Council (2005) European Resuscitation Council Guidelines For Resuscitation. *Resuscitation.* **67**, S171–81.

Hamilton, R. (2005) Nurses' knowledge and skill retention following cardiopulmonary resuscitation training: A review of the literature. *J. Adv. Nurs.* **51**, 288–97.

Handley, A. *et al.* (2005) European Council Guidelines for Resuscitation section 2. Adult basic life support and use of automated external defibrillators. *Resuscitation.* **67**(S1), S7–S23.

http://www.resus.org.uk Decisions relating to cardiopulmonary resuscitation: a joint statement from the BMA, Resuscitation Council (UK) and the Royal College of Nursing (2007).

Hypothermia After Cardiac Arrest Study Group (2002) Mild therapeutic hypothermia to improve the neurological outcome after cardiac arrest. *N. Engl. J. Med.* **346**, 549–56.

Kause, J., Smith, G., Prytherch, D. *et al.* (2004) A comparison of antecedents to cardiac arrests, death, and emergency intensive care admissions in Australia, New Zealand and the UK—ACADEMIA study. *Resuscitation.* **62**, 275–82.

Kloeck, W., Cummins, R.O., Chamberlain, D. *et al.* (1997) Early defibrillation. An advisory statement from the Advanced Life Support Working Group of the International Liason Committee On Resuscitation (ILCOR). *Circulation.* **95**, 2183–4.

McQuillan, P., Pilington, S., Allan, A. *et al.* (1998) Confidential inquiry into quality of care before admission to intensive care. *BMJ.* **316**, 1853–8.

Nadkarni, V.M., Larkin, G.L., and Peberdy, M.A. (2006) First documented rhythm and clinical outcome from in-hospital cardiac arrest among children and adults. *JAMA.* **295**, 50–7.

National Confidential Enquiry into Patient Outcome and Death (2005) An acute problem? *A report of the National Confidential Enquiry into patient Outcome and Death.* National Confidential Enquiry into Patient Outcome and Death, London.

National Patient Safety Agency (2007) Safer care for the acutely ill patient: Learning from serious incidents. The fifth report from the Patient Safety Observatory, London.

NICE (2007) *Acutely Ill Patients in Hospital: Recognition of and Response to Acute Illness in Adults in Hospital.* Clinical Guidence 50, National Institute for Health and Clinical Excellence, London.

Nolan, J.P., Deakin, C., Soar, J. *et al.* (2005) European Resuscitation Guidelines for Resuscitation 2005: Section 4 Adult Advanced Life Support. *Resuscitation.* **675**(S), S39–86.

Nolan, J.P., Soar, J., and Lockey, A. (2006) *Advanced Life Support*. 5th edn. Resuscitation Council (UK), London.

Nolan, J.P., Neumar, R.W., and Adrie, C. *et al.* (2008) ILCOR Consensus Statement: Post cardiac arrest syndrome: Epidemiology, pathophysiology, treatment and prognostication. *Resuscitation.* **79**, 350–79.

Nolan, J.P., Laver, S.R., and Welch, C.A. *et al.* (2007) Outcome following admission to UK intensive care units after cardiac arrest: A secondary analysis of the ICNARC case mix programme database. *Anaesthesia.* **62**, 1207–16.

Paradis, N.A., Martin, G.B., Goetting, M.G. *et al.* (1989) Simultaneous aortic, jugular bulb and right atrial pressures during cardiopulmonary resuscitation in humans. Insights into mechanisms. *Circulation.* **80**, 361–8.

Paradis, N., Halperin, H., Kern, K. *et al.* (2007) *Cardiac Arrest: The Science and Practice of Resuscitation Medicine.* 2nd edn. Cambridge University Press, Cambridge.

Pumphrey, R.S. and Gowland, M.H. (2007) Further fatal allergic reactions to food in the United Kingdom 1999–2006. *J. Allergy Clin. Immunol.* **119**(4), 1018–9.

Rea, T.D. *et al.* (2005) Automated external defibrillators: To what extent does the algorithm delay CPR? *Ann. Emerg. Med.* **46**, 132–41.

Resuscitation Council (UK) (2005) *Guidelines 2005*. Resuscitation Council (UK), London.

Resuscitation Council (UK) (2006a) *Immediate Life Support*. 2nd edn. Resuscitation Council (UK), London.

Resuscitation Council (UK) (2006b) *Advanced Life Support*. 5th edn. Resuscitation Council (UK), London.

Resuscitation Council (UK) (2007) *Decisions relating to Cardiopulmonary Resuscitation*. Resuscitation Council (UK), London.

Resuscitation Council (UK) (2008) *Emergency Treatment of Anaphylactic Reactions: Guidelines for Healthcare Providers*. Resuscitation Council (UK), London.

Royal College of Nursing (2002) *Witnessing Resuscitation: Guidance for Nursing Staff*. Royal College of Nursing, London.

Schwartz, L.B. (2006) Diagnostic value of tryptase in anaphylaxis and mastocytes *Immunol. Allergy Clin. N. Am.* **26**(3), 451–63.

Smith, G.B. (2000) Assessment and stabilisation of the critically ill outside the ICU. *Anaesth. Int. Care Med.* **1**(3), 88–90.

Smith, G.B. (2003) *ALERT: Acute Life-*Threatening *Events Recognition and Treatment*. 2nd edn. University of Portsmouth, Portsmouth.

Twibell, R.S., Siela, D., Riwitis, C. *et al.* (2008) Family presence during cardiopulmonary resuscitation. *Am. J. Crit. Care.* **17**(2), 101–11.

Chapter 14

Transfer of acutely ill patients

Denise Hinge

Chapter contents

In the acute hospital setting patient transfers occur frequently for a variety of reasons. In order to understand how to assess and manage the patient requiring transfer it is essential to have a sound understanding of risk factors involved in transfers and their effect on the individual patient (depending on their acuity and dependency). This chapter will examine:

+ intra- and inter-hospital transfer
+ features of a good hospital transfer
+ physiological changes during transfer
+ preparation for safe transfer
+ clinical assessment before transfer
+ health records
+ clinical skills required during transfer
+ transfer equipment
+ handover
+ medical and legal issues related to transfer.

Learning outcomes

This chapter will enable you to:

+ understand the rationale and challenges in patient transfer
+ understand the decision-making process and nursing responsibilities during transfer
+ analyse the risk of transferring acutely ill patients
+ recognize the need for good communication processes
+ analyse the skills required for escorting personnel
+ evaluate the equipment that may be required to support the patient transfer.

Introduction

+ The transfer of acutely ill patients occurs for many reasons but they can broadly be divided into two main areas: intra-hospital transfers and inter-hospital transfers.

On a daily basis there are many reasons for moving patients around the acute hospital site on intra-hospital transfers, including admission of patients from A&E to the ward, between wards to an area of higher care (e.g. critical care) or for specialist imaging or intervention (X-ray, CT scanner, operating theatre).

Inter-hospital transfers can include transfer for clinical reasons to access more specialist care or between hospital sites within a trust, and for non-clinical reasons due to lack of resources in the referring hospital or repatriation (Lawler 2000a,b; Tillant *et al.* 2000).

Logistically inter-hospital transfers require more organization as they also require the use of the ambulance service (most occur by road) and the transfer of patient information between organizations. This can also be more challenging for the family of the patient if it does not occur in their immediate locality.

Transfers may be elective, facilitating advanced planning and preparation, or may be urgent or an emergency with less time for preparation (which may be associated with increased risk to the patient). Regardless of the reason to transfer it is imperative that a sound assessment is made before moving any patient to reduce patient risk. Making assumptions about a patient's condition can lead to poor clinical decision making. Although this chapter will focus on the needs of the acutely ill patient, the principles of assessment should be applied to all patients. The aim is not to create delay in patient transfers by creating a risk-averse culture but to ensure that patient safety is carefully considered for both the individual patient and the patients in remaining clinical area. It may be challenging to balance the clinical priorities and needs of the patient group but, as with the deteriorating patient, staff should seek advice if unsure how to manage the situation.

There are times when patient transfer is time critical, for example a head-injured patient requiring surgical intervention or the cardiac patient immediately following a myocardial infarction who requires immediate transfer for primary coronary intervention. In these situations rapid decision making and assessment are required (Dunn *et al.* 2006). It is always the aim that before and during the transfer process the patient is adequately oxygenated and perfused (Watson 2007).

The National Health Service Litigation Authority (NHSLA) standards (National Health Service Litigation Authority, updated 2008) require organizations to have robust policies in place, including documentation to outline the process for managing risks associated with patient transfer, including 'out of hours' transfer. Depending on the level of NHSLA standard the organization has achieved (see Table 14.1) the NHSLA assessors will require evidence that the organization is achieving their policy. Consider your own awareness of your organization's transfer policy and your identified responsibilities within this.

There are several national guidelines published on the transfer of critically ill patients. In 2002, the Intensive Care Society published the minimum standards for hospitals that are applicable to the transfer of critically ill level 2 and level 3 patients (see definitions in Chapter 1). These state that the 'standard of care should be at least as good as that at the referring hospital or base unit' and that it must include written documentation of patient status, monitored values, and

Table 14.1 NHSLA risk management standards— transfer of patients

Level 1—policy	Level 2—practice	Level 3—performance
The organization has approved documentation which describes the process for managing risks associated with the transfer of patients	The organization can demonstrate implementation of the approved documentation which describes the process for managing the risks associated with the transfer of patients	The organization can demonstrate that there are processes in place to monitor compliance with the approved documentation which describes the process for managing the risks associated with the transfer of patients

treatment given during transfer. The Association of Anaesthetists (2009) have more recently published their revised guidance on the inter-hospital transfer of patients. The Department of Health publication on the competencies for recognizing and responding to acutely ill patients in hospital outlines the chain of response to patient deterioration, acknowledging that communication and handover of the patient is an essential component of the process (2009). It has a specific section on patient transport and mobility. It is clear that there will be an expectation that staff will need to demonstrate their competence in this aspect of patient care.

The features of a 'good' transfer

+ The patient is involved in the decision making (if possible).
+ Risk is assessed based on the acuity and dependency of the patient.
+ The patient has the appropriately trained escort staff (as identified through above assessment).
+ The patient transfer should be planned, organized, and timely as a delay in the transfer of the patient may result in a delay in gaining timely treatment or a diagnosis.
+ No adverse events occur.
+ The receiving department/hospital is prepared and expecting admission.
+ All relevant patient information is communicated to the receiving team. If more than one person is involved in escorting the patient (if haemodynamically unstable) they should work together as a team and have a clear understanding of each other's role in monitoring the patient.

Other industries and professions have also informed the NHS on the value of process mapping and multiprofessional team work. Cardiothoracic surgeons at Great Ormond Street observed how in motor racing, a Formula One pit stop team worked together to achieve common goal; a complex wheel change and refuel in approximately 7 s. This inspired their study of the patient (paediatric) handover process between cardiac surgery and intensive care (Catchpole *et al.* 2007). The study's aim was to improve the process, quality, and safety. Changes were made to the organization of the paediatric transfer from the operating theatre to the intensive care that improved the process and reduced errors. Both Formula One and aviation industries have a safety culture that focuses on sound risk assessment and learning from serious incidents or 'near misses'. They consider the potential for what could go wrong, what the consequence would be if it did go wrong and what the likelihood is of this happening.

Similarly the Foresight Training programme by the National Patient Safety Agency (National Patient Safety Agency 2008) has been developed to:

> Improve the awareness in nursing and midwifery of the factors that combine to increase the likelihood of patient safety incidents, increase local learning through sharing experiences, improve the understanding of risk prone situations and improve the understanding of situations that could be considered a near miss.

This initiative is based on the work of Reason (2004), which uses foresight for staff to consider:

+ the current safety level the practitioner is working in (**self**)
+ the **context** in which they are working, for example other ward activities/staffing
+ the **task** they are required to do.

He suggests it is the balance between these three aspects of self, context, and task that increases or decreases the risk of a clinical incident or 'near miss' occurring.

A clinical example

Consider this scenario. You have returned to work and are in charge on shift following 2 days off (having just finished nights). You have found it difficult to adjust to a normal sleeping pattern and feel tired (**self**). The ward is busy and staff are dealing with a medical emergency (**context**). You are asked to prepare an intravenous antibiotic for the patient. However, you have only given this drug once previously (**task**) and are interrupted several times during its preparation to answer questions regarding other patients (**context**).

Could this happen? What is the potential for a clinical incident?

Combining all these factors Reason (2004) would consider this to be a high-risk situation but by increasing self-awareness and others awareness the risk can be minimized, for example by asking a second nurse to check the process or take over the intravenous preparation of the drug therapy.

Emergency transfers of patients where rapid decision making is required without clear leadership and clarity over roles of professionals for patient monitoring can create a high-risk environment (**context**). Again, by increased awareness healthcare professionals involved in transfer can minimize the risk to the patient. For example, it should be clear who is monitoring the airway, adequacy of ventilation, and haemodyamic response, and who is documenting the patient's observations.

Changes on physiology during transfer (movement)

The response of the body to a change in movement is governed by the effect of gravitational force (G force). We are under the effect of G force all the time. The effect of acceleration/deceleration is measured in G force. For example, in a large aeroplane the force experienced is approximately 0.25 when we take off and 0.5 G on landing. Surprisingly, in an ambulance, which is excellent at deceleration but not quite so good at acceleration, the G force exerted on the patient on deceleration, i.e. sudden braking, can be as much as 7–8 G (Lawler 2000b). Lawler also cites Waddell *et al.* (1975), who demonstrated that patients reacted to this force unpredictably and that this effect was often prolonged (even after transfer to the receiving department or hospital). The acutely ill patient can therefore become more haemodymamically unstable during the transfer process due the effect of movement on already compensating body dynamics. For the patient in respiratory failure who is spontaneously breathing, sitting in an upright position, and on high-flow oxygen, the physical exertion and any ensuing changes of position (e.g. bed to bed) may alter ventilation/perfusion, which could be enough to cause a physiological deterioration (Lawler 2000a,b).

If the patient requires an inter-hospital transfer the effect of acceleration and deceleration on the patient's vascular system can create more haemodynamic instability. This can occur because of changes in preload that consequently affect cardiac output. Lawler (2000a,b) likens the vascular system to a half-full bath of shifting water. The patient who already has a cardiac problem, for example arrhythmia or ischaemic heart disease, may become more compromised by any change in their cardiac output. Abdominal contents may also move, causing pressure on the diaphragm and a subsequent alteration in ventilation. To minimize the effect of acceleration and deceleration on the acutely ill patient, the patient should be adequately hydrated and may require a fluid challenge before transfer. Clearly this group of patients will also require close continuous monitoring throughout the transfer process.

During the process of transfer between beds essential intravenous (IV) lines can become dislodged, therefore it is crucial that the patient is observed at all stages of movement (Advanced Life Support Group 2002).

The motion of an ambulance can also cause travel sickness for both the patient and susceptible staff. An anti-emetic should be considered. The feeling of nausea for staff may be exacerbated by the limited view (of the horizon) from the vehicle. For some staff, having to document care/monitor values can increase the nausea. It is important that as an escort team it should be established who is documenting monitoring. Some monitoring systems can provide an electronic record summary.

In summary, although the patient transfer may be urgent, to reduce the potentially harmful haemodynamic changes to the patient caused by acceleration/deceleration, the ambulance health-care professional should be advised to proceed as quickly as possible at a steady speed but to avoid excessive acceleration/deceleration. In general, the faster the vehicle travels, the more braking/deceleration will be required to avoid other traffic/obstacles. This will also be exacerbated if travel occurs at times of day where there is more congestion on the roads.

Principles of good practice for the transfer of neurological patients

This must focus on protecting the patient against a secondary brain injury. This can be achieved by:

+ maintaining the cerebral perfusion pressure (cerebral perfusion pressure = systolic blood pressure – intercranial pressure)
+ limiting further ischaemic injury (preventing hypoxia)
+ close monitoring of neurological response.

The actual neurological injury will determine the urgency of the transfer, but delay in transfer could delay essential treatment and lead to a poor neurological outcome for the patient (Association of Anaesthetists 2006; NICE 2007a).

Preparation for safe transfer of the acutely ill patient

In isolation, the process of transfer from one area/facility to another is not a therapy or treatment (Advanced Trauma Life Support for Doctors 2004). As outlined in the above section the process of transfer itself may cause the patient to deteriorate. The environment or context in which personnel may be working can be unfamiliar (e.g. in an ambulance). Team work and preparation are crucial to assist in minimizing this risk to the patient, even if this has to be undertaken rapidly.

The preparation should include:

+ clear documentation of the organization of the transfer, including the referring doctor and team who have accepted the patient (including identified key names and contact numbers)
+ a clinical assessment of the patient
+ identification of the skills the patient requires from the escorting staff
+ identification of who is/are the most appropriate healthcare professional/s to provide those skills and who is available/what is the effect will that have on the remaining service
+ identification of the resources/equipment required for the transfer of the patient
+ recommendation of the monitoring and documentation of patient during transfer (including the frequency of observations)—this should include the identification of who is responsible for different elements of the patient monitoring so that false assumptions are not made.

Clinical assessment before transfer

This should include a comprehensive assessment as outlined in previous chapters. The ABCDE model facilitates a rapid assessment and reassessment if any changes occur in the patient's parameters before and/or during transfer. Patient stability for transfer must be considered carefully. The information gathered should also be assessed against the documented trend and treatment already administered to the patient. This also enables the patient to be prepared and adequately resuscitated before transfer. If stability cannot be achieved and the urgency of transfer is paramount (e.g. neurological transfer), the decision to transfer should be taken by a senior clinician (medical consultant). There may of course be other injuries that are causing the instability.

As with any patient, the patient's preferred method of address (name) should be identified and permission sought to undertake the following assessment. Adherence to privacy and dignity for the patient throughout the assessment is imperative.

Airway: patent airway

The patient's airway should be checked for patency and the patient's position optimized. As most transfers require the patient to be supine for the journey, any patient who has a lowered level of consciousness may be at risk of airway obstruction (usually partial). Assess for any additional sounds, for example snoring. These are of particular concern as they indicate the tongue is causing a partial obstruction. This can be managed by using a simple airway manoeuvre such as head tilt or chin lift, and may necessitate the use of airway adjuncts such a nasopharyngeal or oral airway (depending on the patient's degree of consciousness).

If the patient has a tracheostomy in situ the inner tube should be checked for patency, the stoma inspected, and tracheostomy tapes secured. It is essential that equipment (e.g. tubes, spare inner tube, tracheal dilators) accompany the patient so that if an emergency tube change is required it can be performed without delay (see Chapter 15 for further details).

If the patient with a tracheostomy has audible respiratory secretions and is unable to cough and clear effectively, tracheal suction should be performed. Portable suction should accompany the patient for the transfer (see the section on resources/equipment).

If the patient has a Glasgow Coma Scale of less than 9 they may require intubating to maintain and protect their airway and ensure adequate oxygenation and ventilation. The patient will also need a nasogastric tube to prevent aspiration of gastric fluid.

Cervical/spinal injuries will require immobilization before any movement to protect against any further injury. Airway manoeuvres for airway obstruction in this group of patients initially will require a jaw thrust.

Breathing: adequate oxygenation and ventilation

The work of breathing should be assessed by visual inspection of chest movement, if it is equal and if accessory muscles are being used, the respiratory rate, and depth of breathing. Any confusion or agitation could indicate hypoxia or reduced cerebral perfusion. Oxygen saturation should be assessed and recorded using pulse oximetry. Recent guidance from the British Thoracic Society recommends a target saturation for acutely ill patients (not at risk of hypercapnic respiratory failure) of 94–98% (British Thoracic Society 2008). A target saturation should be identified for the individual patient by their medical team. Oxygen saturation is extremely useful in aiding the clinical assessment, but its use may be limited if the patient is peripherally poorly perfused as the transfer motion can affect the accuracy of the signal. An ear rather than finger probe may provide increased accuracy.

Depending on the inspired oxygen required (which should be recorded in the prescription chart) the appropriate device for administering the oxygen should be obtained: nasal cannulae, simple face mask, venturi mask, or reservoir mask (British Thoracic Society 2008).

If a patient is receiving oxygen via a reservoir mask (which requires a minimum flow of 10–15 L/min) the distance and time for travel should be estimated so that the oxygen required for journey can be calculated. As a guide this figure should be doubled for the journey to allow for any unforeseen delays.

If a patient is requiring non-invasive ventilation, such as BiPAP therapy, the battery backup for the machine should be established as this may impose limitations on transporting the patient.

If respiratory effort is inadequate, supportive ventilation should be instigated immediately using a bag/valve/mask and the patient seen by an anaesthetist urgently regarding a decision to intubate (this should be via the organization's system for rapid response to patient deterioration (NICE 2007b).

If the patient requires intubation a portable mechanical ventilator (with portable oxygen supply) will be required to relieve the anaesthetist from hand ventilating the patient and allow movement around the patient for other clinical activity.

Capnography is an essential monitoring tool used to check the level of carbon dioxide in exhaled air and the adequacy of ventilation (ICS guidelines 2002). It is used to provide a trend of the patient's carbon dioxide levels, but it is not as reliable as blood gas analysis results so results should be viewed with caution.

A chest X-ray will need to be performed to check the position of the endotracheal tube before an inter-hospital transfer to ensure both lungs are adequately ventilating.

Circulation: adequate perfusion

Information on the patient's state of overall perfusion can be gathered using simple physical assessment techniques such as observation of the skin colour, core temperature, and limb temperature, capillary refill time, and any signs of sweating. The pulse rate, regularity, and quality, and the blood pressure should be assessed and compared to previous data. IV access should be reviewed. In general, the patient should have two patent large-bore IV cannulae in situ.

The patient must have an assessment of fluid balance, including:

♦ any response to fluid administered in the previous 24 h

♦ assessing the drugs the patient has received in the last 24 h

♦ if any drugs are due to be given imminently, for example antibiotics

♦ what blood tests/blood cultures have been taken

♦ if there any results from these that need to be obtained before transfer

♦ if there any signs of bleeding

♦ availability of a blood transfusion if appropriate?

♦ what monitoring the patient is currently on

♦ how frequently observations have been undertaken to date

♦ the frequency of observations (including neurological observations) required for the patient during the transfer.

Disability (neurological assessment)

This can be undertaken initially using the patient's response as indicated on the AVPU scale (Alert, Verbal, Pain, Unconscious). A more detailed assessment (Glasgow Coma Score) should be undertaken for patients who are not registering as alert or are showing signs of confusion or disorientation (see Chapter 4 for more detailed neurological assessment). Pupils should be assessed: are they equal and reacting? A blood sugar should also be checked to eliminate hypoglycaemia as a cause of a change in the level of consciousness. Pain assessment (on movement) is important to ensure that the patient receives adequate analgesia before transfer.

Exposure

This allows the patient to be examined thoroughly for any other wounds or injuries, including pressure damage. Any area at risk of pressure damage should be assessed using a risk tool and documented according to the European Pressure Ulcer Advisory Panel Classification System (NICE 2005). Appropriate pressure-relieving devices may include a pressure mattress or a dressing to protect vulnerable skin against further damage.

The abdomen should be examined for signs of distension. If a nasogastric tube or colostomy/ileostomy are in situ, the bags should be emptied before transfer.

IV lines should be inspected and visual IV phlebitis (VIP) score documented. Any IV cannula with a score of 1 or more should be removed and the patient recannulated. The IV lines must be secured to prevent accidental dislodgement during any movement.

The position of the urinary catheter bag is important as it must allow continuous drainage and accurate measurement by being below the level of the bladder, but not cause reflux or contamination (Department of Health 2003). The catheter bag should therefore not be placed on the bed beside the patient, but hung on patient's bed (take care when pushing the bed through doors/lifts). The catheter bag should also be emptied before transfer.

Chest drains are a closed system that should be positioned upright and unobstructed to allow drainage. The patient with a bubbling chest drain or a patient on mechanical ventilation should not have the drain clamped because of the risk of developing a tension pneumothorax (British Thoracic Society 2003). Chest drains must have their collection vessel below the level of the chest at all times and the vessel should have a one-way mechanism to prevent the aspiration of air (this is created by an underwater seal or a flutter valve). Not all patients require suction attached to the drain.

The patient should be prepared and wrapped to limit heat loss but still maintain access to IV lines, etc. The 'mummy wrap' is recommended by the Advanced Life Support Group (2002) as a method of preventing heat loss and in addition preventing the dislodgement of lines, leads, etc. A sheet or insulating blanket is placed underneath the patient and IV lines can be separated from monitor cables (cables to the feet and IV lines to head of patient or vice versa) and the patient wrapped and fastened.

Health records

Other information should be gathered, including the demographic data, relevant patient information, including nursing care, history, drug prescription, allergies, and next of kin information, and number contacts checked. The patient must have an identity band in situ and this should be checked against current health records.

Relevant results, including microbiology results, should be checked and any relevant information regarding infection control status forwarded to the receiving unit before transfer as this may affect their preferred location of the patient on admission.

If the patient is being transferred between organizations, the relevant information from the patient's health records, transfer summary, results, and relevant X-rays/scan results will need to be copied for the receiving organization. Some trusts may be able to send electronic versions of X-rays via trust computer systems otherwise these will need to be copied onto the relevant format.

This is important to prevent the patient from having unnecessary radiation from repeat imaging because the relevant information has not been sent with the patient.

Clinical skills required for patient transfer

The skills required of the health professional will be dependent on the condition of the individual patient (see Figure 14.1). The skills may be provided through a combination of escorting personnel and will include:

1 clinical competence—the ability to perform physical assessment and undertake skills as detailed below

2 clinical knowledge of the illness and individual patient

3 knowledge of the effect of transfer on patient's condition

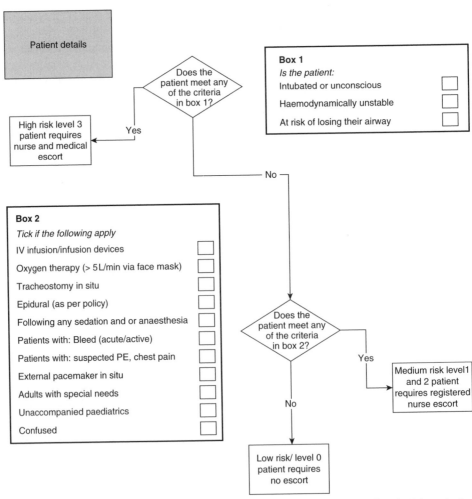

Figure 14.1 A guide to decision making regarding patient escort for the transfer of adult patients. IV, intravenous; PE, pulmonary embolus.

4 the ability to utilize transfer equipment and plan equipment/drugs required for safe transfer

5 the ability to communicate between a range of healthcare professionals, patient, and family.

Clinical competence

Clinical competence is required in a range of clinical activities (as outlined below) depending on the clinical assessment and requirements of the patient. However, the practitioner should also be aware of their own limitations in practice and practice in accordance with their professional role (Good Medical Practice 2006; National Midwifery Council 2008; Department of Health 2009).

Clinical competence should include the ability to problem solve and be proactive and organized in care management (including in unfamiliar environments such as an ambulance). Overall the transfer team's skills should include:

* airway and ventilation management:
  * airway: the ability to intubate (or reintubate) and manage the airway
  * ventilation: the ability to support the patient requiring mechanical ventilation
  * the ability to troubleshoot clinical changes in patients respiratory condition
  * the ability to understand the use of sedation and be able to titrate to maintain patient comfort and facilitate mechanical ventilation
  * the ability to understand use of capnography and interpret results
* cardiovascular management
  * the ability to perform advanced life support including defibrillation
  * the ability to monitor patient and interpret continuous ECG
  * the ability to manage the patient who is haemodynamically unstable
  * the ability to undertake IV cannulation, ability to cannulate if IV lines are dislodged
  * understanding of complex drug and fluid administration, including the use of inotropes; able to titrate inotropes and IV fluids to patients response to maintain mean blood pressure
  * the ability to use non-invasive BP and understand limitations of use in the acutely ill patient
  * the ability to set up and use continuous arterial pressure monitoring
  * the ability to sample and interpret arterial blood gas
  * the ability to set up, use, and troubleshoot infusion devices
* neurological management
  * the ability to assess neurological status of the patient
  * the ability to perform blood sugar checks.

Clinical knowledge of illness and the individual patient

The escorting staff should be familiar with the patient's history, illness, and likely pathway, including the likely potential complications (foreseeable risk).

Knowledge of effect of transfer on patients' condition

The escorting staff should be aware of the effect of movement on the unstable patient and be able to manage changes in the patient's condition.

Staff should be aware of the pressure points on the patient from their position required for transfer and the interface with transfer trolley, and be aware of the patient's risk of developing pressure as the patient must also be secured to the transfer trolley (by five-point patient harness). Staff should be proactive in preventing/limiting potential problems due to pressure damage during transfer.

Ability to utilize transfer equipment

As outlined above, the escorting staff should have a working knowledge of monitoring, mechanical ventilator, defibrillator, suction, infusion devices, and drugs used in the transfer.

Ability to communicate with the patient, their family, and personnel involved in the transfer process

The escorting staff should be calm and good communicators. They should be able to give concise, accurate information, and know the handover plan regarding the patient. If more than one person is involved in the escort of the patient it should be clear who is providing team leadership and coordinating the patient movement. Communication also includes documentation of any care given during the transfer process.

Who can provide these skills?

In order to provide the range of appropriate skills to manage the patient, a combination of health professionals may be required to create a transfer team, each individual providing a different skill set. The escort staff who can potentially be available to transfer the patient are outlined in Table 14.2.

Resources/equipment

This will be dependent on the duration, distance, and mode of transfer (road, sea, air). Even within hospital sites there may be considerable distance to move the patient, involving several lifts. Healthcare professionals must be adequately equipped to manage any reasonable foreseeable situations.

Some organizations may have a dedicated trolley for this purpose incorporating key equipment such as portable ventilator, oxygen, portable monitor, and suction (see Figure 14.2).

Table 14.2 Potential escorting personnel

Hospital staff	Ambulance staff
Anaesthetist	Technician
Intensive care doctor	Paramedic (able to intubate in cardiac arrest situations and give intravenous drugs)
A&E doctor	
Doctor	Emergency care practitioner
Operating department practitioner	Critical care paramedic (a new role within the UK ambulance service)
A&E nurse	
ICU nurse	
Trained nurse (ward based)	
Healthcare assistant	
Clinical site practitioner	
Critical care outreach nurse	

Escorting staff should have training in safe patient transfer.

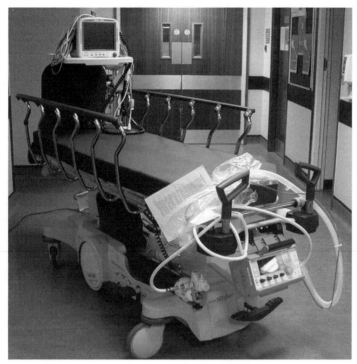

Figure 14.2 Transfer trolley. Supplied with permission from Brighton and Sussex University Hospitals NHS Trust.

Equipment should not be placed on top of the patient (Association of Anaesthetists of Great Britain and Ireland 2009).

Consider:

♦ portable oxygen—calculate oxygen requirements

♦ appropriate oxygen device (and reservoir mask in emergency)

♦ bag–valve–mask, tubing, and connector to oxygen supply

♦ ensure full oxygen cylinder (double the estimated maximum requirement)

♦ type of monitoring required:

• transfer monitor—needs to be robust and lightweight with adequate battery life. Additional batteries may be required for inter-hospital transfer.

• should include continuous ECG, non-invasive BP, pulse oximetry, invasive pressure monitoring (arterial line, CVP) temperature, capnography (if mechanically ventilated)

• alarm limits should be set and alarm volume checked to ensure that they will trigger any change from 'normal' for the patient

• battery status should also be checked and the monitor left on mains supply until ready to transfer

• Non-invasive blood pressure will use up battery faster than any other aspect of monitoring. It is also less reliable when there is additional noise and vibration from vehicle movement.

• for inter-hospital transfers use the ambulance mains adaptor to preserve battery

• defibrillator, including external pacemaker facility, should be available for emergencies.

Transfer bag

Depending on the assessment and acuity of the patient, additional equipment may be required to accompany the patient. Whilst for an inter-hospital transfer much is held on board the ambulance, it is essential that this is also available to and from the vehicle. This includes equipment for intubation, cannulation, nebulizer therapy, emergency drugs, and fluids as well as any items specific to the patient.

Specific circumstances

Ventilated patients

- Mechanical ventilator should be checked before use and once in use left plugged into piped oxygen until ready to transfer to reduce the depletion of the portable oxygen supply.
- Availability of alternative method of ventilation: bag–valve–mask (as outline in above section). In addition, the anaesthetist may require a Mapleson C circuit, as backup for hand ventilating the mechanically ventilated, particularly if the patient is making some spontaneous effort.
- An endotracheal (ET) tube must be secured in position (note position at lip level) and tubing secure to prevent tension on the ET tube.
- A portable suction unit with appropriate suction catheters and a yankuer suction catheter should also accompany the patient. The movement of the patient and motion of an ambulance may mobilize respiratory secretions on both the ventilated and the self-ventilating patient and this may also cause the patient to vomit.

Continuous positive pressure ventilation If a patient is receiving high-flow CPAP, it is important to assess the flow rates the device requires. Most hospital systems use in excess of 100–150 L/min, which makes it exceedingly difficult to transfer a patient due to the supply of oxygen/air mix required to generate the system. Alternatives should be considered, for example would it be safer for the patient be intubated for transfer or could the patient manage on high-flow oxygen via a reservoir mask?

Personal care

If leaving the hospital site for inter-hospital transfer the escort team should consider their own personal requirements (warm clothing, money, refreshments, mobile phone, essential contact numbers). The ambulance service will endeavour to return escorting staff to their base, but when in their locality they may be required to respond to other emergency calls, necessitating the team to travel back by alternative means (with their equipment). Vehicles can occasionally break down, therefore escort staff should have personal protective equipment such as high-visibility jackets as protection.

Moving and handling

The principles of safe patient moving and handling should always be applied in the transfer of all patients using adequate trained personnel and additional devices such as slide sheets/pat slides to assist the process moving of patient between beds/trolleys. This is governed by the Health and Safety at Work Act 1974 (Health and Safety Executive 1974).

The specialist needs of the bariatric patient require consideration to ensure the use of appropriately designed trolley/beds in the transfer process. The weight of any equipment attached to trolleys must also be assessed. Some ambulance services have a dedicated bariatric ambulance that is able to provide the appropriate trolley and moving and handling equipment. Any queries regarding the inter-hospital transfer of the patient with an increased body mass index should be discussed with ambulance control.

Patient handover

Clinical handover has been identified by the World Health Organization as one of the nine areas that could be improved to make a significant difference to patient safety (World Health Organization 2007). Every time there is a handover between personnel, there is a potential for key information to be omitted or poorly communicated. A transfer checklist can aid the effective transfer of information (acting as an aide memoire), including the following:

- key information
- patient demographics, key contact next of kin (and any communications)
- history of present condition
- relevant past medical history
- management plan for the patient
- patient's response to treatment to date, major changes
- care given during transfer
- drug therapy—drugs given/due to be given
- infection control status
- resuscitation status decisions
- results of biochemistry/haematology/microbiology/imaging
- any specific aspects of care that require ongoing assessment and management on admission, for example wound, pressure care, nutrition, mobility
- patient property.

Clinical link activities

The purposes of the following link activities are to encourage the reader to consider how they would manage different situations. They are not exhaustive but reflect some of the varied reasons an acute patient may require transfer. You may reflect on your own experience of a 'good' patient transfer and the features of this.

Clinical link 14.1 (see Appendix for answers)

You are caring for a 65-year-old postoperative patient following over-sewing of bleeding duodenal ulcer. She has become acutely breathless, respiratory rate 36, now requiring 10 L oxygen via a reservoir mask, SpO_2 98% (previously SpO_2 88%). Medical staff suspect a pulmonary embolus (PE) and require the patient to be transferred to CT for a CT pulmonary angiogram to confirm the diagnosis.

    Consider:

Patient escort—who should go?

What are the risks—what could happen during transfer?

What equipment do you require?

What monitoring should the patient have during the transfer?

How should this be documented?

Clinical link 14.2 (see Appendix 14.2 for answers)

You are caring for a patient (78 years old) admitted overnight with pneumonia and a history of COPD. He has become increasingly breathless over the morning shift and the medical team have requested a repeat chest X-ray. He is currently on 35% oxygen via a venturi mask, respiratory rate 28, SpO_2 92%.

Consider:

Patient escort—who should go?

What are the risks—what could happen during transfer?

What equipment do you require?

What monitoring should the patient have during the transfer?

How should this be documented?

Medico legal issues regarding transfer

In inter-hospital transfer the patient remains the responsibility of the parent team until they are in the receiving hospital and handover is complete. If a clinical incident occurs it should be reported and investigated within the organization safety team (see section below). Whether or not the incident involves a medico legal claim will depend on the individual case.

In general, if an allegation of clinical negligence is made, action is taken against the organization rather than an individual unless criminal negligence is alleged (if the action is considered wilful and reckless). As discussed previously, it is crucial that individual healthcare professionals are aware of their own limitations and skills; they should document the care given and be prepared for what is 'reasonably foreseeable'. Clinical negligence may allege that there has been a breach of duty of care where there has been a failure to meet the standard of the ordinary skilled person (exercising and professing to have that special skill). The action of the healthcare professional must be an accepted practice that would withstand logical analysis. For example, it is reasonable

Clinical link 14.3 (see Appendix for answers)

You are working the night shift in an elective hospital site and are caring for a 70-year-old male patient following routine orthopaedic surgery (hip replacement). He has had one episode of fresh vomiting blood earlier in the evening and was uncompromised, but he has a further episode of vomiting blood. The medical team would like to transfer the patient for an emergency oesophogastroduodenoscopy, which can only be undertaken at the main hospital site (10 miles away). The patient must be prepared for immediate transfer. He is currently on 4 L oxygen via nasal cannulae, respiratory rate 24, SpO_2 95%, blood pressure 105/60, pulse 110, temperature 36.0°C. His Hb is 8.0 g/dL and he has had one unit of blood. He has one IV cannula in situ and an infusion of colloid 500 mL in progress over 1 h.

Consider:

Patient escort—who should go?

What are the risks—what could happen during transfer?

What equipment do you require?

What monitoring should the patient have during the transfer?

How should this be documented?

Clinical link 14.4 (see Appendix for answers)

You are working on a head and neck specialist ward and have a 70-year-old patient who has had an emergency tracheostomy in theatre for a stridor. The patient is ready to return to the ward. He is self-ventilating on 35% oxygen via a humidified system. Respiratory rate is 24, SpO_2 96%, blood pressure 130/70, heart rate 100.

You have been asked to collect the patient from theatre and transfer him to the ward.

Consider:

Patient escort—who should go?

What are the risks—what could happen during transfer?

What equipment do you require?

What monitoring should the patient have during the transfer?

to expect that staff transferring a patient requiring high-flow oxygen would have calculated the oxygen required for the journey.

The NHSLA runs schemes for organizations, including personal injury cover. If the organization is part of the NHSLA the level of cover is limited, for example a fixed sum of £20,000 is payable to an employee who suffer serious injury or death whilst performing their professional duty (i.e. on transfers). The employee can also claim against the organization if they consider them responsible. Ahmed & Majeed (2008) highlighted that whilst anaesthetists are usually members of the Association of Anaesthetists of Great Britain and Ireland or the Intensive Care Society (professional organizations which provide personal injury insurance as part of their membership scheme) other members of the escorting team, such as nurses, do not usually have additional cover. Ahmed & Majeed (2008) recommend a national audit of incidents regarding transfers to assess the severity of risk to staff.

Emergency situations

Q: You are escorting a patient on an inter-hospital transfer. The ambulance you are travelling in is also the first on scene to a serious road traffic accident (RTA). Do you have a duty of care to anyone injured in the RTA?

A: Your duty of care is to the patient already entrusted in your care. However, the ambulance personnel may stop and instigate emergency care (radioing for additional help and support) and when that help arrives continue on the inter-hospital transfer.

Q: You are returning from an inter-hospital transfer and the ambulance is required to attend an emergency. Do you have a duty of care to the patient they are attending?

A: Duty of care does not begin until you touch the patient. However, it should be noted that the ambulance personnel are now in their 'normal environment' and will have more skills and experience of working in this scenario. As an escort team you may offer help and be prepared to help if required.

Incident reporting

Organizations who promote incident reporting are associated with having a safer patient safety culture (National Patient Safety Agency 2005; Hutchinson *et al.* 2009). It is therefore essential that if either an actual incident or near miss associated with the patient transfer occurs it should be reported immediately on return so that lessons can be learnt around the process. This enables trending of incidents and importantly will raise questions regarding the process: Does it require change? Other industries (such as the airline industry) view learning from incidents as an essential part of their safety culture.

End of chapter test

It is important that you understand both the theory related to transfer of the acutely ill adult and the practice of transfer skills to safely care for patients whose condition may be deteriorating. In order to test your knowledge and apply this knowledge to clinical practice you should undertake the following assessment with an appropriately trained member of staff in clinical practice. If you are unable to answer any questions it may be helpful to revisit the section in this chapter.

Knowledge assessment

Work with your mentor/supervisor in practice and ask them to test your knowledge in relation to the following. Incorrect answers/lack of knowledge will require further revision/re-reading of this chapter.

- Discuss your organization's policy on patient transfer.
- Discuss situations that may necessitate intra-hospital or inter-hospital transfer.
- Discuss the differences between intra-hospital transfer and inter-hospital transfer.
- Identify the groups of patients who may require inter-hospital transfer and analyse the particular risks of this group of patients.
- Describe the process of risk assessment related to transfer of the patient.
- Discuss which groups of patients may require intubation before transfer and analyse the associated risks.
- Analyse which groups of patients may have additional risk associated with transfer.
- Describe the characteristics of a 'good hospital transfer'
- Discuss the changes in physiology that may be noted during hospital transfer.
- Describe the assessment of the patient that is required before transfer.
- Discuss the role of personnel who may be involved in the transfer.
- Discuss equipment that may be required before transfer.
- Analyse health and safety issues associated with transfer, including:
  - manual handling
  - equipment
  - electrical safety
  - transport of gases
  - appropriate training to use equipment.
- Analyse infection control issues that may occur during transfer.
- Analyse situations where transfer may not be appropriate.
- Discuss how appropriate communication and documentation can enhance transfer.
- Discuss the organization processes involved in inter-hospital transfer (e.g. coordination of ambulance staff).

Skills assessment

Work with your mentor/supervisor in practice and ask her to assess your ability to care for patients who require transfer using the following criteria where appropriate. Note: You may not be able to demonstrate all these skills. Ask your mentor/supervisor to give you feedback on areas that you did well and areas that may require improving.

Intra-hospital transfer

♦ Identifies patient requiring transfer to another area and communicates with other multidisciplinary team members.

♦ Considers which personnel are required to ensure safe patient transfer and ensures that all members are available for a safe transfer.

♦ Conducts an appropriate assessment of the patient's condition and ensures that patient is sufficiently stable to transfer (unless extenuating circumstances, e.g. ruptured aortic aneurysm).

♦ Considers the risks associated with the transfer of the patient and identifies how these risks may be reduced.

♦ Explains the need to transfer to another area to the patient and gains their consent where appropriate.

♦ Reassures patient and tries to reduce any anxiety related to transfer.

♦ Communicates effectively with patient and their family throughout the transfer process.

♦ Contacts patient's relatives and explains need to transfer, giving details of relocated area.

♦ Considers suitability of transferring patient on their bed or the need to move the patient to a transfer trolley.

♦ Considers manual handling risks associated with patient transfer.

♦ Ensures that patient has sufficient IV access and liaises with doctor/senior nurse if more access required.

♦ Ensures appropriate monitoring for transfer is available and attached to patient.

♦ Secures monitoring equipment to reduce risk of injury to the patient or transferring personnel.

♦ Ensures monitoring equipment is charged, has sufficient battery life for transfer, and does not pose safety hazard to patient/accompanying personnel.

♦ Ensures that portable oxygen is available and has sufficient gas for transfer.

♦ Ensures oxygen is secure in oxygen holder and does not pose a health and safety risk.

♦ Ensures that there is sufficient oxygen for duration of transfer.

♦ Ensures that portable suction is available and has sufficient battery life for transfer

♦ Checks that there is appropriate suction equipment, for example emergency suction catheters.

♦ Provides appropriate IV equipment, for example syringe drives/pumps, and ensures that equipment is charged and has sufficient battery life for transfer.

♦ Gives special consideration to the following:
  - patient with deteriorating levels of consciousness
  - patient with unprotected airway (requires intubation)
  - intubated patient (anaesthetist required, portable ventilator, rebreath bag, appropriate oxygen source, end tidal carbon dioxide monitoring, emergency reintubation equipment)
  - patient who is haemorrhaging (sufficient fluid replacement)
  - patient with cardiac arrhythmias (portable defibrillator)

- confused patients (may require sedation, bed rails).
♦ Checks that appropriate emergency equipment and drugs are available during transfer.
♦ Ensures that adequate infection control is in place during transfer and all personnel have appropriate personal protective equipment.
♦ Considers additional risks if patient has known infection control risks, for example MRSA, and follows hospital's infection control procedure.
♦ Liaises with receiving area to confirm timing for transfer.
♦ Communicates effectively with receiving area, providing details of:
  - patient history/reason for admission to hospital
  - reason for transfer
  - patient's medical team
  - who has taken decision to transfer patient
  - whether patient is intubated
  - patient's current condition
  - current medication
  - ongoing treatment
  - any allergies
  - current monitoring required
  - details of next of kin
  - details of infectious status
  - any religious considerations if transfusion likely (Jehovah witness, etc.)
  - time frame of transfer
  - who will be accompanying patient
  - any particular concerns that you have.
♦ Documents the need for transfer in patient's notes and provides a brief account of patient's condition during transfer.
♦ Documents staff involved in transfer and any adverse events that may occur during transfer.
♦ Works well as a team member during transfer and only acts within own level of competence.
♦ Ensures that a senior person is responsible for coordinating the transfer.
♦ Ensures that any accompanying relatives travel to new area separately from the rest of the transfer team.
♦ Introduces patient to new staff and ensures that patient has understood why transfer was required (where appropriate).

Inter-hospital transfer

Inter-hospital transfer carries additional risk for the patient and should only be carried out by staff who are competent and skilled at inter-hospital transfer. Consideration should be given to all the criteria above and in addition to this the practitioner will need to:

♦ explain the need to transfer to another hospital to the patient and their family
♦ liaise with receiving hospital about availability of appropriate bed

- liaise with receiving hospital about timing issues
- liaise with ambulance staff over timing of transfer and requirements of accompanying ambulance personnel
- consider the condition of the patient and liaise with medical team about suitable accompanying personnel
- ensure that there are sufficient staff available to accompany patient
- ensure that accompanying staff are competent to transfer patient
- ensure that the patient's comfort is maintained throughout transfer and temperature is maintained with sufficient clothing/blankets
- provide the next of kin with geographical details of the new hospital and directions for getting to it
- ensure that the receiving hospital is informed when the patient leaves and the estimated time of arrival provided
- handover and documentation (recommended by the Intensive Care Society 2002) should include:
  - transfer details of patient (patient's name, date of birth, next of kin, previous hospital, ward, medical staff, referring doctor, name and status of accompanying personnel)
  - a medical summary (to include reason for admission, past medical history, ongoing procedures and care, patient assessment, medications and fluids, IV access, any recent blood results, MRSA status)
  - nursing summary (to include nursing care, nursing assessment of current status, ongoing care plan)
  - patients status during transfer (vital signs during transfer, medication, fluid status, condition during transfer, any adverse events) (adapted from the University of Brighton skills template, authors Fiona Creed and Denise Hinge)

References

Advanced Life Support Group (2002) *Safe Transfer and Retrieval. The Practical Approach*. BMJ Books, London.

Advanced Trauma Life Support for Doctors (2004) *Course Manual*. 7th edn. American College of Surgeons, Chicago.

Ahmed, I. and Majeed, A. (2008) Risk management during inter-hospital transfer of critically ill patients: Making the journey safe. *Emerg. Med. J.* **25**, 502–5.

The Association of Anaesthetists of Great Britain and Ireland Anaesthesia (2006) Recommendations for the Transfer of Patients with Brain Injury.

Association of Anaesthetists of Great Britain and Ireland (2009) AAGBI Safety Guideline. Interhospital Transfer. http://www.aagbi.org/publications/guidelines.htm

British Thoracic Society (2003) Guidelines for insertion of a chest drain. *Thorax*. **58**, 53–9.

British Thoracic Society (2008) Guideline for emergency oxygen use in adult patients. http://www.brit-thoracic.org.uk/ClinicalInformation/EmergencyOxygen/EmergencyOxygenuseinAdultPatients/tabid/327/Default.aspx

Catchpole, K. de Leval, M., McEwan, A., *et al.* (2007) Patient handover from surgery to intensive care: Using Formula 1 pit-stop and aviation models to improve safety and quality. *Pediat. Anesth.* **17**(5), 470–8.

Department of Health (2003) Winning ways working together to prevent healthcare associated infection in England. http://www.dh.gov.uk/en/Publicationsandstatistics/Publications/PublicationsPolicyAnd Guidance/DH_4064682

Department of Health (2009) Competencies for recognising and responding to acutely ill patients in hospital. http://www.dh.gov.uk/en/Publicationsandstatistics/Publications/PublicationsPolicyAndGuidance/DH_096989

Dunn, M.J., Gwinnutt, C.L., Gray, A.J. *et al.* 2006. Critical care in the emergency department: Patient transfer. http://www.emjonline.com.

Good Medical Practice (2006) *Good Medical Practice.* http://www.gmc-uk.org/guidance/good_medical_practice/how_gmp_applies_to_you.asp.

Health and Safety Executive (1974) Health and Safety at Work Act 1974. http://www.hse.gov.uk/legislation/hswa.htm.

Hutchinson, A., Young, T.A., and Cooper, K.L. (2009) Trends in healthcare reporting and relationship to safety and quality data in acute hospitals: Learning from the National Reporting and Learning System. http://qshc.bmj.com/cgi/content/abstract/18/1/5.

Intensive Care Society (2002) Guidelines for transport of the critically ill adult. http://www.ics.ac.uk/default2.htm.

Lawler, P.G. (2000a) Transfer of critically ill patients: Part 1—preparation for transfer. *Care Crit. Ill.* **16**(2), 61–5.

Lawler, P.G. (2000b) Transfer of critically ill patients: Part 2—preparation for transfer. *Care Crit. Ill.* **16**(3), 94–7.

National Health Service Litigation Authority (2008) Risk management handbook for Acute Trusts.

National Patient Safety Agency (2005) Seven steps to patient safety in primary care. http://www.nrls.npsa.nhs.uk/resources/collections/seven-steps-to-patient-safety/.

National Patient Safety Agency (2008) Improving patient safety. http://www.npsa.nhs.uk/nrls/improvingpatientsafety/humanfactors/foresight/.

National Midwifery Council (2008) The Code. Standards of conduct, performance and ethics for nurses and midwives. http://www.nmc-uk.org/aArticle.aspx?ArticleID=3056.

NICE Clinical Guideline 4 The early management of head injuries, Understanding NICE guidance—information for patients, carers and families, and the public. http://www.nice.org.uk/page.aspx?o=74658.

NICE (2005) Clinical guideline 29. Preventing and treatment of pressure ulcers.

NICE (2007a) Clinical guideline 56. Head injury (partial update of CG 4).

NICE (2007b) Clinical guideline 50. Acutely Ill Patients in Hospital. Recognition of and response to acute illness in adults in hospital.

Reason, J. (2004) Beyond the organisational accident: The need for 'error wisdom' on the front line. *Qual. Safety Healthcare.* **13**, 28–33.

The Neuro Anaesthesia Society of Great Britain (2006) Recommendations for the Transfer of patients with acute head injuries to Neurosurgical Units.

Tillant, D. Baker, D.J., and Carli, P. (2000) Mechanical ventilation during the transport of critically ill patients. *Int. J Int. Care Spring.* 59–67.

Watson, D. (2007) Planning to ensure the safe transfer of hospital patients. *Nurs. Times.* **102**(09), 109.

World Health Organization (2007) Nine safety solutions. http://www.who.int/mediacentre/news/releases/2007/pr22/en/index.html.

Bibliography

Bellingham, G. *et al.* (2000) Comparison of a specialist retrieval team with current United Kingdom Practice for transport of critically ill patients. *Int. Care Med.* **26**, 740–4.

Cohen, A. (2000) The hazards of inter-hospital transfer of patients. *Care Crit. Ill.* **16**(2), 44–5.

Duke, G.J. and Green, J.V. (2001) Outcome of critically ill patients undergoing inter-hospital transfer. *Med. J. Australia.* **174**(3), 122–5.

Knowles, P.R. *et al*. (1999). Meeting the standards for interhospital transfer of adults with severe head injury in the United Kingdom. *Anaesthesia*. **54**(3), 283–8.

Koppenberg *et al*. 2002. Interhospital transport: Transport of critically ill patients. *Curr. Opin. Anaesthesiol*. **15**(2), 211–5.

Sussex Critical Care Network (2003)Transfer Guidelines http://www.sussexcritcare.nhs.uk/documents.asp.

Wallace, P. and Ridley, S. (1999) Transport of critically ill patients. *BMJ*. **319**, 368–72.

Warren, J. *et al*. (2004) Guidelines for the inter and intra hospital transport of the critically ill patients. *Crit. Care Med*. **32**(1), 256–62.

Chapter 15

Caring for the patient post intensive care

Fiona Creed

Chapter contents

The need for a safe transition from the intensive therapy unit (ITU) to ward areas has been stressed (Cutler & Robson 2006; NICE 2007). Problematic transfers may result in discontinuity of care, delayed recovery, adverse health problems, readmission to ITU, and even the death of a patient. There is a need to plan the transfer effectively, provide effective post-ITU care, and understand the complex physical and psychological needs of patients and their families on transfer from ITU.

This chapter will examine:

+ problems with transfer from ITU
+ the physical needs of the patient, including:
    • physical problems post ITU
    • tracheostomy management
+ the psychological needs of the patient, including:
    • the needs of the patient post ITU
    • the needs of the family post ITU
+ appropriate transfer planning
+ preparation for receiving an ITU patient.

Learning outcomes

This chapter will enable you to:

+ understand the vulnerability of the patient post ITU
+ reflect on the physical and psychological problems faced by the patient on transfer from ITU
+ examine the role and needs of the patient's family following transfer from ITU
+ recognize the need for effective monitoring of the patient following transfer from ITU
+ understand the significance of effective planning
+ analyse current recommendations about transfer and discuss how these might impact on practice.

Potential patient problems on transfer from ITU

Patients who have been treated in ITU will be recovering from serious illness and will still require an intensive level of nursing and medical care post discharge from ITU. Although these patients are often classified as 'fit' to be transferred from ITU, they may still be more dependent and require more intensive levels of care than other ward patients. A number of problems have been identified with the transition of care from ITU to the ward that may have an adverse effect on subsequent patient care/patient outcome. This includes problems associated with:

- early discharge
- inadequate planning
- poor communication
- relocation stress
- understanding of patients' needs.

These problems may, at the very least, cause discontinuity of care and delayed recovery. However, several studies have identified a considerable difference between critical care survival and survival to hospital discharge, in some cases the post-ITU mortality rate is as high as 25% (Goldhill & Sumner 1998). Whilst it is not possible to exactly determine the cause of this, a number of problems have been identified that may contribute to the high mortality rate of ITU patients. Reviews of this vulnerable group of patients have suggested there may be a number of contributory factors.

Early transfer

One of the most problematic issues that may lead to increased mortality/morbidity is that of early transfer of the ITU patient. Despite the increase in ITU beds since the publication of comprehensive critical care (Department of Health 2000) there is still a shortage of beds and patients are transferred early from ITU without adequate planning for transfer and subsequent management. Repeated studies have highlighted that early transfer from ITU may lead to an increase in patient mortality and a higher ITU readmission rate (Goldfrad & Rowan 2000). Early transfer at night time appears to be particularly problematic as this is often coupled with a lack of support from critical care outreach teams, who may not offer 24-h cover. Statistically, those patients transferred at night have a higher readmission/mortality rate than those transferred during the day (Duke et al. 2004). Certain physiological variables may also predispose patients to an increased risk of readmission and increased mortality. These include the age of the patient, patients with chronic health problems, level of illness (calculated by acute physiology points), and length of patient stay in ITU (Daly & Chang 2001). Daly's study highlighted that if patients with increased risk stayed in ITU for an additional 48 h after they were deemed fit for transfer the mortality risk was significantly reduced.

Inadequate planning

Inadequate planning has also been shown to have an adverse effect on patient care. It is widely recognized that the patient's transition from ITU to the ward should be planned, as this will ease transition to the ward and reduce the likelihood of readmission to ITU (Watts et al. 2005). The need for seamless, well-planned transfers is stressed throughout the literature and problems with inadequate planning may adversely affect patient care and put patients at increased risk (Cutler & Robson 2006). The need to plan for the patient's transfer, ward care, and management of ward resources is stressed. However, in reality this is often not the case and this may have a detrimental effect on ward staff (Cutler & Robson 2006). The lack of control over transfer of ITU patients to the ward may leave staff feeling stressed about the impact an ITU patient may place on their workload. Whittaker & Ball (2000) highlight that adequate planning enables ward staff to manage their resources more efficiently. In addition, patients and their families/carers may feel increased levels of stress and dissatisfaction if they are unaware of the plan to transfer to a ward (Crocker 2005).

Communication issues

Poor communication between ward staff and ITU staff also impacts on care following transfer from ITU. Whittaker & Ball (2000) explored the communication problems, identifying that some ward staff felt that they had not received enough information to allow them to provide basic care. They argue that ITU staff may fail to address the type of handover that ward staff require, concentrating on the acuity of the patient's illness rather than focusing on the patient's dependence levels and how much care is required (Ball 2005). It is argued that ITU nurses may give excessively detailed handovers in relation to arterial blood gases and little detail about the patient's current status and nursing requirements. The need for clear and effective handover was emphasized as ambiguous terms such as 'the patient has done really well' may indicate that the patient is less dependent than they actually are (Whittaker & Ball 2000). Concerns over ITU nurses' use of unfamiliar terminology was problematic and was viewed as a barrier to understanding the patient's current needs.

It was also felt that ITU nurses sometimes tried to rush the transfer (possibly because the bed was required for another patient). This led to feelings that the ITU nurses lacked empathy in relation to their colleagues' heavy workload and this further perpetuated communication issues. Communication issues were often compounded by problems in accessing written information from patients' notes because either the notes were disorganized or the ward nurses were not familiar with the paperwork.

Relocation stress

The effects of ITU transfer on patients and their carers have been well documented and the concept of relocation stress emphasized in critical care literature. Whilst it is appreciated that not all patients will undergo relocation stress studies suggest that a considerable proportion of ITU patients will exhibit signs of anxiety on transfer to a ward (Cutler & Robson 2006).

Relocation stress is a term used to describe the anxiety a patient may experience when being transferred between care environments. For the acutely ill patient relocation stress may occur when the patient is moved from an ITU area to a ward. It may manifest in physiological or/and psychological disturbances in patients and sometimes their carers. Whilst it is appreciated that many patients view transfer to the ward as a positive step that indicates their condition is improving, others may suffer increased anxiety. A number of factors have been shown to increase relocation stress, including:

+ lack of preparation for transfer
+ significant degree of environmental change
+ sudden reduction in monitoring
+ lack of explanation about differences between ITU and ward
+ insufficient time for 'closure' with ITU staff
+ lack of predictability in new area
+ sudden or abrupt transfer.

Patients often complain of problems associated with the changes in nurse:patient ratio and loss of the close relationship that they may have experienced with the ITU nurse. Haines *et al.* (2001) suggested that relocation stress may manifest as increased requests from the patient that may make them seem very demanding. ITU patients were frequently cited as being 'buzzer happy' or 'institutionalized', seemingly expecting ward nurses 'to do everything for them'. Alongside this relatives may appear overly worried or demanding. The need for adequate preparation for the transition from ITU to ward for the patient is stressed to minimize the effects of relocation stress (Cutler & Robson 2006).

Perception of patient needs

Lack of understanding in relation to the physical/psychological needs of patients has also been highlighted as a problem. McKinney & Deeney (2002) suggest that patients experience many physical and psychological issues post transfer from ITU and these are not always immediately recognized by practitioners. They emphasize the problems with physical weakness, tiredness, difficulty sleeping, and reduced mobility that was still experienced by ITU patients on their return to the ward. Alongside this many patients suffered psychological consequences of acute illness, including psychosis, amnesia, relocation stress, and increased anxiety. There appears to be a perception among patients that nurses on the ward do not always understand their complex needs and have unrealistic expectations about what patients can actually do for themselves (Strahan & Brown 2005). Patients felt that often practitioners lacked understanding about their degree of frailty/physical weakness. Lack of understanding in relation to these patient needs can be seen to further increase the stress of moving to the ward (Cutler & Robson 2006).

It is therefore imperative for practitioners to have an understanding of the complex physical and psychological needs of this vulnerable group of patients in order to deliver safe and effective care.

Physical needs of ITU patients

The physical needs of the patient transferred from ITU will to an extent be dependent on the condition that necessitated ITU admission. Particular vigilance should be used with those patients who have been transferred early from ITU and careful monitoring and assessment of the patient should occur to ensure that any deterioration in condition is picked up and treated in a timely manner to prevent unnecessary readmission to ITU. Ward nurses should work closely with the outreach teams to plan the nursing care of patients post ITU.

Examples of physical problems post ITU include:

+ severe muscle wasting/weakness
+ recovering organ failure
+ postural hypotension
+ joint stiffness/immobility
+ peripheral neuropathy
+ reduced pulmonary reserve/breathlessness
+ management of airway/artificial airway
+ digestive/feeding problems
+ sleep disturbances
+ resistant infections (Griffiths & Jones 1999).

Fatigue and muscle weakness

A universal problem for patients post transfer from ITU is that of muscle weakness. It has been estimated that, because of the catabolic effect of acute illness and the muscle wasting that occurs during prolonged periods of immobility, patients will lose about 2% of their muscle mass per day of critical illness (Griffiths & Jones 1999). Prolonged periods of critical illness may cause patients to lose up to half of their muscle mass. In addition, it may be difficult to ensure adequate nutrition in the critically ill patient because of absorption problems, further contributing to muscle loss. This will clearly impact on the patient's recovery/ability to undertake physical tasks and may lead to such extreme disability that it may take over a year to begin to recover (Griffiths & Jones 1999). This can cause significant problems to patients on transfer to the ward as their ability to physically do anything is severely impaired.

Patients usually present with significant immobility and may struggle to mobilize at all. Often the inability to mobilize is linked to the patient's muscle loss and associated weakness, but other reports highlight that several patients felt that they may have lost the ability to mobilize, walk, or function properly. In some patients the degree of muscle loss is so severe that it impacts on the patient's ability to do anything, for example feeding and simple hygiene tasks are problematic if upper limb wasting is severe (Strahan & Brown 2005).

The muscle weakness is often compounded by feelings of severe fatigue that may worsen the effects of loss of muscle function. Patients have reported either feeling fatigued continuously or becoming fatigued quickly at the slightest effort. Often, because they have no recollection of the severity of their illness, they are unable to comprehend why they are weak and this may heighten their concerns over their weakness/fatigue (McKinney & Deeney 2002). Patients have reported perceptions that ward staff do not appreciate the severity of the weakness and may feel that the patient is being dependent on the nursing staff. It is important that the patient's need for physical support/nursing care and appropriate rest is recognized (Cutler & Robson 2006).

Recovering organ failure

The ITU patient may have experienced either single or multiple organ failure during the period of acute illness and whilst there may be some recovery the patient may still be experiencing some degree of organ dysfunction. Care is likely to be supportive in nature and dependent on the organ involved. Details relating to organ dysfunction/failure should be included in the transfer summary, and current and ongoing care highlighted.

Cardiovascular instability/postural hypotension

Patients who have prolonged periods of bed rest and loss of muscle tone may experience autonomic dysfunction on movement. The nurse should be aware that the risk of postural hypotension in this group of patients is high and that they are in danger of falling if they stand up without sufficient support. It may be advisable to use a tilt table in extreme cases. It is essential that the nurse recognizes that the patient may collapse due to postural hypotension if stood up/asked to mobilize, without adequate assessment.

Neuromuscular problems

Patients may experience neuromuscular problems and the development of critical illness polymyopathy/neuropathy. This will clearly have an effect on neurological functioning and may present with several differing symptoms. Patients may complain of loss of function, loss of movement, weakness, or tingling sensations in affected limbs for a considerable time post ITU (Crocker 2005). They may also experience balance problems when they eventually are able to mobilize. This again may take some time to rectify. In addition, patients may experience stiff joints that cause pain on movement because of prolonged periods of lack of normal body movement.

Airway management

Patients may return to the ward with either an artificial airway or damage to the airway because of long-term/repeated intubation (Adams 2005). Although early tracheostomy placement and low cuff tubes reduce the likelihood of tracheal stenosis, some patients may still present with this problem. Any patients with suspected stenosis should be referred to the ear, nose, and throat team for appropriate management. Stenosis should have been identified by the ITU team but patients may present with breathlessness on exertion/stridor/wheeziness. Muscle wasting may cause problems with the patient's control of upper airways and swallow, and this will put them at increased risk of aspiration and related pneumonia. Patients should be carefully observed for problems with swallowing and any signs of aspiration (coughing, spluttering, etc.), should be referred to the speech and language team and the medical staff.

Tracheostomy

There is also a high likelihood that this group of patients may also still have tracheostomies in situ because they have been weaned from ventilatory support. Ball *et al.* (2003) suggest that this is a significant issue and because of the need for effective tracheostomy management this will be discussed in detail (see section on tracheostomy management).

Communication issues

Patients with cuffed tracheostomies may experience problems communicating because the cuff prevents air passing the vocal cords. In addition, patients who have had the cuff deflated may still experience problems with communicating. It is essential that these patients have an agreed communication plan. This may involve discussion with the speech and language team. Speak valves may be used to facilitate communication, but the patient must have an understanding of how to use these effectively. It is essential that the patient who is unable to communicate verbally has a means of attracting attention if needed and access to a patient call buzzer or bell. Patients should be reassured that they will receive a timely response to the call bell. The inability to communicate effectively may cause the patient to feel vulnerable and isolated. Nurses should explain/reinforce that the inability to communicate is temporary and provide appropriate support (Woodrow 2004).

Reduced respiratory function

Although these patients no longer require respiratory support they are likely to become breathless on slight exertion. The breathlessness may be associated with respiratory damage that has caused a low respiratory reserve or it may be linked to cardiovascular problems (Adams 2005). Muscle wasting to the diaphragmatic and intercostal muscles following prolonged periods of ventilation will further affect respiratory function. Crocker (2005) identifies that this breathlessness may last for some time and ITU patients are often unable to mobilize because of the associated breathlessness. Patients are likely to require oxygen therapy on transfer from ITU and it is important that this is delivered as prescribed and appropriate monitoring available to ensure adequate oxygenation. Patients will also require close respiratory observation and respiratory assessment post transfer from ITU. It has been highlighted that patients with previous respiratory failure are at risk and that the majority (58%) of readmissions is linked to problems with respiratory complications (see Chapter 2 for detailed respiratory assessment/oxygenation).

Digestive/feeding problems

These may be linked to difficulties in swallowing or poor gut function post ITU. Prolonged periods of intubation, insertion of artificial airways, and loss of muscle tone may all lead to difficulties with swallowing. Advice should be sought from the speech and language therapist if there are problems with swallowing or if the patient has an artificial airway in situ. Alongside these difficulties the patients will often have an increased calorific demand because of the need to replace lost muscle mass (Strahan & Brown 2005). Patients' desire to eat and drink may be reduced by changes in mood, taste alterations, reduced stomach capacity, pain, and physical weakness. Patients may experience problems with digestion, especially after periods of prolonged nasogastric feeding and may report feelings of bloating, sickness, and nausea when they begin to eat. This can discourage oral intake and the patient should be encourage to take small amounts of food often. They may also require a specialized diet and review by the dietetic team. It is likely to take time before muscle mass begins to improve, although energy stores may be more rapidly restored, reducing feelings of hunger.

Resistant infections/barrier nursing

Many patients who have been critically ill will return to the ward with a resistant infection for which they will require barrier nursing. Critically ill patients are at particular risk of resistant infection for several reasons, including reduced nutrition, abnormal immune systems, high use of antibiotics, invasive monitoring, decreased resistance to infection, and prevalence of resistant infection in ITU. Adequate transfer planning should ensure that there is provision of an effective barrier nursing environment/side room and local protocol should be followed in relation to treatment for infection and barrier nursing precautions. The psychological effects of resistant infections should be acknowledged and many ITU patients report feelings of stigma and problems with personal cleanliness. Several patients have reported feeling 'dirty' and worried about contaminating their visitors (Crocker 2005). Care should be taken to ensure that patients with resistant infections are treated with sensitivity to avoid worsening the psychological consequences of having a resistant infection. Common infections that require barrier nursing include MRSA, *Clostridium difficle*, and vancomycin-resistant enterococci.

Sleep disturbances

Alongside the muscle weakness and fatigue that patients report they also identify problems with adjusting to day/night sleep patterns. Patients report feelings of extreme tiredness and exhaustion, yet an inability to regulate sleep patterns (Strahan & Brown 2005). Patients have reported problems with re-establishing their sleep patterns and problems with awakening from sleep because of flashbacks, hallucinations, and nightmares. Patients often appear to lose 'normal' night/day patterns and when they do sleep patients often report feelings of having been tortured, trapped, or involved in some sort of disaster (Strahan & Brown 2005). The occurrence of these nightmares is thought to be linked to the patient's illness, the use of opiate and sedative drugs, the unnatural environment of the ITU, and constant sensory overload. Patients who are nursed in an environment where there are no windows or natural light are thought to have even more unpleasant memories of their experience in ITU (Griffiths & Jones 1999). Patients should be encouraged to discuss their fears as inability to discuss issues post ITU has been linked to development of delusional states/psychosis. Physical nursing care for the patient transferred from ITU is summarized in Table 15.1

Tracheostomy care

The importance of appropriate tracheostomy care cannot be over emphasized. It is vital that the patency of the tracheostomy is maintained at all times to prevent respiratory compromise and potential respiratory arrest. Outreach teams comment on the need for adequate understanding of

Table 15.1 Nursing care following transfer from ITU

Problem	Nursing care plan
Airway management	Assess patient's ability to maintain airway Observe patient for signs of airway obstruction Follow emergency protocol if loss of airway Report any problems to medical staff Tracheostomy management (see Tables 15.2 and 15.3)
Reduced respiratory function	Respiratory assessment (see Chapter 2) Ensure those patients with a history of respiratory failure are observed vigilantly since incidence of readmission to ITU is high Score patient's respiratory function using track and trigger system Provide adequate oxygenation and assess oxygenation Report any deterioration in patient's condition quickly Ensure that patient is adequately positioned in bed to optimize ventilation and ensure that patient's position is changed to facilitate effective ventilation Encourage patient to sit out of bed for short periods if able/tolerated Give nebulizers as prescribed Refer to physiotherapist/encourage breathing exercises Observe for signs of chest infection Mobilize patient as able and encourage patient to rest if breathless following exertion
Cardiovascular instability	Cardiovascular assessment (see Chapter 3) CVS monitoring if required on discharge treatment plan: the need and regularity of CVS monitoring should be discussed at handover from ITU staff and may include continuous ECG monitoring, electronic blood pressure recording, and CVP measurement Score patient's CVS status using track and trigger system Report any deterioration in patient's condition quickly Ensure adequate fluid balance/fluid intake Assess for likelihood of postural hypotension Slow mobilization of patient once stable
Organ dysfunction	Care will be dependent on organ involved, ongoing monitoring is essential, and specialist advise may be required
Fatigue and weakness	Accurate assessment of the impact of muscle weakness on functional capacity Provide nursing care as required, gradually increasing patient's involvement in care as patient is able Observe for side effects of prolonged bed rest, including chest infection, DVT, pressure sores Prophylactic DVT treatment Physiotherapy as tolerated Pressure relieving mattresses as indicated Observe for signs of foot drop and other peripheral damage and refer to physiotherapist/occupational therapist Provide psychological support
Neuromuscular problems	Observe for signs of neuropathy/weakness Refer to physiotherapist for appropriate treatment Encourage gentle exercise where tolerated Use splints to support affected limb if required Refer patient to occupational therapist for assessment Provide pain relief as required Refer to neurologist if required

Table 15.1 Nursing care following transfer from ITU *(Continued)*

Problem	Nursing care plan
Communication issues	Ensure that patient has call buzzer/call bell at all times Provide an alternative means of communication, e.g. sign/alphabet boards/writing boards and paper/speech valves (if appropriate)/mouthing words and lip reading Referral to SALT for assessment and appropriate use of aids Encourage patient and their family to communicate to reduce feelings of isolation
Digestive/feeding problems	Complete nutritional assessment. The Malnutrition Universal Screening tool may be useful. This should be completed when the patient returns from ITU and reassessed frequently depending on risk of malnutrition Follow local protocol if patient receiving enteral nutrition Refer to dietician for assessment of nutritional needs Refer to speech and language therapist for assessment of swallow Follow guidance from SALT, observing for any difficulties swallowing/aspiration Use thickening agents in fluids if required Ensure appropriate diet is provided and assistance as required Ensure patient is in an appropriate position to eat safely Ensure nutritional intake is documented and action taken if nutritional needs not met Provide small, frequent meals and observe for nausea/vomiting post meal Provide antiemetic as needed Provide aperients as required and record bowel actions Encourage nutritional supplements
Resistant infections	Assess need for isolation before return to ward (infectious status should always be checked before transfer from ITU to ensure that patient is nursed in a suitable environment) Explain the need for continued barrier nursing to patient Observe for signs of infection and use track and trigger scoring system to monitor patient's temperature Be aware of signs of developing sepsis (see Chapter 8) Ensure adequate barrier nursing is commenced in line with local policy Provide treatment for resistant infection, e.g. antibiotic/nasal cream/appropriate skin washes Provide psychological support to the patient and their family Ensure vigilant monitoring of the post-ITU patient who is being nursed in a side room because of infection
Sleep disturbances	Reorientate to night/day pattern Encourage periods of rest/activity throughout the day Encourage patient to verbalize their worries Observe for signs of distress on awakening from sleep Avoid use of sedatives unless absolutely required Review any medication that may cause sleep disturbances Refer to psychiatrist if exhibiting signs of delusional states/psychosis

ITU, intensive therapy unit; CVS, cardiovascular status; ECG, electrocardiogram; CVP, central venous pressure; DVT, deep vein thrombosis; SALT, speech and language therapists.

tracheostomy management to prevent readmission to ITU. Ball *et al.* (2003) identify that 18% of referrals to their outreach team are related to issues of tracheostomy care. Of these, 10% of referrals relate to assistance with tracheostomy management and 8% relate to assistance with suctioning tracheostomies. It is vital that nurses who accept patients from ITU understand how to manage tracheostmy care appropriately to avoid potential life-threatening problems.

This section will explore:

- the rationale for tracheostomy insertion in ITU patients
- preparing to receive a patient with a tracheostomy
- the need for humidification
- the need for removal of secretions
- maintenance of airway patency/changing inner tubes
- cuff management
- prevention of infection
- emergency procedures for blocked tracheostomy tubes
- removal/decannulation of tracheostomy tubes.

Rationale

Patients in ITU may have a temporary tracheostomy inserted for a number of reasons. Tracheostomies are usually inserted if the patient is mechanically ventilated for more than 7 days because tracheostomies lessen potential damage to the patient's trachea and promote patient comfort. In addition, tracheostomies are used to promote weaning from mechanical ventilation because of their ability to reduce anatomical dead space. When patients are being weaned from ventilatory support it is beneficial to reduce this amount of dead space by making air enter at a lower point (i.e. the trachea rather than the mouth/nose). Tracheostomies have the ability to reduce the anatomical dead space by about 1/3 (Field 2005), significantly reducing the workload of breathing. On return to the ward the ITU patient may still be weak and the tracheostomy is left in situ to reduce the workload of breathing until the patient is more stable. A tracheostomy may be in situ if the patient has copious secretions that they are unable to clear because of physical frailty/inability to cough sufficiently.

Preparing to receive a patient with a tracheostomy

It is important to ask ITU staff about the type and size of tracheostomy the patient has in situ and how long the patient has had the tracheostomy. Communication methods should also be discussed before transfer of the patient. It is vital that sufficient space is available for all of the following equipment:

- wall suction (portable if wall suction not available) and appropriate equipment
- suction catheters/gloves/aprons.
- water and bowl to flush tubing post suction (bowl must be kept dry between procedures)
- oxygen equipment
- tracheostomy disconnection wedge
- equipment to allow emergency replacement of tracheostomy tube if required, including:
  - tracheal dilators
  - tracheostomy tubes (same size and one size smaller)
  - manual ventilation bag/catheter mount/face mask and oxygen source
  - Guerdel airways (if unable to reinsert tracheostomy)
  - scissors (to cut tapes if trachea holder not being used))
  - 10 mL syringe (to deflate tracheostomy cuff)

♦ inner tubes for tracheostomy and appropriate cleaning equipment

♦ call buzzer/bell to summons help if required.

All of this equipment should be available at the patient's bedside and checked each shift for safety reasons. Any missing equipment should be replaced immediately.

The nurse should also have access to the following equipment, although there is no necessity to keep this at the bedside:

♦ equipment for cleaning the tracheostomy site

♦ appropriate dressings for tracheostomy

♦ ties/tapes for securing tracheostomy.

Humidification

The tracheostomy will bypass the nasopharynx and the oropharynx and as a result bypass the normal functions of this area, that is warming, humidifying, and filtering air before it reaches the alveoli. It is important that some sort of humidification device is used to prevent dry, sticky mucous plugs, which may lead to atelectasis (areas where there is alveoli collapse). It is important to ensure that the patient remains well hydrated to ensure moist mucosal membranes and thinner secretions (Field 2005). Most patients will be receiving O_2 via their tracheostomy. This will increase the potential for mucus plug formation and atelectasis as it further dries the airways and may lead to inflammation and ulceration (Adams 2005).

Various methods of humidification exist and the type selected will be dependent on the concentration of oxygen required and patient's need for removal of secretions. Humidification devices include heat moisture exchangers or water humidification.

Heat moisture exchangers

Heat moisture exchangers are commonly used for tracheostomy patients. These are plastic devices that have two 'sponges' either side. Inspired air passes through the sponges, which are warm and moist (from patient's expired air), and this enables air to be warmed and humidified. Some of these devices allow the delivery of a low concentration of oxygen through an additional side port. They are not useful if the patient is requiring more than 4 L of oxygen and in such cases wet humidification should be used instead. Nurses should ensure that these are changed as per manufacturers guidelines (usually every 24 h) as they may become a source for bacterial growth and infection. Care should also be taken to assess the suitability of these for patients with excessive loose secretions that they are able to cough out. Excessive secretions may block the device and necessitate increased frequency of changing. In this situation a water system may be better for the patient and more cost-effective.

Water humidification

In this system oxygen flows via a venturi system (other systems may be used) through a water reservoir. As the oxygen flows through the water, droplets humidify the oxygen. Different types of this humidification system are available which either use a droplet or nebulizer effect to humidify the oxygen. The net effect is moistened/humidified oxygen delivery to the patient. Again manufacturer's recommendations should be followed regarding frequency of humidification/tubing change. Staff should be aware that water vapour may return to its normal state and water may collect in the tubing. Care should be taken with tubing that it does not allow flow of water vapour collection into the patients' lungs. Some ITUs may additionally heat the oxygen as it is humidified as this provides more effective oxygenation and humidification. However, there are risks associated with scalding using heated humidifiers and these should only used when the patient can be closely observed.

Nebulizers

Nebulizers may be used as an adjunct to humidification systems. These deliver aerolized water particles that may be helpful in the clearance of secretions and may be useful in patients with thick secretions (Clotworthy *et al.* 2006). In practice, saline nebulizers (rather than water) may be given alongside other methods. They should not be used without another form of humidification. Again care should be taken to ensure that nebulizer equipment is dried thoroughly before storage and changed in accordance with manufacturer's recommendations to prevent bacterial growth.

Instillation of saline

It should be noted that the direct instillation of saline into the tracheostomy tube is *not indicated* at all. This practice has been used as an attempt to mobilize secretions, but there is no evidence that this is effective and some suggestion that it may increase the likelihood of nosocomial chest infections (bacteria colonized on the inside of the tracheostomy tube may be spread by aerosol on instillation of saline).

Removal of secretions

It may be necessary to suction the patient's tracheostomy to enable removal of secretions. This should only be carried out if necessary and if the patient is unable to cough the secretions out of the tube themselves. It should be remembered that suctioning is an invasive procedure, which may be uncomfortable and frightening for the patient (Field 2005). It should only be carried out following careful assessment of the need for suctioning and should only be undertaken by practitioners who are competent. Patient indications for suctioning may include:

- visible or audible secretions that patient are unable to clear
- patient distress
- increased workload of breathing
- clammy skin or sweating
- increased heart rate/respiratory rate
- reduced oxygen saturations
- reduced airflow at stoma site.

  Assessment for suctioning should include:

- adequate respiratory assessment (see Chapter 2)
- assessment of patient's cough reflex
- assessment of respiratory distress
- assessment of indications for suctioning.

  When suctioning the nurse should ensure that their technique results in a maximum removal of secretions and minimum complications of suctioning. Complications related to suctioning include:

- hypoxia
- laryngospasm

+ trauma to tracheal tissue

+ mucosal damage

+ cardiac arrhythmias/bradycardia/vasovagal stimulation

+ infection

+ hypertension

+ raised intracranial pressure

+ death.

Patients have also reported feelings of pain, suffocation, pressure, choking, and gagging, especially if an unskilled practitioner is undertaking technique. The technique for suctioning is included in Table 15.2. Practitioners should ensure that they are familiar with suctioning equipment as a variety of equipment is available.

Alongside coughing and suctioning it is important to remember that other factors will contribute to the effective removal of secretions, including:

+ effective patient positioning to facilitate mobilization of secretions

+ regular chest physiotherapy to provide enhanced techniques to mobilize and clear secretions

+ deep breathing exercises to minimize atelectasis and mobilization of secretions

+ appropriate humidification and use of nebulizer therapy (Field 2005).

Maintenance of tube patency/changing inner tubes

Although suctioning and effective clearance of secretions will contribute to the maintenance of tube patency, other areas need consideration. The patient should be transferred to the ward with a tracheostomy tube that has a removable inner tube. The inner tube can then be removed and cleaned to reduce the likelihood of tracheostomy obstruction. There are several general recommendations:

+ The inner tube should be cleaned and replaced at least every 4 h (2005). It may be appropriate to reduce this frequency overnight, but careful patient assessment is vital. The inner cannula should usually be changed every 4–12 h (Clotworthy et al. 2006). This may need to be more frequent if the patient has excessive or thick tenacious secretions.

+ The inner tube should be removed and cleaned with normal saline. Brushes are not recommended for the cleaning of inner tubes as they may scratch the surface and increase the colonization of bacteria.

+ The inner tubes should never be soaked or left in any type of fluid as this will increase the likelihood of infection.

+ Once cleaned the inner tube should be replaced immediately. If a temporary inner tube has been used this should be cleaned and stored in a dry clean covering (Clotworthy et al. 2006).

Care should be taken when removing the inner tube as this may cause the patient to cough excessively. Tissues should be available to trap any coughed secretions. If the patient has an ineffective cough it may be of benefit to suction before inner tube changing.

In addition to changing the inner tube the tracheostomy tube will require periodic changing, usually every 7–14 days. The need for this should be assessed individually. It is usual to wait 7 days post tube insertion to allow the stoma to form before attempting to change the tube. Practitioners who undertake this role should ensure an adequate level of competence (further details in the St George's Guidelines for the Management of Patients with Tracheostomy Tubes).

Table 15.2 Trachoestomy suctioning technique

Technique	Rationale
Adequate assessment of patient to ensure that patient is unable to clear own secretions and requires suctioning	To ensure that patient is only suctioned when required
Practitioner's hands should be decontaminated before suction (alcohol gel should suffice) Personal protective equipment for the practitioner (aprons, goggles, visor) should be worn	To reduce risk of infection to the patient and practitioner
Gain consent if patient is able and explain suctioning procedure to patient Close patient's curtains Offer reassurance to the patient	To ensure that informed consent is gained and privacy is maintained throughout procedure Suctioning may also be frightening for other patients to observe Suctioning can be traumatic for patient so reassurance that it will be quick may reduce anxiety
Ensure that all equipment is in place and in working order. This will include: a working suction unit (preferably wall mounted) set at 80–120 mmHg suction catheter(catheter size should be calculated using the formula: (size of tracheostomy tube – 2) × 2 fluid to flush suction tubing	It is important that minimal suction is used to reduce the risk of tracheal damage and lessen the hypoxic effects of suctioning It is important that the suction catheter should not be too large as this will increase the hypoxic effects of suction It will be necessary to flush tubing after suction
Hyperoxygenation is required 3 min. before suctioning is commenced (Note: Take care with COPD patients, they may only require an increase in oxygen concentration of 20%) It will also be necessary to insert a non-fenestrated inner tube if the patient has a fenestrated inner tube	This will reduce the hypoxic effects of suctioning This will prevent trauma to the tracheal mucosa
A non-touch technique should be used and clean disposable gloves applied Each suction catheter should only be passed once If a second attempt is required to clear secretions then a new catheter should be used	Infection control issues
The suction port should be uncovered and the suction catheter should be passed in to just above the carina (about a third of catheter length, the patient should begin to cough) The catheter should be withdrawn whilst suction is applied Suction should be applied continuously as the catheter is withdrawn The total duration of this procedure should be 10–15 s The suction should be released and the catheter should be wrapped up in the practitioner's glove and disposed of in a yellow bag	To minimize the hypoxic effects of suctioning and prevent trauma to tracheal mucosa and to prevent infection
The patient's oxygen should be reapplied immediately The suction tubing should be flushed with water	To maintain oxygenation

Table 15.2 Trachoestomy suctioning technique *(Continued)*

Technique	Rationale
It may be necessary to repeat this procedure, but only three attempts of suctioning should be allowed before a rest (The only exception is if the tube is blocked. The emergency procedure discussed later should then be followed.)	To avoid the occurrence of complications as this may increase with the frequency of suctioning
The patient should be reassessed throughout the procedure to ensure that: secretions have been cleared respiratory assessment is now satisfactory the patient is comfortable there is no sign of respiratory distress	It is important to evaluate the effectiveness of suctioning
Reassurance should be provided to the patient	To reduce the anxiety of the patient if needed
Suctioning and sputum appearance should be documented in patient's notes Colour, consistency, and amount of sputum should be documented Excessive sputum production may indicate the need for more frequent suctioning/referral to physiotherapist/investigations for infection	To ensure accurate documentation and appropriate future interventions
Practitioner to wash hands following suctioning procedure	To reduce risk of infection

Clotworthy et al. (2006)

COPD, chronic obstructive pulmonary disease.

Cuff management

If the cuff is inflated to prevent inhalation of pooled saliva and to maintain airway it is vital that special precautions are taken. Inflated cuffs will place an additional pressure on the tracheal tissue and must be inflated to a correct level (Woodrow 2004).

Although modern trachoestomy tubes have low-pressure cuffs to reduce the likelihood of any damage, the flexibility of these cuffs will be compromised if the cuff is over-inflated, and ulceration and eventual fibrosis of the tracheal tissue will occur. This may lead to impaired respiratory function as the patient recovers and cause chronic respiratory impairment. If the cuff is under-inflated the patient may be at risk of aspiration of any pooled saliva and associated infection. It is vital that tracheostomy cuff pressures are measured in all patients who return to the ward.

A simple manometer can be used to measure cuff pressure. Cuff pressures should be measured at least once per shift. Tracheostomy cuff pressures should be maintained between 10 and 18 mmHg/>25 cm H_2O.

Prevention of infection

The tracheostomy breaches the body's natural defences to bacteria and allows direct entry to the trachea. In addition, the use of humidification and suction has the potential to increase the risk of infection. It is vital that adequate procedures are in place to minimize the risk of infection. The Department of Health (2007) has recently published care bundles as part of the 'Saving lives, reducing infection, delivering clean and safer care' campaign. The care bundle in relation to ventilation has been linked to tracheostomy care. This identifies the need to:

- provide appropriate humidification to prevent thickened secretions
- replace all tracheostomy equipment as per manufacturers' guidelines
- replace any equipment/tubing that is visibly soiled
- prevent condensate from humidifiers from entering the patient's airways
- maintain effective hand-washing or hand decontamination before and after handling tracheostomy/suctioning
- wear gloves when dealing with tracheostomy (these may be clean rather than sterile for suctioning).

In addition to this the nurse should ensure that personal protective equipment (goggles and aprons) are worn when caring for tracheostomy.

The stoma may also become infected. Effective cleaning and dressing of the stoma site is required to prevent the development of localized infection. The tracheostomy should be redressed as required. The stoma site should be checked for signs of infection and cleaned with appropriate solution and a clean dressing applied. Most areas use specially designed trachoestomy dressings. A number of these dressing are available, including charcoal-backed or lyofoam dressings. The dressing and tube should be held in place using a specially designed tracheostomy tube holder. It is essential to have two nurses when dressing a tracheostomy to ensure that accidental displacement does not occur. The patient may cough during dressing changes so adequate assessment of need for suction before dressing change is required (further details in the St George's Guidelines for the Management of Patients with Tracheostomy Tubes).

If chest infection is suspected a sputum specimen should be obtained by either:

- encouraging the patient to expectorate
- using a sputum trap when suctioning.

If the stoma site appears to be infected then swabs should be taken.

Emergency procedure for blocked tracheostomy tubes

Tracheostomy tubes may become blocked if the patient has thick tenacious secretions or if aspects of management of the tracheostomy have been inadequate. Signs of blockage will include:

- respiratory distress
- increased workload of breathing/use of accessory muscles
- possible stridor or no air sounds from tracheostomy
- cyanosis of patient or extreme pallor
- profuse sweating of patient
- no respiratory movement, if completely blocked.

In the initial stages the patient may appear panicked and will require treatment and reassurance to facilitate removal of the obstruction. In later stages the patient's consciousness may be impaired. Initial management will focus on an ABC approach. If the patient is not breathing or does not have a cardiac output then cardiac arrest procedures should be referred to (see Chapter 13). If some respiratory effort is present and the patient has cardiac output then the procedure shown in Table 15.3 should be implemented.

Table 15.3 Procedure for blocked tracheostomy tubes

Procedure	Rationale
Call for immediate help	The patient's condition may rapidly deteriorate and assistance may be required It may be advisable to put out a medical emergency call if problem is not quickly resolved
Assess patient's respiratory function, ensure that saturation monitoring is applied, provide 15 L of oxygen and stop any NG feed that may be in progress	To assess patient's condition quickly and ensure maximum oxygenation
If the tube has an inner tube in situ remove this and assess if this rectifies the situation	The blockage may be in the inner tube and removal will then allow ventilation
Attempt to pass a suction catheter down the tracheostomy tube	This may remove blockage
If this is ineffective use the following procedure: Deflate cuff to allow breathing around the tracheostomy tube If this fails remove occluded tube and either insert new tube if able or assess to see if patient can breath through upper airway (Note: Patients with laryngectomy will not be able to do this) Deliver high-flow oxygen through tracheostomy or face mask (whichever is patent) Await medical assistance	To maintain an adequate airway and oxygenation until help arrives
If respiratory arrest commence BLS protocol	
The patient will require review by medical staff/anaesthetist if tube is changed	To ensure that tube is replaced and positioned correctly

Clotworthy et al. (2006).

BLS, basic life support.

Once airway is re-established the patient should receive frequent respiratory assessment and consideration given to the cause of the blockage, for example increase humidification, increased frequency of suctioning, regular nebulizers.

Removal/decannulation of tracheostomy tubes

Most patients will recover sufficiently to allow removal of tracheostomy. Indicators for tracheostomy removal are:

- the patient is able to cough effectively and maintain their own airway
- the patient has been assessed by the medical staff to ensure that they are free of infection
- the patient's respiratory status is stable and they are receiving less than 40% oxygen (Clotworthy et al. 2006).

However, as the initial rationale for tracheostomy insertion related to reduction of workload of breathing, it should be acknowledged that the patient will increase the workload of breathing by approximately a third when the tracheostomy is removed (Woodrow 2004). The suggested process is to progress from tracheostomy tube to speech valve then decannulation cap then final decannulation, being aware that complications may arise at each stage (Clotworthy et al. 2006).

During decannulation trials it is essential that the patient has close observation and trials should only be attempted when experienced staff are on duty and there are sufficient staff to allow close monitoring of the patient. The decannulation trial should be stopped immediately if the patient exhibits any signs of respiratory distress.

Once the tube has been removed the tracheostomy stoma should be covered with an occlusive dressing and this should be redressed to check for signs of healing (most tracheostomy stomas will heal without further intervention). Occasionally, it may be necessary to suture the site. The patient should be advised that their voice may be hoarse for a few days post decannulation.

Psychological needs of the patient on transfer from ITU

This chapter has so far prioritized and concentrated on the physical needs of the patient post ITU, predominantly because of the need to ensure the physical safety of the patient on return to the

---

Clinical link 15.1: Physical care (see Appendix for answers)

Mrs Smith is a 65-year-old lady who has been a patient on ITU for 24 days. She was admitted with pneumonia and developed type 2 respiratory failure. During her time in ITU she was ventilated and required the insertion of a tracheostomy tube. She has now been breathing without mechanical support for 5 days but still requires oxygen therapy via her tracheostomy tube. Whilst in ITU she developed renal failure and is now recovering from this (her blood results are normal). The ITU staff inform you that she took some time to establish nutritional support and as a result has lost quite a bit of weight. She has now been on bed rest for about 4 weeks and as a consequence feels quite weak. The ITU doctors think there may be some residual respiratory damage following the pneumonia as she becomes breathless on the slightest exertion. She also contracted MRSA in her tracheostomy site. She has not been sleeping well over the last 3 days and has been very anxious about her return to the ward.

- Identify the nursing priorities for this patient.
- Identify how you may prepare the ward area for this patient's transfer.
- Discuss the problems this patient may experience and identify how these may be overcome.

You are called to see Mrs Smith by the student nurse. She is coughing and wheezing but the student does not think she is able to expectorate her secretions. She is looking clammy and pale and is beginning to panic.

- Discuss your immediate assessment of this patient.
- What action may you take?

Mrs Smith is unable to expectorate and suctioning has failed to alleviate the situation as you were unable to pass the catheter into the tracheostomy successfully.

- Identify your immediate priorities.
- What resources will you require to manage this situation?

Mrs Smith's tube is now patent and her breathing is settled.

Identify steps that you may now take to prevent a reoccurrence of this problem.

ward environment. However, it is important to consider the psychological needs of the patient and the detrimental impact poor psychological care can have.

The effects of surviving critical illness often have a profound psychological effect on patients and their families (Adamson *et al.* 2004). Whilst several studies identify that many patients and their families report very positive aspects of their time in ITU (e.g. feelings of trust and security, development of positive relationships between ITU staff and patients/families) the negative psychological effect of critical illness is frequently highlighted (Magarey & McCuthceon 2005). The psychological impact of critical illness has even been linked to post-traumatic stress disorder (Adamson *et al.* 2004). Examination of the literature highlights a number of common psychological themes related to psychological care, including:

- lack of recall/amnesia
- delusions/recurrent nightmares
- fear of dying
- depression
- anxiety/panic attacks
- relationship problems.

Several researchers have undertaken phenomenological research to identify the 'lived experience of the ITU patient'. These studies have identified that often the patient is afraid to talk about their experiences for fear of being labelled and ward staff may not be aware of the impact these psychological problems are having on the patients (Magarey & McCuthceon 2005). The most common problems faced by the patient are:

- confusion and difficulty with reality
- lack of recall/amnesia/flashbacks
- nightmares and hallucinations
- depression.

Reality issues/confusion

Problems with identifying reality have been highlighted by Magarey & McCutcheon (2005), who suggest that patients feel they are moving between reality and non-reality as they struggle to come to terms with their acute illness. Periods of confusion are common post ITU and patients often struggle when attempting to make sense of their situation. McKinney & Deeney (2002) identify that patients struggle to restore meaning and comprehend what has happened to them, and suggest that patients may use discussion with ward staff and family members to attempt to cognitively unpick what has happened to them. Patients described their return to reality and associated this with the beginning of their recovery period.

Lack of recall

Some patients have coherent memories of their critical care stay and demonstrate an ability to recall events (Lof *et al.* 2008). Although this group of patients are often unable to recall events explicitly, they often report feelings of security and impressions that they were in 'safe hands'. However, more commonly patients report either little recollection or recollection of unpleasant experiences.

The reasons behind the lack of recall are complex and have been linked to a number of issues. Adamson *et al.* (2004) argue that lack of recall is compounded by length of stay in ITU rather than amount of sedation given. However, other explanations have also been explored. Some experts maintain that excessive use of benzodiazepines for sedation may cause post-ITU amnesia, whilst others suggest that the lack of recall serves as a protective mechanism that inhibits recollection of bad memories and disturbing events. Despite the lack of evidence to determine the cause it is clear that the lack of recall has a detrimental impact on the patient and means that they are not able to give meaning to the world they find themselves in. Patients have reported having limited recall about the factual events of ITU and any memories that they have tend to be unpleasant and are often persecutory in nature (Rattray & Crocker 2007), many patients have recollections of being subjected to torture or have paranoid delusions (Griffiths & Jones 1999). Patients experience anxiety and frustration in their inability to recall their experience (Hall Smith *et al.* 1997). The lack of recall can often worsen the perception of physical problems as patients are unable to find a reason for their physical symptoms.

Nightmares and hallucinations

ITU patients have also described the devastating effect of flashbacks during their convalescence. During flashbacks patients report experiencing an often negative memory associated with their intensive care stay. The flashbacks are often surreal and memories anxiety provoking and traumatic. Flashbacks have been linked to the development of psychotic states so it is important to discuss the patient's experience of a flashback (Hall Smith *et al.* 1997).

Alongside flashbacks patients often report experiencing disturbing dreams. These dreams can often be a combination of reality and unreal experiences, and patients may be able to recall factual memories about these dreams and hallucinations. Dreams may be persecutory in nature and may lead to thoughts that staff are persecuting the patient and can lead to mistrust between patients and the staff caring for them. Less frequently they may be positive and involve themes of divine intervention and family experiences. It may be useful to discuss dreams with patients to enable them to deal with any issues that arise from these dreams (Pattison 2005).

Depression

Levels of depression post ITU have been shown to be higher than in the ward population (Pattison 2005). Often patients reported perceptions that they were not recovering quickly enough and this enhanced their feelings of anxiety and depression (McKinney & Deeney 2002). Patients reported feeling incapable, worthless, and humiliated, and this, coupled with dependence on nursing staff for even the simplest of care issues, compounded feelings of dejection and despair. Several patients in this study became extremely depressed and despairing of their apparent lack of progress towards recovery. Patients often reported feelings of guilt that they had 'made their relatives suffer', further compounding their negative feelings (Lof *et al.* 2008).

Patients often find it difficult to adapt to physical and psychological changes, and feelings of anxiety and depression are common both in the immediate period after transfer and following discharge home (Strahan & Brown 2005).

Psychological support

The importance of psychological support for the patient cannot be overemphasized. Acknowledgement and assessment of psychological problems is an important step and the patient should be encouraged to discuss feelings and be made aware that psychological problems are common following critical illness. It is beneficial to offer reassurance that psychological issues are normal and transitory. Recuperation for those with psychological issues has implications for care.

Implications for nursing care

At a simplistic level encouraging the patient to discuss and confront the problems they are experiencing may enable them to understand and build a coherent story that enables them to put the experience behind them (Griffiths & Jones 1999). However, there are some important considerations, including family involvement in care, use of booklets to explain potential issues, diaries detailing the patient's ITU experience, and outreach follow-up services. In some patients the use of pharmacological measures, including antidepressants, may be considered (Pattison 2005). These should be used in conjunction with other forms of therapeutic intervention.

Family involvement

Families are often a useful resource for offering emotional support to the patient. It should be recognized that the family may also have some ongoing anxiety issues following the critical illness of their relative and the need for careful assessment and discussion to ensure that the relative is happy to undertake this important role is paramount. Pattison (2005) identifies the potential benefits of involving families in psychological support, emphasizing that the family will be able to offer emotional support on an ongoing basis whereas the professionals may only be able to offer intermittent support. The family may also be useful in trying to fill in memory gaps related to ITU, but this may not always be successful as the family may feel that it will upset the patient to discuss their time in ITU and endeavour to 'protect' the patient from upsetting memories. Relatives may not wish to discuss ITU care in detail as it is reliving a harrowing time for them as well (Griffiths & Jones 1999).

ITU booklets

Information sources form an important part of patient education and it is suggested that booklets highlighting the potential psychological effects of ITU should be provided to patients following or immediately before transfer from ITU. The development of booklets highlighting the potential for relocation stress may be useful in helping to clarify transfer issues and promote realistic expectations about convalescing after a period of illness (Hall Smith et al. 1997).

Patient diaries

The development of patient diaries began in Sweden and is still relatively new in the UK. The purpose of the patient diary is to try to 'fill in the gaps' in relation to the patient's stay in ITU by providing the patient with factual information, written in an easy-to-understand way. The diaries usually include details about activities and events that occurred. They may include photos, written extracts, and details about care and medical and nursing staff, and patients' relatives are all encouraged to contribute to the development of the diary. The diaries are useful but appropriate timing is essential (Robson 2006). It is generally suggested that patients should choose when they view their diaries. This is usually post discharge home when the patient feels able to review their ITU stay. Combe (2005) highlighted that diaries helped patients to:

♦ appreciate how ill they had been
♦ resolve issues that the patient may have about their ITU stay
♦ reorientate back to a 'normal' life by enabling debriefing
♦ facilitate communication channels between family and patient about the critical illness.

Follow-up services

One of the remits of the critical care outreach service is to provide physical and psychological support post transfer from ITU. This may be done immediately on the ward and later at follow-up clinics.

This service may be of value to the ward nurse as the outreach service are able to 'bridge the gap' for the patient in relation to ITU and ward care. They are also skilled in recognition of relocation stress and other psychological issues that the patient may experience (see Chapter 12 on outreach services for more detail on follow-up/rehabilitation).

Psychological issues beyond the ward

It is unlikely that all psychological issues patients may have had post transfer from ITU will be resolved and it should be acknowledged that the patient may have ongoing psychological (and physical) issues for some time after discharge home. Experience from follow-up clinics highlights that often issues relating to depression, anxiety, nightmares, and flashbacks continue for some time and patients are prone to panic attacks and acute anxiety on discharge home (Griffiths & Jones 1999). Patients often feel that the recovery phase of their illness is the most difficult and problems are reported relating to relationship issues, social isolation, and dependence on carers. It is essential that the patient and their family are provided with information relating to length of recovery and potential ongoing psychological issues before they are discharged home.

Needs of the family

The concept of relocation stress and subsequent psychological issues can also affect the family of the ITU patient on transfer to the ward. It is important to remember that the family may have concerns related to ward transfer and this may affect relationships between family members and ward staff. One of the predominant concerns is the reduction in the nurse: patient ratio and many relatives are fearful that the patient may not be closely observed (Robson 2006).

It has been emphasized that stress of transfer to the ward area is reduced in patients and their relatives if the process is planned and the family are encouraged to view this process as positive. Relatives often perceive ITU areas as safe, secure, and familiar, and transfer to the ward area may be viewed negatively (Coyle 2001). Absent, lacking, or untimely information is often perceived as a threat and lack of preparation can result in increased anxiety for the relatives and lead to negative views about the ward transfer.

The stress of relocation may manifest in a number of ways for the patient and their family. Particular symptoms include:

+ insecurity
+ absence of trust
+ need for excessive reassurance
+ unfavourable comparisons between staff
+ anger/outbursts.

Studies suggest it is vital, although not always logistically possible, for adequate planning. It is suggested that transition is eased if sufficient information is provided, reduction in frequency of observation/monitoring has occurred, and a plan is established. Family involvement in the transfer to the ward area and visits to the ward before transfer have been shown to lessen anxiety (Coyle 2001).

Once the patient and family have been settled to the ward area it is likely that relatives will still have a number of needs. Very little has been written in relation to care of the family following transfer to the ward but it is likely that their needs will remain similar to when the patient was in ITU. This area of relatives' needs has been extensively researched and it is probable that these results are transferable to the ward area. ITU literature has identified that relatives and carers appear to have similar needs during periods of acute illness. From this research they have established the critical care family needs inventory (Molter 1979). These needs include:

♦ the need for support

♦ the need for proximity

♦ the need for information

♦ the need for reassurance

♦ the need for comfort (interestingly this is ranked lowest!).

Alongside understanding the needs of the patient it is important to help families to identify coping strategies throughout the illness and convalescence period. A range of coping mechanisms may be exhibited by the relative (Paul & Rattray 2007). Relatives may use mechanisms such as information seeking, gathering resources, and identifying support mechanisms to enable them to cope with the situation. It is important for nurses to assess relatives' coping strategies and offer support where needed.

It is highlighted that the relatives' emotions may impact either positively or negatively on the patient's recovery and it is suggested that the family and their patient are treated holistically (Paul & Rattray 2007). The limited studies that have occurred identify that relatives often have very high anxiety levels even after the patient has been transferred from ITU. It is important that effective mechanisms are put in place to enable the relatives to feel supported, particularly as they are likely to be caring for the patient following discharge home, and that this may be a long and protracted recovery period.

Family's psychological issues beyond the ward

The long-term impact of caring for a patient following an ITU admission may also impact on the family. Family members often take on the role of carer following discharge home and this clearly impacts on their physical and mental well-being. Work by Sharland (2002) identifies that changes in family dynamics, family roles, and relationships may be affected. All of these changes further contribute to the concept of ongoing carer burden following discharge from ITU and may lead to depression and isolation for the carer as well as the patient.

Planning for transfer from ITU

The need for the ward nurse to recognize and deliver appropriate care to the patient following transfer from ITU is stressed throughout the literature. A period of critical illness can, as

Clinical link 15.2 Psychological care (see Appendix for answers)

Mrs Smith is a 65-year-old lady who has been a patient on ITU for 24 days. She was admitted with pneumonia and developed type 2 respiratory failure. She has now been transferred to the ward. The transfer was not planned well as Mrs Smith's bed was urgently needed by another patient from A&E. She was transferred to the ward at 10 o'clock yesterday evening.

The night staff are a little worried about Mrs Smith as she has been acting 'very strangely' overnight. They have told you that she did not sleep well and when she did sleep her sleep was intermittent and she appeared very stressed and anxious on awakening. She is unable to communicate because she has a tracheostomy in situ but she does appear anxious. She appears to be hallucinating.

Discuss your management/intervention.

Clinical link 15.3: Relative care (see Appendix for answers)

At 10 o'clock the next morning Mrs Smith's daughter arrives on the ward area. She is very flustered as she has only just been informed of her mother's transfer. She is very short with the ward clerk and when you see her she appears very demanding.

She wants to know why her mother was moved from ITU. She had been informed that her mother would be there for another 3 days until the tracheostomy was removed and she is very concerned that this will not be properly managed on the ward area. Her mother is in a side ward and does not have her own nurse. Discuss how you will cope with this.

highlighted, have a significant impact on a patient's physical, emotional, and psychological state. It is essential that there is adequate provision to meet the patient's needs on return to the ward. The importance of ensuring continuity of care between the critical care area and the ward is clearly significant (Watts *et al.* 2005), but the 'step down' to ward care can be accompanied by lack of continuity of care and a reduction in the depth and breadth of care provided (NICE 2007). It has been noted that smooth and well-planned transfers may be complex to organize and a number of factors may prevent or impede effective transfer planning, including:

- lack of understanding by ITU staff over the significance of transfer planning and its role in preventing readmission to ITU
- ITU staff not recognizing planning as an important aspect of their role
- transfer planning occurring too late
- lack of ITU beds, causing transfer from ITU to be hurried and unplanned
- inability to involve ward staff in planning because of the busyness of ward nurses (Robson 2006).

In order to make the transfer process more seamless and to reduce the potential problems and significant issues that the ITU patient may experience on transfer to the ward there is now more emphasis on transfer planning and the need to include other practitioners, for example outreach nurses, to ensure appropriate transfer coordination between the ward and the ITU staff. Outreach teams may have several roles in supporting patients on transfer, including educational, planning, and supportive roles. The role of outreach in educating ward nurses about the care required following critical illness is stressed (Cutler & Robson 2006). They may also be instrumental in developing care packages for patient groups post ITU, for example formulating care packages for patients with specific needs, for example patients transferred from ITU with tracheostomies, and offering practical support to ward nurses when caring for these patients (see Chapter 12 on outreach services).

Alongside the expanding role of outreach in enhancing ITU transfer care, NICE (2007) have also been instrumental in encouraging the need to develop effective and seamless transfers from ITU to the ward environment and the report makes a number of key recommendations relating to the timing of transfer and effective planning for post-ITU care.

Transfer timing guidelines

The patient should be transferred out of ITU as early in the day as possible and transfer out of ITU between 22:00 and 07:00 should be avoided where possible. If it is required a clinical risk should be documented as per local protocol.

Planning and support guidelines

Alongside identifying the need for appropriately timed transfers NICE (2007) also consider the impact on the ward and the need for appropriate information for the ward staff when discharging a patient from ITU. The report makes the following recommendations in relation to planning/handover of the patient:

♦ The critical care area transferring team and the receiving ward should take shared responsibility for the care of the patient being transferred. They should ensure:

  • that continuity is encouraged by using structured handovers and care plans
  • that the ward, with support from outreach, can deliver appropriate care.

♦ The need for a structured formal handover of care was identified. This should include:

  • a summary of critical care stay
  • a monitoring and investigation plan
  • a plan for ongoing treatment
  • physical and rehabilitation needs
  • psychological and emotional needs
  • specific communication or language needs.

In order to support effective care post transfer NICE made the recommendation that patients should only be transferred out of ITU if the ward area has the appropriate resources to be able to deliver the agreed care plan. NICE have also emphasized the importance of patient and family/carer involvement in care planning post transfer from ITU.

Whilst the importance of effective planning for transfer of ITU patients and appropriate support on the ward has been emphasized, the question of care delivery for these patients once on the ward has not really been addressed. There is a lack of evidence identifying structures/care delivery that may enhance the care these patients receive and NICE simply identify the need to assess these patients using track and trigger systems so that any deterioration in condition can be quickly identified. Close monitoring is of particular importance for those patients who may have been transferred early from ITU due to pressure on beds. Understanding of the patient's physical and psychological needs and delivering care to meet these needs is also of great importance as is adequate preparation for receiving the patient in the ward area.

Preparation for receiving an ITU patient

A number of steps may be taken to improve the patient's experience of transfer from ITU to the ward and enable the patient and their family to make adjustments to changing care delivery. Some of these steps may occur before the patient leaves ITU and involve ITU and ward staff. Others involve ward staff and outreach teams.

Before transfer to the ward

In a planned ITU transfer a number of important issues may have been addressed before the patient is transferred that may lessen the impact of a changing environment. Cutler & Robson (2006) suggest the following may be useful:

♦ Reduction in monitoring to enable preparation for the ward area where monitoring may be less intense.

♦ Reduction in nurse patient ratio on ITU to prepare the patient for the inevitable reduction following transfer.

- Staff stressing the move to the ward as a positive experience that indicates the patient's condition is improving.
- Introduction to the ward staff before transfer to enable the patient and their family to meet the new staff who will be caring from them.
- Family visit to ward area before transfer.
- Discussion of patients needs/resources required before transfer will enable effective planning and management of ward resources.
- Encouraging the patient to discuss the transfer and to ask questions.
- Ensuring that the bed area and any resources required to care for the patient are prepared before accepting patient. This may include:
  - oxygen/suction equipment
  - tracheostomy equipment
  - any emergency equipment that may be required
  - monitoring equipment if required
  - intravenous pumps and intravenous equipment
  - barrier nursing equipment (if required)
  - special mattresses/special beds
  - nasogastric feeding equipment
  - comfortable chair (if patient is able to sit out of bed)
  - manual handling equipment
  - communication aids/call buzzer
  - fluids/food if able to take oral intake
  - any other additional equipment that may be required.
- Ensuring sufficient staffing levels and skill mix to care for the patient and their family.

Note: Any lack of physical resources/staffing issues should ideally be addressed before accepting patient back to the ward area.

On transfer to the ward

Again a number of factors have been identified that may facilitate the patients transfer once in the ward environment and provide continuity of patient care. These include:

- A welcome and introduction to the ward and ward staff who will be caring for them on arrival on the ward.
- Adequate handover from ITU staff that focuses on the patient's current care needs rather than critical illness.
- An adequate care plan from ITU that highlights the patient's ongoing care planning requirements.
- Settling into the ward area and ensuring patient comfort.
- Introduction to ward routine and layout for patient and their family.
- Explaining patient call system to patient and their family.
- Ensuring that nurses caring for patient are familiar with the complex physical and psychological needs of the patient post transfer from ITU and are familiar with the patient's individualized care requirements.

- Use of a track and trigger system to score physiological observations to enable early detection of any deterioration that may necessitate return to ITU.
- Liaison with outreach team to facilitate smooth transfer and provide support and education to patient and staff.
- Outreach team to visit the patient on the ward to facilitate early identification of any problems.
- Development of clear communication channels between patient, family, and ward staff to ensure continuity of care.

Whilst these suggestions are not exhaustive it is hoped that they will in part, alongside other measures such as effective transfer planning and outreach liaison, improve the continuity of care delivery for the ITU patient and facilitate early detection of those patients who may still deteriorate.

End of chapter test

It is important that you understand both the theory related to patients following transfer from ITU and the practicalities of safely caring for this group of vulnerable patients. In order to test your knowledge and apply this knowledge to clinical practice you should undertake the following assessments with an appropriately trained member of staff in clinical practice. This chapter will test general care for the patient post ITU transfer. A separate assessment is provided for tracheostomy care and should be utilized if you are caring for a patient with a tracheostomy tube in situ. If you are unable to answer any questions it may be helpful to revisit the section in this chapter.

Patient post ITU (general care)

Knowledge assessment

Work with your mentor/supervisor in practice and ask them to test your knowledge in relation to the following. Incorrect answers/lack of knowledge will require further revision/re-reading of this chapter.

- Discuss the rationale for the vulnerability of the patient following transfer from ITU.
- Analyse which groups of patients are particularly at risk following transfer from ITU.
- Evaluate the need for effective transfer planning, highlighting issues that may cause problematic transfer.
- Discuss the need for effective communication and understand some of the barriers that may prohibit this.
- Describe the concept of relocation stress and discuss how patients/carers/family members may exhibit signs of relocation stress.
- Analyse the potential physical needs of patients following transfer from ITU.
- Analyse the potential psychological needs of patients following transfer from ITU.
- Examine the need for follow up and liaison with the outreach services to promote effective care delivery.
- Describe the need of family members/carers following transfer from ITU, highlighting specific issues that may occur.
- Analyse the need for transfer planning and timely transfer from ITU.

Skills assessment

Work with your mentor/supervisor in practice and ask them to assess your ability to care for a patient post ITU using the following criteria where appropriate. Note: You may not be able to demonstrate all these skills. Ask your mentor/supervisor to give you feedback on areas that you did well and areas that may require improving.

- Ensures effective communication between ward and ITU staff before transfer.
- Identifies the need for appropriate resources following liaison with ITU and ensures that all resources (staff and equipment) are available before the patient's admission to the ward.
- Discusses patient needs and care plan with ITU staff and ward team.
- Welcomes patient and their family to ward area and introduces staff member/s responsible for ongoing ward care.
- Ensures that patient is settled into ward area and has call bell available.
- Orientates patient and their family to ward environment.
- Provides appropriate monitoring to ensure assessment needs identified in care plan are met.
- Utilizes track and trigger system to identify any cause of concern and escalates any patient deterioration appropriately.
- Ensures that physical needs are identified and care plan developed to meet patient needs.
- Provides appropriate support for the patient to ensure that their physical needs are met.
- Ensures that psychological needs are identified and care plan developed to meet patient needs.
- Provides appropriate support for the patient to ensure that their psychological needs are met.
- Encourages open communication between patient/family members and ward team.
- Identifies need for frequent ward team review of patient/contact with ITU support services, for example outreach team.

Patient post ITU (tracheostomy care)

Knowledge assessment

Work with your mentor/supervisor in practice and ask them to test your knowledge in relation to the following. Incorrect answers/lack of knowledge will require further revision/re-reading of this chapter.

- Discuss rationale for patient's tracheostomy insertion.
- Describe the altered pathophysiology and associated complications that may occur as a result of altered physiology.
- Analyse the need for two-part tracheostomy tube (inner tube).
- Describe the essential equipment that is needed when caring for a patient with a tracheostomy.
- Examine the need for appropriate humidification and discusses rationale for selected humidification system.
- Analyse rationale for clearance of secretion, discussing potential complications that can occur during suctioning.

- Describe when it is appropriate to use endotracheal suctioning technique and describe how suctioning should be performed.
- Discuss the rationale for close respiratory assessment and methods that may be appropriate to assess the respiratory function of a patient with a tracheostomy tube.
- Explains how tracheostomy blockage may present and discusses management of a patient with a blocked tube.
- Discuss need for appropriate cuff management and complications that may occur if cuff is over- or under-inflated. Analyses recommendations (from the Department of Health Saving lives package) that relate to chest infection prevention.
- Describe how the stoma should be cared for (to include redressing/types of dressing and infection prevention).
- Evaluate the communication problems faced by the patient and examines how these may be overcome.
- Examine the swallowing difficulties of the patient with a tracheostomy.
- Examine the role of the critical care outreach team in managing the patient with a tracheostomy.
- Discuss the rationale and procedure for readiness for decannulation.

Skills assessment

Work with your mentor/supervisor in practice and ask them to assess your ability to care for a patient with a tracheostomy using the following criteria where appropriate. Note: You may not be able to demonstrate all these skills. Ask your mentor/supervisor to give you feedback on areas that you did well and areas that may require improving.

- Ensures all equipment required for caring for patient with tracheostomy tube is available.
- Carries out check for emergency equipment each shift.
- Provides patient with emergency call bell, performs appropriate respiratory assessment, and carefully documents results.
- Assesses need for humidification and selects appropriate system.
- Ensures that humidification system is set up and changed as per manufacturer's guidelines.
- Prevents any condensate from humidification system from entering the patients airways.
- Checks tracheostomy cuff pressure and adds or removes air from cuff if over/under inflated.
- Ensures suctioning equipment is in working order.
- Takes appropriate infection control precautions when carrying out tracheal suctioning.
- Assesses the need for clearance of secretion and evaluates need for suctioning.
- Performs suction technique as per local guidelines and assesses patient for complications associated with suctioning.
- Reassesses patient following suctioning and evaluates need for further intervention.
- Cleans suction equipment and stores appropriately, ensuring suctioning equipment is readily available for next patient suctioning episode.
- Provides psychological support to the patient during suctioning.
- Observes for signs of respiratory distress that may indicate tube blockage and takes appropriate action.

- Changes inner tube as per trust guidelines, ensuring that inner tube is cleaned and stored in a dry clean container.
- Redresses tracheostomy stoma site as per trust guidelines.
- Provides alternative forms of communication/liaises with
- Speech and language therapy team (adapted from the School of Nursing and Midwifery skills template, University of Brighton).

References

Adamson, H., Murgo, M. Boyle, M. *et al.* (2004) Memories of intensive care and experiences of survivors of a critical illness: An interview study. *Int. Crit. Care Nurs.* **20**, 257–63.

Adams, S.K. (2005) *Critical Care Nursing: Science and Practice.* Oxford University Press, Oxford.

Ball, C. (2005) Ensuring a successful discharge from intensive care. *Int. Crit. Care Nurs.* **21**, 1–4.

Ball, C., Kirby, M., and Williams, S. (2003) Effect of the critical care outreach team on patient survival to discharge from hospital and readmission to critical care: non randomised population based study. *BMJ* **327**, 1014–7.

Clotworth, N. et al. and St Georges Health Care Trust (2006) *Guidelines for the care of patient's with tracheostomy tubes.* St Georges Healthcare NHS Trust. Smiths Medical International Limited, Watford.

Combe, D. (2005) The use of patient diaries in an intensive care unit. *Nurs. Crit. Care.* **10**(1), 31–3.

Coyle, M.A. (2001) Transfer anxiety: preparing to leave intensive care. *Int. Crit. Care Nurs.* **17**, 138–43.

Crocker, C.A. (2005) Multidisciplinary follow up clinic after patients' discharge from ITU. *Br. J. Nurs.* **12**(15), 910–4.

Cutler, L. and Robson, W. (2006) *Critical Care outreach.* Wiley, Chichester.

Daly, K. and Chang, R. (2001) Reduction in mortality after inappropriate early discharge from intensive care logistic regression triangle. *BMJ.* **322**, 1274–6.

Department of Health (2000) *Comprehensive Critical Care, a Review of Adult Critical Care Services.* HMSO, London.

Department of Health (2007) *Saving Lives: Reducing Infection, Delivering Clean and Safe Care.* HMSO, London.

Duke, G.J., Green, J.V., and Briedis, J.H. (2004) Night shift discharge from intensive care unit increases the mortality risk of ICU survivors. *Anaesth. Int. Care.* **32**, 697–701.

Field, D. (2005) In: Sheppard, M. and Wright, M. (2005) *Principles and Practice of High Dependency Nursing.* Bailliere Tindall, Edinburgh.

Goldfrad, C. and Rowan, K. (2000) Consequences of discharges from intensive care at night. *Lancet.* **1355**(9210), 1138–42.

Goldhill, D. and Sumner, A. (1998) Outcome of intensive care patients in a group of British intensive care units. *Crit. Care Med.* **26**, 1337–45.

Griffiths, R.D. and Jones, C. (1999) ABC of intensive care. Recovery from intensive care. *BMJ* **319**, 427–9.

Haines, S., Crocker, C., and Leducq, M. (2001) Providing continuity of care for patients transferred from ICU. *Professional Nurse.* **17**(1), 17–21.

Hall Smith, J., Ball, C., and Coakley, J. (1997) Follow up services and the development of a clinical nurse specialist. *Int. Care Int. Crit. Care Nurs.* **13**, 243–8.

Lof, L., Berggren, L., and Ahlstrom, G. (2008) ICU patients recall of emotional reactions in the trajectory from falling critically ill to hospital discharge: Follow ups after 3 and 12 months. *Int. Crit. Care Nurs.* 24, 108–21.

Magarey, J.M. and McCuthceon, H. (2005) Fishing with the dead—recall of memories from the ICU. *Int Crit. Care Nurs.* **21**(6), 344–56.

McKinney, A.A. and Deeney, P. (2002) Leaving the intensive care unit: a phenomenological study of the patients experience. *Int. Crit. Care Nurs.* **18**, 320–31.

Molter, N.C. (1979) Needs of relatives of critically ill patients: a descriptive study. *Heart and Lung.* **8**(2), 332–9.

Moore, T. and Woodrow, P. (2004) *High Dependency Nursing Care: Observation, Support and Practice.* London, Routledge.

NICE (2007) *Acutely Ill Patients in Hospital: Recognition of and Response to Acute Illness of Adults in Hospital.* HMSO, London.

Pattison, N. (2005) Psychological implications of admission to critical care. *Br. J. Nurs.* **13**(13), 708–14.

Paul, F. and Rattray, J. (2007) Short and long term impact of critical illness on relatives: Literature review. *J. Adv. Nurs.* **62**(3), 276–92.

Rattray, J. and Crocker, C. (2007) The intensive care follow up clinic: Current provision and future direction. *Nurs. Crit. Care.* **12**(1), 1–3.

Robson, W. (2006) In: Cutler, L. and Robson, W. (2006) *Critical Care Outreach.* Wiley, Chichester.

Sharland, C. (2002) In: Griffiths, R.D. and Jones, C. (2002) *Intensive Care After Care.* Butterworth Heinemann, Oxford.

Strahan, E. and Brown, R. (2005) A qualitative study of the experiences of patients following transfer from intensive care. *Int. Crit. Care Nurs.* **21**(3), 160–72.

Watts, R., Gardner, H., and Pierson, J. (2005) Factors that impede or enhance critical care nurses discharge planning practices. *Int. Crit. Care Nurs.* **21**(5), 302–14.

Whittaker, J. and Ball, C. (2000) Discharge for intensive care, a view from the wards. *Int. Crit. Care Nurs.* **16**, 135–43.

Woodrow, P. (2004) In: Moore, T. and Woodrow, P. (2004) *High Dependency Nursing Care: Observation, Support and Practice.* London, Routledge.

Chapter 16

Documentation in acute care

Christine Spiers

Chapter contents

Documentation of the health records of our patients is an integral part of nursing practice. It is vital that nurses working in acute care maintain clear, comprehensive, and accurate records of their health interventions. These include not only the records of nursing care, but also all monitoring charts, medication charts, rhythm strips, and records of telephone conversations. This chapter discusses the nurses' professional accountability in relation to their record keeping and the legislative standards that apply to their practice. This chapter will therefore discuss:

- the purpose of documentation and health records
- the principles of good documentation, including content and style of the health record
- common deficiencies identified in health records
- accountability and legal imperatives
- 'Do not attempt resuscitation' orders
- access to health records
- electronic health records
- the audit of documentation/health records.

Learning outcomes

This chapter will enable you to:

- understand the purpose and principles of good record keeping
- discuss the recommended content and style of health records, and consider some common deficiencies in health records
- discuss nurses' professional accountability and consider the legal responsibilities of practitioners in relation to record keeping
- review the principle of access to health records and the statutory provisions which govern this
- consider the benefits and limitations of electronic record systems
- consider the important principles that underpin the implementation of a 'Do not attempt resuscitation' order
- examine the need for auditing patients' records.

Introduction

Clear, comprehensive, and accurate documentation provides a record of the clinical judgement and critical thinking used to provide nursing care. It should provide an account of nursing's unique contribution to the patient's care and may include any written or electronically generated information about patient care or service provision.

Record keeping is a fundamental tool for professional practice. The public (and by implication our patients) expect nurses to maintain high standards of record keeping. The Nursing and Midwifery Council (Nursing and Midwifery Council 2008) state quite clearly that record keeping is *not* an optional extra to be fitted in if circumstances allow.

The aim of good record keeping is to ensure that it is clearly evident in the records what care and treatment has been given, what care is currently being given, any care which may have been omitted (and why), and the aims of future care (Dimond 2005a).

What is a health record?

According to the Data Protection Act (1998), a health record is any electronic or paper document recorded about a person for managing their health care. It includes all sorts of documentation: medical notes, nursing notes, X rays, pathology reports, pharmacy records, observation charts, neurological observation charts, medication cards, and fluid balance charts. Together they form the record of the care given to a patient whilst under your care.

Purpose of documentation

Documentation serves many purposes:

- **Facilitates communication:** Accurate records and documentation enable nurses to communicate about the care provided and to ensure that other nurses and care providers have access to their assessments of the patient, the care delivered, and an evaluation of the care and the results of any interventions given. It should also facilitate dissemination of information between members of the interdisciplinary healthcare team.

- **Early detection of changes in a patient's condition:** In acute care settings, patients may deteriorate very quickly. The institution of appropriate early warning systems or track-and-trigger systems is essential as these systems track changes in physiology and warn of impending physiological collapse. NICE (2007) have recommended that all acute care trusts should implement track-and-trigger scoring systems for all patients in acute hospital wards.

- **Ensures accountability:** Accurate documentation is a valuable tool for demonstrating nursing accountability and giving credit to their professional practice. Nurses' documentation may be used in legal proceedings such as lawsuits, coroner inquests, or disciplinary hearings.

- **Legal requirements:** Nurses are required to make and keep records of patient care, including nursing assessments, care plans, and ongoing notes of care for the patient. The requirements for documentation are drawn from legislation, case law, and standards of practice, and must be adhered to.

- **Ensures high standards of clinical care:** The Nursing and Midwifery Council (2008) state that the quality of the record keeping is a reflection that the practitioner is professional and skilled. An evidence-based care plan forms part of that record. Poor record keeping may be an indication of wider problems with professional practice. Good record keeping is also vital to high-quality care and to the development of nursing research.

Principles of documentation

It is a basic principle that records of care are kept and maintained in an up-to-date state. It is an essential aspect of care for the patient, and records should be sufficiently detailed to show that you have discharged your duty of care to the patient (Dimond 2005a). Nursing documentation should clearly describe:

* an assessment of the patient's health status, including any particular allergies, and relevant past medical, surgical, social, and medication history
* a plan of care, reflecting the needs of the patient and including the medical changes to care as documented in the medical notes
* a record of the nursing interventions carried out and an evaluation of the nursing interventions
* a record of any sudden deterioration in patients and a record of your reaction and outcomes, which should include all relevant assessment data and may also include keeping monitoring strips and records of blood pressure recordings
* any specific information pertaining to the patient, such as resuscitation decisions or advance directives—decisions about care are often taken on a multidisciplinary basis and health records should corroborate the decisions of other team members.

Essentially record keeping serves two functions. Firstly, an accurate record forms an integral part of the nursing management of the patient and allows the patient's progress to be monitored and a clinical history to be developed. Secondly, it serves a very important legal function, helping to protect practitioners if defence of their actions is required (Jevon & Ewens 2007).

The content and style of a health record

Good record keeping is a product of good teamwork and an important tool in promoting high-quality care. The Nursing and Midwifery Council (2008) cite a number of key issues related to good records and record keeping, many of which relate to the content and style of the record. The Nursing and Midwifery Council factsheet (2008) highlights that records should:

* be factual, consistent, and accurate
* be recorded as soon as possible after an event has occurred
* be recorded clearly in such a manner that the text cannot be erased or deleted
* be recorded in such a way that any justifiable alteration or additions are dated, timed, and signed
* be clearly attributable to a named person in an identifiable role, accurately dated, timed, and signed with the signature clearly printed alongside
* not include abbreviations, jargon, irrelevant speculation, offensive, or subjective statements
* be readable when photocopied or scanned.

Common deficiencies in record keeping

Almost every report by the Health Service Commissioner related to complaints in the NHS identifies that record-keeping deficiencies were a key element of the complaint and poor record keeping had hampered the care that was provided and restricted healthcare practitioners' ability to defend their practices (Dimond 2005b).

There are numerous areas where nursing records are found to be woefully lacking. Dimond (2005b) describes an extensive list of potential areas of concern including:

♦ absence of clarity
♦ illegibility
♦ failure to record actions when problems are identified
♦ missing information
♦ spelling mistakes
♦ decimal point errors
♦ inaccurate records
♦ failure to provide contemporaneous record entries
♦ use of jargon and abbreviations
♦ failures in communication between healthcare professionals
♦ failure to document:
  • care given
  • special needs
  • personal conversations and telephone conversations.

Poor nursing documentation does not only relate to nursing records but is evident more widely in relation to the use of various patient assessment forms on acute care wards. The Intensive Care National Audit Research Committee (ICNARC) commissioned a study evaluating track-and-trigger assessment tools (Rowan *et al.* 2007). The study found that poor documentation in relation to track-and-trigger tools was still evident in some areas. The ICNARC study (Rowan *et al.* 2007) found in particular that the lack of impact of track-and-trigger scores and response algorithms or protocols could be attributed to:

♦ lack of completion of track-and-trigger scores
♦ inaccurate scoring of track-and-trigger scores
♦ inaccurate interpretation of track-and-trigger scores.

Whilst this might seem rather negative, the ICNARC study (Rowan *et al.* 2007) highlighted numerous examples where ward nurses had completed track-and-trigger scores appropriately, called the treating team and critical care outreach team, and then initiated appropriate nursing interventions. In some cases ward nurses were frustrated by failure of the junior medical staff to respond to their call for help when the patient was triggering or in some instances whilst junior medical staff had responded effectively, senior medical staff were difficult to contact and did not always respond in a timely fashion. Incidents where medical teams were asked to attend the patient, but failed to respond, *must* be documented in the nursing records.

Clear legible records

It is essential that record entries can be read and understood, and this begins with the clarity of the entry. The use of black ink on white paper is good practice as this provides the greatest contrast and facilitates photocopying if needed. Clear handwritten entries are a requirement of your duty of care to a patient and this legibility also extends to the signature of the person who made the entry.

Records must be clear and unambiguous; care to be implemented and progress recorded should be clearly stated. The use of colloquialisms, for example 'the patient had a good day', or abbreviations must be avoided. There are numerous examples in case law where illegible handwriting has resulted in drug errors or overdose and where misinterpretation of abbreviations has caused errors or even the death of patients (Dimond 2005c). For example, 'PID' as a diagnosis, may imply either 'pelvic inflammatory disease' or 'prolapsed intervetebral disc' and 'CHD' may relate to 'coronary heart disease' or 'congenital heart disease'. Some trusts have an agreed list of abbreviations and these may be utilized, but it is unlikely that there will ever be an agreed list nationally. If abbreviations are to be used, nurses must not include any abbreviations other than those listed in their local trust policy guidelines.

The use of jargon to convey offensive, subjective remarks about patients is also unacceptable and cryptic comments have no place in medical records. Remember in litigation your records will be exposed to intense scrutiny and if records are not professional, the assumption will be that your care is not professional either. The Nursing and Midwifery Council (2008) advises practitioners that they should assume that entries made in a patient's record will at some point be scrutinized and thus maintenance of high standards of record keeping is imperative.

Accurate records

Each entry must be signed with the professional's name together with their position or professional role. Entries should be identified with the date (day, month, year) and time using the 24-h clock. Any alterations may be made by scoring out with a single line so as not to obscure the original entry. The 'erased' error should be dated, timed, and signed. Liquid correcting fluid should not be used.

Records should be written at the time of the event (or as close afterwards as is possible). Such contemporaneous records are vital for ensuring a true, reliable, and accurate record of care given and events encountered; records should also be chronologically arranged. The documentation should allow information to be organized in such a way that it presents a true picture of the patient's needs, the nurse's actions, and the patient's response.

Missing records

The ICNARC report (Rowan *et al.* 2007) highlighted that frequently there was incomplete documentation about a patient's progress recorded in the nursing notes. This was particularly evident when a patient had become acutely unwell and triggered a score requiring escalation of care; this was frequently not documented in the nursing notes. There were also numerous examples where documentation was missing on the track-and-trigger scoring system. Despite numerous research studies pointing to the importance of basic vital signs observations and in particular to the importance of monitoring respiratory rate and fluid balance (Chellel *et al.* 2002; Cretikos *et al.* 2008), these continue to be the most frequently omitted area of nursing documentation. As highlighted in Chapters 2 and 11 the respiratory system provides an important physiological indicator to a deteriorating patient (Cretikos *et al.* 2008). It is therefore alarming that there is strong evidence that monitoring the respiratory rate continues to be the most frequently omitted observation in the early warning scores (EWS) documentation (Rowan *et al.* 2007).

Legislative requirements

Good record keeping helps to protect the welfare of patients, and registrants have a professional and a legal duty of care. Nurses are required to make and keep records, and this is a critical aspect of a nurse's duty of care. Failing to meet these requirements may lead to your name being removed from the professional register. In addition, falsifying a record, breaching patient confidentiality, and providing false statements may also constitute professional misconduct (Nursing and

> ## Box 16.1 Nurse receives 5-year caution order (Nursing and Midwifery Council 2008)
>
> In February 2009, the Nursing and Midwifery Council recorded the case of a nurse who 'failed to assess Patient A before reducing the frequency of observations from 30 min to hourly' on a night shift. The same nurse, who was in charge of the ward at the time, 'failed to ensure that the patient was observed after 20.30 h' by other practitioners on the ward. The patient died unexpectedly at 04:00.
>
> The nurse received a 5-year caution order from the Nursing and Midwifery Council for misconduct.

Midwifery Council 2008). The Nursing and Midwifery Council Fitness to Practise hearings include numerous examples where nurses have received cautions, interim orders, or have been struck off the register for failure to maintain appropriate records. An example is included in Box 16.1.

Patient records are often used in evidence to investigate a complaint at local level, in criminal proceedings, or as evidence by the Nursing and Midwifery Council Fitness to Practise Committee, which considers complaints about registrants. It is essential, therefore, that your records are able to provide a clear audit trail of the care given, decisions made, and communication with other healthcare practitioners, the patient, and their relatives.

Where delegation of record keeping to a healthcare support staff (HCSS) or a student nurse has occurred the registrant should countersign any entry in the records and remain cognisant that they remain accountable for any actions or omissions of the HCSS or student nurse (Nursing and Midwifery Council 2008).

Failure to document actions taken

Courts of law take the approach 'if it has not been recorded, then it has not been done' (Nursing and Midwifery Council 2008). Registered healthcare practitioners are required to use their professional judgement to decide what should be recorded. If a staff nurse on a busy medical assessment unit requests that a medical practitioner attends to a deteriorating patient, but the request is ignored, this *must* be recorded in the nursing notes. Frequently, nurses refer such requests to the critical care outreach team, who are more likely to respond in a timely fashion, but it remains important to document inactions as well as actions (Rowan *et al*. 2007).

Failure to record important items such as failure to administer medications to patients may result in other practitioners administering medications on the following shift, resulting in overdoses for patients. The Nursing and Midwifery Council Fitness to Practise Committee records numerous examples of medication errors and omissions (Nursing and Midwifery Council 2008).

Written communication orders and verbal communications

The National Patient Safety Agency (NPSA) report (National Patient Safety Agency 2007) describes communication difficulties between nurses and doctors as the biggest problem area in the deterioration of events. When a patient is deteriorating nurses may not communicate this clearly to the doctor and appear unable to convey the urgency of the situation. Consequently, the doctors are faced with the difficult decision about how urgently a patient requires help, based on a telephone call. The NPSA report (2007) also gives examples where medical decisions are written

Table 16.1 Areas of communication difficulty in acute care practice (National Patient Safety Agency 2007)

Area of concern	Examples of failure in practice
Incomplete and inadequate written communication	Observations and EWS scores undertaken but not documented Incomplete records such as fluid balance, EWS, and other observation charts Timing of observations not recorded, initials of staff difficult to read, and illegible documentation
Lack of or inadequate communication between doctor and nurse	Doctors do not adequately communicate with nurses regarding patient's plan of care Nurses do not communicate clearly with doctors in a manner which reflects the urgency of the situation
Lack of or inadequate communication between nurses	Poor nursing handovers which include either too much information (overload) or insufficient detail, resulting in lack of prioritization Poorly documented contact details (name and bleep number of doctor responsible for care), resulting in delays in contact during deterioration

EWS, early warning scores.

in the patient's notes, but because nursing and medical documentation is kept in separate folders these orders are not always read by the nursing staff (and vice versa). Where tragedy results in healthcare settings, the inquiry report frequently cites failures in communication, both written and verbal, as the principle reason.

The National Patient Safety Agency (2007) identify three key areas where there are problems with communication in acute care practice (see Table 16.1).

Documenting resuscitation status in patients

It is vital that timely discussions with regard to the status of patients in acute care settings are instituted. 'Do not attempt resuscitation' (DNAR) orders are generally accepted to be appropriate in the following three situations:

- if resuscitation is unlikely to be successful
- if it is known that the patient does not wish to be resuscitated
- if successful resuscitation would not result in an increased length of life or quality of life for the patient.

The Resuscitation Council (UK) (2009) recommends that a DNAR policy should ensure the following:

- effective recording of the DNAR decisions
- effective communication and explanation of DNAR decisions where appropriate to the patient
- effective recording of the DNAR decision to the patient's family and friends, whilst respecting confidentiality as appropriate
- effective communication of DNAR decisions between all healthcare workers involved with caring for the patient.

A recent audit of a district general hospital's policy on DNAR identified disturbingly poor levels of knowledge in a number of areas (Haskett 2008). These included confusion over who should

Box 16.2 Auditing your ward records for DNAR decisions

Clinical issues for consideration: audit your own ward records.

♦ How many patients on your ward have a DNAR order?

♦ Is this clearly noted in the medical and nursing notes?

♦ Are other healthcare professionals, such as physiotherapists and pharmacists, aware of the DNAR decision?

♦ Is the DNAR order signed and dated by the consultant in charge of the patient's care?

♦ Has the DNAR order been discussed with the patient and the relatives if appropriate?

♦ Has the DNAR order been reviewed recently?

♦ Are DNAR decisions revoked on discharge of the patient?

   Discuss this at your ward meeting and with senior members of staff and the multidisciplinary team.

sign the DNAR form and the treatments which should be continued once a DNAR decision was in place. Most importantly, serious concerns were highlighted with regard to documentation issues surrounding DNAR decisions. In his survey Haskett (2008) found that:

♦ only 45% of forms had a Consultant signature

♦ in 58% of cases the names of the relatives with whom the decision was discussed were not recorded

♦ inadequate reasons for the DNAR order were recorded

♦ DNAR decisions were not regularly reviewed

♦ DNAR decisions were not revoked on the patient's discharge from hospital.

Advance directives/advance statements

Advance statements are founded on the principles of patient choice and informed consent (see Chapter 9). An advanced directive allows a patient's wishes about possible future treatment to be stated in advance. It allows patients to decide, when competent, the level of treatment they might wish to receive in the event of loss of capacity (Jones & Jones 2007). For example, if a patient has stated, in an advanced directive, that in the event of a cardiac arrest they would not wish to be resuscitated, this decision must be respected. Advance directives are legally binding documents that allow healthcare professionals to take into account the patient's known wishes. If a patient has an advanced directive in place all members of the healthcare team must be made aware of this and it must be clearly documented in the patient's notes.

Security and confidentiality

All staff have a duty to act in accordance with the Data Protection Act (1998) and to protect the confidentiality of the patient record at all times. All staff should ensure that:

♦ records are stored in a safe and secure place

♦ records are filed in a systematic manner to allow for easy retrieval

♦ electronic records are protected by the use of secure passwords.

Access to health records

There are several statutory provisions that relate to the disclosure of records and privacy rights, namely the Access to Health Records Act (1990), the Data Protection Act (1998), the Freedom of Information Act (2000), and the Records Management: NHS Code of Practice (2006).

♦ The Access to Health Records Act (1990) allows patients the right to access their manually maintained health records. Access to the health records of a deceased person is also governed by the Access to Health Records Act (1990).

♦ The Data Protection Act (1998) gives patients the rights to access their computer-generated health records.

♦ The Freedom of Information Act (2000) was established to give the general public the right to obtain information held by public authorities (including the NHS).

♦ Records Management: NHS Code of Practice (Department of Health 2006) is a guide to the required standards of practice in the management of records for those who work in the NHS.

Patients have the right to be informed about personal data held about them and they have rights of access to their health records. Patients may request access to their health data under the provisions of the Data Protection Act (1998). Requests for access are made in writing to the person in charge of keeping the record—the data controller. It is likely that patients may require help from a health professional when accessing their notes to facilitate understanding. There are, however, some instances when information cannot or will not be disclosed, for example:

♦ information that would breach another patient's confidentiality (Nursing and Midwifery Council 2008)

♦ access may not be granted to any information that, in the opinion of the appropriate health professional, might cause serious harm to the patient or another person

♦ there are specific exemptions for children

♦ access to records of deceased patients (access to these records is granted within the provisions of the Access to Health Records Act 1990).

Patient involvement

Patients should be equal partners in the creation of their health records. The Nursing and Midwifery Council (2008) assert that the best health record is one that is the product of consultation and discussion between all members of the multidisciplinary healthcare team, the patient, and their carers. The success of patient-held records in areas such as antenatal care reflects this philosophy.

Electronic record systems

The NHS is currently seeking to standardize and improve its communication and record-keeping systems by implementing a new integrated information technology system. However, in many areas of practice there is evidence of electronic record keeping that improves patient care. The standards of documentation remain the same whether nurses use manual (paper) or electronic (computer) record systems. If using electronic records nurses remain accountable for ensuring:

♦ the accuracy, comprehensiveness, and timeliness of the entries

♦ the use of electronic signatures and dates

- the use of an electronic correction system that allows for changes to be made without deleting the original entry

- the maintenance of confidentiality of patient information by using passwords and having a reasonable belief that the record is safe and secure.

Audit

Audit is an essential tool in ensuring the quality of health care and there is evidence that auditing record keeping can have a real impact on the quality of clinical records and on the valuing of those records (Darmer et al. 2006). By auditing records the standard can be evaluated and the process of undertaking the audit can raise awareness of the need to improve practice (Griffiths et al. 2007). Furthermore, areas for education and staff training will be highlighted and enhancements to existing systems can be implemented.

Audit should be used to serve the needs and interests of the patients, rather than to benefit the organization. Confidentiality of patient's records applies throughout the audit and a system of peer review may be helpful (Nursing and Midwifery Council 2008).

Competencies for care

The Department of Health (2009) competencies for recognizing and responding to acutely ill patients in hospital clearly identifies the importance of accurate documentation. All staff are responsible for clear, legible documentation, and for ensuring that management plans are in place.

Healthcare records should include notes of the event, date, time, name, and contact details of staff attending the patient. Frequency of observations and ongoing management plans for those requiring escalation of care should also be clearly documented and handover to the next shift of carers must be coordinated and include communication with the multidisciplinary team. Patients who are not improving and those in whom there is further cause for concern must be clearly highlighted and calls for help initiated via the appropriate in-hospital mechanisms (Department of Health 2009).

Box 16.3 Principles of good documentation/record keeping

Clinical issues for consideration: audit your own ward records.

- Are your nursing records factual, accurate, and contemporaneous?
- Are all nursing records legible, signed, and dated?
- Are the patient records clearly written, free of jargon and abbreviations?
- Are there any areas where care given has not been documented?
- Are telephone conversations with doctors recorded in the nursing notes?
- Are DNAR orders and advance directives clearly documented in the medical and nursing notes?
- Are there any errors/deletions in the nursing notes—are these amended appropriately with signatures, dates, and times?
- Are EWS charts, fluid balance charts, and care plans completed correctly and maintained regularly?

Conclusion

Good record keeping is vital to high-quality patient care and to the maintenance of patient safety. Patient confidentiality should be maintained, and legal and professional imperatives observed. Where tragedy results in healthcare settings, the inquiry report frequently cites failures in communication, both written and verbal, as the principle reason. Audit can play a vital role in ensuring the quality of care delivered to patients and good quality record keeping is vital to safe and efficient patient care.

References

Chellel, A., Fraser, J., and Fender, V. (2002) Nursing observations on ward patients at risk of critical illness. *Nurs. Times.* **99**(46), 36–9.

Cretikos, M., Bellano, R., Hillman, R. *et al.* (2008) Respiratory rate as an indicator of acute illness. *Med. J. Australia.* **188**(11), 657–9.

Darmer, M.R., Ankersen, L., Neilsen, B.G. *et al.* (2006) Nursing documentation audit—the effect of VIPS implementation programme in Denmark. *J. Clin. Nurs.* **15**(5), 525–34.

Department of Health (2006) *Records Management: NHS Code of Practice.* The Stationary Office, London.

Department of Health (2009) *Competencies for Recognising and Responding to Acutely Ill Patients in Hospital.* The Stationary Office, London.

Dimond, B. (2005a) Exploring the principles of good record keeping in nursing. *Br. J. Nurs.* **14**(8), 460–2.

Dimond, B. (2005b) Exploring common deficiencies that occur in record keeping. *Br. J. Nurs.* **14**(10), 568–70.

Dimond, B. (2005c) Abbreviations: The need for legibility and accuracy in documentation. *Br. J. Nurs.* **14**(12), 665–6.

Griffiths, P., Debbage, S., and Smith, A. (2007) A comprehensive audit of nursing record keeping practice. *Br. J. Nurs.* **16**(21), 1324–7.

Haskett, G. (2008) Staff knowledge survey of hospital Do Not Attempt Resuscitation (DNAR) policy: Is this policy effective and is the documentation completed accurately? *Resuscitation* **77**(suppl. 1), May S525.

http://www.nmc-uk.org Nursing and Midwifery Council—Fitness to Practise procedures.

http://www.opsi.gov.uk The Access to Health Records Act 1990.

http://www.opsi.gov.uk The Data Protection Act 1998.

http://www.opsi.gov.uk The Freedom of Information Act.

Jevon, P. and Ewens, B. (2007) *Monitoring the Critically Ill Patient.* 2nd edn. Blackwell Publishing, Oxford.

Jones, S. and Jones, B. (2007) Advance directives and implications for emergency departments. *Br. J. Nurs.* **16**(4), 220–3.

National Patient Safety Agency (2007) *Recognising and Responding Appropriately to Early Signs of Deterioration in Hospitalised Patients.* National Patient Safety Agency, London.

NICE (2007) *Acutely Ill Patients in Hospital: Recognition of and Response to Acute Illness of Adults in Hospital.* HMSO, London.

Nursing and Midwifery Council (2008) *NMC Record Keeping.* Nursing and Midwifery Council, London.

Resuscitation Council (UK) (2009) *Recommended Standards for Recording 'Do not Attempt Resuscitation' DNAR Decisions.* Resuscitation Council (UK), London.

Rowan, K., Adam, S., Ball, C. *et al.* (2007) *Evaluation of Outreach Services in Critical Care: Intensive Care National Audit and Research Committee (ICNARC).* ICNARC, London.

Chapter 17

Continuing education and acute care delivery

Helen Stanley

Chapter contents

The purpose of this chapter is to help you understand and plan your continuing professional education (CPE) to meet your statutory professional body, the Nursing and Midwifery Council, requirements, and your personal and professional responsibilities to maintain and develop your practice as an acute care nurse.

Learning outcomes

This chapter will enable you to:

♦ consider the purpose of CPE for your role as an acute care nurse

♦ reflect on your professional responsibilities with regard to maintaining your knowledge and skills for practice

♦ discuss the benefits of CPE and work-based learning (WBL) and develop your personal portfolio to reflect the key elements of contemporary strategic documents

♦ analyse the need for life-long learning, clinical supervision, and reflection on practice

♦ consider the role of simulation and e-learning in acute care education

♦ discuss the impact of education on care delivery and benefits of various in-trust and university programmes to direct your future education and career pathway.

Introduction

Working in acute care involves complex decision making and skilled communication with a range of patients, carers, and healthcare professionals. The increasing complexity of health care, the ageing population, and shorter length of stay in hospital all contribute to patients in hospital needing a higher level of care than ever before (Department of Health 2008a,b).

There is a body of evidence of a lack of preparation to assess and manage the needs of the acutely ill patient outside of the critical care setting, which points to educational needs not being met (McQuillian *et al.* 1998; Goldhill 2001; NCEPOD 2005; NPSA 2007). The development of evidence-based recommendations such as the National Institute for Health and Clinical Excellence guidelines (NICE, 2007) on the recognition and management of acute illness in acute hospitals and the Department of Health (2009) Competencies for Recognising and Responding to Acutely Ill patients in Hospital, offer frameworks to support the development of key skills and knowledge in this area. The Department of Health (2009) competencies are currently out for national consultation and discussion, and the final version should be available shortly. A range of educational initiatives have been designed to address some of the shortcomings identified in the reports in the delivery of acute care.

Purpose of continuing professional education

The role of CPE has never been more crucial to high standards of acute patient care and job satisfaction for practising nurses. CPE is a complex concept that has evolved over time from mandatory education, life-long learning, and continuing professional development. The most significant implication of continuing education is its ability to enhance practice and promote the health of the public, and therefore the impact of CPE must be fully recognized in government policy, by professional bodies, health service agencies, and educators understanding the importance of accessibility and to provide more opportunities for nurses to attend CPE throughout their career (Gallagher 2007).

A number of important Department of Health and Nursing and Midwifery Council documents have driven the CPE agenda forward and these are briefly summarized here to show the key issues that need to be considered when planning your CPE and nursing career.

The *Working Together—Learning Together* framework for life-long learning for the NHS (Department of Health 2001) devised a number of general principles that should apply across the spectrum of post registration and continuing education, suggesting that CPE should:

+ be patient centred
+ be delivered in partnership with stakeholders
+ be aligned with the requirements of regulatory bodies for re-registration and be relevant to the individual's working environment and to the job they actually do
+ meet local service needs as well as the individual's personal and professional development needs
+ be increasingly work based
+ use a full range of development approaches and methods, rather than rely mainly on formal courses
+ link with clinical governance and the quality agenda
+ develop a research-aware workforce.

A task group convened by the Chief Nursing Officer (Department of Health 2004) examined post registration development for nurses and midwives and identified four categories for learning beyond registration:

1 Ad hoc training—study days, organizational training, such as required for health and safety purposes, as moving and handling and risk reduction such as infection control.

2 Continuing professional development—to update and refresh professional knowledge and skills and to maintain competence in the current sphere of practice.

3 More formalized education and training for additional knowledge, skills, and professional competencies of an advanced nature, intended to enable the practitioner to move from their current sphere and scope of practice to more advanced professional activity.

4 Education, training, and development—generic and relevant to professional practice, such as a leadership development programme or degree/masters' qualifications.

Within the profound changes taking place in the healthcare arena of the NHS, there was a need to create flexible, diverse, and rewarding nursing careers that are fit for purpose. The Modernising

Nursing Careers Report (Department of Health 2006) identified four key priority areas that needed to be addressed:

+ develop a competent and flexible nursing workforce
+ update career pathways and career choices
+ prepare nurses to lead in a changed healthcare system
+ modernize the image of nursing and nursing careers.

These priorities were taken forward for consultation to support a new post-registration careers framework for nursing (Department of Health 2007). The main proposals were that careers in nursing should be structured with five pathways:

+ child, family, and public health
+ first contact, access, and urgent care
+ supporting long-term care
+ acute and critical care
+ mental health and psychosocial care.

It was identified that these pathways would have clear standards and corresponding levels of education for the newly registered through to advanced practice. There would be core competencies defined for each stage of practice so that nurses could move more flexibly between different clinical areas, with the boundaries between community and hospital nursing becoming less distinct.

Nurses would 'major' in one pathway, such as acute and critical care, moving from novice to expert, but be able to intervene at a level appropriate to the situation and degree of competence in cross-cutting themes, such as health promotion, preventative long-term conditions, safeguarding vulnerable groups, end of life care, and holistic care. There were to be common elements for all nurses: practice; education, training, and development; quality and service development; leadership, management, and supervision; and research.

The consultation response report (Department of Health 2008b) supported the need for change and the career pathway approach, identifying that nurses would need support during the transition to a new system, and job titles, responsibility, and educational attainment should be aligned. There was a call for the regulation of advanced practice, which was seen as a necessary step in enforcing compliance and investment in education to ensure the safety of the public. This is currently under review by the Nursing and Midwifery Council, working with the Health Professions Council across all professions.

Following on from these reports, the NHS Next Stage Review (Department of Health 2008a) reaffirmed the importance of the role of the nurse, particularly in improving the quality of nursing care, and supported a foundation period of preceptorship. This would enable nurses at the start of their careers to apply the knowledge, skills, and competencies acquired as students in their area of practice and was advocated as laying a solid foundation for life-long learning.

Professional responsibilities for continuing professional education

There needs to be a strong partnership between individual's needs, the context in which they work, the nature of the CPE undertaken, and the professional body to which they belong (Lawton & Wimpenny 2003). However, accessing CPE can be fraught with issues and tensions, and in one study (Munro 2008), the nature and type of CPE seemed to be determined by the individual or their employer, rather than occurring as an integral part of professional activity within the workplace, which can lead to a mismatch between personal and organizational goals.

Some employers will both fund CPE and support time for study, but with the infinite demand on a finite resource, increasingly staff 'donate' their own time (days off or annual leave) to attend courses, pay at least some of their own fees and travel, and may be restricted to in-trust mandatory training. Competence development in an organization is dependent on a number of different factors, technology, people, the structure of the organization, and culture, as well as the economic means to support development (Munro 2008).

Take a moment to reflect on your professional responsibilities with regard to maintaining your knowledge and skills for practice (Activity 17.1).

You may have thought about a trust study day you attended, positive and negative experiences you have had on your acute ward, or a journal article you read recently. They can all be useful and appropriate forms of CPE and enable you to keep abreast of current practice. In terms of out-of-date practice, the Nursing and Midwifery Council Code (Nursing and Midwifery Council 2008a) has been revised with the central message to ensure that practitioners' knowledge and skills are up to date and reflect post-registration education and practice (Prep) requirements.

The requirements of the Nursing and Midwifery Council Code are:

♦ to deliver care based on the best available evidence or best practice and, where applicable, validated research

♦ to ensure that any advice given is evidence based if suggesting healthcare products or services

♦ to ensure that the use of complementary or alternative therapies is safe and in the best interests of patients.

To keep skills and knowledge up to date, the practitioner must:

♦ have the knowledge and skills for safe and effective practice when working without direct supervision

♦ recognize and work within the limits of their competence

♦ keep their knowledge and skills up to date throughout their working life

♦ take part in appropriate learning and practice activities that maintain and develop their competence and performance.

The Nursing and Midwifery Council's Prep requirements

The Nursing and Midwifery Council have designed a set of Prep standards and guidance (Nursing and Midwifery Council 2008b) to help practitioners provide a high standard of practice and care through a framework for CPE, which, although not a guarantee of competence, acts as a key component of clinical governance. This framework is designed to support the practitioner keep

---

Activity 17.1 Think about the ways in which you currently keep up to date

♦ How effective are they for your learning?
♦ How effective are they for your patients/unit/trust?
♦ What are the implications if your practice is out of date?

up to date with new developments in their clinical speciality, think and reflect for themselves, demonstrate to their patients, colleagues, and employers that they are up to date and developing their practice, and, ultimately, provide a high standard of skilled nursing care.

There are two Prep standards which affect the practitioners' registration (Nursing and Midwifery Council 2008b: 4):

♦ The Prep (practice) standard

The practitioner must have worked in some capacity by virtue of their nursing or midwifery qualification during the previous 3 years for a minimum of 450 h or have successfully undertaken an approved return-to-practice course within the last 3 years.

♦ The Prep (continuing professional development) standard

The practitioner must have undertaken and recorded their CPE over the 3 years before the renewal of their registrations. The practitioner must undertake at last 35 h of learning activity relevant to their practice, maintain a personal professional profile, and comply with any request from the Nursing and Midwifery Council to audit how they have met these requirements.

Practitioners are required to provide a signed notification of practice form and declare that they have met the Prep requirements and are of good health and good character when they renew their registration. If a practitioner is not registered with the Nursing and Midwifery Council, they cannot be employed to practise as a nurse or midwife in the UK.

The Nursing and Midwifery Council do not define how a practitioner should meet the standards and believe that each individual practitioner should decide for themselves what learning activities they need to undertake. *The Prep Handbook* (Nursing and Midwifery Council 2008b) offers a range of helpful case examples.

Types of acute care educational opportunities

Within the acute care setting, the learning activity for Prep (Nursing and Midwifery Council 2008b) might be:

♦ structured formal learning, such as undertaking an accredited module or pathway in acute care or mentorship preparation, or attending a study day, such as Basic or Advanced Life Support (BLS), or the Acute-Life Threatening Emergencies-Recognition and Treatment (ALERT™) course. BLS can be taught locally within trusts and is mandatory for all hospital employees. Algorithms are endorsed by the Resuscitation Council UK. ALERT™ is a 1-day multiprofessional course using a structured and prioritized system of patient assessment and management to assist in treating the acutely unwell (Smith *et al.* 2002).

♦ informal learning, such as reflecting on practice and observations with nurses from the outreach team (Plowright *et al.* 2006); undertaking a literature search on tracheostomy management; reading and reviewing an intravenous infusions policy document; exploring a topic of interest and relevance to acute care practice; or shadowing an experienced colleague from the high dependency unit

♦ other innovative ways of experiencing CPE, such as secondments, in-house teaching, project learning opportunities, coaching, networking with peers, journal clubs, practice development forums, WBL initiatives, and internet discussion groups (Price 2007).

The Department of Health (2009) Competencies for Recognising and Responding to Acutely Ill patients in Hospital do not endorse any programme in particular, but generally support the need for education and training for staff to improve the care of acutely ill patients. Short skills courses such as Advanced Life Support (Resuscitation Council (UK) 1998) and, more recently, the ALERT™ course have been put in place alongside former English National Board for Nursing,

Midwifery and Health Visiting (ENB) courses such as Intensive Care Nursing in response to concern about acute care.

Wood *et al.* (2004) undertook a project to identify the education and training needs of healthcare professionals in assessing and managing acutely physically ill hospital patients. They found that the core educational needs were:

+ assessment of patients' physical needs, including knowledge of anatomy and physiology of body systems

+ common pathologies (e.g. respiratory distress, 'shock'), and use and limitations of equipment (e.g. pulse oximetry)

+ hydration status, e.g. urine output, fluid balance, and recognition of pulmonary oedema; interpretation of investigations results

+ use of relevant 'at-risk' assessment tools (e.g. patients at risk (PAR), modified early warning score (MEWS))

+ skills needs for patient assessment (airway status, respiratory, cardiovascular and neurological function, recognizing when a patient is deteriorating)

+ skills and knowledge for patient management; communication skills (confidence and referral skills)

+ interprofessional working (awareness of roles and responsibilities in the 'management' of acutely ill patients)

+ resource issues (equipment, documentation, use of scoring systems, outreach teams)

+ prioritization issues; terminology and definitions (e.g. levels of care).

Wood *et al.* suggested an urgent need for post-registration preparation in the assessment and management of acutely ill patients across all professional groups: alongside funding for practitioners to undertake short courses such as ALERT™, local education centres to become providers of these courses. One example of this has been the acute care pathway within the BSc (Hons) Acute Clinical Practice degree at the University of Brighton.

Example: Acute care pathway

This clinical pathway is aimed at the increasing number of practitioners who work with acutely ill patients. It provides practitioners with the diverse skills and knowledge they require to care for the acutely ill adult in a variety of clinical settings and enables them to deliver timely and appropriate acute care. The pathway has been designed with great flexibility to ensure that nurses will study the aspects of acute care that are pertinent to their own working environment and each student will be encouraged to select clinical modules that will be useful for their own areas of clinical practice. Each student will be able to devise their own learning package in agreement with the module leader.

At the end of the pathway, each student will have developed an insight into the care needs of the acute patients in their clinical environment and an understanding of the distinct nature of acute care delivery. Completion of a clinical pathway will enable practitioners to develop towards enhanced career status. The majority of practitioners who undertake these pathways continue to work in the chosen area of practice after completion.

Students are free to identify areas in which they wish to study and select appropriate modules following discussion with the pathway leader. Two examples of pathways are included below but numerous other packages may also be devised.

+ Staff nurse working in a general medical ward:
  - Care of the acutely ill adult (20 credits)

- Acute coronary syndromes (20 credits)
- Cardiac arrhythmias (10 credits)
- Heart failure (10 credits)
- Staff nurse working in a neuroscience centre:
  - Care of the acutely ill adult (20 credits)
  - Neurological patient care (20 credits)
  - Physical assessment of adults (20 credits)

Care of the acutely ill adult module

Practitioners who are new to acute care nursing will be strongly encouraged to undertake the Care of the acutely ill adult module. This module aims to provide a foundation and an in-depth introduction to acute care through increased theoretical knowledge and improved decision-making skills, and enable practitioners to provide care to the acutely ill patient. The content reflects the syllabus advocated by the Department of Health (2009) and Wood *et al.* (2004), and is taught using a range of teaching and learning strategies, including lectures, guided study packages, case studies, and simulation exercises, and the students are encouraged to reflect on and share their work-based experiences from the disciplines of nursing and midwifery. The module is assessed by a theoretical reflective essay examining the management of an acutely ill patient who has been cared for by the student (50%) and practical assessment of six related clinical skills, including the key problem-solving skill of management of the acutely ill patient, which is assessed using simulation in the skills room at the university.

Courses for continuing professional education

Some nurses wish to further develop their education by undertaking formal courses leading to diplomas, degrees, and even masters and doctorates, and there has been a massive expansion in CPE to meet this demand (Stock 2002). There is emerging evidence that quality healthcare education and training can directly and substantially benefit patient care (Mackinnon 2007). In addition, many studies have identified how further post-registration study can also increase self-awareness and self-confidence, as well as enhancing clinical skills and career prospects (Davey & Robinson 2002; Bahn 2007).

Many courses offer a combination of traditional modular university-based and flexible approaches, utilizing work-based, online, distance, and open learning, which can enable nurses to work in a demanding acute environment in addition to caring for their families (Presho 2006). However, an effective staff and student support network, including lecturers, family, and work colleagues, is required as the personal and professional challenges on the part-time post-registration journey to becoming a graduate nurse can be stressful (Stanley 2003).

Continuing professional education careers advice

There has been a vast expansion in the range of CPE programmes available and at times it is hard for nurses to find their way through the labyrinth of choices and identify which programme best fits their current and future educational needs. In a number of universities, a CPE careers service is offered, where nurses can access independent advice to navigate the various options open to them to make best use of their previous educational experiences and be signposted to the most appropriate module, pathway, or course for their individual needs. Increasingly, nurses can gain credit for their learning through flexible learning, including accreditation of prior learning (APL) or accreditation of past experiential learning (APEL) or recognition of work-related learning (RAWL) opportunities. This may allow them to make best use of their professional development. For examples of this type of role, access your local university website or the useful NHS careers website http://www.nhscareers.nhs.uk.

Flexible learning opportunities

A flexible learning framework provides a number of ways to undertake post-registration qualifications and CPE, all of which are designed to suit the needs of nurses and employers. Flexible learning is knowledge that is derived from, for, and about the learner's workplace. The University of Brighton has worked with employers to design a framework that enables healthcare workers to develop academic abilities and professional competencies to meet personal, professional, and workforce needs. Flexible learning can be retrospective (AP(E)L and RAWL) or prospective learning (WBL).

Accreditation of past experiential learning/recognition of work-related learning

Nurses often bring previous academic study and a wealth of experience from practice when they enrol on courses. It is important that this prior achievement is recognized and valued. It may reduce both the duration and the assessment load of the course and can avoid repetitious learning. There are processes for accrediting past learning (APL) and past experiential learning (APEL). APL enables nurses to transfer credits gained in one higher education institution (HEI) to another, if that credit can be matched to the learning outcomes of modules of learning within their current programme of study and/or course outcomes. Credit is normally achieved within the last 3–5 years or, if not, evidence of currency is required using APEL processes. APEL enables nurses to gain credit for relevant prior experience in the workplace. The nurse provides documentary evidence of prior learning in the workplace that can be matched against their current programme of study.

Recognizing and accrediting work-related learning (RAWL) is a concept similar to AP(E)L but refers to prior learning of a more recent nature. It is likely to follow on from a quality approved in-house event. Nurses can demonstrate the scope of their learning in their work organization from the recent past—normally 1 year. The credit claimed is not linked to an award but can be transferred to an award at a later stage if course-specific regulations allow.

Work-based learning

WBL modules are a modern way of learning for busy professionals, who respond well to the rapidly changing skill and knowledge needs of nurses. The 'empowerment' model of WBL is ideally suited to professional practice and development of better skilled, more qualified, and more flexible workers to enable modernization of the NHS (Rounce & Workman 2005). There are successful examples of work-based approaches to acute and critical care modules, such as one developed jointly by service and HEI staff in Scotland for post-registration nurses (Rattay et al. 2006).

WBL modules are flexible and responsive to individual learning requirements and they achieve this because they are 'empty' modules that enable the nurse to design their own learning programme with a diploma, degree, and postgraduate course. It may also be possible to take a WBL module as a discrete module to meet CPE needs.

WBL modules are ideal for facilitating development in the following areas:

♦ exploration of new roles

- change in role focus
- to improve the quality of healthcare service delivery
- extending knowledge and skills in a particular area of practice
- mapping knowledge and skills development to competency frameworks
- developing effective project management skills.

The nurse takes a central role in the construction of this type of learning; they have to develop aspects of curriculum design, for example define appropriate learning outcomes and methods of assessment. They need to learn how to negotiate learning contracts, study time, and access to opportunities, and some students lack confidence in their skills to 'identify the right thing' to study.

Overall, there is wealth of educational opportunities in acute care that can be undertaken by a variety of learning approaches. The next exercise is to help you prepare yourself for future study see Activity 17.2.

By careful consideration of the above, nurses should be in a better position to articulate their career plans and direction, and have all the information required to make a successful application for their chosen route, be that a course, WBL, or developing their skills in acute care for their Prep requirements.

Personal and professional responsibility

Personal professional profiles

Practitioners are required as part of their Prep requirements to maintain a personal profile to record their learning activity for re-registration purposes (Nursing and Midwifery Council 2008c). This profile is a personal document and does not belong to the Nursing and Midwifery Council or to the practitioners' employer, and employers and managers cannot demand to see it.

The profile has two key functions:

- it contributes to practitioners' professional development by helping them recognize and appreciate their abilities, achievements, and experiences
- it provides an information source to which practitioners can refer to in order to collect material about standards of education.

There are a number of benefits to maintaining a profile:

- it helps to assess practitioners' current standards of practice

---

Activity 17.2 Preparing to study

Undertaking a SWOT (Strengths, Weaknesses, Opportunities and Threats) analysis may be a good starting point:

- Think about your practice—what are your *strengths* and *weaknesses*—in practice and academic learning? Which skills do you have and which do you need to develop?
- What are the *opportunities* available? Will it be a trust study day, workshop, module, pathway, course, or a diploma/degree?
- What are the *threats* to your CPE? Do you have support from your manager, workplace colleagues, family, and friends? How much will it cost? What commitment will be required?

- it helps to develop practitioners' analytical skills through reflection on their experience
- it enables review and evaluation of past experience and learning to help inform future career planning
- it provides effective and current information when practitioners apply for jobs or courses
- it demonstrates experiential learning, which may allow practitioners to obtain credit towards further qualifications.

There are no set procedures for building a profile, but three broad, inter-related steps have been suggested by the Nursing and Midwifery Council (2008c) for practitioners to consider:

Step 1: Review experience to date, including areas of practice most enjoyed and where there is scope for improvement, what has been done to improve practice and performance, and how they intend to continue to do so for the next 3 years.

Step 2: Self-appraisal of practice, examining performance and standards of knowledge and practice, focusing on one event, which may be positive or negative, and analysing critically the experience, considering areas for development highlighted by the event. This process can be facilitated by a colleague, manager, or supervisor, especially for those new to the reflective process.

Step 3: Set goals and action plans to begin to identify learning needs from Steps 1 and 2.

The self-appraisal process should be a continuing one and linked to the life-long learning principle (Jarvis 1998). Ways of supporting life-long learning through approaches such as clinical supervision and reflection are described below.

Life-long learning, clinical supervision, and reflection on practice

The professional career of the registered nurse in the ever-changing environment of acute care should encompass the principles of life-long learning to maintain high standards of patient care and to keep abreast of the increasing technological advances in treatment, continuing reorganization, and the redirection of resources. This requires nurses to demonstrate responsibility for their own learning through the development of a personal portfolio of learning and practice (including their personal professional profile for Prep) and to be able to recognize when further learning and development may be required (Nursing and Midwifery Council 2002).

Life-long learning

The government document *Working Together—Learning Together: a Framework for Life-long Learning* (Department of Health 2001) advocates life-long learning and development as key to delivering the NHS plan (Department of Health 2000) to modernize the NHS and supporting changes in patient care. Life-long learning as a concept has evolved over time with the changing focus towards adult education principles and student-centred rather than teacher-centred approaches (Jarvis 1998). As far back as 1994, the English National Board identified the characteristics of life-long learners, which still resonates with the situations in which acute care nurses practice today. Life-long learners are:

- *innovative* in their practice
- *flexible* to changing demand
- *resourceful* in their methods of working
- able to work as *change agents*
- able to share *good practice*
- *adaptable* to changing healthcare needs

+ *challenging* and *creative* in their practice
+ *self-reliant* in their way of working
+ *responsible* and *accountable* for their work.

From the description above, it seems that life-long learning is more than simply keeping up to date, but requires a constantly enquiring approach to the practice of nursing as well as to the issues that impact on that practice (Nursing and Midwifery Council 2002). Through maintaining a process of CPE linked to the registration renewal process through the Prep standards, the acute care nurse can enjoy a stimulating career that builds on the learning achieved in their pre-registration programme of preparation and is carried throughout a lifetime.

There are some initiatives that, alongside workshops, study days, and courses, can support the nurse in acute care with their life-long learning journey. These include a period of preceptorship when newly qualified, use of reflective practice, and support through clinical supervision.

Preceptorship

The concept of a period of consolidation after qualifying as a nurse is not new (Nursing and Midwifery Council 2006a) but this has only recently been formally endorsed by the Department of Health and Nursing and Midwifery Council (Department of Health 2008a; Nursing and Midwifery Council 2008c). Mandatory preceptorship is to follow initial registration and has been agreed in principle but is subject to further exploration of issues relating to objectives, the period required, protected learning time, nature of assessed outcome, and potential links to first renewal of registration.

Research into the experiences of newly qualified nurses demonstrated how the need for structured, constructive, and positive feedback about competence and performance had a crucial role in learning for improving skills and confidence, maintaining people's interest in their jobs and enabling them to cope with new challenges (Blackman *et al.* 2006). Other studies of preceptorship have identified an overwhelming demand for this form of support for the staff nurse in their first job (Hardy & Hickey 2001). One useful model suggested for acute care, in common with medicine and physiotherapy, is a period of post-registration consolidation to take place the year after qualifying, with nurses' rotation to recognized acute care areas, to share good practice, build individual's confidence, and hone assessment and management skills in the acutely ill setting (Wood *et al.* 2004).

Clinical supervision

Clinical supervision allows a nurse to receive professional supervision by a skilled supervisor in the workplace (Nursing and Midwifery Council 2006b). Clinical supervision enables nurses to:

+ identify solutions to their practice problems
+ increase their understanding of professional issues
+ improve standards of patient care in the acute setting
+ further develop their skills and knowledge
+ enhance their understanding of their own practice.

A review of the literature on clinical supervision suggests it can act as a strategy to enhance other models of support, such as preceptorship or mentorship, to positively influence the recruitment and retention of newly qualified nurses (Cummins 2008).

Clinical supervision may be offered in small groups and often away from the work setting to enable nurses to reflect on their practice, analyse their responses to situations, and evaluate their performance to contribute to their professional development, within a supportive environment.

Many trusts are now realizing the positive benefits of a robust clinical supervision policy and how the time and resource commitment can have a very real effect on sickness absence and retention of staff. The need for resilient nurses in acute care facilitated by skilled staff can help prevent burn out or disillusionment in practitioners. Clinical supervision may help staff cope with the demands of the current challenges in this fast paced healthcare setting (Scholes 2008).

Mentorship and practice educators

Other support roles in clinical practice include mentorship and practice educators/teachers, and these roles are now more clearly defined by the recent Nursing and Midwifery Council Standards (Nursing and Midwifery Council 2008d). A mentor facilitates learning, and supervises and assesses students in a practice setting and although the Standards to Support Learning and Assessment in Practice are primarily focused at support for student nurses, they also apply to post-registration nurses undertaking educational programmes. some acute care units have invested in practice educator/teacher roles to facilitate practice development and assess skills and competencies such as those found in the Department of Health (2009) framework (Department of Health 2009).

The role of reflective practice

Many nurses are now familiar with models of reflection as they form a part of their pre-registration educational programme or they may have used some of the concepts in other post-registration modules. However, there are a number of books available to guide the novice to develop these skills, which are crucial to developing practice and life-long learning, for example Rolfe *et al.* (2001). The use of a model of reflection, where a critical incident is examined, analysed, and learning extracted, can be an empowering process to 'unpack' a clinical experience and gain professional and personal development (Gustafsson & Fagerberg 2004). Some acute care units may offer action learning sets to support reflective learning strategies to enhance practice.

There seem to be tensions in acute care education, where perhaps empirical knowledge and behaviourist approaches prevail. Randall *et al.* (2007) argued for an approach whereby 'critical questioning', which they define as purposeful questioning or co-creating dialogue, serves as a trigger for thinking, rather than an opportunity for the regurgitation of content or depositing of specific facts. By initiating critical questioning with a mentor or clinical supervisor, nurses' experiences are critically analysed, enabling them to re-form their experiences and learn.

Alongside formal courses, the role of reflection and experiential learning in the workplace has been advocated in acute care. A study in Canada of acute care nurses found learning from one's own experiences and the experiences of others, with importantly learning from mistakes, errors, and misjudgements, to be significant learning experiences (Jantzen 2008). She argued for nurses to value and utilize shared workplace experiences as a form of professional development. Another study suggested that nurses calling for emergency assistance in the acute care setting be provided with the opportunity to debrief after the event (Cioffi 2000).

The processes of preceptorship, mentorship, and clinical supervision described above can all contribute to both the life-long learning and well-being of the nurse in the acute care setting see Activity 17.3.

Teaching methods: objective structured clinical examinations, simulation, and e-learning

Although most of the research has been undertaken in the pre-registration area of nurse education, as skills rooms return and more use is made of techniques such as simulation using sophisticated manikins and objective structured clinical examinations (OSCEs) as a form of assessment,

Activity 17.3 Support for clinical practice

Think about the forums for support which currently exist within your place of work:

♦ Are they formal or informal?

♦ Do they occur on a regular basis?

♦ Are they supported by management?

♦ What records, if any are made?

♦ Are these records supportive of your professional development?

Do these forums enable you to address:

♦ professional issues

♦ clinical practice/skills development

♦ educational needs

♦ workload management

♦ emotional support?

Where else might you go for professional support in the workplace?

the role of these innovative teaching methods is emerging in acute care programmes. The chance to learn the practical skills in a safe environment with a skilled facilitator can be beneficial and can develop high levels of clinical reasoning, and there has been a return in the UK to the use of simulation (Thompson *et al.* 2005; McCallum 2007). There are, however, some criticisms of the learning of practice skills in the classroom related to the artificial nature of the situation without the unique nuances of practice.

Simulation and objective structured clinical examination

There has recently been a resurgence in the use of this type of learning approach in an attempt to enable student nurses to develop competence in the clinical skills required for fitness for award, practice, and purpose. Nurses need to be prepared adequately for OSCEs and there are issues concerning the parity of workstations and the reliability and validity of the examination process, but they have a valuable part to play in their contribution to professional education (Rushforth 2007).

As part of a study exploring using designated practice hours for simulation, commissioned by the Nursing and Midwifery Council (Moule *et al.* 2008), students attended five simulation sessions including BLS, manual handling, infection control, and clinical decision making. Students completed pre and post tests in BLS, and vignettes and OSCEs. Simulation was reported as a positive experience for both student and mentors, and offered scope for interprofessional application.

A review by McCallum (2007) examined the advantages and disadvantages of using simulation education in pre-registration adult education. She found that students' experiences are generally positive, especially in light of shorter clinical placements and increasing student confidence in performing clinical skills. Simulation has to reflect reality, which is referred to as fidelity and with current technology simulators can now reflect very sophisticated engineering and psychological fidelity.

There is a lack of research into the use of technology-based learning tools such as human patient simulation, but a critical examination of behaviourist approaches in the development of psychomotor clinical skills and constructivist approaches to the development of clinical decision making, problem solving, collaboration, and group processes argue that a blended philosophy of learning can be effective in nurse education to maximize the potential benefits for the modern nursing student, who may expect more 'high tech' approaches in this digital age (Parker & Myrick 2009). The teaching of ECG interpretation has offered challenges to the traditional methods in use in many university programmes, and one study explored ways of making this more realistic for learning life-saving procedures such as thrombolysis administration (Alunier *et al.* 2006).

A training programme for qualified health professionals, the North West Strategic Health Authority Acute Illness Management (AIM) course, was adapted for student nurses in their adult branch year of the Diploma programme in the School of Nursing, Midwifery and Social Work at the University of Manchester (Steen & Costello 2008). This provided students with an introductory programme before placements in acute and critical care areas, when most students had limited awareness of AIM. A structured approach to assessment was introduced, using case histories and manikins in a clinical skills laboratory, utilizing the AIM assessment tool: the airway, breathing, circulation, disability, and exposure (ABCDE) model. The study found a positive correlation between theoretical learning and practical application, with a clear perception that the programme enhanced clinical practice and awareness of the needs of the acutely ill patient in hospital. The programme did not focus exclusively on *how* intervention occurs, but rather on *when* intervention should occur and *what* is the most appropriate form of intervention. Although further quantitative research is necessary, by exposing pre-registration student nurses to this sort of programme the indications are that incorporating acute illness assessment into the theoretically orientated curriculum has the potential for more effective interventions to take place in practice.

E-learning

E-learning has become more widely used in nurse education, with the use of technology and virtual learning environments to facilitate learning and offer stimulating resources. In the acute care setting, computer programs to examine nurses' use of clinical information when diagnosing hypovolaemic shock have highlighted how the processing of clinical information is not well understood (Thompson *et al.* 2005). Other initiatives for nurses include the development and evaluation of an e-learning scenario, using computer technology to support learning due to a shortage of critical care placements for nursing students (Tait *et al.* 2008). The positive attitude of student nurses to the scenario strongly supported its use in helping learners to acquire knowledge and awareness when real-life placements are not available and to extend their knowledge after meeting similar situations in practice.

Impact of education on care delivery and benefits of in-Trust and university programmes and future planning

Why education is important in the delivery of acute care

Studies have found a generally positive perception of CPE (Stanley 2003; Hughes 2005) and the current focus is on how effectively these programmes impact on the care delivered to patients, and not solely on the satisfaction of the nurse as a student (Jordan 2000). The ALERT™ course was evaluated and found to have beneficial effects in the confidence levels and attitudes of healthcare staff in the recognition and management of acutely ill patients (Featherstone *et al.* 2005). There is a paucity of research in the emerging field of acute care education, but studies of other critical care settings have found that courses do impact on practice (Armstrong & Adam 2002) but other approaches, such as extensive orientation with in-service educational programmes, can also be effective (Tennant & Field 2004).

Activity 17.4 Planning your CPE

The following areas may offer some triggers to consideration of your CPE:

♦ Think 'out of the box'—does it have to be a course/study day/workshop?

♦ What previous study have you undertaken or experiences have you achieved that could be accredited?

♦ How do you like to learn? What will encourage and support you? What motivates you and why?

♦ What do you enjoy about your job? Think about your role/work/job description, short- and long-term career plans. Where do you see yourself working in 1, 2 or even, 5 years' time?

♦ Consider the workplace/unit/trust strategic plans—this can be helpful to map to your requests, for example to undertake a degree.

♦ Use your personal development plan and appraisal—this should help you and your manager identify your CPE needs.

♦ Study leave and funding—you will need to negotiate this so follow your employer's study leave policy and check the university application process.

♦ Talk to your manager/link lecturer/local HEI careers advice service/careers fairs/access the NHS careers website.

With the changes to an all-graduate profession for nurses planned by the Nursing and Midwifery Council in the near future (Nursing and Midwifery Council 2009), there may be even more pressure for diplomats and nurses who trained some time ago to seriously consider their future CPE and perhaps completing their own degree level studies may be a timely option. It could be argued that in times of turbulent change in health care and reductions in educational budgets for CPE, it is not appropriate to consider further learning but even when faced with such challenges, it is important to prioritize education and take advantage of any career opportunities that emerge to ensure that the maximum potential for both patient care and possible promotion is achieved (Price 2007). Activity 17.4 and Activity 17.5 case studies may be helpful to prepare you for the complex web of choices available to the acute care nurse of today who wants to have a successful and fulfilling career in this exciting sphere of nursing.

Activity 17.5 CPE case study exercises

Plan your application for a place at a study day that you really want to attend on acute care assessment skills at the local university.

♦ What factors would you include in your application form to make a good impression?

♦ How could you utilize and share this knowledge back in the workplace?

You have completed your pre-registration Diploma in Nursing and after a year of consolidation working in an acute care medical ward you feel ready to complete your degree and you want to apply for study leave and funding.

♦ Which course would you apply for and why?

♦ How would you go about securing a place on the course?

♦ What issues would you have to negotiate in the workplace and with your trust?

Activity 17.5 CPE case study exercises *(continued)*

You see an opportunity on the surgical assessment unit notice board for an international nursing conference in Europe on Developments in Acute Care. You would really like to go and the surgeons have offered to fund a delegate and require a supporting statement for how this would benefit the unit.

♦ What would you include in your statement to make a sound case?

♦ How could you demonstrate the learning achieved by such an opportunity in your personal profile?

You are an acute care ward manager with a very limited CPE budget and in their recent appraisal, it was identified that a member of your staff wants to develop their leadership and management skills.

♦ How might they develop these skills via WBL in the ward setting?

♦ What other opportunities could you consider to support this staff member?

As a newly qualified nurse in a newly opened high dependency unit that has just introduced the Department of Health (2009) Competencies for Recognising and Responding to the Acutely Ill in Hospital, you wish to include your assessment into your Prep profile as evidence of achievement from your period of preceptorship.

♦ What aspects of the competencies would you utilize and why?

♦ How could you demonstrate your competence in acute care?

References

Alunier, G., Gordon, R., Harwood, C., and Hunt, W. (2006) 12-Lead ECG training: the way forward. *Nurse Educ. Today.* **26**, 87–92.

Armstrong, D. and Adam, J. (2002) The impact of a postgraduate critical care course in nursing practice. *Nurse Educ. Prac.* **2**, 169–75.

Bahn, D. (2007) Reasons for post registration learning: Impact of the learning experience. *Nurse Educ. Today.* **27**, 715–22.

Blackman, C., Miller, C., and Cabellero, C. (2006) LiNEA–R Retaining Nurses in the Workforce. Brighton and Sussex University Hospitals and Medical School and University of Brighton, Brighton. Available on-line at http://www.brighton.ac.uk/snm/research/cnmr/projects/pedagogy/Linear-RExecutiveSummary.pdf (accessed 26.3.09).

Cioffi, J. (2000) Nurses' experiences of making decisions to call emergency assistance to their patients. *J. Adv. Nurs.* **32**(1), 108–14.

Cummins, A. (2008) Clinical supervision: The way forward? A review of the literature. *Nurse Educ. Prac.* In press, doi:10.1016/jnepr.2008.10.009.

Davey, B. and Robinson, S. 2002. Taking a degree after qualifying as a registered general nurse: constraints and effects. *Nurse Educ. Today.* **22**, 624–31.

Department of Health (2000) *The NHS Plan.* Department of Health, London.

Department of Health (2001) *'Working Together – Learning Together': A Framework for Lifelong Learning for the NHS.* Department of Health, London.

Department of Health (2004) *Post Registration Development—A Framework for Planning, Commissioning and Delivering Learning Beyond Registration for Nurses and Midwives.* Department of Health, London.

Department of Health (2006) *Modernising Nursing Careers—Setting the Direction.* Department of Health, London.

Department of Health (2007) *Towards a Framework for Post Registration Nursing Careers*. Department of Health, London.

Department of Health (2008a) Roles and education and training pathways. In: *A High Quality Workforce— NHS Next Stage Review*. Department of Health, London, Ch. 2.

Department of Health (2008b) *Towards a Framework for Post Registration Nursing Careers: Consultation Response Report*. Department of Health, London.

Department of Health (2009) *Draft Acute Care competencies for Recognising and Responding to the Acutely Ill Adult in Hospital*. Department of Health, London.

Featherstone, P., Smith, G., Linnell, M. *et al.* (2005) Impact of a one-day inter-professional course (ALERT) on attitudes and confidence in managing critically ill adult patients. *Resuscitation.* 65(2005), 329–36.

Gallagher, L. (2007) Continuing education in nursing: a concept analysis. *Nurse Educ. Today.* 27(5), 466–73.

Goldhill, D. (2001) The critically ill: Following your MEWS. *QJM Int. J. Med.* 94(10), 507–10. Available on-line at: http:qjmed.oxfordjournals.org/cgi/content/full/94/10/507 (accessed 4.11.08).

Gustafsson, C. and Fagerberg, I. (2004) Reflection, the way to professional development? *J. Clin. Nurs.* 13, 271–80.

Hardy, R. and Hickey, G. (2001) What do newly-qualified nurses expect from preceptorship? Exploring the perception of the preceptee. *Nurse Educ. Today.* 21, 58–64.

Hughes, E. (2005) Nurses' perceptions of continuing professional development. *Nurs. Standard.* 19(43), 41–9.

Jantzen, D. (2008) Reframing professional development for front-line nurses. *Nurs. Inq.* 15, 21–9.

Jarvis, P. (1998) The emergence of lifelong learning. *The Theory and Practice of Learning*. Kogan Page, London, Ch 1.

Jordan, S. (2000) Educational input and patient outcomes: exploring the gap. *J. Adv. Nurs.* 31(2), 461–71.

Lawton, S. and Wimpenny, P. (2003) Continuing professional development: a review. *Nurs. Standard* 17(24), 41–4.

McCallum, J. (2007) The debate in favour of using simulation education in pre-registration adult nursing. *Nurse Educ. Today.* 27, 825–31.

McQuillian, P., Pilkington, S., Allan, A. *et al.* (1998) Confidential inquiry into quality of care before admission to intensive care. *BMJ.* 316, 1853–8.

Mackinnon Partnership (2007) A Literature Review of the Relationship between Quality Health Care Education and Quality of Care. Available on-line at: http://www.skillsforhealth.org.uk/~/media/Resource-Library/Word/LiteratureReviewoftherelationshipbetweeneducationandcare.ashx (accessed 23.10.09).

Moule, P, Wilford, A., Sales, R., and Lockyer, L. (2008) Student experiences and mentor views of the use of simulation for learning. *Nurse Educ. Today.* 28, 790–7.

Munro, K. (2008) Continuing professional development and the charity paradigm: Interrelated individual, collective and organisational issues about continuing professional development. *Nurse Educ. Today.* 28, 953–61.

National Confidential Enquiry into Patient Outcome and Death (2005) *An Acute Problem? A Report of the National Confidential Enquiry into Patient Outcome and Death*. Executive summary. Available on-line at http://www.ncepod.org.uk/2005report/summary.html.

National Patient Safety Agency (2007) *Safer Care for the Acutely Ill Patient: Learning From Serious Incidents*. National Patient Safety Agency, London.

NICE (2007) *Acutely Ill Patients in Hospital: Recognition of and Response to Acute Illness of Adults in Hospital*. National Institute for Health and Clinical Excellence, London.

Nursing and Midwifery Council (2002) *Supporting Nurses and Midwives Through Lifelong Learning*. Nursing and Midwifery Council, London.

Nursing and Midwifery Council (2006a) Preceptorship Guidelines. NMC Circular 21/2006. Available on line at: http://www.nmc-uk.org/aDisplayDocument.aspx?DocumentID=2088 (accessed 25.1.09).

Nursing and Midwifery Council (2006b) *Clinical Supervision A-Z advice sheet*. Available on line at http://www.nmc-uk.org/aframeDisplay.aspx?DocumentID=4022 (accessed 25.1.09).

Nursing and Midwifery Council (2008a) *The Code: Standards of Conduct, Performance and Ethics for Nurses and Midwives*. Nursing and Midwifery Council, London.

Nursing and Midwifery Council (2008b) *The Prep Handbook*. Nursing and Midwifery Council, London.

Nursing and Midwifery Council (2008c) *Profiles A-Z Advice Sheet*. Nursing and Midwifery Council, London.

Nursing and Midwifery Council (2008d) *Standards to Support Learning and Assessment in Practice*. 2nd edn. Nursing and Midwifery Council, London. Available on line at http://www.nmc-uk.org/aArticle. aspx?ArticleID=2649 (accessed 25.1.08).

Nursing and Midwifery Council (2009) *Review of Pre-registration Nursing Education—Phase 2*. Available on line at http://www.nmc-uk.orgt/aArticlePrint.aspx?ArticleID=3566 (accessed 24.3.09).

Parker, B. and Myrick, F. (2009) A critical examination of high-fidelity human patient simulation within the context of nursing pedagogy. *Nurse Educ. Today*. **29**(3), 322–9.

Plowright, C.J., Fraser, S., Buras-Rees, L. *et al*. (2006) Perceptions of critical care outreach within a network. *Nurs. Times*. **102**, 29, 36–42.

Price, B. (2007) Professional development opportunities in changing times. *Nurs. Standard*. **21**(25), 29–33.

Presho, M. (2006) Earning and learning: recruitment and retention in post registration nurse education. *Nurse Educ. Today*. **26**, 511–8.

Randall, C., Tate, B., and Lougheed, M. (2007) Emancipatory teaching-learning philosophy and practice education in acute care: navigating tensions. *J. Nurs. Educ*. **46**(2), 60–4.

Rattay, J., Paul, F., and Tully, V. (2006) Partnership working between a Higher Education Institution and NHS Trusts: developing an acute and critical care module. *Nurs. Crit. Care*. **11**(3), 111–7.

Rounce, K. and Workman, B. (2005) *Work*-based *Learning in Health Care*. Kingsham, Chichester.

Rolfe, G., Freshwater, D., and Jasper, M. (2001) *Critical Reflection for Nursing and the Helping Professions: A User's Guide*. Palgrave, Basingstoke.

Rushforth, H. (2007) Objective structured clinical examination (OSCE): Review of literature and implications for nursing education. *Nurse Educ. Today*. **27**, 481–90.

Scholes, J. (2008) Why health care needs resilient practitioners. *Nurs. Crit. Care*. **13**(6), 281–5.

Smith, G., Osgood, V., Crane, S. ALERT Course Development Group (2002) ALERT—a multiprofessional training course in the care of the acutely ill adult patient. *Resuscitation*. **52**(2002), 281–6.

Stanley, H. (2003) The journey to becoming a graduate nurse: a study of the lived experience of part-time post-registration students. *Nurse Educ. Prac*. **3**, 62–71.

Steen, C. and Costello, J. (2008) Teaching pre-registration student nurses to assess acutely ill patients: An evaluation of an acute illness management programme. *Nurse Educ. Prac*. **8**, 343–51.

Stock, J. (2002) Demand for graduate education set to rise. *Employing Nurses Midwives*. **December/ January**, 7–8.

Tait, M., Tait, D., Thornton, F., and Edwards, M. (2008) Development and evaluation of a critical care e-learning scenario. *Nurse Educ. Today*. **28**, 971–81.

Tennant, S. and Field, R. (2004) Continuing professional development: Does it make a difference? *Nurs. Crit. Care*. **9**(4), 167–72.

Thompson, C., Foster, A., Cole, I., and Dowling, D. (2005) Using social judgement theory to model nurses' use of clinical information in critical care education. *Nurse Educ. Today*. **25**, 68–77.

Wood, I., Douglas, J., and Priest, H. (2004) Education and training for acute care delivery: A needs analysis. *Nurs. Crit. Care*. **9**(4), 159–66.

Useful websites

The Nursing and Midwifery Council http://www.nmc-uk.org.

Royal College of Nursing http://www.rcn.org.uk.

University of Brighton http://www.brighton.ac.uk/snm.

Department of Health http://www.dh.gov.uk.

NHS careers http://www.nhscareers.nhs.uk.

Basic life support course http://www.resus.org.uk.

Appendix: Clinical link answers

This section contains suggested answers to the clinical link activities for each chapter. These are not exhaustive; you may have additional considerations depending on your own role and organization. You are reminded that you must always adhere to local policy and national guidance, and act within the Nursing and Midwifery Council code of professional conduct whenever patient care is being delivered.

Chapter 2

Clinical link 2.1a

This patient has a respiratory acidosis, with a pH of 7.3 and an increased $PaCO_2$. She also has a lower than normal oxygen level (hypoxia) and there are no signs of compensation. The treatment would include:

- ensuring airway is maintained
- increasing the FiO_2 in line with the British Thoracic Society 2008 guidelines (possibly high flow until she is awake)
- conducting a neurological assessment (AVPU)
- considering reducing analgesia until patient is more awake and reviewing analgesia with your medical colleagues
- the patient should be encouraged to take deep breaths

  Note: If the patient is very drowsy you should seek medical attention and consider administering opiate reversal drugs (once reviewed by medical team).

Clinical link 2.1b

This patient has a severe metabolic acidosis. The pH is 7.31 and the bicarbonate is 20. He has a history of diabetes (and has developed diabetic keto acidosis). This should be considered a medical emergency and urgent help should be summoned. His ability to maintain an airway should be assessed whilst you await help arriving and high flow oxygen administered as he is hypoxic. It may be necessary to move this patient to a higher care level where he will require:

- frequent blood glucose monitoring
- frequent assessment
- urgent blood electrolyte evaluation
- insulin (and accompanying dextrose) using a sliding scale
- fluid and electrolyte replacement
- close observation
- possibly mechanical ventilation and cardiovascular support.

Clinical link 2.1c

This patient has a type 2 respiratory failure. Her blood gas indicates respiratory acidosis with some partial compensation. The patient is hypoxic and has CO_2 retention. This requires:

+ adequate positioning of the patient
+ increased oxygen in line with British Thoracic Society 2008 guidelines to maintain saturations at 88–92%
+ close observation
+ repeat blood gases.

Urgent medical review is required and the following may be requested:

+ urgent chest X-ray
+ intravenous antibiotics
+ Non-invasive ventilation
+ nebulizers
+ physiotherapy.

Clinical link 2.2

This patient has type I respiratory failure with a low oxygen but a normal pH and carbon dioxide as indicative of her obstructive lung disease. Her carbon dioxide is a little low because her respiratory rate is high but the metabolic parameters are within normal limits. She has acute asthma and her vital signs indicate that she is critically ill because she is still wheezing and still desaturated on supplemental oxygen.

The main priorities are:

+ Calculate a risk score using a track-and-trigger system if available and follow the recommended escalation process as indicated.
+ Carry out an urgent medical review because of failure to improve.
+ Repeat nebulized bronchodilators according to prescription.
+ Increase her oxygen saturation.
+ Close observation of her respiratory function to ensure early detection of any deterioration. She has a high respiratory rate and is already using her accessory muscles but is desaturated on 35% oxygen. If she becomes tired, she will move to type II respiratory failure and alveolar hypoventilation. A rising carbon dioxide is a cause for concern and an indication of deterioration in an asthmatic patient but this is not detectable by pulse oximetry. Frequent observations of vital signs every 30 min should be initiated and clinical signs to watch for an increase in respiratory rate, more shallow apical breathing, and decreasing ability to manage speech. Peak expiratory flow rates before and after nebulizers should be rigorously recorded.
+ Ensure that this patient receives the prescribed nebulizers to relieve the bronchospasm. This is the treatment required to alleviate her symptoms and should not be delayed.
+ Reassure the patient so that she keeps the mask on long enough for her nebulizers to work. This means phoning her husband to ensure that her children are safely collected from school. She will not settle until she knows that this has been arranged. Do not leave the patient behind closed curtains, reassure her that you will watch her closely.

The following actions are required:

- Request urgent medical review giving clear indication of the patient's respiratory condition. State clearly the respiratory rate, use of accessory muscles, and desaturation to explain why you are concerned. An increase in inspired oxygen to 50–60% is needed to bring the saturations up and request repeat arterial blood gas analysis to monitor the carbon dioxide.

- Ensure that a treatment plan is in place and discuss this with senior medical staff. If this patient does not improve, admission to the intensive therapy unit (ITU) for intubation and ventilation is likely. Close liaison between nursing and medical staff is needed.

- Ensure that the patient's family are aware of her admission and the severity of her illness. Remain calm and reassuring and position the patient with enough pillows to maintain a comfortable sitting position to facilitate ventilation.

Clinical link 2.3

This patient has type II respiratory failure with a low oxygen and a high carbon dioxide and a low pH. His arterial blood gas analysis indicates a respiratory acidosis with metabolic compensation because the metabolic parameters indicate alkalosis but the pH is still low. The pyrexia and expectoration of thick green sputum indicate that he has an infective exacerbation of chronic obstructive pulmonary disease (COPD).

The main priorities are:

- Ensure that nebulizer and antibiotic medication is given as prescribed to treat this infective exacerbation of his COPD.

- Reach target saturations of 88% for this patient by changing from nasal specs which are unsuitable for mouth breathers to a white Venturi mask at 5 L per minute to deliver 28% oxygen in keeping with British Thoracic Society guidelines (2008a).

- Reposition the patient to facilitate ventilation.

- Encourage oral intake of fluid and maintain a strict fluid balance chart. He is dehydrated (as shown by urine colour, dry mouth, and viscous sputum). This will make it more difficult for him to expectorate.

The following actions are required:

- Contact medical team to discuss oxygen prescription.

- Sit the patient up in a comfortable position well supported with pillows and tilt the foot of the bed up a little to prevent him slipping back down.

- Oral fluids must be increased to maintain oral hygiene and increase urine output. Find out what he likes to drink and ask his daughter to bring it in. Ensure that the nursing team are aware of the need to increase his oral intake and provide drinks that are acceptable to the patient.

- Ensure that physiotherapists visit the patient to assist with expectoration and mobility if necessary.

- Ensure that the patient is well supported with pillows in a sitting position to facilitate ventilation.

- Encourage diet and refer to dietician for food supplements to prevent further weight loss. Discuss diet with the patient and his daughter, who does the shopping.

- This patient may be depressed as he has recently been bereaved and may be feeling lonely and isolated. Discuss this with the patient and his daughter and try to encourage a positive outlook.
- Discharge planning should ensure that the community team, for example the community matron, is contacted with regard to case management to prevent repeated admissions and improve the patient's ability to manage his disease.

Clinical link 2.4

This patient has type I respiratory failure and a partially compensated metabolic acidosis secondary to probable sepsis. The pH and metabolic parameters (standard bicarbonate and base excess) and high lactate indicate metabolic acidosis and the patient is compensating with an increased respiratory rate, which has reduced the carbon dioxide to raise the pH.

- This patient is seriously ill and a track-and-trigger score should be calculated if available and escalation initiated.
- Urgent medical review is required and admission to ITU is likely (see chapter on track-and-trigger systems and chapter on sepsis). Anaesthetic review and transfer to ITU should be discussed immediately with the surgical specialist registrar.
- High-flow oxygen and intravenous fluids should be prescribed and administered as a matter of urgency.
- The patient's designated next of kin should be contacted and informed of his deteriorating condition.

Clinical actions should be:

- Request urgent medical review.
- Initiate high-flow oxygen.
- Initiate quarter hourly monitoring of vital signs and saturations.
- Initiate hourly monitoring of urine output and fluid balance.
- Ensure peripheral venous access.
- Ensure that the patient's next of kin has been informed that his condition has deteriorated.
- Inform senior nursing staff of the patient's critical illness and discuss possibility of transfer to ITU.

Clinical link 2.5

This patient has type I respiratory failure with a low oxygen and normal pH and carbon dioxide. He remains desaturated and tachypnoeic on high-flow oxygen. The history of sudden onset of symptoms and his height and body shape are suggestive of a spontaneous pneumothorax.

The main priorities are:

- Expedite the chest X-ray to confirm diagnosis and ensure that medical staff are aware of the delay.
- Liaise with the medical registrar and ensure that the chest X-ray is reviewed as soon as possible to facilitate early medical intervention, which is likely to be the insertion of an underwater seal chest drain.
- Maintain close observation of the patient's respiratory function. Vital signs, especially respiratory rate and saturations, should be recorded half hourly.

The clinical actions should be:

+ Organize the chest X-ray as soon as possible.
+ Inform medical staff of the patient's improvement in response to oxygen but emphasize that he remains breathless and desaturated.
+ Ensure adequate pain relief.
+ Reassure the patient and explain what is happening.
+ Prepare equipment and trolley for insertion of chest drain.

Chapter 3

Clinical link 3.1

+ Systematic analysis of the arrhythmia, including diagnosis:
  + rate—fast, variable: using R-R interval method, rate varies from 125/min to 214/min
  + rhythm—irregularly irregular
  + P–QRS ratio—no p-waves are discernible
  + P–R interval—impossible to measure P–R interval as no p-waves evident
  + QRS complex—narrow, normal duration
  + ST segment—ST segment is deviated 2 mm below the isoelectric line, indicative of myocardial ischaemia
  + T waves—positive, normal.
  + Diagnosis: This arrhythmia is a fast, irregularly irregular rhythm indicative of atrial fibrillation. The patient appears to have some degree of myocardial ischaemia secondary to the atrial fibrillation and the tachycardia indicated by the ST segment depression.
+ Nursing actions for the next 10 min:
  + Reassure Mrs Jones. Sudden onset of atrial fibrillation is a very frightening experience as the patient is often aware of the fast, irregular palpitations in their chest. In addition, extreme anxiety will exacerbate her breathlessness and potentially make the tachycardia faster. Assure Mrs Jones that you will stay with her.
  + Alert medical staff and senior nurse on the ward that assistance is required.
  + Check Mrs Jones' vital signs:
    + Establish continuous ECG monitoring.
    + Record and compare radial and apical heart rate.
    + Record blood pressure in both arms.
    + Record respiratory rate.
    + Attach oxygen saturation probe and monitor O_2 saturation.
    + Establish baseline and record 15-min recordings as above.
  + Position patient appropriately—if blood pressure will tolerate, sit patient in upright position, and administer prescribed high-flow oxygen.
  + Record a 12-lead ECG to check for evidence of myocardial ischaemia/infarction.
  + Prepare emergency equipment at bedside. Ensure that patient has an intravenous line in situ for administration of emergency drugs.

- Potential medical interventions:
  - Sudden onset of atrial fibrillation with haemodynamic compromise requires urgent medical treatment. The most likely option is to aim to restore sinus rhythm as quickly as possible by electrical cardioversion under anaesthetic.
  - Direct current cardioversion is performed under general anaesthetic with either 200 J monophasic or 120 J biphasic current.
  - Intravenous heparin will be commenced before cardioversion to protect against potential thromboembolism.
  - 12-Lead ECG should be examined for any indication of myocardial infarction or ischaemia.

Clinical link 3.2

- Priorities for this patient with justifications for actions:
  - Assessment of chest pain: using PQRST approach to establish the potential cause. Assess severity of pain using numeric pain scale and to establish pattern and evolution of pain. Aim is to rule in or rule out causes of cardiac chest pain. Reassure the patient that the aim is to relieve the pain as quickly as possible. Anxiety may exacerbate the existing pain.
  - Repeat 12-lead ECG to see whether there is any evidence of new myocardial ischaemia (ST segment depression or T-wave inversion) or myocardial infarction (ST segment elevation). Myocardial ischaemia evolves slowly and may not be immediately apparent on the ECG recorded in A&E. The pulse is now irregular so look for evidence of ventricular extrasystoles and/or atrial fibrillation.
  - Review the medication card and administer sublingual GTN, intravenous morphine with an anti-emetic if prescribed. Be cautious with doses as blood pressure is low. It is important to relieve the chest pain, but care should be taken with nitrates and opiates in the presence of a low blood pressure.
  - Sit patient upright and administer high-flow oxygen—this will improve myocardial perfusion and improve oxygen saturation.
  - Advise the medical staff of the current vital signs given in the scenario and of the deteriorating vital signs. Advise medical staff of the low blood potassium which, in conjunction with the irregular pulse, requires administration of potassium supplements.
- What interventions from the doctors would you anticipate?
  - Review of 12-lead ECG:
  - Cardiovascular examination to reveal any evidence of heart failure, shock, myocardial infarction.
  - Review of urea and electrolytes, administration of potassium supplements for low K^+ (3.2 mmol/L).
  - Arterial blood gases to evaluate reasons for breathlessness.
- What type of assessment and monitoring will you continually undertake?
  - Chest pain assessment to evaluate effectiveness of pain relief.
  - Continuous ECG recording, using continuous ST segment monitoring if available.
  - Vital signs every 15 min:
    - heart rate

- blood pressure
- respiratory rate
- oxygen saturations
- capillary refill.

♦ What are the potential differential diagnoses for this presentation? Give rationales for your answers.

- n-STEMI. The troponin result is not yet available and whilst the 12-lead is normal, the patient still has a dull ache in his chest and left arm.
- Atrial fibrillation secondary to acute cardiac event (n-STEMI). Patient has a fast and irregular pulse.
- Early left ventricular failure and/or poor cardiac output due to either n-STEMI or atrial fibrillation or both. Patient has poor capillary refill, is peripherally cool and pale and has a tachycardia, low blood pressure and fast respiratory rate.

Clinical link 3.3

♦ Immediate actions and why?

- Reassure the lady, but explain that you need to record some more investigations.
- You suspect sudden onset of atrial fibrillation the pulse rate is fast and irregular. Record a synchronized radial and apex beat and record a 12-lead ECG.
- You suspect sudden onset left ventricular failure as she is hypoxic and breathless, her capillary refill is prolonged. Ask for medical staff to attend to review this lady.
- It is possible that she has re-infarcted—review 12-lead ECG against last recording.

♦ Other investigations by doctor and why?

- Check medications—some drugs in combination can cause hypotension (β-blockers and ACE inhibitors). Similarly β-blockers can cause left ventricular failure, especially immediately post-myocardial infarction.
- Review 12-lead ECG as above.
- Conduct a thorough cardiac and respiratory physical examination; sudden onset heart failure may present with bilateral crackles at both lung bases and the addition of a third heart sound (S3) to the normal heart sounds S1 and S2.
- Request U&Es, cardiac markers (Troponins, CK), FBC.
- Request a chest X-ray to review for possible pulmonary oedema.

♦ Potential problems.

- Atrial fibrillation secondary to recent acute myocardial infarction (AMI).
- Left ventricular failure secondary to recent AMI and possible atrial fibrillation.
- Possible further myocardial infarction.

Chapter 4
Clinical link 4.1

♦ Frequency of observations

This patient's GCS was 15 on admission so following the NICE (2007) guidance observations have been recorded quarter hourly for 2 h, but the observations were inadvertently reduced to hourly after 2 h. In the light of this patient's deterioration it would be more appropriate to:

- keep the observations quarter hourly until the GCS returns to 15
- consider increasing to quarter hourly as this man's condition is deteriorating within 6 h of injury (the most common time for deterioration to occur).

♦ Trigger for medical review

This patient is deteriorating and help should be sought. The initial drop to 14 could just be attributed to the patient feeling sleepy, but at 12:00 the following changes occurred:

- new confusion (this should prompt quick medical intervention)
- unequal pupils (this should always prompt quick medical intervention).

At 13:00 the patient's GCS has dropped to 12. The NICE guidance highlights the need for urgent attention if there is a drop in GCS of greater than 2 points. In addition, the continued pupil changes are a cause for great concern as are the limb changes. The patient has developed a left-sided weakness.

From a physiological perspective you will note that there is an increasing blood pressure and decreasing pulse. These point to the start of the Cushings triad and further patient deterioration is likely to be rapid.

♦ Significance of drop

Any change in level of consciousness and changes in motor function should receive prompt intervention. These changes all point to increasing intracranial pressure. The injury is likely to be on the right side of the brain (ipsilateral pupil changes/contralateral limb changes). This patient requires urgent intervention/scanning to exclude an extradural/subdural haematoma.

Clinical link 4.2

♦ Potential nursing problems and associated management

This patient is likely to have a number of problems related to his left-sided stroke. The potential problems and their associated management include:

- *Airway maintenance*: He is dribbling and spluttering and will require urgent assessment of his ability to maintain his airway. He may require insertion of an artificial airway or careful positioning to ensure that his airway is not compromised.
- *Respiratory compromise/risk of aspiration*: He may be susceptible to aspiration because of his airway/swallowing difficulties. Vigilance for signs and symptoms of respiratory distress is essential. Further neurological compromise may cause reduced respiratory function (CNS control). Again adequate assessment of respiratory function is needed. Saturations should be monitored and oxygen given if saturations fall below 94% (routine oxygen is not provided). Suction equipment should be available at all times as should airway adjuncts. Chest auscultation/chest X-ray may be required if condition deteriorates. The patient should be made nil by mouth until his swallow assessment has been performed to reduce the likelihood of aspiration pneumonia. Close monitoring for development of chest infection is vital.
- *Blood pressure*: He is hypertensive and blood pressure and pulse should be closely monitored alongside neurological observations. Blood pressure is not routinely reduced because of the risk of reduced cerebral perfusion. Blood pressure parameters should be set by medical staff and urgent intervention if blood pressure continues to rise. Blood pressure and

pulse should be closely monitored for signs of Cushing's triad (increased blood pressure, decreased HR, respiratory changes) as these may indicate increasing intracranial pressure. Cardiac monitoring and continuous blood pressure recordings may be advisable.

- *Neurological deterioration*: Neurological observations should be recorded at regular intervals (at least half hourly). Any deterioration in condition should be quickly reported. Neurological deficits should be identified and monitored for any changes and any deterioration should be reported immediately to medical staff. Further CT scans may be indicated if condition deteriorates. Neurological assessment may be difficult in this man if his speech centres have been affected (left-sided stroke patients are at risk of dysphasia as speech centres are located in left brain for most people). Limb assessment should use objective grading criteria. Care should be taken with patient positioning to ensure any affected limbs are positioned appropriately and supported with pillows.

- *Dehydration*: This patient must be nil by mouth until he has been assessed by an appropriate person. He should be commenced on intravenous fluids (preferably isotonic, e.g. normal saline. Five per cent dextrose should be avoided because it may increase blood glucose and it may further increase cerebral oedema as it is a free fluid). A fluid balance chart is essential and careful recording of input/output. Reduced urine output may indicate dehydration, increased urine output may indicate rising intracranial pressure.

- *Poor nutrition/blood glucose instability*: This patient will require blood glucose monitoring. Stress of stroke may cause a physiological increase in blood glucose and a growing body of evidence suggests this is detrimental. Current stroke guidelines highlight the need to maintain blood glucose between 4 and 11 mmol. Monitoring for hypoglycaemia should also occur as the patient's nil by mouth status may make him susceptible to low blood glucose. The patient may require enteral nutrition. It is essential to check the position of the nasogastric tube before commencing feed. Again any feed should be recorded and advice sought from a dietician.

- *Risk of falling safety issues*: This man's right-sided weakness and potential communication difficulties/potential confusion puts him at risk of falling. Care should be taken with positioning this patient; cot sides may be required (in line with local policies). Communication aids and call buzzer should be available at all times. Patient should remain on bed rest until assessed by physiotherapist.

- *Need for anticoagulation*: Aspirin should be administered as per guidance within first 24 h. Care should be taken with those patients who have a history of gastric problems and it may be necessary to provide supplemental proton pump inhibitors. Patients who are allergic to aspirin should be provided with a suitable alternative, as prescribed by the medical staff.

- Nursing priorities

In line with the ALERT framework care should be prioritized using the ABC system. This patient's priorities are:

- **A**irway assessment and maintenance
- **B**reathing assessment and oxygenation
- **C**ardiovascular assessment and monitoring of blood pressure
- **D**isability/neurological assessment, monitoring for any changes
- **E**verything else
- Multidisciplinary involvement

- Speech and language team (SALT): to assess speech and language problems and swallow.
- Dietician: to assess nutritional intake and requirements for enteral nutrition.
- Physiotherapist: chest assessment/to assess mobilization.
- Occupational therapist: to assess need for splints to prevent contractions.
- Medical staff: review of treatment/ongoing monitoring.
- Radiographer: imaging if required.

Clinical link 4.3

This patient is awake and has a GCS of 15 so airway will not be compromised. Breathing should be assessed but is unlikely to be problematic (ensure smoking history recorded as smokers are more at risk of SAH and subsequent chest infections).

- Nursing priorities for this patient include:

  - *Cardiovascular assessment*: Blood pressure and pulse should be recorded at least hourly. Hypertension increases the likelihood of rebleeding so should be avoided if excessively high. Hypotension should also be avoided as this can worsen the ischaemic side effects of SAH. Treatment is dependent on consultation with the neurosurgeons, but any antihypertensive should be used with caution as blood pressure should not be lowered too much as this may worsen ischcaemia. The patient should be kept adequately hydrated to maintain blood pressure and intravenous fluids may be required. Bed rest is essential.

  - *Neurological assessment*: It is vital that this patient's neurological observations are recorded at least hourly. Specific attention should be paid to any focal deficiencies as these may indicate worsening of her condition. SAH patients are at risk of rebleeding so bed rest should be enforced and patient nursed at 30° (avoid sitting up). Any changes in neurological condition should be reported immediately and action taken.

  - *Pain control*: Pain is likely to be very severe and difficult to control, the patient is also likely to feel nauseated and may be vomiting due to the effects of menigeal irritation. Pain should be assessed and appropriate medication offered. Analgesia may be opiate based, but care should be taken to avoid suppressing neurological status with analgesia. The patient may also require additional analgesia and this should be given as per hospital protocol. Overstimulation should be avoided and the patient should be encouraged to rest as much as possible. Laxatives may be required to prevent constipating effects of analgesia. Antiemetic may be required to reduce emetic effect of analgesia (these should be offered with analgesia).

  - *Potential dehydration due to nausea/vomiting*: Dehydration will worsen complications of SAH and should be avoided. Intravenous isotonic fluid should be given (preferably saline). The patient should be commenced on a fluid balance chart and held at a slightly positive or neutral fluid balance. Oral fluids should be encouraged if tolerated. Electrolyte balance should be monitored at least daily.

  - *Drug therapy*: The Cochrane review suggests that nimodopine should be administered provided it does not have a negative effect on the patient's blood pressure (it may be necessary to reduce dose/route of administration if blood pressure falls). Nimodopine should be given as per manufacturer's guidance in line with local neurosurgical protocol. Aggressive treatment of SAH (e.g. triple H therapy) will not commence until the aneurysm has been secured.

- Anxiety

This is understandably common in both patient and family. SAH patients will have most likely been informed of their diagnosis and subsequent potential management and implications/complications of SAH. This will clearly add to their anxiety, which is often also exacerbated by their physical symptoms. Reduction of anxiety will require:

- understanding of the patient/family fears
- honest explanation of impending treatment
- maintenance of open communication channels
- appropriate advice to relieve anxiety
- reduction of physical symptoms
- encouragement of relaxation (if possible)

♦ Transfer and treatment

Treatment will usually involve referral to a neurological centre for further assessment and treatment. Treatment options include:

- coiling or clipping of the aneurysm to prevent rebleeding (other techniques are being developed for management of aneurysm, but these are the most common).

The patient is still at risk of deterioration/disability/death even after the aneurysm has been treated. Treatment is dependent on site and size of aneurysm so it may be best to discuss potential options but highlight that this decision will be discussed further at the neurological centre. It may be possible to open communication channels with neurological centre and patient before transfer.

Clinical link 4.4

Part 1 Assessment of this patient will be difficult due to his aggression. However, assessment is vital and needs to be undertaken. Assessment will also be made difficult by the presence of alcohol (although it is vital not to assume that this man is drunk, his aggression and agitation could be as a result of head injury). Assessment during the initial period following head injury (6 hours) is very important (NICE 2007).

It may be helpful to explain quietly and carefully to this man the need for neurological observation. His aggression and agitation may be worsened by pain so adequate pain assessment and pain control is vital. Observations should be recorded at least half hourly as his GCS is below 15 (NICE 2007). Any changes should be reported and acted on immediately. Care should be taken by the nurse to ensure that he/she is not harmed whilst recording observations. Increasing aggression/agitation may be a sign of worsening head injury and should be dealt with immediately.

Care should be taken to maintain the safety of this patient.

Part 2 His GCS is now 12 (E2, V4, M6). Although he is less agitated it is worrying that he now needs painful stimuli to awaken him. His ovoid sluggish pupils are also a worrying sign as this may indicate a raising intracranial pressure. In accordance with the NICE (2007) guidance immediate help should be sought as he:

♦ has new neurological symptoms (pupil changes)

♦ has a drop in GCS.

Whilst awaiting assistance, neurological observation frequency should be increased to quarter hourly. It may be of benefit to check a blood glucose level. If further deterioration occurs whilst awaiting medical review urgent assistance should be sought.

This patient will require medical examination, a more in-depth neurological assessment by the doctor, and possibly a CT scan.

Clinical link 4.5

Your immediate action would be to ensure that the patient cannot be harmed during this seizure. Any optical glasses should be removed from the patient. Any objects/furniture that may hurt the patient should be removed and the area around the patient should be cleared as much as possible.

You will need to time and observe the seizure so an accurate estimation of how long the seizure lasted and what occurred during the seizure should be noted. Things to observe include:

- any aura or warning (not likely in this case)
- which parts of the body are moving, what sort of movement, the spread of movement, and the amount of time in the tonic and clonic phases
- whether patient becomes cyanosed
- whether patient stops breathing
- whether there is any incontinence (urinary and faecal)
- pupil changes (once seizure stopped)
- post ictal state.

Seizures will normally limit themselves, but this patient's seizure appears to be progressing into status epilepticus (a series of seizures with little or no recovery of consciousness between seizures). This is a *medical emergency* and immediate help is required. You should ensure that someone stays with patient and intubation equipment and monitoring is bought to the patient (crash trolley). Drugs should be available for the doctors arrival (this includes benzodiazepines—these may be given rectally or intravenously if access is available). Oxygen via a non rebreathe mask should be applied (10–15 L) until the anaesthetist arrives and assesses need for intubation.

Should this patient require an ITU bed then hospital policy for transfer of level 2/3 patient should be followed. This usually necessitates the need for a trained nurse and doctor to accompany the patient (see Chapter 14).

Chapter 5

Clinical link 5.1

Mr T has a variety of problems that need to be prioritized. He should be recovering from musculoskeletal pain but instead his condition is aggravating quickly. His early warning score would suggest that he has become acutely ill with pyrexia, possible acute kidney injury, and possible bowel obstruction. He needs an urgent medical review, if that is not possible you should contact the outreach team. Mr T should be catheterized for hourly monitoring of urinary output, be asked to fast, and have a peripheral cannula inserted to commence intravenous fluids, with possible addition of potassium to correct hypokalaemia. An urgent blood sample for urea and electrolytes should be taken as soon as possible, together with a blood culture sample. Intravenous antibiotics will be needed as Mr T has a urinary infection, as suggested by the presence of leucocytes at the urinalysis. A mid-stream urine sample should be taken after catheterization for microbiology culture. You should monitor urinary output hourly, maintain a fluid balance chart, and consider naso-gastric intubation for gastric drainage. In Mr T's case acute kidney injury may be caused by urinary sepsis, prostatic obstruction, or cancer metastasis.

Clinical link 5.2

- Lydia may be developing pulmonary oedema. You should sit Lydia upright to encourage ventilation, you should also commence prescribed oxygen therapy

- Pulmonary oedema is present; this is evident in Lydia's sense of impending doom, her fast respiratory rate and 'bubbly' breathing.
- The medical team need to be contacted urgently and taking an electrocardiogram prior to their arrival is necessary. The medical team prescribe furosemide intravenously which initially improves her breathing. She is catheterised and fluid balance carefully monitored.

Clinical link 5.3

- For Lydia, sepsis may have caused acute kidney injury, or it may be the result of the nephrotoxicity of vancomycin on silent chronic kidney failure (Lydia has had long-standing hypertension). Lydia is now acutely ill and needs urgent medical attention. She has incipient pulmonary oedema and acute kidney failure.
- The high potassium is due to acute kidney failure and this may exacerbate cardiac dysfunction and cause cardiac arrhythmias.
- The medical team need to take cognisance of the incipient heart failure whilst managing the acute kidney failure. The most pressing problem is the hyperkalaemia and Lydia will have glucose 5% intravenous fluid infusion prescribed. The glucose triggers a surge in insulin release, which in turn pushes potassium molecules back into the intracellular space. The medical staff also need to replace fluid, but in the presence of incipient pulmonary oedema, this is dangerous and they will therefore insert a central venous catheter prior to commencing fluid replacement therapy and you will be advised to monitor the central venous pressure regularly, maintaining it within prescribed limits. If Lydia does not respond to the fluid replacement management, the hyperkalaemia may worsen, causing cardiac arrhythmias and in addition the pulmonary oedema may escalate. You need to maintain regular monitoring of Lydia's vital signs and seek assistance from the nurse in charge and from the outreach team.

Clinical link 5.4

Calcium gluconate given intravenously increases the arrhythmia threshold and has a cardiac protective effect against hyperkalaemia. Insulin changes cell permeability to potassium and causes a shift to the intracellular space, immediately improving the hyperkalaemia risk to the cardiac muscle. However, if you give Lydia insulin, she needs glucose to prevent hypoglycaemia. Please note that only human insulin can be given intravenously.

Once the hyperkalaemia emergency is averted, the focus changes to address the life-threatening pulmonary oedema. Urgent fluid reduction is needed, but this cannot be too sudden as blood pressure is low and therefore haemodiafiltration is the optimal choice for solute and fluid removal.

Chapter 6

Clinical link 6.1

- Priorities for this patient
  - Check to see if dysphagia is due to airway obstruction: observe for obstruction.
  - Evaluate swallowing reflex (if you are competent to do so) by placing your fingers along the thyroid notch and instructing the patient to swallow. If you feel the larynx rise, the reflex is functioning. If uncertain follow local protocol and refer to (SALT) for swallowing assessment.
  - Ask patient to cough to assess the cough reflex.
  - If certain that both the swallowing and the cough reflex are present assess the gag reflex.
  - Look at the face and listen to the speech for signs of muscle weakness.

- Ask whether solids or liquids are more difficult to swallow.
- Ask whether the symptoms disappear after trying to swallow a few times. Is the swallow affected by the position in bed or chair?

◆ What actions will you take to ensure her nutritional and fluid needs are met?

- Ensure that patient is sitting up and able to reach food.
- Ensure that patient has a clean, moist mouth and if present, correctly fitting dentures. This will aid the formation of a bolus which will assist swallowing.
- Ensure that patient has a soft diet avoiding use of mixed foods such as soup and breakfast cereals. Foods that contain both liquids and solids are more difficult to swallow.
- If patient is unable to consume large volumes of food offer supplements or snacks between meals.
- Monitor intake of food and fluids, recording amount consumed on a food and fluid chart.
- Repeat nutritional screening tool according to local protocol.
- Refer to dietician in accordance with local policy.
- Refer to SALT in accordance with local policy.

◆ What signs might indicate that she has a problem with swallowing?

- Drooling of saliva from the mouth.
- Inability of the patient to poke her tongue out.
- Drooping to left side of face and mouth.
- Patient has aphasia or dysarthria.
- When attempting to speak voice sounds 'wet'.

Clinical link 6.2

◆ What actions will you take to plan the nutritional support for Eva during the acute phase of her illness?

- Complete the MUST screening tool.

Eva is elderly and has multiple fractures, both these factors increase her risk of being malnourished before and during this period of hospitalization.

- Using a pragmatic approach calculate her energy requirement $59 \times 1.25 \times 30 = 2655$ calories.

Although dieticians would normally calculate the energy requirements of a patient, using a pragmatic approach nurses can have some idea as to how much energy should be consumed.

- Monitor how long Eva is nil by mouth. If it exceeds 6 h ensure a plan is in place for when eating and drinking can resume.

Evidence has indicated that elderly orthopaedic patients can be nil by mouth for excessive periods of time. They are often malnourished and under-hydrated before surgery and as a result their recovery from the operation could be further compromised.

◆ What actions will you take to ensure that Eva's nutritional status is not compromised during this period?

- Review intravenous regimen.

Eva is having an intravenous infusion of normal saline but is having no calories. Discuss with the medical team about reviewing the intravenous regimen. Intravenous 5% dextrose contains 5 g/100 mL fluid, 20 kcal/100mL fluid. A volume of 1 L of 5% dextrose will supply 200 kcal, which may help to conserve skeletal muscle.

♦ Record intake of food and fluids.

- Encourage small frequent intakes of liquid such as water; milk based drinks.
- Encourage small, easily digested, energy dense meals

If Eva is still not able to consume an adequate intake consider complete liquid supplementation.

- Monitor fluid output.

Increased fluid intake will replace fluid loss associated with the operation and filtration by the kidney. As fluid loss is replaced urine output will increase. Elderly patients are susceptible to fluid overload due to reduced kidney function.

Clinical link 6.3

♦ Critically discuss the actions you will take before commencing the feed.

- Ensure George is in a position to facilitate gastric emptying.

Although George is on traction he is able to be positioned at an angle no less than 30° and no greater than 45°. This will facilitate gastric emptying by gravity and reduce the risk of reflux occurring.

- Check position of feeding tube using pH indicator paper.

The position of a feeding tube must be checked after insertion and before commencing each feed using pH indicator paper. The HCL released from the oxyntic cells reduces the pH to between 1 and 3. The use of proton pump inhibitors and histamine-2 receptor antagonists reduces the amount of HCL present in the stomach. The gold standard for checking position of a feeding tube is an X-ray.

- Flush nasogastric tube with a minimum of 20 mL of clean water or sterile water (according to local protocol).

Feeding tubes must be flushed before and after each feed. The volume of water used must be recorded on a fluid chart.

- Ensure that giving set has been in place no longer than 24 h.

Formula feed provides an ideal environment for bacteria, and although tubes are flushed before and after a feed they are at high risk of being contaminated.

- Ensure that a clean procedure is adopted in the preparation of the formula feed and connection to the feeding tube.

Washing hands before and after connecting the formula feed, and ensuring that the tip of the feeding tube and the formula feed container are not touched will reduce the risk of contamination of the feed by bacteria.

- Ensure that feeding rate is correctly set.

The formula feed is prescribed to ensure that George receives adequate nutrition and fluids over each period of 24 h. Ensuring that the feed rate is correct will ensure that the correct volume of feed is administered and reduce the risk of complications associated with incorrect feeding.

♦ After 8 h George complains of feeling sick and nauseous. What actions will you take?

- Check that George is in the correct position.
- Check the feed rate.

If these checks are satisfactory it may be of benefit to administer anti-emetics (if they are prescribed).

Chapter 7

Clinical link 7.1

- What would your priorities be for this patient? Justify your actions.
- Assess intravenous access sites to ensure that they are intact.
- Evaluate rate of current infusions (crystalloid and insulin therapy) and ensure that they are infusing well via a pump/syringe driver.
- Begin fluid balance chart.
- Liaise with doctor regarding prescription for fluids, electrolytes, and insulin because these are the three key features of diabetic ketoacidosis management.
- Recheck blood glucose because insulin infusion had been commenced before coming to the high dependency unit.

- What interventions from the doctors would you anticipate?
  - Intravenous infusion—rapid fluid replacement needed to correct fluid loss.
  - Potassium replacement—although potassium is within normal range, it will probably continue to drop as insulin therapy progresses.
  - Insulin therapy—aim to reduce blood glucose by 2–3 mmolL/h.
  - Anti-emetic for nausea and vomiting.

- What types of assessment and monitoring will you continually undertake?
  - Blood glucose and electrolytes.
  - Vital signs.
  - Urine output.
  - ECG monitoring.
  - Level of consciousness and ability to maintain airway.
  - Early warning score.

- Why would the lactate be elevated and how can this be resolved?
  - If tissue perfusion has been compromised from the fluid deficit, the tissues will be starved of oxygen and needing to rely on anaerobic metabolism which produces lactate.
  - As the intravenous fluid therapy replacement progresses, tissue perfusion will improve and help to resolve the high lactate.

- Identify possible causes for this episode of DKA and how the clinical picture fits the diagnostic criteria for DKA.
  - Potential causes: infection, errors with insulin injections, stress, trauma.
  - Diagnosis of DKA would have been made by the doctor based on the high blood glucose, ketones in urine, acidosis, high osmolarity, polyuria, ketonic breaths, and high respiratory rate.

- What type of shock is occurring? Rationalize your answer.
  - Hypovolaemic shock because there are signs and symptoms of intravascular fluid deficit: thirst, tachycardia, hypotension, dry mucous membranes, cool peripheries, and prolonged capillary refill.
  - It is more likely to be hypovolaemic shock compared with other types of shock because of clinical picture of diabetic ketoacidosis, which leaves patients with severe dehydration.

Clinical link 7.2

- What would be your next immediate actions and why?
  - Look for signs of external bleeding (dressing, drains, and nasogastric drainage) because clinical signs are indicating postoperative bleeding.
  - Call for the doctor to come and assess the patient immediately in order to confirm postoperative bleeding or another cause for the abnormal clinical findings.
  - Apply pressure to site of bleeding if this becomes obvious.
  - Inform the nurse in charge because you may need more support to care for this patient or other patients you are responsible for that shift.
- What other signs and symptoms would indicate that postoperative bleeding is occurring?
  - Abdominal distension, drop in haemoglobin, reduced urine output, increased lactate.
- If active bleeding was ruled out, what other reasons could be causing these abnormalities?
  - Sepsis, hypotension from epidural infusion, or cardiogenic shock.
- If active bleeding was confirmed, how would you coordinate care of the patient, including interaction with the nurse in charge and surgical team?
  - Pass on to the nurse in charge and another nurse colleague key information about other patients you are for caring that will need to be delegated to another nurse while you are busy with this patient.
  - Liaise with surgical team about if/when patient will return to theatres and make suitable arrangements with porters and attach patient to monitoring equipment.
  - Administer blood products as prescribed.
  - Continue to monitor vital signs and level of consciousness.

Clinical link 7.3

- Identify all the potential causes for fluid and electrolyte deficit with this patient.
  - Confusion, which may be impairing his oral intake of food and fluids.
  - Large amounts of watery stools.
  - Urine output may be low from poor oral intake of fluids or from renal failure, which could be altering sodium and water excretion.
- How would you manage the diarrhoea?
  - Faecal collection bag to protect skin, promote dignity for the patient, and prevent patient from having to be cleaned and moved as frequently.

- Skin care, including barrier cream/sprays after cleaning patient for diarrhoea if faecal collection bag becomes detached.
- Monitor colour, amount, frequency, and consistency of stool.

♦ How would you manage improving the fluid input?
- Encourage oral intake.
- If oral intake insufficient, liaise with doctor regarding the need for an intravenous infusion.

♦ What investigations and treatments does this patient appear to need?

- Blood tests: full blood count, urea, creatinine, electrolytes.
- Stool sample for culture and sensitivity to identify any infection.
- Urine sample for culture and sensitivity to rule out urine infection.
- Full physical assessment to identify potential causes for confusion besides infection.

Clinical link 7.4

♦ Explain why hypotension due to hypovolaemia may occur with this patient, who has both peripheral oedema and ascites.
- There is an excess amount of fluid in the body but this is in the interstitial space rather than intravascular.
- Low albumin from liver failure reduces the oncotic pressure within the blood, which then causes fluid to leak out of vessels into interstitum.
- Low intravascular volume (hypovolaemia) then occurs, although excess fluid rests in the interstitial space.

♦ What impact does the excessive fluid in the peritoneal space have on other body systems?
- Abdominal distension may prevent normal expansion of the lungs because the larger abdomen pushes up into diaphragm restricting ventilation.
- Ascites may cause discomfort and prevent normal mobility due to the excessively large abdomen.

♦ Why was an albumin infusion prescribed?

- If a large amount of ascitic fluid is removed, there can be clinically significant fluid shifts resulting in a drop in intravascular volume.
- The aim of the albumin infusion is to prevent hypovolaemia and to increase the oncotic pressure from the large albumin molecules to prevent further movement of fluid into the interstitial space.
- Although the use of albumin as a colloid for fluid resuscitation has not been supported by research (Finfer *et al.* 2004; Perel & Roberts 2007), there remains debate on the value of albumin following drainage of a large amount of ascites.

Clinical link 7.5

Iatrogenic intravenous fluid overload

♦ What other signs and symptoms would indicate to you that this patient has become hypervolaemic?

- Positive fluid balance, high respiratory rate, and low oxygen saturation.

♦ What would be your immediate actions and why?

- Administer oxygen and sit patient up in bed.
- Inform doctor to have immediate medical review.
- Inform nurse in charge for further support and to keep up to date.
- Discuss with doctor need for diuretics if hypervolaemia is confirmed to remove excess intravascular fluid.

♦ What medical investigations would help to confirm whether the patient has hypervolaemia?

- Chest X-ray to assess for pulmonary oedema.
- Advanced cardiovascular assessment to assess for acute heart failure.

♦ Provide an explanation for why the patient has a reduced urine output despite having an increase in total blood volume.

- If there is hypervolaemia, normally the compensation response would be to increase urine output to remove excess water although this requires normal functioning kidneys and cardiovascular system.
- This patient could potentially have renal failure, heart failure, or in fact both, which has resulted in a decrease in urine output (in which case providing more intravascular fluid when the circulating blood volume is already high has caused further hypervolaemia).

Chapter 8

Clinical link 8.1

Septic shock is sometimes defined as a 'distributive' shock because it is the distribution of circulating plasma fluid between the cellular, interstitial, and intravascular compartments that becomes problematical in sepsis. A disproportionate amount of fluid moves from the intravascular space into the interstitium due to endothelial 'leakiness'. This fluid normally stays in the vasculature and helps maintain blood pressure—without it the patient experiences shock.

Septic hypovolaemia is referred to as 'relative' because unlike situations where blood losses are 'absolute'—such as haemorrhage—the volume of fluid is still in one of the fluid compartments—albeit in the wrong one.

Clinical link 8.2

Early sepsis is sometimes called 'hot' or 'warm' sepsis because of vasodilation and increased cardiac output states bringing a lot of blood and therefore metabolic warmth to the skin surface. Also because of the presence of pyrexia in response to invading organisms.

Later sepsis is sometimes called 'cold' or 'cool' sepsis because these states are when the compensation mechanisms have failed, but also because there is frequently the development of oedema globally, resulting in 'water-logged' skin, which often feels cold to touch.

Clinical link 8.3

♦ Reservoir:

- prohibiting flowers in water being left on wards

- use of disinfectants for ward cleaning
- personal hygiene is maintained (e.g. oral care)
- suction containers/drainage bottles are disposed of as needed and per local protocol.

♦ Portal of exit:
  - minimize talking and breathing *directly* over exposed wounds
  - do not come into work if you are poorly with an infectious disease or illness.

♦ Mode of transmission:
  - hand washing
  - aseptic techniques
  - universal precautions—use of personal protective equipment
  - antiseptic skin preparations before inserting a cannula
  - dispose of soiled linen and clinical waste in appropriately colour-coded plastic bags
  - disposal of used sharps is in accordance with local policy.

♦ Portal of entry:
  - invasive lines used in accordance with care bundles
  - soiled/wet dressings changed
  - single use/disposable items.

♦ Susceptible host:
  - barrier nursing
  - isolation/use of side rooms
  - promote good diet
  - health education/promotion to encourage uptake of immunization, where offered.

♦ Infectious agent:
  - antibiotics/anti-fungals, etc.
  - sterilization of equipment.

Clinical link 8.4

♦ Which risk factors for developing sepsis does John have?

John is somewhat elderly and may have a weaker immune system than a younger person. He has had recent surgery and we know his gut has been perforated by an ulcer. He has a peripheral cannula still in use and a urinary catheter in situ. These are both invasive devices and may be a route for infection.

♦ What suggests to you that John is possibly developing sepsis? How advanced is this development?

The increase in respiratory rate is nearly always a sign of deterioration. His temperature and falling blood pressure are actually quite developed signs of sepsis—John is moving noticeably into severe sepsis. Note that it is the diastolic pressure especially that is falling. The increasing heart rate is a compensatory mechanism and, again, is a fairly advanced sign that John is being compromised by the developing sepsis. The fact that his urine output has been poor for several hours will be indicative of poor perfusion pressure and this will all need to be relayed to the surgeons. John's complaint of queasiness is non-specific but often the patient will only identify rather general symptoms before becoming extremely unwell.

♦ What possible sources for the infective agent might there be that are identified in the scenario?

The cannula or the catheter. John has had recent surgery. Signs of inflammation would be apparent on the cannula site. Urine may be discoloured in appearance or offensive in odour, urinalysis may be abnormal.

♦ What other possible causes of infection might you follow up to find the cause of a possible infection?

John's wound site and the state of his dressings need reviewing. There is no mention of John's respiratory function besides the tachypnoea—as a smoker he is more liable to a chest infection than a non-smoker.

♦ Which of John's recent laboratory results will the surgical team be particularly interested in, in relation to your findings?

The white cell count—a rise would indicate infection. Any MC&S sample results that have come back as positive would also be important in terms of treating the source of infection. The doctors would also review the CRP and lactate.

♦ What would your course of action be in response to your findings for John?

John requires an urgent review by his doctors. It would be important to handover the key physiological findings and also alert them to positive MC&S results and white cell results if they have been received on the ward or hospital information system after the ward round, for example. Generally, the sepsis six guidelines are the ones to follow:

- 100% oxygen via rebreathe mask.
- Blood cultures: even if you are not able to perform venepuncture, the necessary equipment can be ready to expedite this.
- Intravenous antibiotics: these will probably be 'broad spectrum' antibiotics at this point unless a sample has been positive from MC&S.
- Intravenous fluids: John already has some 0.9% saline running but will need more fluid as he is becoming cardiovascularly compromised. These fluids will need to be prescribed—is his cannula patent—does he need a new cannula?
- Lactate and haemoglobin levels: lactate can be measured using a blood gas analyser or hand-held device. Failing this, a sample may be sent to the laboratory, as can a full blood count if haemoglobin levels have not been taken recently.
- Measure and improve urine output. John has a catheter so monitoring is easier—his observations show inadequate renal function which will need to be prioritized.

The HCA would need to be encouraged to report these findings earlier but also explanation as to what the signs of deterioration were.

Chapter 9

Clinical link 9.1

♦ Identify aspects from the health history and assessment findings which indicate that this patient may be experiencing delirium, dementia, and/or depression.

- Delirium
  - Acute onset of confusion.
  - Agitated, restless, and disoriented to place and time.
  - Urinary tract infection appears likely which could be the cause of the delirium.
- Dementia
  - There is no direct indication that this patient suffers from dementia although a full health history has not yet been established (patient unable to provide a health history at this time and the information passed on by the neighbour is brief).
  - Potential signs of dementia could be how the patient is no longer caring for the outside of the house and previous episodes of forgetfulness and poor short-term memory, although these things may be due to other reasons
- Depression
  - At risk for depression because of age and living alone.
  - Potential for social isolation if physical health deteriorates.
  - Unclear from scenario whether patient has any chronic disease but this would further increase the risk for depression.
- What investigations, treatments, and ongoing monitoring does this patient appear to need?
  - Urine testing to confirm urinary tract infection and assess for dehydration.
  - Fluid balance assessment, including close attention to renal output and ability to take in oral fluids.
  - Full blood count to ensure that adequate haemoglobin and to monitor white blood cells for infection.
  - CRP to monitor for infection.
  - Urea and creatinine to assess for adequate renal function.
  - Electrolytes to assess for renal function and dehydration.
  - Antibiotics to treat urinary tract infection.
  - Encourage oral fluids if swallowing not impaired and discuss with doctor need for intravenous fluid replacement.
  - Discuss with doctor reasons why pedal oedema is present and need for further cardiovascular investigations/treatment.
  - Ongoing monitoring of vital signs, keeping in mind that the elderly do not always present with a fever when there is an infection.
  - Ongoing monitoring of neurological status, reporting to the doctor any further deterioration in cognitive functioning.
  - Ongoing monitoring for signs and symptoms of sepsis.
  - Respiratory, abdominal, and skin assessment did not indicate any other causes of infection but ongoing monitoring of the respiratory and abdominal systems will help to confirm there is no other internal infections.
  - Ongoing monitoring for signs and symptoms of respiratory infection—potential for respiratory infection present due to reduced mobility while hospitalized, confusion, risk for pulmonary aspiration from impaired cognitive functioning.

- Ongoing monitoring of patient's ability to see and hear well—hearing aid and glasses indicate a potential for sensory impairment, which could exacerbate delirium further.

♦ How would you support the psychosocial needs of the patient?

- Contact son to inform him that his mother has been hospitalized and establish who is the next of kin with contact details clear in the patient's notes.
- Obtain a more detailed psychosocial history from the son to establish a baseline of the patient's normal cognitive functioning and ability to achieve activities of daily living.
- Provide education to son about patient condition.
- Assess whether patient would like to be support by chaplain/spiritual care services.
- Assess whether patient would benefit from having a volunteer visitor.
- Prior to discharge, refer to other healthcare services to ensure that patient is discharged to a safe environment with adequate support in place as necessary (e.g. social worker, occupational therapist, and district nursing).

Chapter 10

Clinical link 10.1

It is vital that this patient's clinical symptoms are considered alongside his blood results as this enables an accurate diagnosis and facilitates appropriate intervention.

This patient's clinical observations suggest he is in the compensatory stages of hypovolaemic shock. He is tachycardic and has an increased respiratory rate, yet his blood pressure is being stabilized by the release of sympathetic hormones (adrenaline and noradrenaline). His CVP is low further indicating hypovolaemia.

His blood results indicate:

♦ High sodium: the most common cause of a high sodium is dehydration and fits this patient's history of prolonged episodes of vomiting. He may additionally report a dry mouth and have dry mucous membranes.

♦ Normal potassium: this is normal, but regular repeats should be performed as excessive vomiting may lower potassium concentrations.

♦ A high urea: this is high and possibly linked to his dehydration. His blood pressure should be sufficiently high to maintain renal perfusion. However, if this patient has a history of hypertension this may be a low blood pressure for him and may alter renal perfusion. This should be closely monitored. It is worth considering catheterization in this patient to enable close observation of renal output.

♦ A high creatinine: this is normal (but highest end of normal). Care should be taken to monitor renal function as this may be an early indicator of hypovolaemic shock and poor tissue perfusion.

This patient clearly needs fluid replacement and appropriate fluid replacement should be discussed with the doctor. Frequent repeat bloods will be necessary to check electrolyte balance. This patient should be closely monitored for further complications. Anti-emetics may be useful to decrease fluid and electrolyte loss from vomiting. Urgent tests should be undertaken to establish the cause of the vomiting.

Clinical link 10.2

Again it is vital that this patient's clinical symptoms are considered alongside her blood results as this enables an accurate diagnosis and facilitates appropriate intervention.

This patient's clinical observations suggest she is in the initial stages of sepsis. Her blood pressure is normal (but diastolic pressure is low because the mediators of sepsis cause marked vasodilatation). Her heart rate and respiratory rate are high, indicating shock and her temperature is 38.6 C (indicating infection). The surviving sepsis campaign (2008) highlighted the need for urgent blood investigations to include blood cultures if the core temperature is above 38.5 C. It would be useful to assess this patient's peripheral temperature; it is likely to be warm in early stages of sepsis but may begin to cool as shock worsens.

Her blood results indicate:

♦ A high lactate: this can be attributed to the development of sepsis and is an indicator that anaerobic metabolism is occurring. The surviving sepsis campaign highlights that urgent action should be taken if the lactate exceeds 2 mmol/L.

♦ A high CRP: this is an increase in an inflammatory marker, indicating the possibility of sepsis in this patient. CRP is released as part of the complement cascade released during inflammatory processes. The increased CRP alongside the patient's other symptoms is indicative of infection.

♦ A high white cell count (leucocytosis): again this is an indicator of inflammation. White cells increase to protect the body from infection, and the increased white cell count, alongside the other symptoms, is indicative of infection.

This patient will require:

♦ An urgent medical review.

♦ Urgent blood cultures and consideration of any other source of infection, for example sputum specimen.

♦ The surviving sepsis campaign (2008) indicates the need for urgent broad spectrum intravenous antibiotics (within 1 h of initial diagnosis, these should not be delayed).

♦ Other treatment will be required. This is detailed in care of the septic patient in Chapter 8.

Clinical link 10.3

Again it is vital that this patient's clinical symptoms are considered alongside his blood results as this enables an accurate diagnosis and facilitates appropriate intervention.

This patient's clinical observations suggest he is in the compensatory stages of hypovolaemic shock. He is tachycardic and has an increased respiratory rate, yet his blood pressure is being stabilized by the release of sympathetic hormones (adrenaline and noradrenaline) but there is a decreasing pulse pressure suggesting vasoconstriction caused by these compensatory mechanisms.

His blood results show:

♦ Decreased red blood cell count, which may indicate a number of clinical diagnosis, however, given this patient's other symptoms and presentation, bleeding is the most likely cause.

♦ Decreased haemoglobin, which again is indicative of many conditions but the most probable cause in this case is recent/active bleeding.

♦ Decreased haematocrit again may indicate recent/active bleeding.

This patient will require:

♦ urgent referral to the medical staff.

♦ volume replacement to correct fluid loss. (Note: This may further reduce his Hb due to effects of dilutional anaemia.) Blood transfusion is probably not necessary as this is generally only given if HB below 8 because of associated risks.

- urgent clotting to establish whether coagulation problems are the cause of bleeding
- urgent review by surgeons
- close nursing observation.

Chapter 13

Clinical link 13.1

Part A

- Immediate actions
  - Call for help—senior nurse on ward initially for support.
  - Re-assess **A**—**Airway**: look, listen, and feel. This is important to ensure that she is still maintaining her own airway (the sedative agents she had been given for her endoscopy have made her very sleepy).
  - Administer high-flow oxygen via non rebreathe mask with reservoir at 15 L as O_2 saturations are only 86%. Call 2222 (or appropriate local number) for medical emergency call if senior nurse help not immediately available. When O_2 saturations are this low they are inadequate and are unable to supply enough oxygen to the tissues, and is a sign of critical illness and a potential for cardiorespiratory arrest.
  - It is really important to turn her onto her side because if she vomits this will help to protect her airway and prevent choking and/or aspiration.
  - Reassess **B**—**Breathing**: look, listen, and feel. This is important to see if O_2 saturations are improving with high-flow oxygen. Also assess if there is a problem identified with breathing as a cause for inadequate O_2 saturations. Are both sides of the chest moving equally? Check rate and depth of breathing as well.
  - O_2 saturations improve to 100% and then are maintained at 95% on 3 L O_2 via nasal specs. Your colleague leaves you but will be available if needed.
- Other assessments
  - After **A & B** reassessment check **C**—**Circulation**: colour, pulse, blood pressure, 12-lead ECG, check adequate intravenous access. If so check it is patent with a 5 mL saline flush. If not, a cannula will be required. Check recent blood results.
  - **D**—**Disability** (neurological) assessment: AVPU. Are pupils equal and reactive to light (PEARL)? Blood sugar check. Can she move all four limbs? Obey commands? GCS score?
  - **E**—**Exposure** to perform a quick top to toe assessment. Check abdomen is soft, check calves for signs of deep vein thrombosis and perfusion to limbs and feet. Check for any evidence of bleeding. Check for rashes. Take central temperature.
  - It is also important to check fluid balance charts. Check all prescription charts, especially looking at the endoscopy procedure information, to see what she had been given for sedation and how much.

Part B You go to get help so she can be turned onto her side. She is cyanosed and noises are radiating from her airway.

- Priorities:
  - Call for help! Pull bedside buzzer.
  - Assess **ABC**—look, listen, feel for 10 s only.

Patient is breathing regular respirations and noise and cyanosis disappears with head tilt chin lift. Colour improves. She has a rapid regular central pulse. She is not moving and does not resist head tilt chin lift.

- Other actions/interventions
  - Call 2222 medical emergency number (or appropriate local number).
  - Maintain airway opening manoeuvre. Reapply high-flow O_2 with non-rebreathe and reservoir at 15 L. Check O_2 saturations and colour. Remember: *simple manoeuvres will almost always open an obstructed airway.*
  - Ask for suction (bedside) to be turned on and ensure yankeur suction available.
  - Call for resuscitation trolley so equipment is near to hand for you and for when the team arrive.
  - With A being maintained, reassess B and C. (Because of the patient's deterioration it is vital a repeat of ABCDE is carried out so nothing is missed.) Remember: *Even though the tubing has been attached to the O2 cylinder confirm it HAS been turned on and the reservoir bag is moving in and out with the patient's breathing.* Then reassess D and E again.
  - Anticipate the need for simple and advanced airway equipment so ensure that your colleague is preparing this when the trolley arrives.
  - Consider obtaining antidotes (if known) to sedatives given to patient, that is naloxone for morphine overdose. This will save important time for when the doctors arrive.

- Signs of airway obstruction

  Complete:
  - Absent breath sounds at mouth/nose.
  - Use of accessory muscles.
  - Paradoxical chest movements ('see–saw' breathing).
  - Central cyanosis may not be evident initially as it can be a late sign.

  Partial:
  - Air entry diminished.
  - Noisy breathing depending on cause of obstruction, that is gurgling may be blood or vomit, snoring noise due to tongue partially occluding the airway.

Clinical link 13.2

Part A

- Course of action/nursing care
  - Call for more help immediately.
  - Give the patient lots of reassurance.
  - Ask for the emergency equipment to be near by if needed and obtained equipment to assess vital signs.
  - **A—Airway**: look, listen, and feel. Patient is still communicating audibly despite swollen face and lips. He has hives all over his arms and chest/neck and some around his hairline.
  - **B—Breathing**: he appears to have difficulty breathing using all accessory muscles and a rate of 36. SaO_2 91%. Assess whether chest expansion is equal on both sides.

- Call 2222 medical emergency number (or appropriate local number).
- Apply high-flow O_2 15 L via non-rebreathe mask with reservoir. Keep monitoring oxygen saturations and reassess **A** and **B**.

On initial findings it appears he may be suffering from an anaphylactic reaction. A colleague arrives to inform you that she had just given him intravenous flucloxacillin 10 min previously. He has no known allergies.

The medical emergency team arrive.

- ◆ Anticipated interventions from the doctor

  - To reassess **A** and **B** (as above).

  - Perform a thorough **C—circulation** assessment. Pulse, blood pressure. Connect to heart monitor once stable enough to move back to his bed space. Check adequate intravenous access.

  - Assessing whether the anaphylaxis criteria are met? In this patient YES.

    Criteria for Anaphylaxis (Resuscitation Council 2008):

  Sudden onset and rapid progression of symptoms
  Life-threatening airway and/or breathing and/or circulation problems
  Skin and/or mucosal changes: flushing, urticaria, angiodema

  - If tolerated by the patient lie him down.
  - Give immediate intramuscular adrenaline 0.5 mg (0.5 mL 1:1000).
  - Prescribe intravenous fluids (500–1 L) crystalloid fluid challenge.
  - Reassess **A**, **B** and **C**, repeat adrenaline after 5 min if symptoms do not improve.
  - Continue assessment and complete **D** and **E**.
  - Review antibiotics(discontinue flucloxacillin)/discuss with microbiology.
  - Documentation and appropriate referral/follow-up

Part B

- ◆ Differentiation between analphylaxis and panic attack

Anaphylaxis	Panic attack
Anxious	Anxious
Hypotension	Hypertension
Wheezy	Breathless
Swollen airway	Hyperventilation
Urticaria, erythema	Flushed and/or erythematous rash

Chapter 14

Clinical link 14.1

- ◆ Patient escort—who should go?

At least one healthcare professional with advanced life support skills, for example experienced trained nurse, doctor.

- ◆ What are the risks—what could happen during transfer?

This is an acute event, the patient is already symptomatic before any movement and at this stage diagnosis not confirmed. Due to the requirement for the patient to change position, to lie horizontal for transfer to imaging table and for CT itself, they are at high risk of becoming more hypoxic and therefore breathless and anxious. If the patient has a pulmonary embolus and the embolus large enough it could potentially lead to cardiopulmonary arrest. Escorting staff need to be prepared for complications and ensure adequate intravenous access before transfer. It is also imperative that any movement is carefully controlled and patient lies flat for the least amount of time possible. Escorting staff also should provide continual reassurance to the patient explaining each stage of movement. During the actual CT scan the patient is usually left alone (to reduce risk of radiation to healthcare staff) therefore monitoring needs to be positioned to allow staff to view both visual and audible alarms. It is important that the patient understands that they are still being monitored, that the time in the CT will be brief and that they can still communicate with staff in the control room.

♦ What equipment do you require?

Oxygen (adequate supply consider oxygen may need to be increased to 15 L/min), cardiac monitor, 'emergency bag' with access to intubation equipment, bag/valve/mask, emergency cardiac drugs, intravenous administration equipment, ABG syringe.

♦ What monitoring should the patient have during the transfer?

Respiratory rate, work of breathing, cardiac monitor, including pulse oximetry (SpO2), continuous ECG, non-invasive blood pressure and alarms set appropriately, level of consciousness (any signs of increasing respiratory distress or confusion). CT scanner will usually have CCTV to allow vision of patient and communication with patient. The screen should be closely observed to monitor during procedure.

♦ How should this be documented?

Take observation charts (useful to trend patient response and in addition facilitate documentation at regular intervals (every15 min). Trend of track-and-trigger score.

Clinical link 14.2

♦ Patient escort—who should go?

At least one healthcare professional with advanced life support skills and who is familiar with patients with acute or chronic illness, for example experienced trained nurse.

However, if this patient is becoming more unwell consideration should be given to the patient having a portable chest X-ray to avoid the additional movement/transfer. Although a portable chest X-ray is not same quality as that of an X-ray taken in the imaging department it should be adequate for this purpose. This needs to be balanced against the risk of using portable imaging, therefore radiation in the ward area. The medical team should make this decision urgently.

If an advance decision has been made regarding the patient's resuscitation status that information must be transferred with the patient and the imaging department briefed (whilst ensuring patient confidentiality).

♦ What are the risks—what could happen during transfer?

Patient will be sitting upright for imaging procedure. This is an acute event and patient could become more hypoxic and breathless depending on the requirement to move/change position. The patient should have clear management plan for the administration for oxygen therapy, target SpO2, so that staff can titrate oxygen accordingly if there are changes in the patient parameters. The patient should also have adequate intravenous access before transfer.

+ What equipment do you require?

Oxygen plus additional venturi™ devices as appropriate, portable pulse oximeter, 'emergency bag'.

+ What monitoring should the patient have during the transfer?

Respiratory rate, work of breathing, pulse oximetry, level of consciousness (any signs of increasing respiratory distress or confusion).

+ How should this be documented?

Take observation charts (useful to trend patient response and in addition facilitate documentation at regular intervals (every15 min). Trend of track-and-trigger score.

Clinical link 14.3

+ Patient escort—who should go?

As an unplanned inter-hospital transfer the decision should be made by the consultant responsible for the patient. At least one healthcare professional with advanced life support skills, ability to prescribe fluids, manage the changing patient haemodynamics, for example doctor/anaesthetist.

+ What are the risks—what could happen during transfer?

This is an acute event and the patient is at high risk of further bleeding. Vomiting blood could cause a compromised airway through aspiration particularly if there is a reduction in conscious level due to haemodynmic instability (consider anti-emetic). Hypovolaemia (due to blood loss) and ensuing haemodynamic instability (if not adequately fluid resuscitated) could potentially lead to cardiopulmonary arrest. The patient must have adequate intravenous access before transfer with two large cannulae and be optimized with fluid replacement, consider urinary catheterization to assess response to fluid resuscitation.

If the patient has a distended abdomen this could cause pressure on diaphragm, reduced lung expansion.

+ What equipment do you require?

Oxygen, cardiac monitor (adequate battery life), 'emergency bag' with access to intubation equipment, bag/valve/mask, emergency cardiac drugs, intravenous fluids administration, ABG syringe. Portable suction. Blood and crossmatch information. All health records, including recent blood results.

+ What monitoring should the patient have during the transfer?

Respiratory rate and evaluation of work of breathing. Cardiac monitor, including pulse oximetry, continuous ECG, non-invasive blood pressure and alarms set appropriately, level of consciousness (any signs of increasing respiratory distress or confusion). Response to intravenous fluids. Trend of track-and-trigger score.

+ How should this be documented?

Use hospital transfer, document at regular intervals (every15 min).

Clinical link 14.4

+ Patient escort—who should go?

One healthcare professional with advanced life support skills, including tracheostomy skills, for example experienced trained nurse.

+ What are the risks—what could happen during transfer?

As a patient with a newly formed tracheostomy the main risks are dislodgement of the tube and blockage due to bronchial secretions or bleeding. The tube should have an inner cannula, which should be checked for patency before transfer. Tube tapes should be checked to ensure that they are adequately secure. Cuff should be examined (this is usually inflated post procedure to reduce risk of aspiration). Bleeding could also occur around the stoma site therefore this should be checked to gain baseline information. The patient's target SpO2 should be determined by medical team before the patient's return to the ward to enable titration of oxygen therapy.

♦ What equipment do you require?

Humidified oxygen, portable suction, depending on the patient's respiratory status portable pulse oximetry may be required. Equipment for the emergency change of a tracheostomy, spare tracheostomy tube/inner cannula, tracheostomy dilators, tapes.

♦ What monitoring should the patient have during the transfer?

Respiratory rate and evaluation of work of breathing, level of consciousness (any signs of increasing respiratory distress or confusion). SpO2 if using pulse oximeter.

♦ How should this be documented?

Document on return to ward, observations should be rechecked, including track-and-trigger score.

Chapter 15

Clinical link 15.1

Nursing priorities

Nursing priorities and preparation for this patient can be identified using the ALERT framework.

A: Airway

♦ Ensure that all equipment required to nurse patient with a tracheostomy is by the bedside before transfer.

♦ Liaise with ITU re type and size of tracheostomy and any particular requirement.

♦ Ensure that communication system available as patient will require barrier nursing.

♦ Ensure staff on duty familiar with tracheostomy equipment and competent to manage care.

♦ Communicate with outreach if support needed.

♦ On arrival back to the ward ensure patient's tracheostomy is patent and discuss suctioning/clearance of secretion with ITU staff. Introduce yourself to the patient.

♦ Ensure O_2 and humidification set up as required.

♦ Conduct respiratory assessment.

B: Breathing

♦ Conduct full respiratory assessment.

♦ Record baseline observations.

♦ Ensure frequency of monitoring is discussed with ITU staff.

♦ Ensure saturation monitor in situ and alarms set with appropriate range.

♦ Ensure that patient is positioned to optimize ventilation.

♦ Report any changes immediately.

C: Circulation

- Assess cardiovascular status.
- Record baseline observations.
- Ensure frequency of monitoring In discussion with ITU staff.
- Set up haemodynamic monitoring if in isolation and set alarms appropriately.
- Check fluid balance.
- Ensure that fluid replacement is adequate.

D: Disability

- Ensure that patient is comfortable and well supported by pillows.
- Conduct assessment of neurological function and record any deficits to enable a baseline to be recorded.
- Advise patient to rest as much as possible.
- Provide assistance as required, remembering the loss of muscle function/fatigue that this group of patients may experience.
- Liaise with physiotherapist as needed.
- Liaise with occupational therapist if limb support needed.

Other considerations

Resistant infection:

- Hospital protocol in relation to MRSA should be adhered to.
- Frequent observation of this patient and visible nursing presence will be required if she is nursed in a side ward.
- Communication should be ensured and buzzer/call bell accessible.
- Eradication and rescreening for MRSA should be conducted in line with protocol.

   Recovering organ failure:

- Baseline blood results should be available.
- Hourly fluid balance charting to check input/output.
- Report any concerns to medical staff.

Nutrition and weight loss:

- Conduct MUST assessment on return to ward.
- Discuss diet/enteral nutrition with ITU staff.
- Monitor weight at least three times a week.
- Encourage supplements as required.
- Ensure that any dietary restrictions re-renal failure are adhered to.

Immobility:

- Pressure areas should be assessed on admission to ward.
- Special mattress should be used in line with hospital protocol.

Sleep disturbance:

- Encourage rest as much as possible.

- Try to establish a night/day routine for patient.
- Discuss patient worries, etc.
- Assess whether patient is experiencing nightmares/flashbacks, etc.

Anxiety:

- If possible visit patient in ITU before transfer and plan for transfer to ward.
- Settle patient to ward.
- Ensure that patient and family know how to ask for help.
- Frequent nurse presence during initial stages.
- Orientate to environment.
- Discuss concerns with patient/family.

Tracheostomy problems

Mrs Smith appears to be having difficulty with her airway. This requires:

- Immediate nursing assessment to include:
  - assessment of airway
  - assessment of respiratory function
  - assessment of need to suction/clear secretions/unblock tracheostomy.
- The protocol in Table 15.3 should be followed if tube is blocked/partially blocked or if respiratory distress is apparent.

Once tracheostomy patency is ensured the nurse should:

- ensure frequent changing of inner tube
- ensure adequate humidification of O_2
- ensure adequate and frequent suctioning
- ensure frequent nebulizers are given.

Clinical link 15.2

Nightmares and hallucinations are common after long periods of intensive care but it is vital to ensure that adequate support is provided to Mrs Smith.

Before caring for Mrs Smith's psychological needs, it is essential to ensure that these problems do not have an organic root and her respiration/saturations should be reviewed to ensure that she is not hypoxic and bloods taken to ensure renal function is adequate as build up of urea and creatinine can cause confusion.

Having ensured that there is no organic cause to this, Mrs Smith will require support. She should be encouraged to:

- discuss any nightmares, etc. if she is able to recall them and try to alleviate any concerns that she may have
- identify whether she has had any flashbacks, etc. which may be adding to her anxiety/state of confusion

If the patient is having flashbacks and hallucinations additional assessment may be required as these are closely linked to development of psychotic states. It may be of benefit to liaise with outreach to enable appropriate support for this patient. Outreach teams will be used to developing strategies to help patients overcome psychological problems.

Clinical link 15.3

Mrs Smith's daughter is likely to be concerned over the unplanned transfer of her mother and may have some concerns about this, especially if she was expecting her mother to remain in ITU for a few more days and the transfer occurred without her knowledge. Staff should remember that relatives may not have good memories of ward areas (as often this is where patient's condition deteriorated before ITU). Appropriate support and reassurance is often required as the relative also experiences a degree of relocation stress, often manifested in the 'demanding' relative role.

Her daughter should be:

- orientated to the ward area
- encouraged to meet the staff caring for Mrs Smith
- provided with reassurance over changes in nurse:patient ratio
- reassured that she will be able to visit her mother
- reassured that her mother is being cared for appropriately.
- provided with information related to early transfer and her mother's improving condition.

Staff should:

- ensure that all the daughter's questions are answered honestly
- encourage the daughter to discuss issues arising with the nurses and multidisciplinary team
- encourage the family to view transfer to the ward as a positive outcome, i.e. Mrs Smith's condition is improving.

Index

Note: Subjects are indexed under their non-abbreviated form. A list of abbreviations appears on pp. xi–xiv.